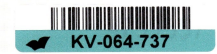
Winter's **BASIC CLINICAL PHARMACOKINETICS**

Sixth Edition

Paul M. Beringer, PharmD

Associate Professor
Department of Clinical Pharmacy
University of Southern California
Los Angeles, California

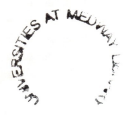

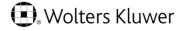

Wolters Kluwer

Philadelphia · Baltimore · New York · London
Buenos Aires · Hong Kong · Sydney · Tokyo

Acquisitions Editor: Matt Hauber
Development Editor: Andrea Vosburgh
Editorial Coordinator: Jennifer DiRicco
Editorial Assistant: Brooks Phelps
Marketing Manager: Mike McMahon
Production Project Manager: Joan Sinclair
Design Coordinator: Elaine Kasmer
Manufacturing Coordinator: Margie Orzech
Prepress Vendor: S4Carlisle Publishing Services

Sixth Edition

9 8 7 6 5 4 3 2 1

Printed in China

Library of Congress Cataloging-in-Publication Data

Names: Beringer, Paul, author.
Title: Winter's basic clinical pharmacokinetics / Paul Beringer, PharmD,
  Associate Professor, University of Southern California, Los Angeles, CA.
Other titles: Basic clinical pharmacokinetics
Description: Sixth edition. | Philadelphia : Wolters Kluwer Health, [2018] |
  Revised edition of: Basic clinical pharmacokinetics / Michael E. Winter.
  5th ed. 2010. | Includes bibliographical references.
Identifiers: LCCN 2017035249 | ISBN 9781496346421
Subjects: LCSH: Pharmacokinetics. | Pharmacokinetics—Problems, exercises,
  etc.
Classification: LCC RM301.5 .W56 2018 | DDC 615.7076—dc23 LC record available at
  https://lccn.loc.gov/2017035249

RRS1708

I would like to dedicate this edition to my wife, Annie Wong-Beringer, PharmD, who is a constant source of inspiration both personally and professionally.

Contributors

Timothy J. Bensman, PharmD, PhD
Post-doctoral Fellow
Systems Pharmacology &
    Pharmacometrics
Department of Biomedical
    Engineering
University of Southern California
Los Angeles, California

Paul M. Beringer, PharmD
Associate Professor
Department of Clinical Pharmacy
University of Southern California
Los Angeles, California

Maureen S. Boro, PharmD
Clinical Professor
Department of Clinical Pharmacy
UCSF School of Pharmacy
Pharmacokinetics and Pharmacy
    Informatics Program Manager
Pharmacy Service
San Francisco VA Health Care System
San Francisco, California

Julie A. Dopheide, PharmD, BCPP, FASHP
Professor of Clinical Pharmacy
Department of Clinical Pharmacy
University of Southern California
Psychiatric Pharmacist Specialist

Department of Psychiatry
Los Angeles County + USC Medical
    Center
Los Angeles, California

Thomas C. Dowling, PharmD, PhD
Assistant Dean
Director of Research
Ferris State University
Grand Rapids, Michigan

**Mary H. H. Ensom, PharmD,
BS(Pharm), FASHP, FCCP, FCSHP,
FCAHS**
Professor
Faculty of Pharmaceutical
    Sciences
The University of British Columbia
Vancouver, BC, Canada
Clinical Pharmacy Specialist
Pharmacy Department
Children's & Women's Health Centre
    of British Columbia
Vancouver, BC, Canada

Reginald F. Frye, PharmD, PhD
Professor and Chair
Pharmacotherapy and Translational
    Research
University of Florida
Gainesville, Florida

Emily Han, PharmD, BCPS

Assistant Professor
Department of Clinical Pharmacy
University of Southern California
Clinical Pharmacist
Department of Pharmacy
Keck Medical Center of USC
Los Angeles, California

Tony K. L. Kiang, PhD, BSc(Pharm), ACPR

Clinical Instructor
The Faculty of Pharmaceutical
    Sciences
The University of British Columbia
Clinical Pharmacy Specialist
Department of Pharmacy
St. Paul's Hospital & Vancouver
    General Hospital
Vancouver, BC, Canada

Erin D. Knox, PharmD, BCPP

Clinical Pharmacist in
    Psychiatry
Department of Pharmacy
Keck Hospital of USC
Los Angeles, California

Russell E. Lewis, PharmD, FCCP

Associate Professor of Medicine
Department of Medical and Surgical
    Sciences
University of Bologna
Clinical Pharmacologist
Operative Unit-Infectious Diseases
Sant Orsola-Malpighi Hospital
Bologna, Italy

John E. Murphy, PharmD, BS(Pharm)

Professor and Associate Dean
Department of Pharmacy Practice &
    Science
The University of Arizona College of
    Pharmacy
Tucson, Arizona

Laura F. Ruekert, PharmD, BCPP, BCGP

Associate Professor of Pharmacy
    Practice
Department of Pharmacy Practice
College of Pharmacy and Health
    Sciences
Butler University
Clinical Pharmacist Specialist,
    Psychiatry
Pharmacy Department
Community Health Network
Indianapolis, Indiana

Irving Steinberg, PharmD

Associate Professor
Department of Pediatrics and Clinical
    Pharmacy
Keck School of Medicine and
    Pharmacy
University of South California
Director, Division of Pediatric
    Pharmacotherapy
Department of Pediatrics
Los Angeles County + USC Medical
    Center
Los Angeles, California

Timothy W. Synold, PharmD

Professor
Department of Cancer Biology
Beckman Research Institute of the
    City of Hope
Duarte, California

Jeanne H. VanTyle, PharmD

Professor of Pharmacy Practice
College of Pharmacy and Health
    Sciences
Butler University
Indianapolis, Indiana

Michael E. Winter, PharmD

Professor Emeritus
Department of Clinical Pharmacy
UCSF School of Pharmacy
San Francisco, California

Preface

Since the publication of the first edition of *Basic Clinical Pharmacokinetics* more than 30 years ago, the use of serum drug concentrations as a guide for monitoring drug therapy has continued to gain increased acceptance. The use of pharmacokinetic and biopharmaceutical principles in predicting plasma drug concentrations, as well as the changes in plasma drug concentrations that occur over time, is now widely accepted as useful adjuncts in patient care. With the continued advancement of analytical technology, every health care institution and practitioner has access to a wide range of drug assays, and monitoring serum drug concentrations has become the standard of practice for many drugs. As we continue to gain more knowledge about both the limitations and applications of drug concentrations and their correlation with either efficacy or toxicity, concentration sampling strategies change. Appropriate use of serum drug concentrations, however, continues to be a major problem in the clinical setting. Basic pharmacokinetic principles must be applied rationally to specific patients.

Patient care continues to trend toward value-based care. This includes everything from minimizing and streamlining drug therapy and laboratory testing to the increased use of automation. The use of serum drug concentrations is not immune to the pressure of doing more with less. It is my hope that this sixth edition of *Basic Clinical Pharmacokinetics* will help the clinician in the rational application of pharmacokinetics and therapeutic drug monitoring to patient care and help to ensure that drug concentration monitoring is focused in an optimal way on the most appropriate patients.

A number of physiologic and mathematical assumptions have been made. This is a common practice in the clinical setting because of the dosing strategies and the limited number of concentrations sampled. An attempt has been made to alert the reader to these assumptions. There are a large number of texts and articles that present a much more detailed and in-depth analysis and explanation of the physiologic and pharmacokinetic principles being discussed. It is not the intent of this book to explore all of these issues. Rather, the goal of this book is to simplify pharmacokinetics so that it can be more easily understood and visualized by practitioners, and, as a consequence, the use of pharmacokinetics can become part of their professional practice.

Although plasma drug concentrations are useful in evaluating drug therapy, they constitute only one source of information. They should not, therefore, be used as the sole criterion on which treatment is based. Pharmacokinetic calculations should be considered only as an adjunctive guide to the determination of dosing regimens.

If a calculated dosing regimen seems unreasonable, reevaluation is essential since sampling or assay errors, an inaccurate dosing history, or a mathematical error are always a possibility. Another problem inherent in these calculations is that the literature or assumed pharmacokinetic parameters utilized may be inappropriate for the patient under consideration. Many of the pharmacokinetic parameters available in the literature are based upon a relatively small number of patients or normal volunteers. Therefore, values obtained from these experimental data are, at best, estimates for any given patient. If the basic underlying pharmacokinetic assumptions are not applicable to the particular patient, even the most elegant calculation will be invalid.

Review articles and some texts commonly list pharmacokinetic parameters for a number of drugs and are a good initial source of pharmacokinetic information. However, the reader is encouraged to seek out the original literature to evaluate the methodology and data from which this information was derived. Some factors that should be considered in scrutinizing these studies include the number and type of subjects, type and specificity of drug assay, degree of inter- and intrasubject variability, statistical analysis of the data, and whether the drug was studied prospectively or retrospectively. The potential problems associated with using the literature data to predict disposition of a drug within a specific patient emphasize the need to obtain accurate plasma-level measurements. Clearly, the literature can serve as a guide to make initial a priori clinical decisions, but even with the best predictions, significant variance does exist. Therefore, only with a complete dosing history, appropriate drug sampling, accurate and specific assay procedures, and logical pharmacokinetic analysis can patient-specific parameters be derived that will be useful adjuncts to providing optimal patient care and improving clinical outcomes.

ORGANIZATIONAL PHILOSOPHY

The book is divided into two parts: Part I reviews basic pharmacokinetic principles and Part II illustrates the clinical application of pharmacokinetics to specific drugs through the presentation and step-by-step solutions of common clinical problems. The reader is strongly urged to read each section in the order it appears in the book because many of the concepts discussed in the latter portions of the book are based on an understanding of those presented earlier. The appendices from previous editions—Nomograms for Calculating Body Surface Area, Common Equations Used Throughout the Text, Algorithm for Evaluating and Interpreting Plasma Concentrations, and Glossary of Terms and Abbreviations—are also included and have been updated as appropriate.

Part I

As in previous editions, Part I is divided into sections that describe major pharmacokinetic parameters and their clinical applications. Equations that express the relationships between the various parameters and the resultant plasma concentrations are presented and discussed. Many individuals feel overwhelmed by the apparent complexity of some of the equations used to describe pharmacokinetic behavior of drugs. Therefore, extensive explanations that emphasize major concepts accompany the more complex equations. Figures continue to be useful to help the reader visualize the concepts that are being reviewed. The principles discussed in Part I gives the clinician the basis for manipulating the dosing regimens and interpreting plasma concentrations for the drugs discussed in Part II of this book.

In this sixth edition, the authors and I have attempted to maintain a simple clinical approach to the application of pharmacokinetic principles to patient care. A number of sections in Part I have been expanded; including new chapters on drug dosing in renal disease, pediatric considerations, and pharmacogenomics.

Part II

Most of the chapters on drugs in Part II now contain cases that address pediatric considerations and pharmacogenomics information where relevant. The drugs discussed in Part II were selected because they represent the most commonly monitored drugs in the clinical setting, assays are widely available, and an understanding of their pharmacokinetic and biopharmaceutical properties can substantially aid clinicians in dosing these drugs more rationally and safely. The updates include new information on the clinical use of serum drug concentrations, and, where appropriate, new cases and examples have been added to further expand and exemplify the use of pharmacokinetics in clinical practice.

Over the years, some drugs have been deleted for a variety of reasons. In some cases, the drugs have been replaced by safer, more efficacious agents that do not require drug concentration monitoring. There have been few new drugs that have gained acceptance as requiring concentration monitoring. The reasons for this vary, but, in most cases, plasma concentration monitoring is limited to those drugs that have either a narrow therapeutic index and/or when toxicity or lack of efficacy is clinically unacceptable. Nonetheless, the basic pharmacokinetic principles about drug accumulation, selecting dosing intervals, and when to monitor for either efficacy or toxicity continue to be important considerations in clinical practice. In this edition, we have added a new chapter on antifungals and expansion of the cytotoxic and immunosuppressant therapies in response to new data supporting TDM of these agents.

For each of the drugs in Part II, examples of the most common pharmacokinetic manipulations, such as calculation of a loading dose and maintenance dose, are presented. An example of the process used to interpret a reported plasma concentration is also given. In addition, pathophysiologic factors and drug–drug interactions that influence the pharmacokinetics of these drugs and their significance are discussed. Examples of the most common problems encountered in clinical practice are also given to help the reader recognize when caution should be exercised in making patient care decisions based upon serum drug concentrations and pharmacokinetic principles. Ultimately, the goal is for the reader to recognize the fundamental principles that are being applied to each of the drugs. As confidence and skill in using pharmacokinetics as a clinical tool are developed, it is hoped that the reader will then be able to apply these same principles to new drugs and situations not covered in this book.

ONLINE RESOURCES

Basic Clinical Pharmacokinetics, sixth edition, includes an image bank for instructors that is available on the book's companion website at http://thePoint.lww.com/Beringer6e.

ACKNOWLEDGMENTS

The completion of the sixth edition of *Basic Clinical Pharmacokinetics* would not have been possible without the support of my family, friends, and colleagues. I am grateful to the highly professional coauthors who lent their expertise, knowledge, and skill to contribute new chapters and provide important updates to the individual chapters on drugs.

I would also like to recognize and thank the many students, residents, and colleagues who have provided feedback about what helps them understand and apply pharmacokinetics to their professional practice.

Most of all, I would like to thank Dr. Michael Winter for introducing me to the field of clinical pharmacokinetics, serving as a role model for education in pharmacy, and for providing the opportunity to contribute to this important textbook.

Contents

Contributors...vii

Preface...ix

PART I Basic Principles

1   Pharmacokinetic Processes and Parameters...3

2   Selecting the Appropriate Equation and Interpretation
of Measured Drug Concentrations...57

3   Drug Dosing in Kidney Disease and Dialysis..98

4   Pediatrics...129

5   Pharmacogenetics...154

PART II Drug Monographs

6   Aminoglycoside Antibiotics...163

7   Antifungal Agents: Triazoles..213

8   Carbamazepine..241

9   Cytotoxic Anticancer Drugs: Methotrexate and Busulfan...........................256

10   Digoxin...281

11   Immunosuppressants: Cyclosporine, Tacrolimus,
Sirolimus, and Mycophenolic Acid...320

12   Lithium...358

13   Phenobarbital...371

14   Phenytoin..398

15   Valproic Acid..446

16   Vancomycin..467

APPENDICES

Appendix 1: Nomograms for Calculating Body Surface Area 497
Appendix 2: Common Equations Used Throughout the Text 499
Appendix 3: Algorithm for Evaluating and Interpreting Plasma
Concentrations 505
Appendix 4: Glossary of Terms and Abbreviations 510

Index 515

BASIC PRINCIPLES

The goals and objectives in Part I, Basic Principles, should be used in concert with the goals and objectives in Part II, Drug Monographs.

GOAL

To understand and be able to apply the basic pharmacokinetic principles to the specific drugs in Part II. The learner needs to not only be able to "say the words" and write the equations that are outlined in Part 1 but, just as importantly, develop an understanding of the principles and equations so that when presented in a different way, the principle can be recognized and applied. This second step is not an easy one to take. Pharmacokinetics is a language and to truly understand the equations and become "fluent" requires patience, practice, and time. As an example, if asked "how much drug is remaining after one half-life," most can immediately answer "half". However, if asked what is the value of e^{-Kt}, where t is one half-life, most have to ponder the question for some time before arriving at the same answer.

The following set out the goals for Part I: Basic Principles

1. Understand and appreciate the meaning of the factors that can influence drug absorption into the body.
2. Understand and be able to assign a dosing rate.
3. Appreciate the influence of plasma protein binding on the total, bound, and unbound drug concentration and the influence of altered plasma biding on the desired or target drug concentration.
4. Understand the concept of the "apparent volume of distribution" and the clinical utility of volume of distribution with regards to calculating a dose that would rapidly achieve a desired plasma concentration.
5. Understand how clearance can be used to calculate dug loss and maintenance dosing regimens and the importance of renal and hepatic function in determining clearance.
6. Understand the first-order rate constant (K) and half-life with regard to drug elimination and accumulation and how drug concentrations will change with time. In addition, given a set of variables the learner should be able to determine what additional pharmacokinetic parameters or information can be calculated.

7. Understand the relationship between [(S)(F)(Dose)]/V, the dosing interval, the drug half-life, and the maximum and minimum plasma concentrations.

8. Given a set of pharmacokinetic parameters and a drug dosing history, be able to draw to approximate scale a plasma concentration-versus-time curve. Conversely, given a plasma concentration-versus-time curve, be able to write the equations that represent the curve.

9. Given a patient's dosing history, plasma drug concentration(s), and the literature estimates of the drug's pharmacokinetic parameters, be able to determine if it is likely that the measured drug concentration represents steady state or non–steady state and then select the model to revise the proper pharmacokinetic parameter(s).

10. Describe the key drug clearance mechanisms in the kidney, and estimate creatinine clearance in various patient populations including CKD, AKI, pediatrics, obesity and elderly.

11. To obtain an appreciation for the types of dialysis (intermittent hemo, continuous renal replacement, and peritoneal) and to know how each is likely to affect drug elimination and dosing strategies.

12. Appreciate the need for specific pediatric pharmacokinetic studies and clinical application concepts, and differences between children and adults.

13. To understand how genetic variation in drug-disposition proteins affects therapeutic efficacy and toxicity.

PHARMACOKINETIC PROCESSES AND PARAMETERS

Paul M. Beringer and Michael Winter

Learning Objectives

By the end of the basic principles chapter, the learner shall be able to:

Bioavailability (F)

1. Define bioavailability and list the typical conditions necessary for absorption into the systemic circulation, following oral administration (e.g., stability in GI fluids, proper lipid vs. water solubility, etc.).
2. Define dosage form and salt form (S) and list two or more drugs that are administered as different dosage and/or salt forms.
3. Define first-pass effect with regard to hepatic metabolism and what influence it can have on oral bioavailability if there is a significant first-pass effect.
4. Describe the relationship between the oral and parenteral dose of a drug that has a significant first-pass effect.

Administration Rate (R_A)

1. Define dose and dosing interval.
2. Describe the difference between a continuous infusion and an intermittent dosing regimen.
3. Explain how the units for dosing interval are usually assigned for drugs that are administered on a regular but intermittent basis.

Desired Plasma Concentration (C)

1. Define fraction unbound (fu).
2. Explain saturable plasma binding and at what concentrations most drugs might show saturable binding. List one drug that is known to have saturable plasma binding.

3. Describe the impact of a decrease in the plasma protein on the:
   a. Total plasma concentration.
   b. Bound plasma concentration.
   c. Unbound plasma concentration.
4. Explain the effect on the desired plasma concentration necessary to give a normal therapeutic response when plasma binding is decreased.
5. List two or more drugs that have a fu of 0.1.
6. Know the plasma protein to which drugs that are weak acids bind most frequently.
7. Describe the effect of end-stage renal failure on the total, bound, and unbound phenytoin concentration.
8. List two reasons why assays for unbound drug concentrations would be desirable and two reasons why not.

Volume of Distribution (V)

1. Define with an equation the relationship between volume of distribution, total amount of drug in the body, and the assayed plasma concentration.
2. List two conditions or factors that would increase the apparent volume of distribution and two factors that would decrease the apparent volume of distribution.
3. Demonstrate with an equation how to calculate an initial loading dose necessary to achieve a desired plasma concentration.
4. Demonstrate with an equation how to determine the loading dose if the patient has an initial plasma concentration.
5. Explain the significance of two-compartment modeling when the end organ for response (receptors) behaves as though they are in the first compartment. Consider the rapid onset and the initial rapid decline in pharmacologic effect relative to administration of the loading dose. List at least two drugs that behave this way.
6. Explain the significance of two-compartment modeling when the end organ for response (receptors) behaves as though they are in slower equilibrating tissue compartment. List at least two drugs that behave this way.
7. Why do almost all drugs display two-compartment modeling when given IV but not when given orally? Name two drugs that are an exception and the distribution phase can be seen following oral administration.
8. Explain for a drug with a large volume of distribution, that is, the majority of drug is in the tissue, the impact of a decrease in plasma binding on the loading dose of a drug.

Clearance (Cl)

1. Use an equation to "define" clearance relative to a dosing regimen [(S)(F)(Dose/τ)] and the Css ave.
2. Select the proper units (volume/time) for clearance, given a dosing regimen and Css ave.
3. Calculate the third if any two of the three (dosing regimen, Css ave, and clearance) are given.
4. Approximate a patient's body surface area if weight is given.
5. Explain why, when plasma protein binding is decreased, the Css ave of the unbound drug almost always remains unchanged. The learner shall also be able to give at least one example.
6. Calculate clearance and dosing rate adjustment factors that can be used to calculate a dose for a patient with compromised renal or hepatic function, given the renal clearance and metabolic clearance (or fractions eliminated renally and metabolically).
7. List at least four factors that can influence or alter clearance.

Elimination Rate Constant (K) and Half-Life (t½)

1. Define K with regard to Cl and V and be able to identify which of the variables (K, Cl, or V) are dependent and which are independent.
2. Perform a unit analysis and select units that are consistent for K, Cl, and V.
3. Calculate the expected drug concentration (C_2) after a given time interval (t), given an initial drug concentration (C_1) and K value.
4. Calculate the K value, given two drug concentrations (C_1 and C_2) and the time interval between the two.
5. Explain why the time interval between C_1 and C_2 should be a minimum of one half-life in order to make a reasonable estimate of K or t½.
6. Know the number of half-lives necessary to achieve 90% of steady state and explain why in clinical practice many use four or five half-lives as the time necessary to assure steady state has been attained.
7. Calculate a non–steady-state drug concentration (C_1) t_1 hours after initiating a constant infusion and the drug concentration (C_2) t_2 hours after ending the infusion.

Maximum and Minimum Plasma Concentrations

1. Write the equations representing the maximum or minimum concentration, assuming instantaneous absorption and an intermittent, fixed dosing interval.
2. Draw a graph of the steady-state plasma concentrations that is approximately to scale, given a dosing interval and drug half-life. For example, if the dosing interval is equal to the half-life, the peak should be two times the trough and the line connecting the peak and trough should be slightly convexly curved.
3. Explain why, if the dosing interval is much less than the drug half-life, the Css trough can be used as Css ave to calculate clearance.

Bioavailability (F)

DEFINITION

Bioavailability is the percentage or fraction of the administered dose that reaches the systemic circulation of the patient. Examples of factors that can alter bioavailability include the inherent dissolution and absorption characteristics of the administered chemical form (e.g., salt, ester), the dosage form (e.g., tablet, capsule), the route of administration, the stability of the active ingredient in the gastrointestinal (GI) tract, and the extent of drug metabolism before reaching the systemic circulation. Drugs can be metabolized by GI bacteria, the GI mucosa, and the liver before reaching the systemic circulation.

To calculate the amount of drug absorbed, the administered dose should be multiplied by a bioavailability factor, which is usually represented by the letter "F." For example, the bioavailability of digoxin is estimated to be 0.7 for orally administered tablets.[1-3] This means that if 250 mcg (0.25 mg) of digoxin is given orally, the effective or absorbed dose can be calculated by multiplying the administered dose by F:

$$\text{Amount of Drug Absorbed or Reaching the Systemic Circulation} = (F)(Dose) \qquad \textbf{(Eq. 1.1)}$$

$$\text{Amount of Drug Absorbed or Reaching the Systemic Circulation} = (F)(Dose)$$
$$= (0.7)(250 \text{ mcg})$$
$$= 175 \text{ mcg}$$

It should be emphasized that this factor does not take into consideration the rate of drug absorption; it only estimates the extent of absorption. Although the rate of absorption can be important when rapid onset of pharmacologic effects is required, it is not usually important when a drug is administered chronically. The rate of absorption is important only when it is so slow that it limits the absolute bioavailability of the drug, or when it is so rapid that too much drug is too quickly absorbed. "Dose dumping" can occur under certain conditions with some sustained-release preparations.[4,5] In addition, incomplete absorption of sustained-release dosage forms should be considered in patients who have a short GI transit time. GI transit times of 24 to 48 hours are probably average, but patients with bowel disease may have transit times of only a few hours. A lower-than-average bioavailability should be considered in these patients, especially when the duration of absorption is extended.

DOSAGE FORM

As noted previously, bioavailability can vary among different formulations and dosage forms of a drug. For example, digoxin elixir has a bioavailability of approximately 80% (F = 0.8), whereas the soft gelatin capsules have a bioavailability of 100% (F = 1.0). This is in contrast to the tablets, which have a bioavailability of 70% (F = 0.7).[2,6,7] When drugs are administered parenterally, the bioavailability is usually considered to be 100% (F = 1.0). Equation 1.1 can be rearranged to calculate equivalent doses of a drug when a patient is to receive a different dosage form of the same drug.

$$\frac{\text{Dose of New}}{\text{Dosage Form}} = \frac{\begin{array}{c}\text{Amount of Drug Absorbed}\\\text{From Current Dosage Form}\end{array}}{\text{F of New Dosage Form}} \qquad \textbf{(Eq. 1.2)}$$

For example, if a patient who has been receiving digoxin 250 mcg (0.25 mg) in the tablet dosage form, with a bioavailability of 0.7, needs to receive digoxin elixir, an equivalent dose of the elixir would be calculated as follows:

$$\text{Dose of Elixir} = \frac{(0.7)(250\,\text{mcg})}{0.8}$$
$$= \frac{175\,\text{mcg}}{0.8}$$
$$= 219\,\text{mcg}$$

If the soft gelatin capsules of digoxin were to be administered, the bioavailability or F of the new dosage form would have been 1.0, and the equivalent dose would have been 175 mcg.

The bioavailability of parenterally administered drugs is usually assumed to be 1.0. Drugs which are administered as inactive precursors that must then be converted to an active product are an exception to this rule. If some of the inactive precursor is eliminated from the body (renally excreted or metabolized to an inactive compound) before it can be converted to the active compound, the bioavailability will be <1.0.

For example, parenteral chloramphenicol is given as the succinate ester, and this chloramphenicol ester must be hydrolyzed to the active compound. The bioavailability of the parenterally administered chloramphenicol succinate ranges from 55% to 95% because from 5% to 45% of the chloramphenicol ester is eliminated renally before it can be converted to the active compound.[8-10] Generally, for those drugs with nearly complete absorption (F > 0.8), bioavailability is usually consistent. For those drugs with a low oral bioavailability (F < 0.5), there is often a large variation in the extent of absorption. This is not a hard and fast rule because any drug under the right conditions can have an altered bioavailability.

CHEMICAL FORM (S)

The chemical form of a drug must also be considered when evaluating bioavailability. For example, when a salt or an ester of a drug is administered, the bioavailability factor (F) should be multiplied by the fraction of the total molecular weight that the active drug represents. If "S" represents the fraction of the administered dose that is the active drug, then the amount of drug absorbed from a salt or an ester form can be calculated as follows:

$$\text{Amount of Drug Absorbed or Reaching the Systemic Circulation} = (S)(F)(Dose) \qquad \text{(Eq. 1.3)}$$

The "S" factor should be included in all bioavailability equations as a constant reminder of its importance in assessing bioavailability of the active drug form. When a drug is administered in its parent or active form, the "S" for that drug is 1.0.

Equation 1.2 can now be expanded to consider the salt factor and the bioavailability when calculating the dose of a new dosage form:

$$\text{Dose of New Dosage Form} = \frac{\text{Amount of Drug Absorbed from Current Dosage Form}}{(S)(F) \text{ of New Dosage Form}} \qquad \text{(Eq. 1.4)}$$

Aminophylline and phenytoin are examples of this principle (Fig. 1.1). Aminophylline is the ethylenediamine salt of the pharmacologically active moiety, theophylline. For this salt, 80% to 85% (by weight) is theophylline so that the "S" for aminophylline is approximately 0.8. Uncoated aminophylline tablets are considered to be completely (100%) bioavailable; the bioavailability factor (F) for this dosage form is, therefore, 1.0. It is important to consider the salt form in determining the amount of theophylline absorbed from an aminophylline tablet. When Equation 1.3 is applied to this situation,

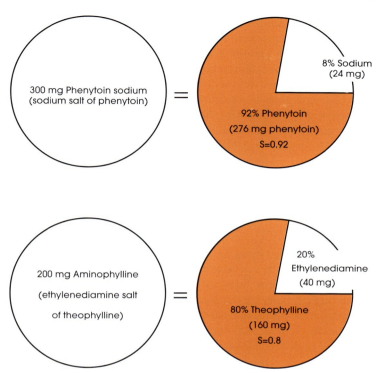

FIGURE 1.1   The effect of the chemical drug form on bioavailability. The examples above emphasize the importance of considering the chemical form when calculating the amount of active drug actually administered. The amount of active drug administered may represent only a fraction (S) of the salt, ester, or other chemical form of the drug contained in the formulation. The bioavailability (F) of the dosage form itself must also be considered when drugs are administered by the oral route.

it can be demonstrated that 160 mg of theophylline is absorbed from a 200-mg aminophylline tablet:

$$\text{Amount of Drug Absorbed or Reaching the Systamic Circulation} = (S)(F)(\text{Dose})$$

$$= (0.8)(1)(200 \text{ mg Aminophylline})$$

$$= 160 \text{ mg Theophylline}$$

Similarly, 300 mg of phenytoin sodium with an S of 0.92 represents only 276 mg of phenytoin reaching the systemic circulation, assuming complete absorption (F = 1).

$$\text{Amount of Drug Absorbed or Reaching the Systemic Circulation} = (S)(F)(\text{Dose})$$

$$= (0.92)(1)(300 \text{ mg Phenytoin Sodium})$$

$$= 276 \text{ mg Phenytoin}$$

In some cases, the labeled amount of drug has already taken into account the amount of active drug. Valproate sodium, the sodium salt of valproic acid, is manufactured and labeled with the amount of valproic acid and, therefore, a value of 1 would be appropriate for S. Fosphenytoin sodium is the sodium salt of the phosphate ester of phenytoin. Although fosphenytoin sodium is only 61% phenytoin, the manufacturers have labeled the drug as phenytoin sodium equivalents or P.E. Therefore, to calculate the amount of phenytoin in 100 mg of fosphenytoin P.E., an S value of 0.92 would be used.

The important concept is to understand and be able to calculate the amount of the labeled drug that will be available to the patient as active drug. To do this, both the fraction of the dose that is active drug (S) and the bioavailability or fraction of administered dose that will reach the systemic circulation (F) needs to be considered when calculating doses and dosing regimens.

FIRST-PASS EFFECT

Because orally administered drugs are absorbed from the GI tract into the portal circulation, some drugs may be extensively metabolized by the liver before reaching the systemic circulation. The term "first pass" refers to metabolism by the liver because the drug passes through the liver via the portal vein following absorption. This "first-pass effect" can substantially decrease the amount of active drug reaching the systemic circulation and thus its bioavailability (Fig. 1.2).

Propranolol is an example of a drug that has a significant portion of an orally administered dose that does not reach the systemic circulation because it is metabolized as it passes through the liver following absorption from the GI tract. Because of this "first-pass effect," oral bioavailability is low, and orally administered doses are much larger than doses administered intravenously (IV). However, the propranolol issue is further complicated by the fact that one of the metabolites, 4-hydroxy-propranolol, is pharmacologically active.[11] Lidocaine is an example of a drug with a first-pass effect that is so great that oral administration is not practical as a route of administration if systemic effects are desired.[12] In addition, some drugs are extensively metabolized by cytochrome enzymes, primarily CYP3A4, that are located in the gut wall. As an example, the low and variable bioavailability ($F \approx 0.3$) of cyclosporine is in part because of metabolism by CYP3A4 in the gut wall.[13]

Administration Rate (R$_A$)

The administration rate is the average rate at which absorbed drug reaches the systemic circulation. This is usually calculated by dividing the amount of drug absorbed (see Equation 1.3) by the time over which the drug was administered (dosing interval). The dosing interval is usually represented by the symbol, tau (τ).

$$\text{Administration Rate } R_A = \frac{(S)(F)(\text{Dose})}{\tau} \qquad \textbf{(Eq. 1.5)}$$

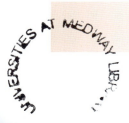

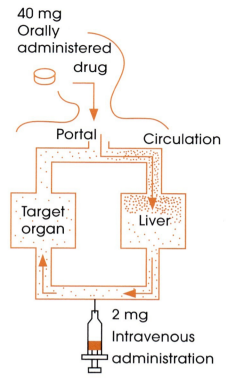

FIGURE 1.2   First-pass effect. When drugs with a high "first-pass effect" are administered orally, a large amount of the absorbed drug is metabolized before it reaches the systemic circulation. If the drug is administered intravenously, the liver is bypassed and the fraction of the administered dose that reaches the circulation is increased. Parenteral doses of drugs with a high "first pass" are much smaller than oral doses necessary to produce equivalent pharmacologic effects.

When drugs are administered as a continuous infusion, the dosing interval can be expressed in any convenient time unit. For example, the theophylline administration rate resulting from aminophylline infused at a rate of 40 mg/hr is calculated using Equation 1.5 as follows:

$$\text{Administration Rate } R_A = \frac{(S)(F)(Dose)}{\tau}$$
$$= \frac{(0.8)(1)(40 \text{ mg})}{1 \text{ hr}}$$
$$= 32 \text{ mg/hr}$$

or

$$\text{Administration Rate } R_A = \frac{(S)(F)(Dose)}{\tau}$$
$$= \frac{(0.8)(1)(40 \text{ mg})}{60 \text{ min}}$$
$$= 0.53 \text{ mg/min}$$

When drugs are administered at fixed dosing intervals, the calculated administration rate is an average value. For example, the average administration rate of digoxin resulting from an oral dose of 250 mcg of digoxin given orally as tablets every day would be calculated using Equation 1.5 as follows:

$$\text{Administration Rate } R_A = \frac{(S)(F)(\text{Dose})}{\tau}$$

$$= \frac{(1)(0.7)(250 \text{ mcg})}{1 \text{ day}}$$

$$= 175 \text{ mcg/day}$$

or

$$\text{Administration Rate } R_A = \frac{(S)(F)(\text{Dose})}{\tau}$$

$$= \frac{(1)(0.7)(250 \text{ mcg})}{24 \text{ hr}}$$

$$= 7.29 \text{ mcg/hr}$$

Although each digoxin tablet is actually absorbed over 1 to 2 hours, the average "administration rate" is calculated over the entire dosing interval. Although the administration rate of 7.29 mcg/hr and 175 mcg/day are equivalent, most clinicians think of the dosing rate that is consistent with how the drug is administered. In this case, the usual interval would be 1 day because digoxin is most commonly administered once each day. In the section on clearance, we consider how the drug administration rate, drug clearance, and the usually reported units for drug concentration all need to be consistent for the purposes of performing pharmacokinetic calculations.

Desired Plasma Concentration (C)

PROTEIN BINDING

Most clinical laboratory reports of drug concentrations in plasma (C) represent drug that is bound to plasma protein plus drug that is unbound or free. It is the free or unbound drug that is in equilibrium with the receptor site and is, therefore, the pharmacologically active moiety. Thus, in the case of a drug with significant plasma binding, the reported plasma drug concentration indirectly reflects the concentration of free or active drug (Fig. 1.3).

Some disease states are associated with decreased plasma proteins or with decreased binding of drugs to plasma proteins.[14-17] In these situations, drugs that are usually highly protein bound have a larger percentage of free or unbound drug present in plasma. Therefore, a greater pharmacologic effect can be expected for any given drug

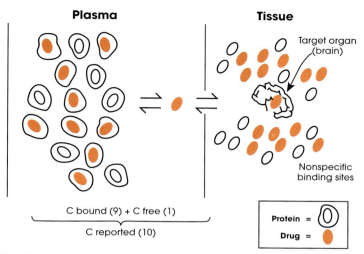

FIGURE 1.3   Plasma concentration of a highly protein-bound drug: normal plasma protein concentration. The plasma drug concentration reported by the laboratory represents a total of both "bound" and "free" drug. It is the "free" drug that is in equilibrium with the target organs and is the pharmacologically active moiety. In this illustration, fu (or the fraction of free drug to total drug concentration) is 0.1.

concentration in plasma (C). Clinicians must always consider altered protein binding and whether the fraction of free drug concentration or fraction unbound (fu) is altered when interpreting or establishing desired plasma drug concentrations.

$$fu = \frac{\text{Free Drug Concentration}}{\text{Total Drug Concentration}}$$

$$fu = \frac{\text{C free}}{\text{C bound} + \text{C free}} \qquad \textbf{(Eq. 1.6)}$$

The fraction of drug that is unbound (fu) does not vary with the drug concentration for most drugs that are bound primarily to albumin. This is because the number of protein binding sites far exceeds the number of drug molecules available for binding. When the plasma concentrations for drugs bound to albumin exceed 25 to 50 mg/L, however, albumin binding sites can start to become saturated. As a result, fu, or the fraction of drug that is free, will change with the plasma drug concentration. For example, valproic acid can saturate plasma protein binding sites when plasma concentrations exceed 25 to 50 mg/L.[18] For those drugs that do not reach serum concentrations capable of saturating protein binding sites, the plasma protein concentration (in many cases, this is albumin) and the binding affinity of the drug for the plasma protein are the two major factors that control the fu.

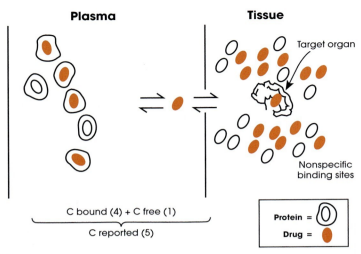

FIGURE 1.4 Effect of decreased plasma protein concentration on plasma drug concentration. Compare this figure with Figure 1.3. The decreased protein concentration decreases the plasma drug concentration reported by the laboratory. In this situation, the concentration of free, or active, drug remains the same because free drug that is released as a result of the lowered plasma protein concentration is taken up by nonspecific tissue binding sites and/or cleared from the body. For this reason, the pharmacologic effect, which can be expected from the reported C of 5, will be the same as that produced by the reported C of 10 in Figure 1.3. In this illustration, fu (or the fraction of free drug to total drug concentration) is increased to 0.2 because of the decrease in the bound concentration.

LOW PLASMA PROTEIN CONCENTRATIONS

Low plasma protein concentrations decrease the plasma concentration of bound drug (C bound); however, the concentration of free drug (C free) generally is unaffected. Therefore, the fraction of drug that is free (fu) increases as plasma protein concentrations decrease. Free or unbound drug concentrations are not significantly increased because the free drug that is released into plasma secondary to low plasma protein concentrations equilibrates with the tissue compartment (compare Fig. 1.4 with Fig. 1.3). Therefore, if the volume of distribution (V) is relatively large (e.g., phenytoin 0.65 L/kg), only a minor increase in C free will result (also see Volume of Distribution [V]).

The relationship between the plasma drug concentration and the plasma protein concentration can be expressed as follows:

$$\frac{C'}{C_{\text{Normal Binding}}} = (1 - fu)\left[\frac{P'}{P_{NL}}\right] + fu \qquad \textbf{(Eq. 1.7)}$$

This equation can be used to estimate the degree to which an altered plasma protein concentration will affect the desired therapeutic drug concentration. C' represents the patient's plasma drug concentration, and P' represents the patient's plasma protein concentration. $C_{\text{Normal Binding}}$ is the plasma drug concentration that would be expected if the patient's plasma protein concentration were normal (P_{NL}). Note that fu is the free fraction associated with "normal plasma protein binding." The $C_{Normal\ Binding}$ for any given drug can be calculated by rearranging Equation 1.7 as:

$$C_{Normal\ Binding} = \frac{C'}{(1-fu)\left[\dfrac{P'}{P_{NL}}\right] + fu} \qquad \text{(Eq. 1.8)}$$

For example, a patient with a low serum albumin of 2.2 g/dL (normal albumin, 4.4 g/dL) and an apparently low plasma phenytoin concentration of 5.5 mg/L still has a therapeutically acceptable plasma drug concentration when it is adjusted for the low serum albumin. When the normal free fraction (fu) for phenytoin of 0.1 is substituted into Equation 1.8, an adjusted phenytoin plasma concentration of 10 mg/L is calculated.

$$C_{Normal\ Binding} = \frac{C'}{(1-fu)\left[\dfrac{P'}{P_{NL}}\right] + fu}$$

$$= \frac{5.5 \text{ mg/L}}{(1-0.1)\left[\dfrac{2.2 \text{ g/dL}}{4.4 \text{ g/dL}}\right] + 0.1}$$

$$= \frac{5.5 \text{ mg/L}}{(0.9)(0.5) + 0.1}$$

$$= 10 \text{ mg/L}$$

The phenytoin concentration that would have been reported from the laboratory if the patient's albumin concentration was "normal" would be approximately 10 mg/L. This calculation is based on the assumption that phenytoin is primarily bound to albumin and that an average normal albumin concentration is 4.4 g/dL (range: 3.5 to 5.5 g/dL). Although Equation 1.8 could be used to adjust for any drug significantly bound to albumin, the degree to which the drug concentration will be adjusted or "normalized" for the alteration in serum albumin between 3.5 and 5.5 g/dL will be minimal and is generally unwarranted.

Many other drugs are bound primarily to globulin rather than albumin. Adjustments of plasma drug concentrations for these drugs based on serum albumin concentrations would, therefore, be inappropriate. Unfortunately, adjustments for changes in globulin binding are difficult, because drugs usually bind to a specific globulin that is only a small fraction of total globulin concentration. In general, acidic drugs (e.g., phenytoin, most of the antiepileptic drugs, and some neutral compounds) bind primarily to albumin; basic drugs (e.g., lidocaine and quinidine) bind more extensively to globulins.[15,19–22]

ELEVATED PLASMA PROTEIN CONCENTRATIONS

The fu value (fraction of total drug concentration that is free or unbound) for selected drugs is provided in Table 1.1. Because increases in serum albumin are uncommon in

TABLE 1.1   Drugs and fu Values for Plasma Protein Binding

DRUG	fu VALUE
Amitriptyline	0.04[a]
Carbamazepine	0.2
Chlordiazepoxide	0.05
Chlorpromazine	0.04[a]
Cyclosporine	<0.1[b]
Diazepam	0.01
Digoxin	0.70
Digitoxin	0.10
Ethosuximide	1.0
Gabapentin	0.97
Gentamicin	0.9
Imipramine	0.04[a]
Lidocaine	0.30[a]
Lithium	1.0
Methadone	0.13[a]
Methotrexate	0.5
Nafcillin	0.10
Nelfinavir	0.02
Phenobarbital	0.5
Phenytoin	0.10
Propranolol	0.06[a]
Quinidine	0.20[a]
Salicylic acid	0.16[c]
Valproic acid	0.15[c]
Vancomycin	0.9
Warfarin	0.03

[a]Basic drugs that are bound significantly to plasma proteins other than albumin.[14,19,20,23]
[b]Bound to lipoproteins and other blood elements.[24,25]
[c]Concentration-dependent plasma protein binding (see Chapter 15).
fu, unbound fraction.

the clinical setting, the use of Equation 1.8 for high serum albumin would be rare. Many basic drugs, however, are bound to the acute phase reactive protein,[26,27] α_1-acid glyco-protein (AAG). This plasma protein has been known to be significantly decreased and increased under certain clinical conditions. For example, increases in plasma quinidine concentrations have been observed following surgery or trauma.[19,28] The change in the quinidine concentration is the result of increased concentrations of the plasma binding proteins (AAGs) and increased bound concentrations of quinidine. There appears to be little or no change in the free quinidine level because re-equilibration with the larger tissue stores occurs. In this situation, there would be a decrease in fu, and the therapeutic levels of free or unbound drug should correlate with higher-than-usual drug concentration (C bound + C free). Other basic compounds with significant binding to AAGs would be expected to be similarly affected. Unfortunately, AAG concentrations are seldom assayed in the clinical setting, thereby making it difficult to evaluate the relationship between the total drug concentration and the fu. For this reason, evaluation of plasma levels for basic drugs that are significantly protein bound is often difficult. A careful evaluation of the patient's clinical response to a measured drug level, as well as an evaluation of any concurrent medical problems (such as surgery, trauma, or inflammatory disease) that could influence plasma protein concentrations and drug binding, is required.

Patients with cirrhosis vary considerably in their plasma protein binding characteristics. Some patients have significantly elevated binding capabilities, whereas others have significantly decreased binding capabilities. This variation probably reflects the fact that some cirrhotic patients have a strong stimulus for the production of AAGs, whereas others with more serious hepatic disease are unable to manufacture these binding proteins.[26,28,29]

BINDING AFFINITY

The binding affinity of plasma protein for a drug can also alter the fraction of drug that is free (fu) (compare Fig. 1.5 with Fig. 1.3). For example, the plasma proteins in patients with uremia (severe end-stage renal failure) have less affinity for phenytoin than that in nonuremic individuals.

As a result, the fu for phenytoin in uremic patients is estimated to be in the range of 0.2 to 0.3 in contrast to the normal value of 0.1.[22,30] The "effective" or free drug concentration can be calculated by rearranging Equation 1.6:

$$\text{fu} = \frac{\text{C free}}{\text{C bound} + \text{C free}}$$

$$= \frac{\text{C free}}{\text{C total}}$$

$$\text{C free} = (\text{fu})(\text{C total}) \qquad \textbf{(Eq. 1.9)}$$

According to Equation 1.9, the concentration of free phenytoin in uremic patients is comparable to that in nonuremic patients—despite lower phenytoin

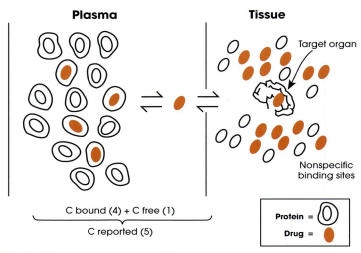

FIGURE 1.5 The effect of decreased binding affinity on plasma drug concentration. Compare this figure with Figure 1.3. Although the protein concentration is normal, the decreased binding affinity of the drug for protein has decreased the reported drug concentration. The concentration of free, or active, drug remains the same because drug that is released from the plasma binding sites as a result of this decreased affinity is taken up by nonspecific binding sites in the tissue and/or cleared from the body. Thus, the pharmacologic effect that can be expected from the reported C of 5 will be the same as that produced by the reported C of 10 in Figure 1.3. In this illustration, fu (or the fraction of free drug to total drug concentration) is increased to 0.2 because of a decrease in the bound concentration.

plasma concentrations (C total). In the uremic patient, the fu is increased because the bound concentration is decreased, and as a result, the C total is decreased. The important point is that the unbound concentration is not increased. The uremic patient with an fu of 0.2 and a reported phenytoin concentration of 5 mg/L would have the same free drug concentration (and same pharmacologic effect) as a patient with normal renal function who has a reported phenytoin concentration of 10 mg/L (using Equation 1.9):

$$C \text{ free} = (fu)(C \text{ total})$$

$$\begin{aligned}
&C \text{ free} \\
&\text{(in a Uremic Patient)} = (0.2)(5 \text{ mg/L}) \\
&\qquad\qquad\qquad\quad = 1 \text{ mg/L}
\end{aligned}$$

$$\begin{aligned}
&C \text{ free} \\
&\text{(in a Patient with} \quad = (0.1)(10 \text{ mg/L}) \\
&\text{Normal Renal Function)} \\
&\qquad\qquad\qquad\quad = 1 \text{ mg/L}
\end{aligned}$$

In summary, any factor that alters protein binding becomes clinically important when a drug is highly protein bound (i.e., if fu is <0.1 or 10% unbound). For example, if fu is increased from 0.1 (10% free) to 0.2 (20% free), the concentration of free or active drug *for any given value of* C (bound + free) would be double the usual values, that is:

$$C \text{ free} = (\text{fu})(C \text{ total})$$
$$= (0.1)(10 \text{ mg/L})$$
$$= 1 \text{ mg/L}$$
$$\text{vs.}$$
$$= (0.2)(10 \text{ mg/L})$$
$$= 2 \text{ mg/L}$$

While, in the above example, it is true that the patient with altered binding had a higher unbound concentration, the increase in the unbound concentration was not owing to or caused by the decrease in binding. The unbound concentration of 2 mg/L is the result of a larger amount of drug in the body from either a loading or maintenance dose.

If, on the other hand, the fu for a drug is ≥0.5 (50% free), it is unlikely that changes in plasma protein binding will be of clinical consequence. As an illustration, if the fu for a drug is increased from a normal value 0.5 (50% free) to 0.6 (60% free) because of decreased protein concentrations, the concentration of free active drug (assuming the same total concentration) would actually be increased by only 20%.

$$C \text{ free} = (\text{fu})(C \text{ total})$$
$$= (0.5)(10 \text{ mg/L})$$
$$= 5 \text{ mg/L}$$
$$\text{vs.}$$
$$= (0.6)(10 \text{ mg/L})$$
$$= 6 \text{ mg/L}$$

As a general rule, if fu is increased in any given situation, the clinician should reduce the desired C by the same proportion.[14] That is, if fu is increased twofold, the desired C or "therapeutic range" should be reduced to one-half the usual value.

What is often misunderstood is that for drugs with significant plasma protein binding, changes in plasma binding will have a profound effect on the plasma drug concentration, because the bound concentration has been altered but generally the unbound concentration is unchanged. As a consequence, the fu of drug in plasma is altered. Again, the unbound drug concentration is, in most cases, relatively unaffected.[31] When considering changes in binding, it should be kept in mind that the fu is the ratio of unbound drug concentration to total drug concentration, as outlined in Equation 1.6.

$$\text{fu} = \frac{C \text{ free}}{C \text{ bound} + C \text{ free}}$$

As depicted in Equation 1.6, fu is dependent on the binding characteristics and is not the "cause" of the free or unbound drug concentration as might be suggested in Equation 1.9.

$$\text{C free} = (\text{fu})(\text{C total})$$

As an example, let us consider four patients, the first two with phenytoin concentrations of 10 and 20 mg/L, respectively. If both these patients had normal plasma binding (fu = 0.1), their respective C free phenytoin concentrations would be 1 and 2 mg/L. The increased potential effect of the C total phenytoin concentration of 20 mg/L with a C free of 2 mg/L seems intuitively obvious. The fact that the drug concentration (C bound and C free) is higher in the second patient is probably the result of either higher-than-average doses or decreased elimination.

Now let us consider two other patients each with a phenytoin concentration of 10 mg/L. However, in this case, the first patient has normal plasma binding and an fu of 0.1. The second patient has decreased plasma binding and, as a result, an fu of 0.2. In this situation, the first patient with a normal binding fu of 0.1 and C total of 10 mg/L would have a C free of 1 mg/L. The second patient with an altered binding fu of 0.2 and a C total of 10 mg/L would have a C free of 2 mg/L. It is important to recognize that although both patients have a phenytoin concentration of 10 mg/L, the second patient would be expected to have an increased drug effect because of the higher C free or unbound drug concentration. The reason that the second patient has an increased C free is not because of altered binding, but probably because the patient has been given higher-than-average doses or their metabolism is less than average.

MONITORING FREE OR UNBOUND PLASMA CONCENTRATIONS

Although many clinicians believe that monitoring free or unbound plasma concentrations is desirable, it is not common in general clinical practice. The reasons are several and include the fact that assay procedures for free or unbound drug are not commercially available for many compounds. Furthermore, the assay procedures available for free drug concentrations are more expensive and increase the cost of providing patient care. In addition, most patients exhibit reasonably normal binding characteristics; therefore, monitoring unbound drug concentrations would not add significantly to the evaluation of their clinical status. Whereas, in theory, monitoring unbound drug concentrations should be clinically superior, there is little evidence demonstrating that monitoring unbound drug levels improves the correlation between the plasma concentration and the pharmacologic effect or therapeutic outcome.

If unbound drug concentrations are to be used in clinical practice, the clinician must be aware of factors that can alter the relationship between in vitro and in vivo plasma binding characteristics. For example, the method used to determine the free drug level (equilibrium dialysis, ultrafiltration, saliva sampling, etc.) and the conditions under which the sample is obtained can alter the in vitro assay results. This in turn can result in an inaccurate estimate of the in vivo binding characteristics.[17,32–35] For these reasons, the use of unbound or free plasma level monitoring is not the standard of practice and is used in only a limited number of clinical settings. If unbound serum drug concentrations are used infrequently, the results should be carefully evaluated and compared to both the expected free drug level and the clinical response of the patient.

Volume of Distribution (V)

The volume of distribution for a drug or the "apparent volume of distribution" does not necessarily refer to any physiologic compartment in the body.[1,36] It is simply the size of a compartment necessary to account for the total amount of drug in the body if it was present throughout the body at the same concentration found in the plasma (Fig. 1.6A). The equation for the volume of distribution is expressed as follows:

$$V = \frac{Ab}{C}$$

(Eq. 1.10)

where V is the apparent volume of distribution, Ab the total amount of drug in the body, and C the plasma concentration of drug.

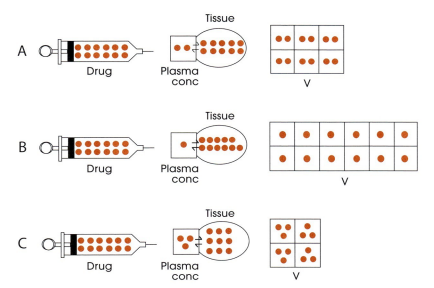

FIGURE 1.6   Volume of distribution. (**A**) The administration of a drug into the body produces a specific plasma concentration. The apparent volume of distribution (V) is the volume that accounts for the total dose administration based on the observed plasma concentration. (**B**) Any factor that decreases the drug plasma concentration (e.g., decreased plasma protein binding) will increase the apparent volume of distribution. (**C**) Conversely, any factor that increases the plasma concentration (e.g., decreased tissue binding) will decrease the apparent volume of distribution.

The plasma volume of the average adult is approximately 3 L. Therefore, apparent volumes of distribution that are larger than the plasma compartment (>3 L) only indicate that the drug is also present in tissues or fluids outside the plasma compartment. The actual sites of distribution cannot be determined from the V value. For example, a drug with a volume of distribution similar to total body water (0.65 L/kg) does not indicate that the drug is equilibrated equally throughout the total body water. The drug may or may not be bound in or excluded from certain tissues. However, the average binding results in an apparent volume of distribution that is approximately equal to that of total body water. Without additional specific information, the actual sites of a drug's distribution are only speculative.

The apparent volume of distribution is a function of the lipid versus water solubilities and of the plasma and tissue protein binding properties of the drug. Factors that tend to keep the drug in the plasma or increase C (such as high water solubility, increased plasma protein binding, or decreased tissue binding) tend to reduce the apparent volume of distribution. It follows then that factors which decrease C in plasma (such as decreased plasma protein binding, increased tissue binding, and increased lipid solubility) tend to increase the apparent volume of distribution.

LOADING DOSE

Because the volume of distribution is the factor that accounts for all of the drug in the body, it is an important variable in estimating the loading dose necessary to rapidly achieve a desired plasma concentration:

$$\text{Loading Dose} = \frac{(V)(C)}{(S)(F)}$$

(Eq. 1.11)

where V is the volume of distribution, C the desired plasma level, and (S)(F) the fraction of the dose administered that will reach the systemic circulation (Fig. 1.7).

For example, if one wishes to calculate an oral loading dose of digoxin (i.e., using digoxin tablets) for a 70-kg man that produces a plasma concentration of 1.5 mcg/L, Equation 1.10 can be used. If S is assumed to be 1.0, F to be 0.7, and V to be 7.3 L/kg,[1,3,37] the loading dose will be 1,095 mcg or 1.095 mg based on the following calculation:

$$\begin{aligned}
\text{Loading Dose} &= \frac{(V)(C)}{(S)(F)} \\
&= \frac{(7.3 \text{ L/kg})(70 \text{ kg})(1.5 \text{ mcg/L})}{(1)(0.7)} \\
&= 1{,}095 \text{ mcg or } 1.095 \text{ mg}
\end{aligned}$$

A reasonable approximation of this dose would be 1 mg given orally as tablets. The usual clinical approach is to give the loading dose in divided doses (0.25 mg per dose every 6 hours). The patient is observed and evaluated for therapeutic response, and digoxin toxicity before each successive dose is administered. In addition, some clinicians

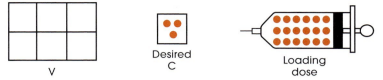

FIGURE 1.7 Loading dose. The volume of distribution is the major determinant of the loading dose. If the V for a drug is known, the loading dose that produces a specific concentration can be calculated (see Equation 1.11).

use a bioavailability factor >0.7 (e.g., 0.75 or 0.8), which would further decrease the chance of exceeding the desired drug concentration.

Equation 1.11 can also be used to estimate the loading dose that will be required to achieve a higher plasma concentration than the present concentration (Fig. 1.8). This new formula is derived by replacing the C in Equation 1.10 with an expression that represents the increment in plasma concentration that is desired.

$$\frac{\text{Incremental}}{\text{Loading Dose}} = \frac{(V)(C_{desired} - C_{initial})}{(S)(F)} \qquad \textbf{(Eq. 1.12)}$$

For example, if the previous patient had a digoxin level of 0.5 mcg/L and the desired concentration was 1.5 mcg/L, the loading dose would have been:

$$\frac{\text{Incremental}}{\text{Loading Dose}} = \frac{(V)(C_{desired} - C_{initial})}{(S)(F)}$$

$$= \frac{(7.3 \text{ L/kg})(70 \text{ kg})(1.5 \text{ mcg/L} - 0.5 \text{ mcg/L})}{(1)(0.7)}$$

$$= 730 \text{ mcg or } 0.73 \text{ mg}$$

A reasonable incremental loading dose in this case would be about 0.75 mg.

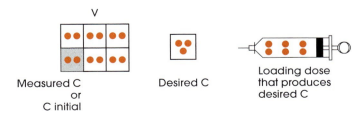

FIGURE 1.8 Loading dose to produce an increment in plasma level. If the V and initial plasma concentration for a drug are known, the incremental loading dose that produces a higher desired plasma concentration can be calculated (see Equation 1.12).

FACTORS THAT ALTER VOLUME OF DISTRIBUTION (V) AND LOADING DOSE

In analyzing Equation 1.11, it becomes clear that any factor that alters the volume of distribution will theoretically influence the loading dose.

Decreased tissue binding of drugs in uremic patients is a common cause of a reduced apparent volume of distribution for several agents (Fig. 1.6C).[38,39] Decreased tissue binding will increase the C by allowing more of the drug to remain in the plasma (Fig. 1.6C). Therefore, if the desired plasma level remains unchanged, a smaller loading dose will be required. Digoxin is an example of a drug whose loading dose should be altered in uremic patients. This is discussed in Chapter 10.

Decreased plasma protein binding, on the other hand, tends to increase the apparent volume of distribution because more drug that would normally be in plasma is available to equilibrate with the tissue and the tissue binding sites (Fig. 1.6B). Decreased plasma protein binding, however, also increases the fraction of free or active drug so that the desired C that produces a given therapeutic response decreases. To summarize, diminished plasma protein binding increases V and decreases C in Equation 1.11, resulting in no net effect on the loading dose.

$$\overset{\leftrightarrow}{\text{Loading Dose}} = \frac{(\uparrow V)(C \downarrow)}{(S)(F)}$$

This is based on the assumption that the majority of drug in the body is actually outside the plasma compartment and that the amount of drug bound to plasma protein comprises only a small percentage of the total amount in the body.

This principle is illustrated by the pharmacokinetic behavior of phenytoin in uremic patients. Plasma phenytoin concentrations in uremic patients are frequently one-half of those observed in normal patients given the same dose. The lower plasma levels, however, produce the same free or pharmacologically active phenytoin concentration as levels twice as high in nonuremic patients because the fu is increased from 0.1 to 0.2 in these individuals, indicating that the target plasma concentrations (bound + free) in uremics should be about half of the usual target concentration. Furthermore, a loading dose of phenytoin that produces a normal therapeutic effect is the same for both uremic and nonuremic patients, because the volume of distribution increases by approximately twofold (0.65 to 1.44 L/kg) in uremic individuals.[27] Equation 1.11 indicates that there would be no change in the loading dose if the volume of distribution is increased by a factor of 2 and the desired drug concentration is decreased by a factor of ½.

$$\overset{\leftrightarrow}{\text{Loading Dose}} = \frac{(2 \times V)(1/2 \times C)}{(S)(F)}$$

TWO-COMPARTMENT MODELS

Pharmacokinetic parameters

If one thinks of the body as a single compartment, pharmacokinetic calculations are relatively simple. However, there are some situations in which it is more appropriate to conceptualize the body as two, and occasionally, more than two compartments when thinking about drug distribution, elimination, and pharmacologic effect. The first compartment can be thought of as a smaller, rapidly equilibrating volume, usually made up of plasma or blood and those organs or tissues that have high blood flow and are in rapid equilibrium with the blood or plasma drug concentration. This first compartment has a volume referred to as V_i or initial volume of distribution. The second compartment equilibrates with the drug over a somewhat longer period. This volume is referred to as V_t or tissue volume of distribution.[36,40] The half-life for the distribution phase is referred to as the alpha (α) half-life, and the half-life for drug elimination from the body is referred to as the beta (β) half-life. The sum of V_i and V_t is the apparent volume of distribution (V). Drugs are assumed to enter into and be eliminated from V_i. That is, any drug that distributes into the tissue compartment (V_t) must re-equilibrate into V_i before it can be eliminated (Fig. 1.9).

Effects of a two-compartment model on the loading dose and plasma concentration (C)

Because some time is required for a drug to distribute into V_t, a rapidly administered loading dose calculated on the basis of V ($V_i + V_t$) would result in an initial C that is higher than predicted, because the initial volume of distribution (V_i) is always smaller than V. The consequences of a higher than expected C depends on whether the target organ for the clinical response behaves as though it were located in V_i or V_t.

Drugs such as lidocaine, phenobarbital, and theophylline exert therapeutic and toxic effects on target organs that behave as though they are located in V_i. In these instances, when loading doses are calculated based on the total volume of distribution, the concentration of drug delivered to the target organs could be much higher than expected and produce toxicity if the loading dose is not administered appropriately. This problem can be circumvented by first calculating the loading dose based on the total volume of distribution (V), and then administering the loading dose at a rate slow enough to allow for drug distribution into V_t. This approach is common in clinical practice, and the guidelines for rates of drug administration are often based on the principle of two-compartment modeling, with the receptors for clinical response (toxic or therapeutic) responding as though they were located in V_i. A second approach is to administer the loading dose in sufficiently small individual bolus doses such that the C in V_i does not exceed some predetermined critical concentration.[41,42]

Although not commonly discussed in pharmacokinetic terms, potassium is a good example of a drug that follows this principle of two-compartment modeling with the end organ being located in V_i. Potassium is primarily an intracellular electrolyte, but its cardiac effects parallel the plasma concentration. In addition, there is a slow equilibrium between plasma and tissue potassium concentrations. When potassium is given IV, the rate of administration must be carefully controlled as serious cardiac

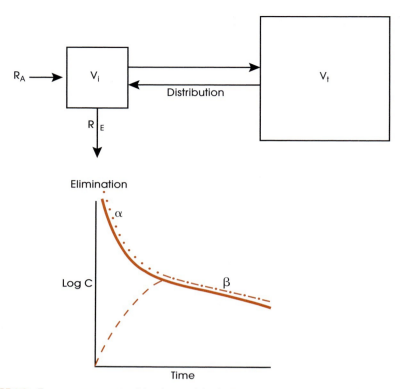

FIGURE 1.9 Two-compartment model: volumes of distribution. V_i is the initial volume of distribution. Drug administration (R_A) and elimination (R_E) are assumed to occur in V_i. The lower graph shows that, following rapid administration of drug into V_i, the plasma concentration (*solid line*) follows a biphasic decay pattern. The initial decay half-life ($\alpha t\frac{1}{2}$) is usually primarily because of drug distribution into V_t. The second decay half-life ($\beta t\frac{1}{2}$) is usually because of drug elimination from the body. The dotted line (*dotted line*) represents the drug effect when the end organ for effect is located in V_i. Note that drug effect parallels the plasma concentration at all times. The dashed line (*dashed line*) represents the drug effect when the end organ for effect is located in V_t. Note that initially when all of the drug is in V_i, there is no drug effect. However, as distribution takes place, the drug effect increases and begins to parallel the plasma concentration only in the elimination phase after distribution is complete.

toxicity and death can occur if the patient experiences excessive potassium concentrations in the plasma (V_i).

This concept of two-compartment modeling is also important in evaluating the offset of drug effect. For drugs with the end organ for clinical response located in V_i, rapid achievement of a therapeutic response followed quickly by a loss of the therapeutic response may be the result of drug being distributed into a larger volume of distribution rather than drug being eliminated from the body (see Chapter 10).

When the drug's target organ is in the second or tissue compartment, V_t (e.g., digoxin, lithium), the high C, which may be observed before distribution occurs, is not dangerous. However, plasma concentrations that are obtained before distribution is complete will not reflect the tissue concentration at equilibrium. Therefore, these plasma samples cannot be used to predict the therapeutic or toxic potential of these drugs.[43,44] For example, clinicians usually wait 1 to 3 hours after an IV bolus dose of digoxin before evaluating the effect and 4 to 6 hours before obtaining a digoxin concentration. This delay allows the digoxin to distribute to the site of action (myocardium) so that the full therapeutic or toxic effects of a dose can be observed (see Chapter 10 and Fig. 10.1).

Slow drug distribution into the tissue compartment can pose problems in the accurate interpretation of a drug concentration when a drug is given by the IV route. It is not generally a problem when a drug is given orally because the rate of absorption is usually slower than the rate of distribution from V_i into V_t. Nevertheless, digoxin and lithium are exceptions to this rule. Even when these drugs are given orally, several hours are required for complete absorption and distribution.

Plasma samples obtained less than 6 hours after an oral dose of digoxin or less than 12 hours after an oral dose of immediate-release lithium are of questionable value. For these two drugs, the receptors in the end organs behave as though they are located in the more slowly equilibrating tissue compartment or V_t. Plasma concentrations obtained during the distribution phase (before equilibrium with the deep tissue compartment is complete) will be increased, and the pharmacologic response will be much less than the plasma concentration would indicate.

As a general rule, sampling of drug concentrations during the absorption/distribution phase should be avoided because these concentrations are changing very rapidly and are difficult to interpret.

Drugs with significant and nonsignificant two-compartment modeling

As illustrated in Figure 1.9, the α phase for most drugs represents distribution of drug from V_i into V_t, and relatively little drug is eliminated during the distribution phase. Drugs that behave in this way are generally referred to as "nonsignificant" two-compartmental drugs. The term "nonsignificant" means that if the patient is not harmed by the initially elevated drug concentration in the α phase and no drug samples are taken in the α phase, then the drug can be successfully modeled as a one-compartment drug (i.e., only the elimination or β phase is considered). It is important to recognize that for some drugs, increased drug plasma concentrations during the α phase can be clinically significant because the patient may experience serious toxicity if the end organ behaves as though it lies within the initial volume of distribution (V_i). These drugs are considered to exhibit "nonsignificant" two-compartmental modeling only after the α phase or distribution has been completed. That is, plasma samples are obtained for pharmacokinetic modeling only during the β or elimination phase.

Drugs with "significant" two-compartment modeling are those that are eliminated to a significant extent during the initial α phase. For these drugs (e.g., methotrexate), the α phase cannot be thought of simply as distribution because significant elimination occurs as well. Two drugs that border on having significant two-compartment modeling are lithium and lidocaine. When a one-compartment model is used for drugs that exhibit significant drug elimination in the α phase, the actual trough concentrations will be lower than those predicted by the one-compartment model.

Some clinicians have suggested that these drugs could be more successfully monitored by use of two-compartmental model pharmacokinetics. The complexity of these models, however, as well as the number of plasma samples required for patient-specific dose adjustments, usually limits the use of two-compartmental modeling techniques.

Two-compartment computer models are available for therapeutic drug monitoring. Usually, the value of these two-compartment computer models is that they can compensate or adjust for drug samples that have been obtained in the distribution phase. If care is taken to avoid obtaining samples in the distribution phase, very similar pharmacokinetic interpretations are usually arrived at using the simpler one-compartment model.

Clearance (Cl)

Clearance can be thought of as the intrinsic ability of the body or its organs of elimination (usually the kidneys and the liver) to remove drug from the blood or plasma. Clearance is expressed as a volume per unit of time. It is important to emphasize that clearance is not an indicator of how much drug is being removed; it only represents the theoretical volume of blood or plasma which is completely cleared of drug in a given period. The amount of drug removed depends on the plasma concentration of drug and the clearance (Fig. 1.10).

At steady state, the rate of drug administration (R_A) and rate of drug elimination (R_E) must be equal (also see Elimination Rate Constant [K] and Half-Life [t½]: Elimination Rate Constant [K]).

$$R_A = R_E \tag{Eq. 1.13}$$

Clearance (Cl) can best be thought of as the proportionality constant that makes the average steady-state plasma drug level equal to the rate of drug administration (R_A):

$$R_A = (Cl)(Css\ ave) \tag{Eq. 1.14}$$

where R_A is $(S)(F)(Dose)/\tau$ (see Equation 1.5), and Css ave the average steady-state drug concentration.

If an average steady-state plasma concentration and the rate of drug administration are known, the clearance can be calculated by rearranging Equation 1.14 as:

$$Cl = \frac{(S)(F)(Dose/\tau)}{Css\ ave} \tag{Eq. 1.15}$$

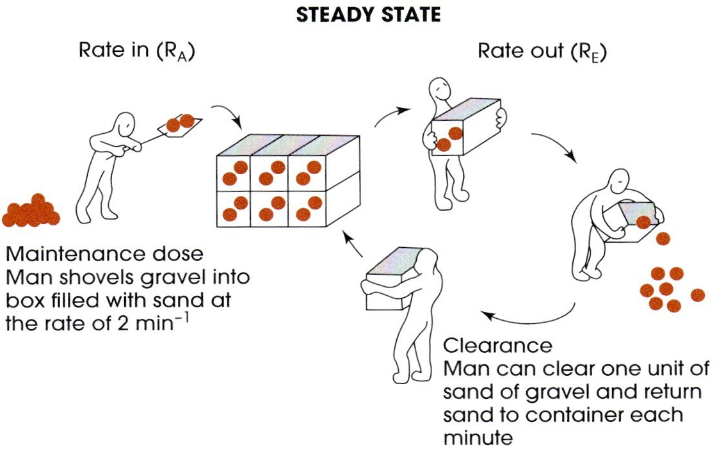

STEADY STATE

Rate in (R_A)   Rate out (R_E)

Maintenance dose
Man shovels gravel into
box filled with sand at
the rate of 2 min^{-1}

Clearance
Man can clear one unit of
sand of gravel and return
sand to container each
minute

FIGURE 1.10   Steady state, maintenance dose, clearance, and elimination rate constant. At steady state, the rate of drug administration (R_A) is equal to the rate of drug elimination (R_E), and the concentration of drug remains constant. In this example, the man on the left is able to shovel gravel or "drug" into a container of sand at the rate of 2 min^{-1}. The man on the right is able to remove one unit of sand containing gravel or "drug" from the container, dump the gravel, and return the sand to the container each minute. The amount of gravel or "drug" removed per unit of time (rate of elimination) will be determined by the concentration of gravel per unit of sand as well as the clearance (volume of sand cleared of gravel). The elimination rate constant (K) can be thought of as the fraction of the total volume cleared per unit of time. In this case, K would be equal to ⅙ or 0.17 min^{-1}.

For example, if IV lidocaine is infused continuously at a rate of 2 mg/min and if the concentration of lidocaine at steady state is 3 mg/L, the calculated lidocaine clearance using Equation 1.15 would be 0.667 L/min:

$$Cl = \frac{(S)(F)(Dose/\tau)}{Css\ ave}$$

$$= \frac{(1)(1)(2\ mg/min)}{3\ mg/L}$$

$$= 0.667\ L/min$$

or a clearance of 40 L/hr if the administration rate of lidocaine was expressed as 120 mg/hr.

$$Cl = \frac{(S)(F)(Dose/\tau)}{Css\ ave}$$

$$= \frac{(1)(1)(120\ mg/hr)}{3\ mg/L}$$

$$= 40\ L/hr$$

F is considered to be 1.0 because the drug is being administered IV. S is also assumed to be 1.0 because the hydrochloride salt represents only a small fraction of the total molecular weight for lidocaine and correction for the salt form is unnecessary.

MAINTENANCE DOSE

If an estimate for clearance is obtained from the literature, the clearance formula (Equation 1.15) can be rearranged and used to calculate the rate of administration or maintenance dose that produces a desired average plasma concentration at steady state:

$$\text{Maintenance Dose} = \frac{(\text{Cl})(\text{Css ave})(\tau)}{(\text{S})(\text{F})} \qquad \textbf{(Eq. 1.16)}$$

For example, using the literature estimate for theophylline clearance of 2.8 L/hr, the rate of IV administration for theophylline that produces a steady-state plasma theophylline concentration of 10 mg/L is given in the following equation:

$$\begin{aligned}
\text{Maintenance Dose} &= \frac{(\text{Cl})(\text{Css ave})(\tau)}{(\text{S})(\text{F})} \\
&= \frac{(2.8\ \text{L/hr})(10\ \text{mg/L})(1\ \text{hr})}{(1)(1)} \\
&= 28\ \text{mg given qh}
\end{aligned}$$

Because τ is 1 hour, the rate of administration is 28 mg/hr. If the theophylline was to be given every 12 hours, the dose would be 336 mg or 12 times the hourly administration rate to maintain the same average steady-state concentration.

$$\begin{aligned}
\text{Maintenance Dose} &= \frac{(\text{Cl})(\text{Css ave})(\tau)}{(\text{S})(\text{F})} \\
&= \frac{(2.8\ \text{L/hr})(10\ \text{mg/L})(12\ \text{hr})}{(1)(1)} \\
&= 336\ \text{mg to be given q12h}
\end{aligned}$$

The units for volume and time in clearance are somewhat arbitrary but must be consistent with the units for the drug administration rate and drug concentration.

Administration rate	Mass/time
Drug concentration	Mass/volume
Clearance	Volume/time

As an example, if the drug administration rate is in mg/hr and concentration is in mg/L, then clearance would be in L/hr. Conversely, if the administration rate was mg/day and concentration in mg/L, then clearance be in L/day. Again, the units are somewhat arbitrary, but clinicians usually use values that are consistent with how the drug is used in clinical practice.

In some cases, conversions need to be made. Digoxin is usually prescribed as milligrams (e.g., 0.25 mg) given once daily. The plasma concentration is usually reported as mcg/L (ng/mL). Therefore, the units of clearance would be either L/day or L/hr depending on whether the dosing interval is thought of as daily or every 24 hours. Another example is methotrexate that is usually administered as grams or milligrams, but methotrexate concentrations are reported as mcg/L (ng/mL) (see Chapter 9). Care should be taken to ensure that the appropriate units and conversions are used when performing pharmacokinetic calculations.

FACTORS THAT ALTER CLEARANCE (Cl)

Body surface area

Most literature values for clearance are expressed as volume/kg/time or as volume/70 kg/time. There is some evidence, however, that drug clearance is best adjusted on the basis of body surface area (BSA) rather than weight.[45–50] BSA can be calculated using Equation 1.16 or it can be obtained from various charts and nomograms[51–53] (see Appendix II).

$$\text{BSA in m}^2 = \left(\frac{\text{Patient's Weight in kg}}{70 \text{ kg}} \right)^{0.7} (1.73 \text{ m}^2) \qquad \textbf{(Eq. 1.17)}$$

The value of a patient's weight divided by 70 taken to the 0.7 power is an attempt to scale or size a patient as a fraction of the average 1.73 m^2 or 70-kg individual. Weight divided by 70 taken to the 0.7 power has no units and should be thought of as the fraction of the average-size person.

As an example, a 7-kg patient has a weight ratio relative to 70 kg of 0.1 and, therefore, may be thought of as having a size and thus a metabolic and renal capacity that is one-tenth of the average 70-kg person.

$$\left(\frac{7 \text{ kg}}{70 \text{ kg}} \right) = 0.1$$

If the same weight individual was compared to the 70-kg standard using weight to the 0.7 power, the ratio becomes 0.2 or 20% the size and clearance capacity of the standard 70-kg or 1.73-m^2 individual.

$$\left(\frac{7 \text{ kg}}{70 \text{ kg}} \right)^{0.7} = 0.2$$

In the example above, the difference between 0.1 and 0.2 is large. However, when patients do not differ significantly from 70 kg, the difference between using weight versus weight to the power 0.7 or BSA becomes less significant.

It is also important to remember that the 0.2 has no units and represents the fraction of the average-size (1.73 m² or 70 kg) individual. Occasionally, the value of 0.2 is mistaken for the surface area or size of the patient in square meters. This is not correct and can lead to dosing errors.

The following formulas can be used to adjust the clearance values reported in the literature for specific patients. There are other equations one can use depending on units used in the literature for clearance.

$$\text{Patient's Cl} = \text{Literature Cl/m}^2)(\text{Patient's BSA}) \qquad \textbf{(Eq. 1.18)}$$

$$\text{Patient's Cl} = \left(\text{Literature Cl/70 kg}\right)\left(\frac{\text{Patient's BSA}}{1.73\text{ m}^2}\right) \qquad \textbf{(Eq. 1.19)}$$

$$\text{Patient's Cl} = \left(\text{Literature Cl/70 kg}\right)\left(\frac{\text{Patient's Weight in kg}}{70\text{ kg}}\right) \qquad \textbf{(Eq. 1.20)}$$

$$\text{Patient's Cl} = (\text{Literature Cl/kg})(\text{Patient's Weight in kg}) \qquad \textbf{(Eq. 1.21)}$$

Equations 1.20 and 1.21 adjust clearance in proportion to weight, whereas Equations 1.18 and 1.19 adjust clearance in proportion to BSA.

The underlying assumption in using weight or surface area to adjust clearance is that the patient's liver and kidney size (and hopefully function) vary in proportion to these physical measurements. This may not always be the case; therefore, clearance values derived from the patient populations having a similar age and size should be used whenever possible. If the patient's weight is reasonably close to 70 kg (BSA = 1.73 m²), the patient's calculated clearance will be similar whether weight or BSA is used to calculate clearance. If, however, the patient's weight differs significantly from 70 kg, then the use of weight or surface area is likely to generate substantially different estimates of the patient's clearance. When a patient's size is substantially greater or less than the standard 70 kg, or 1.73 m², a careful assessment should be made to determine whether the patient's body stature is normal, obese, or emaciated. In obese and emaciated patients, neither weight nor surface area is likely to be helpful in predicting clearance, because the patient's body size will not reflect the size or function of the liver and kidney (Table 1.2).

Plasma protein binding

For highly protein-bound drugs, diminished plasma protein binding is associated with a decrease in reported steady-state plasma drug concentrations (total of unbound and free drug) for any given dose that is administered (see Figs. 1.4 and 1.5 and Desired Plasma Concentration [C], this part). According to Equation 1.15, a decrease in the denominator, Css ave, increases the calculated clearance.

$$Cl = \frac{(S)(F)(Dose/\tau)}{Css\text{ ave}}$$

TABLE 1.2   Factors that Alter Clearance (Cl)

Body weight
Body surface area
Cardiac output
Drug–drug interactions
Extraction ratio
Genetics
Hepatic function
Plasma protein binding
Renal function

It would be misleading, however, to assume that because the calculated clearance is increased, the amount eliminated per unit of time has increased. Equation 1.15 assumes that when Css ave (total of bound and free drug) changes, the free drug concentration, which is available for metabolism and renal elimination, changes proportionately. In actuality, the free or unbound fraction of drug in the plasma generally increases (even though Css ave decreases) with diminished plasma protein binding.[15,54] As a result, the amount of free drug eliminated per unit of time remains unchanged.[28] This should be apparent if one considers that at steady state, the amount of drug administered per unit of time (R_A) must equal the amount eliminated per unit of time (R_E). If R_A has not changed, R_E must remain the same.

In summary, when the same daily dose of a drug is given in the presence of diminished protein binding, an amount equal to that dose will be eliminated from the body each day at steady state despite a diminished steady-state plasma concentration and an increase in the calculated clearance. This lower plasma concentration (C bound + C free) is associated with a decreased C bound, no change in C free, and as a result, there is an increase in the fraction of unbound drug (fu).

$$\uparrow \text{fu} = \frac{\text{C free}}{\downarrow \text{C bound} + \text{C free}} \qquad \textbf{(Eq. 1.22)}$$

Therefore, the pharmacologic effect achieved will be similar to that produced by the higher serum concentration observed under normal protein binding conditions. This example re-emphasizes the principle that clearance alone is not a good indicator of the amount of drug eliminated per unit of time (R_E) (Figs. 1.11 and 1.12).

This principle is illustrated by comparing phenytoin in a uremic and nonuremic patient at steady state. As noted previously in the discussion of desired plasma concentration, the steady-state unbound plasma phenytoin concentration (C free) will be the same in both the uremic and nonuremic individual receiving the same daily dose and having the same metabolic capability. However, owing to decreased protein binding, C bound and, therefore, C total will be lower in the uremic than that in the nonuremic patient.

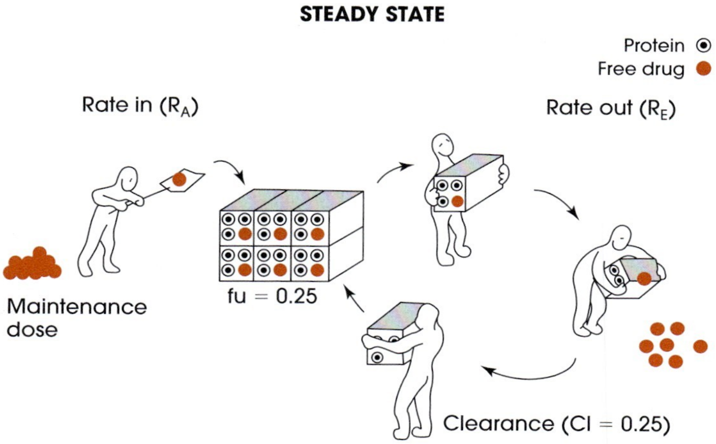

STEADY STATE

Protein ◉
Free drug ●

Rate in (R$_A$)   Rate out (R$_E$)

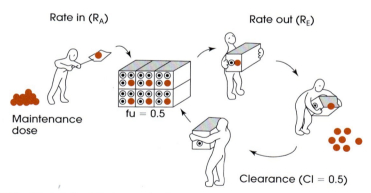

Maintenance
dose

fu = 0.25

Clearance (Cl = 0.25)

FIGURE 1.11 Clearance (Cl) of a highly protein-bound drug with a low extraction ratio. The free or unbound drug is available for clearance. Protein-bound drug is returned to the container so that the actual volume cleared of drug is one-fourth of the total volume removed by the man and presented to the clearing organ (e.g., kidney or liver). (Compare with Fig. 1.10.)

STEADY STATE

Rate in (R$_A$)   Rate out (R$_E$)

Maintenance
dose

fu = 0.5

Clearance (Cl = 0.5)

FIGURE 1.12 Effect of diminished protein binding on clearance (Cl) of a highly protein-bound drug that has a low extraction ratio. Compare this figure with Figure 1.11. The plasma concentration of drug has decreased, but the free concentration remains the same (fu is increased) (see Fig. 1.4). The volume cleared of drug has increased (½) compared to that cleared in Figure 1.11, even though the unbound concentration and amount of drug cleared per unit of time remained unchanged. This illustrates the principle that the amount of a highly protein-bound drug cleared per unit of time or rate of elimination (R$_E$) remains the same if the increase in clearance is owing to a decrease in plasma binding and the intrinsic metabolism or renal elimination remains unchanged.

As an example, consider two patients with the same metabolic capability receiving phenytoin 300 mg/day. The first patient is nonuremic with a phenytoin concentration of 10 mg/L and normal plasma binding (fu = 0.1). The second patient is uremic with a phenytoin concentration of 5 mg/L and decreased plasma binding (fu = 0.2). If these two patients were to have their clearance calculated using Equation 1.15, it would appear as though the uremic patient has a higher clearance.

$$Cl = \frac{(S)(F)(Dose/\tau)}{Css\ ave}$$

Nonuremic:

$$Cl = \frac{(S)(F)(Dose/\tau)}{Css\ ave}$$
$$= \frac{(1)(1)(300\ mg/day)}{10\ mg/L}$$
$$= 30\ L/day$$

Uremic:

$$Cl = \frac{(S)(F)(Dose/\tau)}{Css\ ave}$$
$$= \frac{(1)(1)(300\ mg/day)}{5\ mg/L}$$
$$= 60\ L/day$$

Although the calculated clearance for the uremic patient is higher than that for the nonuremic patient (60 vs. 30 L/day), the amount of drug cleared per day (300 mg) is the same because, at steady state, the rate of drug administration (R_A) is equal to the rate of drug elimination (R_E) for both the uremic and nonuremic patient.

$$R_A = R_E$$
$$300\ mg/day = 300\ mg/day$$

When protein binding is decreased, the increase in calculated clearance is generally proportional to the change in fu. Although the calculated clearance may be used to estimate a maintenance dose, careful selection of the plasma level that will produce the desired unbound or free plasma level and pharmacologic effect is critical to the determination of a therapeutically correct maintenance dose.

Extraction ratio

The direct proportionality between calculated clearance and fu does not apply to drugs that are so efficiently metabolized or excreted that some (perhaps all) of the drug bound to plasma protein is removed as it passes through the eliminating organ.[28,47,55] In this situation, the plasma protein acts as a "transport system" for the drug, carrying it to the eliminating organs, and clearance becomes dependent on the blood or plasma flow to the eliminating organ. To determine whether the clearance for a drug with significant plasma binding will be influenced primarily by blood flow or plasma protein binding, its extraction ratio is estimated and compared to its fu value.

The extraction ratio is the fraction of the drug presented to the eliminating organ that is cleared after a single pass through that organ. It can be estimated by dividing the blood or plasma clearance of a drug by the blood or plasma flow to the eliminating organ. If the extraction ratio exceeds the fu, then the plasma proteins are acting as a transport system and clearance will not change in proportion to fu. If, however, the extraction ratio is less than fu, clearance is likely to increase by the same proportion that fu changes. This approach does not take into account other factors that may affect clearance such as red blood cell binding, elimination from red blood cells, or changes in metabolic function.

Renal and hepatic function

Drugs can be eliminated or cleared as unchanged drug through the kidney (renal clearance) and by metabolism in the liver (metabolic clearance). These two routes of clearance are assumed to be independent of one another and additive.[36,40]

$$Cl_t = Cl_m + Cl_r \qquad \text{(Eq. 1.23)}$$

where Cl_t is total clearance, Cl_m the metabolic clearance or the fraction cleared by metabolism, and Cl_r the renal clearance or the fraction cleared by the renal route. Because the kidneys and liver function independently, it is assumed that a change in one does not affect the other.

Most pharmacokinetic adjustments for drug elimination are based on renal function (see Chapter 3) because hepatic function is usually more difficult to quantitate. Elevated liver enzymes do reflect liver damage but are not a good measure of function. Hepatic function is often evaluated using the prothrombin time, serum albumin concentration, and serum bilirubin concentration. Unfortunately, each of these laboratory tests is affected by variables other than altered hepatic function. For example, the serum albumin may be low owing to decreased protein intake or increased renal or GI loss, as well as decreased hepatic function. Although liver function tests do not provide quantitative data, pharmacokinetic adjustments must still take into consideration liver function because this route of elimination is important for a significant number of drugs.

Cardiac output

Cardiac output also affects drug metabolism. Hepatic or metabolic clearances for some drugs can be decreased by 25% to 50% in patients with congestive heart failure.

For example, the metabolic clearances of theophylline[56] and digoxin[45] are reduced by approximately one-half in patients with congestive heart failure. Because the metabolic clearance for both of these drugs is much lower than the hepatic blood or plasma flow (low extraction ratio), it would not have been predicted that their clearances would have been influenced by cardiac output or hepatic blood flow to this extent. The decreased cardiac output and resultant hepatic congestion must, in some way, decrease the intrinsic metabolic capacity of the liver. The effect of diminished clearance on plasma drug concentrations is illustrated in Figure 1.13 (compare with Fig. 1.10).

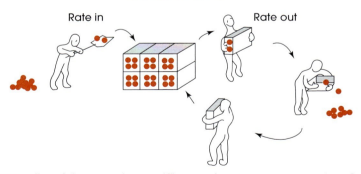

NON–STEADY STATE

Rate in

Rate out

Maintenance dose

Clearance (Cl = 0.5)

Gravel accumulation

NEW STEADY STATE

Rate in

Rate out

FIGURE 1.13 Effect of changes in clearance (Cl) on steady-state serum concentrations. Compare this figure with Figure 1.10. In this illustration, the maintenance dose or amount of gravel added to the container per unit of time remains the same; however, the volume of sand cleared of gravel (clearance) has been halved. Initially, the amount of gravel or "drug" cleared per unit of time is less than the maintenance dose; the concentration of gravel in the container increases until a new steady state is reached. At this point, the rate at which gravel is added to the container again equals the rate at which gravels is eliminated from the container. If clearance had increased, the concentration of gravel would have decreased until the amount removed per unit of time (R_E) again equaled the rate of administration (R_A).

Elimination Rate Constant (K) and Half-Life (t½)

It is often desirable to predict how drug plasma levels will change with time. For drugs that are eliminated by first-order pharmacokinetics, these predictions are based on the elimination rate constant (K). The key characteristic of first-order elimination is that both clearance and volume of distribution do not vary with dose or concentration.

FIRST-ORDER PHARMACOKINETICS

First-order elimination pharmacokinetics refers to a process in which the amount or concentration of drug in the body diminishes logarithmically over time (Fig. 1.14).

The rate of elimination (R_E) is proportional to the drug concentration; therefore, the amount of drug removed per unit of time (R_E) will vary in direct proportion to drug concentration. The fraction or percentage of the total amount of drug present in the body (Ab) that is removed at any instant in time, however, will remain constant and independent of dose or concentration. That fraction or percentage is expressed by the

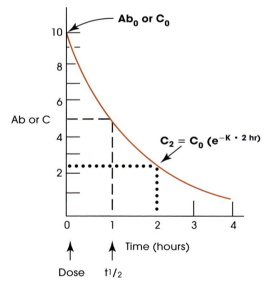

FIGURE 1.14   First-order elimination C versus time. The initial amount (Ab_0) or concentration (C_0) diminishes logarithmically over time. The half-life (t½) is the time required to eliminate one-half of the drug. The concentration at the end of a given time interval (in this example, 2 hours) is equal to the initial concentration times the fraction of drug remaining at the end of that time interval ($e^{-K \cdot 2 hr}$). The amount or concentration of drug lost in each 1-hour interval diminishes over time (5, 2.5, and 1.25); however, the fraction of drug that is lost in each unit of time remains constant (0.5). For example, over the first hour (0 to 1 hour), of the total amount of drug in the body (10), one-half was lost (5). In the next time interval (1 to 2 hour), of the amount of drug that remained (5), one-half was lost (2.5).

elimination rate constant, K. The equations that describe first-order elimination of a drug from the body are as follows:

$$Ab = (Ab_0)(e^{-Kt})$$

(Eq. 1.24)

or

$$C = (C_0)(e^{-Kt})$$

(Eq. 1.25)

where in Equation 1.24, Ab_0 and Ab represent the total amount of drug in the body at the beginning and end of the time interval, t, respectively; and e^{-Kt} is the fraction remaining at time t. In Equation 1.25, C_0 and C are the plasma concentrations at the beginning and end of the time interval, respectively. Because the drug concentration diminishes logarithmically, a graphic plot of the logarithm of the plasma level versus time yields a straight line (Fig. 1.15).

This type of graphic analysis of declining plasma drug concentrations is often used to determine whether a drug is eliminated by a first-order process. The key element is that the drug concentration decay curve when plotted as C versus time is a concave curve (see Fig. 1.14) and when plotted as log C versus time is a straight line (see Fig. 1.15). One important assumption in this analysis is that there is no additional drug being absorbed or placed into the body during the decay process.

Because first-order drugs have a volume of distribution and clearance that are constant (assuming no change in a patient's clinical status), many but not all the dose-to-concentration relationships are proportional. As an example, the average steady-state concentration will be proportional to the dosing rate. Therefore, the steady-state concentration can be adjusted by altering the drug dosage rate in proportion to the desired change in concentration (Fig. 1.16).

Equation 1.25 can also be thought of as any initial drug concentration C_1 that is decayed over some time interval t_1 to calculate the subsequent drug concentration C_2.

$$C_2 = (C_1)(e^{-Kt_1})$$

(Eq. 1.26)

ELIMINATION RATE CONSTANT (K)

The elimination rate constant, K, is the fraction or percentage of the total amount of drug in the body removed per unit of time and is a function of clearance and volume of distribution.

$$K = \frac{Cl}{V}$$

(Eq. 1.27)

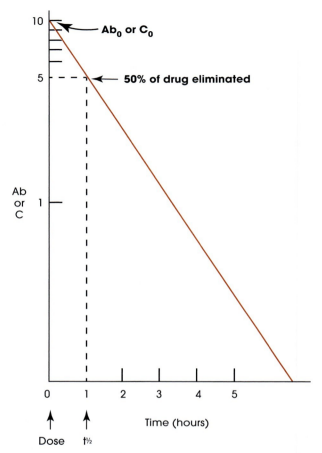

FIGURE 1.15 First-order elimination log C versus time. A graph of the log of Ab or C versus time yields a straight line. The half-life is the time required for Ab or C to decline to one-half the original value.

As Equation 1.27 shows, K can also be thought of as the fraction of the volume of distribution that will be cleared of drug per unit of time (see Fig. 1.10). For example, a drug with a clearance of 10 L/day and a V of 100 L would have an elimination rate constant of 0.1 day^{-1}.

$$K = \frac{10\,L/day}{100\,L}$$

$$= 0.1\,day^{-1}$$

The elimination rate constant of 0.1 day^{-1} indicates that in 1 day, the volume cleared is 1/10 or 10% of the total volume of distribution. The value of K is based on the units used for clearance and volume of distribution and is somewhat arbitrary. As an example, using the same clearance of 10 L/day expressed as 0.417 L/hr (10 L/day divided

NON-STEADY STATE

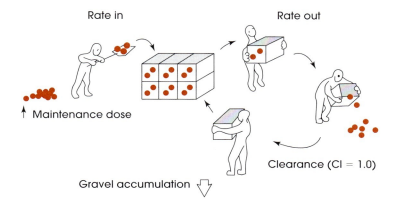

NEW STEADY STATE

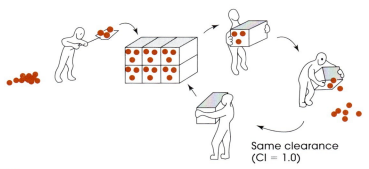

FIGURE 1.16 Effect of changes in maintenance dose on steady-state plasma concentrations. Compare this figure with Figure 1.10. In this illustration, the clearance or volume of sand cleared of gravel remains the same; however, the maintenance dose or the amount of gravel added to the container per unit of time has been increased from 2 to 3 min^{-1}. Therefore, the concentration of gravel or "drug" increases until a new steady state is reached. At this point, the rate at which gravel is added to the container again equals the rate at which gravel is eliminated from the container. If the maintenance dose decreased, the concentration of gravel would have gradually decreased until a new steady state had been achieved.

by 24 hr/day) and the V of 100 L, the corresponding K value would be 0.00417 hr^{-1} or 0.417% of the total volume of distribution cleared in 1 hour. As previously discussed, the units chosen for clearance and volume of distribution should be consistent with the units used to report the dose, concentration, and dosing interval (see Clearance [Cl]: Maintenance Dose).

Because the drug elimination rate constant is the slope of the natural log or ln C versus time plot, two plasma concentrations measured during the decay or elimination phase (i.e., between doses or following a single dose) can be used to calculate the K for a specific patient. The equation used to calculate K is a rearrangement of Equation 1.26:

$$C_2 = (C_1)(e^{-Kt})$$

$$\frac{C_2}{C_1} = e^{-Kt}$$

$$\ln\left(\frac{C_2}{C_1}\right) = -Kt$$

$$\ln\left(\frac{C_1}{C_2}\right) = Kt$$

$$\frac{\ln\left(\dfrac{C_1}{C_2}\right)}{t} = K$$

or

$$K = \frac{\ln\left(\dfrac{C_1}{C_2}\right)}{t} \qquad \textbf{(Eq. 1.28)}$$

where C_1 is the first or higher plasma concentration, C_2 is the second or lower plasma concentration, and t is the time interval between the plasma samples. For example, if C_1 is 5 mg/L and C_2 is 2 mg/L, and the time interval between the samples is 8 hours, the elimination rate constant (K) will be 0.115 hr^{-1}.

$$K = \frac{\ln\left(\dfrac{C_1}{C_2}\right)}{t}$$

$$= \frac{\ln\left(\dfrac{5\ \text{mg/L}}{2\ \text{mg/L}}\right)}{8\ \text{hr}}$$

$$= 0.115\ \text{hr}^{-1}$$

One of the key issues in using Equation 1.28 is that to estimate K accurately, the time between C_1 and C_2 should be at least one half-life (see Elimination Rate Constant [K] and Half-Life [t½]: Half-Life [t½]). In other words, C_2 should be equal to or less than half of C_1. This time interval of one half-life is a minimum, and an interval of longer than a half-life is desirable. Whereas K can be calculated from any two drug concentrations during a decay phase, when the interval is less than one half-life, assay error alone results in highly variable and inaccurate estimates of K.

HALF-LIFE (t½)

The elimination rate constant is often expressed in terms of a drug's half-life, a value that is more conveniently applied to the clinical setting. The half-life (t½) of a drug is the time required for the total amount of drug in the body or the plasma drug concentration to decrease by one-half (see Fig. 1.15). It is sometimes referred to as the β t½ to distinguish it from the half-life for distribution (α t½) in a two-compartment model, and it is a function of the elimination rate constant, K.

$$t\,\tfrac{1}{2} = \frac{0.693}{K} \qquad \textbf{(Eq. 1.29)}$$

If the K used in Equation 1.29 is derived from plasma concentrations obtained during the decay phase, then the time interval in which the samples are drawn should span at least one half-life as previously mentioned (see discussion of Equation 1.28).

Because the dosing interval is frequently equal to or shorter than the usual half-life for many drugs, it is often impractical to obtain peak and trough levels within a dosing interval to determine the half-life (e.g., theophylline, digoxin, and phenobarbital).

If the volume of distribution and clearance for a drug are known, the half-life can be estimated using Equation 1.30. The half-life, like K, is dependent on and determined by Cl and V. This relationship is illustrated in Equation 1.30, which was obtained by substituting Equation 1.27 into Equation 1.29:

$$t\,\tfrac{1}{2} = \frac{0.693(V)}{Cl} \qquad \textbf{(Eq. 1.30)}$$

The dependence of t½ or K on V and Cl is emphasized because the volume of distribution and clearance for a drug can change independently of one another and, thus, affect the half-life or elimination constant in the same or opposite directions. Another caution is appropriate at this point. It is a common misconception that because Equation 1.27 can be rearranged to

$$Cl = (K)(V) \qquad \textbf{(Eq. 1.31)}$$

that clearance is determined by K (or t½) and V; however, this is incorrect considering the physiologic model that is used in the application of pharmacokinetics to the clinical setting. Instead, K and t½ depend on clearance and the volume of distribution. Therefore, caution should be used when making any assumptions about the volume of distribution or clearance of a drug based solely on knowledge of its half-life. For example, if the half-life of a drug is prolonged, the clearance may be increased, decreased, or unchanged depending on corresponding changes in the volume of distribution. As a general principle, however, when the half-life is longer than the usual value for that drug, it is more likely owing to a decrease in clearance than an increase in volume of distribution. This is because the variability in both renal and hepatic function (i.e., clearance) is more likely to be altered than is the plasma and tissue distribution characteristics (volume of distribution) of a drug. However, there are situations when the volume of distribution is significantly altered and should be considered when using pharmacokinetics in the clinical setting (see Chapters 6 and 10).

CLINICAL APPLICATION OF ELIMINATION RATE CONSTANT (K) AND HALF-LIFE (t½)

Time to reach steady state

Half-life is an important variable to consider when answering questions concerning time such as "How long will it take a drug concentration to reach steady state on a constant dosage regimen?" or "How long will it take for the drug concentration to reach steady state if the dosage regimen is changed?" (For clinical application of half-life, see Table 1.3).

When drugs are given chronically, they accumulate in the body until the amount administered in a given period (maintenance dose) is equal to the amount eliminated in that same period, that is, rate in equals rate out. When this occurs, drug concentrations in the plasma will plateau and will have reached "steady state" (see Figs. 1.10 and 1.16). The time required for a drug concentration to reach steady state is determined by the drug's half-life. It takes 1 half-life to reach 50%, 2 half-lives to reach 75%, 3 half-lives to reach 87.5%, 3.3 half-lives to reach 90%, and 4 half-lives to reach 93.75% of steady state. With each additional half-life, the residual fraction from steady state diminishes, and at some point (usually ≤10%), this residual is considered negligible, and steady state is assumed to have been achieved. In most clinical situations, the attainment of steady state can be assumed after 3 to 5 half-lives (Fig. 1.17).

TABLE 1.3   Clinical Application of the Elimination Rate Constant (K) and Half-Life (t½)

1. Estimating the time to reach steady-state plasma concentrations after initiation or change in the maintenance dose
2. Estimating the time required to eliminate all or a portion of the drug from the body once it is discontinued
3. Predicting non–steady-state plasma levels following the initiation of an infusion
4. Predicting a steady-state plasma level from a non–steady-state plasma level obtained at a specific time following the initiation of an infusion
5. Given the degree of fluctuation in plasma concentration desired within a dosing interval, determine that interval; given the interval, determine the fluctuation in the plasma concentration

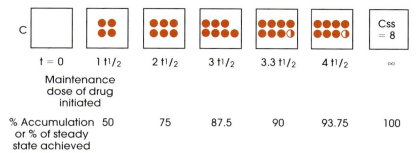

FIGURE 1.17   First-order accumulation. When a maintenance dose is initiated, it takes 3 to 5 half-lives to reach steady-state plasma levels; 3.3 half-lives represent 90% of steady state. This example assumes that the maintenance dose administered will produce an average steady-state level (Css ave or Css) of 8.

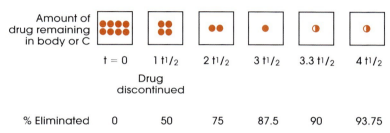

FIGURE 1.18   First-order elimination: amount of drug remaining in the body after one to four half-lives have passed. The amount of drug eliminated per unit of time diminishes over time, but the fraction eliminated in each time interval (in this case, 0.5 as the interval is 1 t½) remains the same; 3.3 t½ represents 90% eliminated or only 10% remaining.

Time for drug elimination

The half-life can also be used to determine how long it will take to effectively eliminate all the drug from the body after the drug has been discontinued. It takes 1 half-life to eliminate 50%, 2 half-lives to eliminate 75%, 3 half-lives to eliminate 87.5%, 3.3 half-lives to eliminate 90%, and 4 half-lives to eliminate 93.75% of the total amount of drug in the body. Again, in most clinical situations, it can be assumed that all the drug has been effectively eliminated after 3 to 5 half-lives (Fig. 1.18).

Prediction of plasma levels following initiation of an infusion

Often, when drugs are given by constant infusion, it is useful to predict the plasma concentrations that will be achieved at a specific period (Fig. 1.19). The rate at which a drug approaches steady state is also governed by the elimination rate constant; therefore, this parameter can be used to calculate the fraction of steady state that is achieved at any time after initiation of the infusion (t_1):

$$\text{Fraction of Steady State Achieved at Time } t_1 = 1 - e^{-Kt_1} \qquad \textbf{(Eq. 1.32)}$$

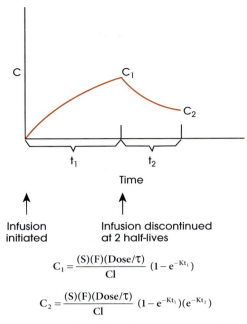

FIGURE 1.19   Graphic representation of an infusion that is discontinued before steady state. C_1 is a concentration that is achieved any time (t_1) after the infusion is initiated, and C_2 is a concentration that results any interval of time (t_2) after the infusion has been discontinued.

$$C_1 = \frac{(S)(F)(Dose/\tau)}{Cl}\,(1 - e^{-Kt_1})$$

$$C_2 = \frac{(S)(F)(Dose/\tau)}{Cl}\,(1 - e^{-Kt_1})(e^{-Kt_2})$$

The average plasma concentration at steady state (Css ave) can be calculated by rearranging the clearance formula (Equation 1.15) as:

$$Cl = \frac{(S)(F)(Dose/\tau)}{Css\ ave}$$

$$Css\ ave = \frac{(S)(F)(Dose/\tau)}{Cl} \qquad \textbf{(Eq. 1.33)}$$

The expected plasma concentration (C_1) at a specific time (t_1) after initiation of the infusion can be calculated by multiplying the average steady-state concentration (Css ave) by the fraction of steady state achieved at t_1.

$$C_1 = (Css\ ave)\left(\begin{array}{c} \text{Fraction of Steady State} \\ \text{Achieved at } t_1 \end{array} \right) \qquad \textbf{(Eq. 1.34)}$$

By substituting the appropriate parts of Equations 1.32 and 1.33 into Equation 1.34, a new equation for plasma concentration C_1 at t_1 is derived:

$$C_1 = \frac{(S)(F)(Dose/\tau)}{Cl}\,(1 - e^{-Kt_1}) \qquad \textbf{(Eq. 1.35)}$$

All the units in Equation 1.35 must be consistent (e.g., time in τ, Cl, and t_1; volume in Cl, V, and C; mass in dose and C). According to Equation 1.35, as the duration of the infusion (t_1) approaches three to five half-lives, the fraction of steady state achieved approaches 1, and, for all practical purposes, the patient is at steady state. Conversely, if a drug plasma concentration (C_1) was obtained before steady-state concentration was attained, the approximate steady-state concentration that should eventually be achieved can be estimated through rearrangement of Equation 1.35 and substituting Css ave for $[(S)(F)(Dose/\tau)]/Cl$:

$$\text{Css ave} = \frac{C_1}{1 - e^{-Kt_1}} \qquad \text{(Eq. 1.36)}$$

If the predicted steady-state concentration is unacceptably high, side effects or toxicities might be avoided by reducing the maintenance infusion before the achievement of steady state.

Prediction of plasma levels following discontinuation of an infusion

The plasma concentration any time after an infusion is discontinued (C_2) can be estimated by multiplying the measured or predicted plasma concentration (C_1) at the time the infusion is discontinued by the fraction of drug remaining at t_2 hours from the end of the infusion (Fig. 1.19).

$$\frac{\text{Fraction of Drug}}{\text{Remaining at } t_2} = e^{-Kt_2} \qquad \text{(Eq. 1.37)}$$

$$C_2 = (C_1)(e^{-Kt_2}) \qquad \text{(Eq. 1.38)}$$

If the right side of Equation 1.35

$$C_1 = \frac{(S)(F)(Dose/\tau)}{Cl}(1 - e^{-Kt_1})$$

is substituted for C_1 in Equation 1.38, the plasma concentration (C_2) at any time (t_2) after an infusion is discontinued is as follows:

$$C_2 = \frac{(S)(F)(Dose/\tau)}{Cl}(1 - e^{-Kt_1})(e^{-Kt_2}) \qquad \text{(Eq. 1.39)}$$

(see Fig. 1.19).

Although Equation 1.39 may look complicated, it is really a series of simpler equations linked together to model the continuous infusion that was discontinued before steady state (Equation 1.35) followed by a first-order decay (Equation 1.37).

Calculation of a theophylline concentration, which will be expected 8 hours after a theophylline infusion of 80 mg/hr is discontinued, can be used to illustrate this principle. Assume that theophylline has been administered for 16 hours to a patient with a theophylline clearance of 2.8 L/hr and a half-life of 8 hours (K of 0.087 hr^{-1}). The calculations can be accomplished step by step as follows:

1. The expected steady-state theophylline concentration resulting from a theophylline infusion of 80 mg/hr to a patient with a theophylline clearance of 2.8 L/hr and an assumed S and F of 1 can be calculated using Equation 1.33:

$$
\begin{aligned}
\text{Css ave} &= \frac{(S)(F)(\text{Dose}/\tau)}{Cl} \\
&= \frac{(1)(1)(80 \text{ mg}/1\text{ hr})}{2.8 \text{ L/hr}} \\
&= 28.6 \text{ mg/L}
\end{aligned}
$$

2. The expected concentration after 16 hours of infusion (t_1) can be calculated using Equation 1.35:

$$
\begin{aligned}
C_1 &= \frac{(S)(F)(\text{Dose}/\tau)}{Cl}(1-e^{-Kt_1}) \\
C_1 &= 28.6 \text{ mg/L } (1-e^{-(0.087 \text{ hr}^{-1})(16 \text{ hr})}) \\
&= 28.6 \text{ mg/L } (1-e^{-1.392}) \\
&= 28.6 \text{ mg/L } (1-0.25) \\
&= 21.45 \text{ mg/L}
\end{aligned}
$$

3. The expected concentration 8 hours after the end of the infusion can be calculated using Equation 1.38:

$$
\begin{aligned}
C_2 &= (C_1)(e^{-Kt_2}) \\
C_2 &= 21.45 \text{ mg/L } (e^{-(0.087 \text{ hr}^{-1})(8 \text{ hr})}) \\
&= 21.45 \text{ mg/L } (e^{-0.696}) \\
&= 21.45 \text{ mg/L } (0.5) \\
&= 10.7 \text{ mg/L}
\end{aligned}
$$

Of course, these three steps could have been combined by using Equation 1.39, where t_1 would be 16 hours and t_2 would be 8 hours.

$$
C_2 = \frac{(S)(F)(\text{Dose}/\tau)}{Cl}(1-e^{-Kt_1})(e^{-Kt_2})
$$

Whether the stepwise or single combined equation is used depends on how the sequence of events is visualized and, therefore, how the problem or equation is expressed (see Fig. 1.19).

Dosing interval (τ)

The half-life can also be used to estimate the appropriate dosing interval or tau (τ) for maintenance therapy when a drug is administered intermittently and the absorption or input into the body is relatively rapid. For example, if the goal of therapy is to minimize plasma fluctuations to no more than 50% between doses, the dosing interval τ should be less than or equal to the half-life. The maintenance dose can be calculated using Equation 1.16:

$$\text{Maintenance Dose} = \frac{(\text{Cl})(\text{Css ave})(\tau)}{(\text{S})(\text{F})}$$

If τ is less than or equal to the half-life of a drug, the calculated maintenance dose will produce plasma concentrations that will fluctuate by ≤50% during that dosing interval. The plasma levels will be above the average steady-state plasma level for the first half of the dosing interval and below the average steady-state plasma level during the second half of the dosing interval (Fig. 1.20).

If the approximate half-life and dosing interval are known, the degree of change in plasma drug concentration that will occur over a dosing interval can be determined. Once the degree of fluctuation is known, one can then determine whether the primary determinant of plasma levels between dosing intervals is the volume of distribution or the clearance or in some cases both volume and clearance.

In certain situations, the dosing interval is much longer than the half-life and, for practical purposes, all the drug is eliminated before the next dose. Therefore, each new dose is essentially a new loading dose. In this situation, each new peak concentration will be determined primarily by the volume of distribution because almost no drug remains from the previous dose.

Antibiotics are commonly dosed in this manner. The therapeutic index for antibiotics is usually so large that wide fluctuations in plasma levels are acceptable and perhaps even desirable.[57,58] Furthermore, the therapeutic effect may require a plasma level that is above the minimal bactericidal or inhibitory concentration for only a brief period relative to the dosing interval.[59]

When the dosing interval is much shorter than the half-life, the plasma concentration fluctuates very little throughout the dosing interval. In this case, the plasma concentration will be primarily determined by clearance. Digoxin and phenobarbital given orally and any drug administered by a constant infusion or as a sustained-release dosage form that releases the drug over the entire dosing interval are good examples of such a situation (also see Maximum and Minimum Plasma Concentrations, this part).

Determining the parameter that primarily affects plasma concentration for any given dosage regimen (when τ is longer or shorter than t½) is important because one then knows which parameters can be calculated reliably from the reported steady-state plasma concentrations. For example, if a patient who has been taking a dose of 0.375 mg of digoxin daily has a reported steady-state trough plasma

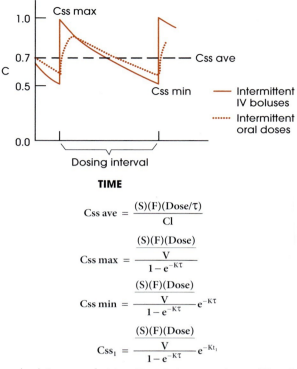

FIGURE 1.20   Plasma level–time curve for intermittent dosing at steady state. When the dosing interval is equal to the half-life, plasma concentrations are above the average steady-state plasma concentration (Css ave) approximately 50% of the time. Oral administration dampens the curve, and the maximum concentration at steady state (Css max) occurs later and is lower than that produced by IV bolus. The minimum concentration at steady state (Css min) is greater than that produced by IV bolus doses because of the effect of absorption. In the equations above, τ is the interval between doses and t_1 is the time from the theoretical peak concentration following a dose to the time of sampling. IV, intravenous.

concentration of 3.8 mcg/L, one can reliably calculate the digoxin clearance for this patient using Equation 1.15.

$$Cl = \frac{(S)(F)(Dose/\tau)}{Css\ ave}$$

Because the dosing interval is much shorter than the half-life, the trough concentration is a good approximation of the Css ave, and, therefore, clearance is the major determinant of the patient's plasma concentration. One cannot reliably use the reported plasma concentration to calculate a patient-specific V because the average steady-state concentration is only a function of clearance (see Maximum and Minimum Plasma Concentrations, page 51).

With a new revised clearance value, one can estimate a new maintenance dose. Loading doses are based on the volume of distribution and would require a literature estimate, because no patient-specific information about V can be determined from this drug level. In addition, using the value of V from the literature and our revised clearance, a new estimate of K (Equation 1.27) or t½ (Equation 1.30) can be obtained:

$$K = \frac{Cl_{revised}}{V_{assumed}}$$

$$t\,\tfrac{1}{2} = \frac{0.693(V_{assumed})}{Cl_{revised}}$$

Of course, the confidence in this new K or t½ would depend on the confidence in the assumed value of V derived from the literature.

Maximum and Minimum Plasma Concentrations

It is often important to estimate the maximum (Css max or peak) and minimum (Css min or trough) plasma drug concentrations produced by a given dose of drug within the dosing interval at steady state (see Fig. 1.20). For example, whereas it is critical in gentamicin therapy to achieve an acceptable peak concentration for efficacy, it is also important that the trough level be below a specified concentration to minimize concentration-related toxicity.

For drugs with a narrow therapeutic index (e.g., theophylline), it is useful to determine the degree of fluctuation in plasma drug concentration that will occur between doses. This can be particularly important if the dosing interval is longer than the half-life (i.e., fluctuations will be large) and Css min levels are being used to monitor therapy.

Most frequently, plasma samples for drug assays are drawn as a trough or just before a dose because Css min levels are the most reproducible. The reported plasma drug concentrations for these samples are often considered to be average steady-state concentrations (Css ave). However, when the dosing interval approaches or exceeds the drug's half-life, a patient's pharmacokinetic parameters can be more accurately estimated using an equation that describes Css min rather than Css ave (see Maximum and Minimum Plasma Concentrations: Minimum Plasma Drug Concentration [Css min]).

MAXIMUM PLASMA DRUG CONCENTRATION (Css max)

The maximum plasma drug concentration can be calculated from Equation 1.41 if the dose, salt form (S), bioavailability (F), volume of distribution (V), and elimination rate constant (K) are known:

$$\text{Css max} = \frac{\Delta C}{\text{Fraction of Drug Lost in } \tau} \qquad \textbf{(Eq. 1.40)}$$

or

$$\text{Css max} = \frac{\dfrac{(S)(F)(Dose)}{V}}{1 - e^{-K\tau}} \qquad \textbf{(Eq. 1.41)}$$

where ΔC and $(S)(F)(Dose)/V$ represent the change in drug concentration that occurs over the dosing interval, and $(1 - e^{-K\tau})$ represents the fraction of drug that is eliminated in the dosing interval.

Some pharmacokineticists have chosen to describe the fraction lost in a dosing interval $(1 - e^{-K\tau})$ as the "accumulation factor" and express it as

$$\frac{1}{1 - e^{-K\tau}}$$

and the Css max equation as

$$\text{Css max} = \left(\frac{(S)(F)(Dose)}{V} \right) \left(\frac{1}{1 - e^{-K\tau}} \right)$$

This equation is the same as Equation 1.41 expressed in a slightly different format.

Equation 1.41 assumes that drug absorption and distribution rates are rapid in relation to the drug elimination half-life and the dosing interval. This assumption is valid as long as drug concentrations are not sampled during the absorption and distribution phases. Following IV injection, the absorption and distribution phases are relatively short compared to the dosing interval and half-life for most drugs. When drugs are administered orally, the primary concern is with the absorption phase because the distribution component associated with two-compartment modeling is usually negligible. Digoxin and lithium are two notable exceptions in that a distribution phase continues for several hours after oral administration.

For digoxin, the observed peak concentration following oral administration will be greater than that predicted by Equation 1.41 for Css max because drug distribution into tissue requires a minimum of 6 hours. When theophylline is dosed every 6 to 8 hours as an immediate-release product, the observed peak concentration will be slightly lower than that predicted by Equation 1.41 because absorption is relatively slow compared to the dosing interval and the half-life of the drug. This tends to blunt or dampen the peak and trough level fluctuations of theophylline because elimination begins before the entire drug enters the body. For most drugs, following oral administration as an immediate-release product, the time required to reach peak concentrations after oral administration is between 1 and 2 hours.

MINIMUM PLASMA DRUG CONCENTRATION (Css min)

The minimum plasma drug concentration can be estimated by subtracting ΔC or the change in plasma concentration in one dosing interval from the maximum plasma concentration:

$$\text{Css min} = \text{Css max} - \Delta C \qquad \textbf{(Eq. 1.42)}$$

or

$$\text{Css min} = \text{Css max} - \left(\frac{(S)(F)(\text{Dose})}{V} \right) \qquad \textbf{(Eq. 1.43)}$$

Alternatively, Css min can be calculated by multiplying Css max by the fraction of drug that remains at the end of the dosing interval $(e^{-K\tau})$.

$$\text{Css min} = \text{Css max}\, (e^{-K\tau}) \qquad \textbf{(Eq. 1.44)}$$

Substituting Equation 1.41 for Css max into Equation 1.44 enables one to calculate Css min if the dose, elimination rate constant (K), volume of distribution (V), salt form (S), and bioavailability (F) are known.

$$\text{Css min} = \frac{\dfrac{(S)(F)(\text{Dose})}{V}}{1 - e^{-K\tau}} e^{-K\tau} \qquad \textbf{(Eq. 1.45)}$$

If a steady-state sample is obtained at some time other than the peak or trough, the concentration can be calculated by the following equation as follows:

$$\text{Css}_1 = \frac{\dfrac{(S)(F)(\text{Dose})}{V}}{1 - e^{-K\tau}} e^{-Kt_1} \qquad \textbf{(Eq. 1.46)}$$

where t_1 is the number of hours since the last dose, and Css_1 is the steady-state plasma concentration "t_1" hours after the last dose or Css max, which is "assumed" to occur at the time of dose administration (i.e., absorption or drug input is assumed to be instantaneous). Note that although steady state has been achieved, not all plasma concentrations within the dosing interval represent the average concentration or Css ave. If the dosing interval (τ) is short compared to the half-life, the plasma concentration changes very little within the dosing interval and all concentrations are a close approximation of Css ave (see Figs. 1.20 and 2.11).

Note that when a slow absorption rate significantly dampens the plasma drug concentration versus time curve (e.g., sustained-release dosage forms), the Css min can usually be assumed to be a close approximation of the average steady-state concentration (Css ave) and Equation 1.15,

$$Cl = \frac{(S)(F)(Dose/\tau)}{Css\ ave}$$

is used to calculate the patient's pharmacokinetic parameter (i.e., clearance) (see Figs. 1.20 and 2.11). This assumption is also applicable when the dosing interval is short relative to the half-life. Although it would not be incorrect to use Equation 1.46,

$$Css_1 = \frac{\dfrac{(S)(F)(Dose)}{V}}{1 - e^{-K\tau}} e^{-Kt_1}$$

when the dosing interval is much shorter than the drug half-life, the complexity of the equation tends to obscure the fact that all drug concentrations within the dosing interval are essentially an approximation of Css ave. In addition, if pharmacokinetic revisions are made by manipulating K and/or V in Equation 1.46, it should be kept in mind that it is the product of K times V or clearance that has the most value or accuracy from the revision process. Again, when the dosing interval is much shorter than the half-life, peak and trough plasma levels are about equal to the average concentration and are, therefore, primarily determined by clearance. Although the product of the V and K obtained by manipulating Equation 1.46 may closely approximate clearance, there is less confidence in the V and K values.

REFERENCES

1. Huffman DH, Manion CV, Azarnoff DL. Absorption of digoxin from different oral preparations in normal subjects during steady state. *Clin Pharmacol Ther.* 1974;16:310.
2. Lisalo E. Clinical pharmacokinetics of digoxin. *Clin Pharmacokinet.* 1977;2:1.
3. Mooradian AD. Digitalis. An update of clinical pharmacokinetics: therapeutic monitoring techniques and treatment recommendations. *Clin Pharmacokinet.* 1988;15:165–179.
4. Weinberger M, Hendeles L, Bighley L. The relation of product formulation to absorption of oral theophylline. *N Engl J Med.* 1978;299:852.
5. Hendeles L, Weinberger M, Milavetz G, et al. Food-induced dose dumping from a once-a-day theophylline product as a cause of theophylline toxicity. *Chest.* 1985;87:758.
6. Mallis GI, Schmidt DH, Lindenbaum J. Superior bioavailability of digoxin solution in capsules. *Clin Pharmacol Ther.* 1975;18:761.
7. Marcus FI, Dickerson J, Pippin S, et al. Digoxin bioavailability: formulations and rates of infusions. *Clin Pharmacol Ther.* 1976;20:253.
8. Nahata MC, Powell DA. Bioavailability and clearance of chloramphenicol after intravenous chloramphenicol succinate. *Clin Pharmacol Ther.* 1981;30:368.

9. Burke JT, Wargin WA, Sherertz JR, et al. Pharmacokinetics of intravenous chloramphenicol sodium succinate in adult patients with normal renal and hepatic function. *J Pharmacokinet Biopharm*. 1982;10:601–614.

10. Kramer WG, Rensimer ER, Ericsson CD, et al. Comparative bioavailability of intravenous and oral chloramphenicol in adults. *J Clin Pharmacol*. 1984;24:181–186.

11. Niles AS, Shand DG. Clinical pharmacology of propranolol. *Circulation*. 1975;52:6.

12. Boyer RN, Scott DB, Jebson PJ, et al. Pharmacokinetics of lidocaine in man. *Clin Pharmacol Ther*. 1971;12:105.

13. Fahr A. Cyclosporin clinical pharmacokinetics. *Clin Pharmacokinet*. 1993;24:472–495.

14. Koch-Weser J, Sellers EM. Binding of drugs to serum albumin. *N Engl J Med*. 1976;294:311.

15. Levy RH, Shand D, eds. Clinical implications of drug-protein binding. *Clin Pharmacokinet*. 1984;9(suppl):1.

16. Levine M, Chang T. Therapeutic drug monitoring of phenytoin. Rationale and current status. *Clin Pharmacokinet*. 1990;19:341–358.

17. Barre J, Didey F, Delion F, et al. Problems in therapeutic drug monitoring: free drug level monitoring. *Ther Drug Monit*. 1988;10:133–143.

18. Perucca E. Pharmacological and therapeutic properties of valproate: a summary after 35 years of clinical experience. *CNS Drugs*. 2002;10:695–714.

19. Fremstad D, Bergerud K, Haffner JF, et al. Increased plasma binding of quinidine after surgery: a preliminary report. *Eur J Clin Pharmacol*. 1976;10:441.

20. Tucker GT, Boyes RN, Bridenbaugh PO, et al. Binding of anilide-type local anaesthetics in human plasma. *Anesthesiology*. 1970;33:287.

21. Borgå O, Piafsky KM, Nilsen OG. Plasma protein binding of basic drugs. *Clin Pharmacol Ther*. 1977;22:539.

22. Adler DS, Martin E, Gambertoglio JG, et al. Hemodialysis of phenytoin in a uremic patient. *Clin Pharmacol Ther*. 1975;18:65.

23. Thummel KE, Shen DD. Appendix II: design and optimization of dosage regimens: pharmacokinetic data. In: Hardman JG, ed. *Goodman and Gilman's The Pharmacologic Basis of Therapeutics*. 10th ed. New York, NY: McGraw-Hill; 2001:1917–2023.

24. LeMarie M, Tillement JP. Role of lipoproteins and erythrocytes in the in vitro binding and distribution of cyclosporin A in the blood. *J Pharm Pharmacol*. 1982;34:715–718.

25. Niederberger W, LeMaire M, Maure G, et al. Distribution and binding of cyclosporine in blood and tissue. *Transplant Proc*. 1983;15:2419–2421.

26. Piafsky KM. Disease-induced changes in the plasma binding of basic drugs. *Clin Pharmacokinet*. 1980;5:246.

27. Pike E, Skuterud B, Kierulf P, et al. Binding and displacement of basic drugs, acidic and neutral drugs in normal and orosomucoid deficient plasma. *Clin Pharmacokinet*. 1981;6:367.

28. Edwards DJ, Lalka D, Cerra F, et al. Alpha-1-acid glycoprotein concentration and protein binding in trauma. *Clin Pharmacol Ther*. 1982;31:62.

29. Routledge PA, Shand DG, Barchowsky A, et al. Relationship between alpha-1-acid glycoprotein and lidocaine disposition in myocardial infarction. *Clin Pharmacol Ther*. 1981;30:154.

30. Odar-Cederlöf I, Borgå O. Kinetics of diphenylhydantoin in uremic patients: consequence of decreased protein binding. *Eur J Clin Pharmacol*. 1974;7:31.

31. Benet LZ, Hoener BA. Changes in plasma protein binding have little clinical relevance. *Clin Pharmacol Ther*. 2002;3:115–121.

32. Svensson CK, Woodruff MN, Baxter JG, et al. Free drug concentration monitoring in clinical practice. Rationale and current status. *Clin Pharmacokinet*. 1986;11:450–469.

33. Booker HE, Darcy B. Serum concentrations of free diphenylhydantoin and their relationship to clinical intoxication. *Epilepsia*. 1973;14:177–184.

34. Conford EM, Pardridge WM, Braun LD, et al. Increased blood–brain barrier transportation of protein-bound anticonvulsant drugs in the newborn. *J Cereb Blood Flow Metab*. 1983;3:280–286.

35. Tozer TN, Gambertoglio JG, Furst DE, et al. Volume shifts and protein binding estimates using equilibrium dialysis: application to prednisolone binding in humans. *J Pharm Sci*. 1983;12:1442–1446.

36. Rowland M. Drug administration and regimens. In: Melmon K, Morelli H, eds. *Clinical Pharmacology and Therapeutics.* 2nd ed. New York, NY: Macmillan; 1978:25–70.

37. Reuning RH, Sams RA, Notari RE. Role of pharmacokinetics in drug dosage adjustment: I. Pharmacologic effect kinetics and apparent volume of distribution of digoxin. *J Clin Pharmacol.* 1973;13:127.

38. Gibaldi M, Perrier D. Drug distribution and renal failure. *J Clin Pharmacol.* 1972;12:201.

39. Kappel J, Calissi P. Nephrology: 3. Safe drug prescribing for patients with renal insufficiency. *CMAJ.* 2002;1664:473–477.

40. Rowland M, Tozer TN. *Clinical Pharmacokinetics: Concepts and Applications.* 2nd ed. Philadelphia, PA: Lea & Febiger; 1989.

41. Benowitz N. Clinical application of the pharmacokinetics of lidocaine. In: Melmon K, ed. *Cardiovascular Drug Therapy.* Philadelphia, PA: FA Davis; 1974:77–101.

42. Mitenko PA, Ogilvie RI. Rapidly achieved plasma concentration plateaus, with observation on theophylline kinetics. *Clin Pharmacol Ther.* 1972;13:329.

43. Walsh FM, Sode J. Significance of non–steady state serum digoxin concentrations. *Am J Clin Pathol.* 1975;63:446.

44. Shapiro W, Narahara K, Taubert K. Relationship of plasma digitoxin and digoxin to cardiac response following intravenous digitalization in man. *Circulation.* 1970;42:1065.

45. Sheiner LB, Rosenberg B, Marathe VV. Estimation of population characteristics of pharmacokinetic parameters from routine clinical data. *J Pharmacokinet Biopharm.* 1977;5:445.

46. Barot MH, Grant RH, Maheendran KK, et al. Individual variation in daily dosage requirement for phenytoin sodium in patients with epilepsy. *Br J Clin Pharmacol.* 1978;6:267.

47. Vogelstein B, Kowarski A, Lietman PS. The pharmacokinetics of amikacin in children. *J Pediatr.* 1977;91:333.

48. FDA Drug Bulletin. IV guidelines for theophylline products. *FDA Drug Bull.* 1980;10:4–6.

49. Lack JA, Stuart-Taylor ME. Calculation of drug dosage and body surface area of children. *Br J Anaesth.* 1997;5:601–605.

50. Sawyer M, Ratain MJ. Body surface area as a determinant of pharmacokinetics and drug dosing. *Invest New Drugs.* 2001;2:171–177.

51. Diem K, Lentner C, eds. *Documenta Geigy: Scientific Tables.* 7th ed. Switzerland: Ciba-Geigy; 1972.

52. Gunn VL, Nechyba C, eds. *The Harriet Lane Handbook: A Manual for Pediatric House Officers.* 16th ed. Chicago, IL: Mosby; 2003.

53. Taketomo CK, ed. *Pediatric Dosage Handbook.* 9th ed. Hudson, OH: LexiComp; 2002.

54. Ohnhaus EE, Spring P, Dettli L. Protein binding of digoxin in human serum. *Eur J Clin Pharmacol.* 1972;5:34.

55. Pang KS, Rowland M. Hepatic clearance of drugs: I. Theoretical considerations of a "well-stirred" model and a "parallel tube" model. Influence of hepatic blood flow, plasma and blood cell binding and hepatocellular enzymatic activity on hepatic drug clearance. *J Pharmacokinet Biopharm.* 1977;5:625.

56. Powell JR, Vozeh S, Hopewell P, et al. Theophylline disposition in acutely ill hospitalized patients. *Am Rev Respir Dis.* 1978;118:229.

57. ter Braak EW, de Vries PJ, Bouter KP, et al. Once-daily dosing regimen for aminoglycoside plus β-lactam combination therapy for serious bacterial infection: comparative trial with netilmicin plus ceftriaxone. *Am J Med.* 1990;89:58–66.

58. Nicolau D, Freeman CD, Belliveau PP, et al. Experience with a once-daily aminoglycoside program administered to 2,184 adult patients. *Antimicrob Agents Chemother.* 1995;39:650–655.

59. Craig WA, Vogelman B. The post antibiotic effect [editorial]. *Ann Intern Med.* 1987;106:900–902.

2

SELECTING THE APPROPRIATE EQUATION AND INTERPRETATION OF MEASURED DRUG CONCENTRATIONS

Paul M. Beringer and Michael Winter

By the end of the selecting the appropriate equation and interpretation of measured drug concentrations chapter, the learner shall be able to:

Selecting the Appropriate Equation

1. Draw to approximate scale a plasma concentration versus time curve, given a set of pharmacokinetic parameters and a drug dosing history. Write the equations that represent the curve, given a plasma concentration versus time curve.

Loading Dose or Bolus Dose

1. Calculate the initial drug concentration and subsequent drug concentration at any time t_1 following the loading dose, given the salt form, bioavailability, elimination rate constant, volume of distribution, and a loading dose.

Continuous Infusion to Steady State

1. Calculate the steady-state drug concentration and the drug concentration at any time t_1 following the discontinuation of the infusion, given the salt form, bioavailability, clearance, elimination rate constant, and an infusion or input rate.

Initiation and Discontinuation of Infusion before Steady State

1. Calculate the drug concentration as it accumulates toward steady state at t_1 or t_{in} hours after initiating the infusion and the drug concentration at any time t_2

following the discontinuation of the infusion, given the salt form, bioavailability, clearance, elimination rate constant, and an infusion or input rate.

2. Explain when the instantaneous input or bolus versus short infusion model can be used, and given a set of pharmacokinetic parameters and the duration of drug input, the learner shall also be able to select the simplest model that will approximate the drug concentrations with 10% error.

3. Describe the different pharmacokinetic functions of t_{in} in $[(S)(F)(Dose)]/t_{in}$ versus $1 - e^{-Kt_{in}}$ for the short infusion model, that is, which one is used to determine "rate" and which to determine "duration" of the infusion.

Loading Dose Followed by Infusion

1. Calculate the expected concentration C_1 at any time t_1 following a loading dose and immediate initiation of a continuous infusion, given the pharmacokinetic parameters S, F, dose, volume of distribution, clearance, and K.

Intermittent Administration at Regular intervals to Steady State

1. Predict steady-state peak and trough concentrations and the drug concentration at any time t_1 following the steady-state peak concentration, given the pharmacokinetic parameters S, F, dose, volume of distribution, and K.

Series of Individual Doses

1. Predict a drug concentration at any time after the administration of a series of individual doses given at irregular intervals by summing the concentration remaining for each of the individual doses, given the pharmacokinetic parameters S, F, dose, volume of distribution, clearance, and K.

2. Predict a drug concentration at any time after the administration of a series of individual doses (N doses) given at regular intervals, given the pharmacokinetic parameters S, F, dose, volume of distribution, clearance, and K.

Sustained-Release Dosage Forms

1. Define the conditions that allow the use of a continuous uninterrupted infusion model for sustained-release oral dosage forms (i.e., $\tau - t_{in}$ vs. drug $t\frac{1}{2}$), assuming zero-order input, and recognize when the continuous uninterrupted infusion model would not be appropriate, given a set of pharmacokinetic parameters.

Algorithm for Choosing the Appropriate Equation

1. Determine whether steady state has or has not been achieved, given a set of pharmacokinetic parameters and a dosing history.

2. Determine whether steady state has been achieved:
   a. If a continuous or intermittent input model is required to predict plasma concentrations.

    b. If an intermittent input model is required to determine whether it is the bolus model or short infusion model that would be most appropriate to predict plasma concentrations.

3. Determine whether steady state has not been achieved:

    a. Whether a series of individual bolus or short infusion models would be required to predict the drug concentrations if dose and τ are not consistent.

    b. Whether a non–steady-state continuous infusion, non–steady-state bolus, or non–steady-state short infusion model would be required to predict the plasma concentrations if dose and τ are consistent.

Interpretation of Plasma Drug Concentrations

1. Determine whether it is likely that the measured drug concentration represents steady state or non–steady state and then select the model to revise the proper pharmacokinetic parameter(s), given a patient's dosing history, plasma drug concentration(s), and the literature estimates of the drug's pharmacokinetic parameters.

Plasma Sampling Time

1. Explain why, in most cases, trough drug samples are preferred over peak drug samples.

2. Recognize whether or not the drug sample is likely to have been obtained in the absorption/distribution phase when given a dosing history and drug sampling time(s).

Revising Pharmacokinetic Parameters

1. Define the conditions with regard to drug input (absorption and distribution) and the time interval (absorption and decay) that must be met in order to be able to revise volume of distribution.

2. Explain why the average steady-state concentration is determined by clearance.

3. Explain when a steady-state trough concentration can be substituted for steady-state average concentration to revise clearance.

4. Recognize when the change in the literature or predicted versus revised pharmacokinetic parameter is much different than the change in predicted versus measured drug concentration when performing pharmacokinetic revisions.

5. Identify and explain why volume, clearance, or neither volume nor clearance can be revised, given a patient's dosing history, drug sampling times, and the literature estimates of the drug's pharmacokinetic parameters.

Choosing a Model to Revise or Estimate a Patient's Clearance at Steady State

1. Determine, by comparing $[(S)(F)(Dose)]/V$ versus Css min, the approximate relationship between τ and the drug t½.

2. Choose the simplest equation necessary to revise clearance using a single Css trough concentration when:
    a. $\tau \le \frac{1}{3} t\frac{1}{2}$
    b. $\tau \le t\frac{1}{2}$
    c. $\tau > t\frac{1}{2}$
3. Know the conditions required for (2) and, given a patient dosing history and time of drug sampling, recognize when one or more of the conditions have not been met.
4. Explain why confidence in the revised clearance increases when $\tau \le t\frac{1}{2}$ and decreases as τ increases beyond $t\frac{1}{2}$.

Non–Steady-State Revision of Clearance (Iterative Search)

1. Recognize which equations can be rearranged to solve directly for clearance and which cannot.
2. Explain why it is important, when performing non–steady-state revisions, for the change in the predicted relative to the revised clearance to approximate the change in the predicted relative to the measured drug concentration. That is, sensitivity analysis.
3. Recognize when the percentage change in the literature or predicted versus revised clearance is very much different from the percentage change in the predicted versus measured drug concentration.

Non–Steady-State Revision of Clearance (Mass Balance)

1. Use the mass balance approach to calculate a revised clearance, given two non–steady-state drug concentrations, a literature estimate of volume of distribution, and the drug dosing history between the two concentrations.
2. Know the conditions required for using the mass balance approach, time interval in $t\frac{1}{2}$s between the two concentrations, the allowable change from the first to the second concentration, and consistency of the dosing rate.
3. Recognize when one or more of the above conditions have not been met, for example, compare the interval between the two concentrations to the revised $t\frac{1}{2}$ as calculated from the predicted volume of distribution and the mass balance revised clearance.

Single-Point Determination of Clearance

1. Demonstrate graphically the impact on the drug concentration decay from a single bolus dose when clearance is held constant and volume of distribution is increased or decreased.
2. Explain why, while in principle, the single-point determination of clearance is appealing, but its clinical use is limited.

Bayesian Analysis

1. Explain the basic concepts of Bayesian analysis and why this type of approach will help to avoid "making too much out of too little" when performing pharmacokinetic revisions.

2. Give at least one example of where Bayesian analysis would help to avoid making an inappropriate revision of a pharmacokinetic parameter.

Assay Specificity

1. List at least two factors that may make a reported drug concentration inaccurate.
2. Recognize that drug assay procedures are often changed, so that knowledge of the specific assay used is the only way to know for sure whether there is likely to be conditions that alter the utility of the reported drug concentration.
3. List at least two drugs that have active metabolites.

Selecting the Appropriate Equation

It is often difficult to determine which of the many equations should be used to solve specific clinical problems. A technique used by this author to avoid the use of inappropriate equations is to draw a graphic representation of the plasma drug concentration versus time curve that would be expected on the basis of the dosage regimen the patient is receiving. Once the graph is drawn and the plasma concentration visualized, mathematical equations that describe the drug's pharmacokinetic behavior are selected. To facilitate this process, a series of typical plasma level–time curves and their corresponding formulas is presented in Figures 2.1 to 2.7.

LOADING DOSE OR BOLUS DOSE

When a loading dose or a bolus of drug has been administered (Fig. 2.1), the initial plasma concentration (C) can be determined by rearranging the "loading dose" equation (see Equation 1.11):

$$C = \frac{(S)(F)(\text{Loading Dose})}{V} \qquad \textbf{(Eq. 2.1)}$$

A subsequent plasma level (C_1) any time (t_1) after the dose has been administered can be calculated by using a variation of Equation 1.26 that describes first-order elimination:

$$C_2 = (C_1)(e^{-Kt_1})$$

where C_1 is replaced by $C = \dfrac{(S)(F)(\text{Loading Dose})}{V}$ and C_2 is replaced by C_1.

$$C_1 = \frac{(S)(F)(\text{Loading Dose})}{V}(e^{-Kt_1}) \qquad \textbf{(Eq. 2.2)}$$

C_1 now represents the concentration remaining t_1 hours after the loading dose.

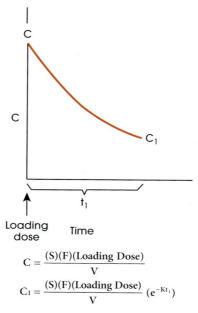

$$C = \frac{(S)(F)(\text{Loading Dose})}{V}$$

$$C_1 = \frac{(S)(F)(\text{Loading Dose})}{V} (e^{-Kt_1})$$

FIGURE 2.1 Graphic representation of the change in plasma level that occurs over time following a loading dose. C represents the initial concentration immediately following the administration of a loading dose, and C_1 represents the concentration at any interval of time (t_1) after the dose has been administered. Assume a one-compartment model and rapid absorption if the drug is given orally.

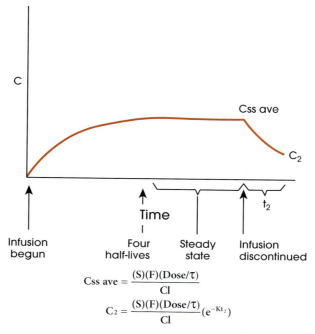

$$\text{Css ave} = \frac{(S)(F)(\text{Dose}/\tau)}{Cl}$$

$$C_2 = \frac{(S)(F)(\text{Dose}/\tau)}{Cl} (e^{-Kt_2})$$

FIGURE 2.2 Graphic representation of the plasma concentration versus time curve that results when an infusion is continued until steady state is reached and then discontinued. Css ave is the steady-state concentration, and C_2 is the concentration at any interval of time (t_2) after the infusion has been discontinued.

CONTINUOUS INFUSION TO STEADY STATE

The plasma concentration versus time curve produced by a continuous infusion, which has been administered until steady state has been achieved, is represented by Figure 2.2. The average steady-state concentration (Css ave) that will be produced by the infusion can be calculated using Equation 1.33.

$$\text{Css ave} = \frac{(S)(F)(\text{Dose}/\tau)}{\text{Cl}}$$

DISCONTINUATION OF INFUSION AFTER STEADY STATE

The curve representing a change in plasma concentration after the infusion has been discontinued is also represented in Figure 2.2. The concentration (C_2) produced any time (t_2) after the infusion has been discontinued can be calculated using a variation of the first-order elimination equation (Equation 1.26):

$$C_2 = (C_1)(e^{-Kt_1})$$

where C_1 is replaced by Css ave and t_1 by t_2:

$$C_2 = (\text{Css ave})(e^{-Kt_2}) \qquad \textbf{(Eq. 2.3)}$$

or substituting for Css ave gives:

$$C_2 = \frac{(S)(F)(\text{Dose}/\tau)}{\text{Cl}}(e^{-Kt_2}) \qquad \textbf{(Eq. 2.4)}$$

INITIATION AND DISCONTINUATION OF INFUSION BEFORE STEADY STATE

When an infusion is initiated and discontinued before steady state is achieved (<3 to 5 $t\frac{1}{2}$), the plasma concentration versus time curve can be described, as depicted in Figure 1.19. In this situation, the concentration (C_1) that occurs at any time (t_1) after the infusion has been initiated and the concentration (C_2) that occurs any time (t_2) after the infusion was discontinued can be approximated by Equation 1.35:

$$C_1 = \frac{(S)(F)(\text{Dose}/\tau)}{\text{Cl}}(1 - e^{-Kt_1})$$

and Equation 1.39:

$$C_2 = \frac{(S)(F)(\text{Dose}/\tau)}{\text{Cl}}(1 - e^{-Kt_1})(e^{-Kt_2})$$

The input model for Equations 1.35 and 1.39 is an infusion model. Whether a bolus or an infusion model is used to represent the input or absorption of drug into the body depends on the relationship between the duration of drug input relative to the drug's half-life. For example, if a drug is administered rapidly as an intravenous (IV) bolus or if an orally administered drug is absorbed rapidly relative to the drug's half-life, very little drug will be cleared or eliminated during the administration or absorption process. Therefore, absorption can be thought of as instantaneous, and the bolus model can be used. If, however, a drug is absorbed over a long time relative to its half-life, a significant amount of drug will be eliminated during the input or absorption period, and the plasma-level concentrations resulting from oral administration would resemble those resulting from an infusion model. As a general rule, if the drug input time (t_{in}) is less than one-tenth its half-life, then it can be successfully modeled as a bolus dose; however, if the drug input time is greater than one-half its half-life, it is more appropriate to use an infusion model. When the duration of drug input falls between one-tenth and one-half of its half-life, an arbitrary choice can be made between a bolus dose and an infusion model.

As a clinical guideline, the author uses one-sixth of a drug half-life as an arbitrary break point. That is, for those drugs that are absorbed over a period equal to one-sixth of a half-life or less, the bolus model is used; for those drugs absorbed over a period that is greater than one-sixth of the half-life, the short infusion model is used. Whereas the one-sixth of a half-life "rule" is arbitrary, it was selected because the difference in the calculated plasma concentrations when using the bolus or short infusion model is <10% (see Fig. 2.4).

If there is any uncertainty about which model is more appropriate, the short infusion model should be used because it more closely approximates the actual absorption and plasma concentration curve during drug absorption and elimination. Figure 2.3 represents the plasma concentration obtained at the end of a short infusion, as calculated by Equation 2.5.

$$C_{t_{in}} = \frac{(S)(F)(Dose \, / \, t_{in})}{Cl}(1 - e^{-Kt_{in}}) \qquad \text{(Eq. 2.5)}$$

Note, in the above equation, that t_{in} represents the duration of drug input and $1 - e^{-kt_{in}}$) represents the fraction of steady state that would be achieved during the infusion time. This concentration (C_{tin}), therefore, represents the peak level at the end of the infusion.

Conceptually, it is useful to compare Equation 2.5 with Equation 1.35.

$$C_1 = \frac{(S)(F)(Dose/\tau)}{Cl}(1 - e^{-Kt_1})$$

Both equations represent the process of multiplying a steady-state average concentration by the fraction of steady state achieved. The dosing interval (τ) and duration of infusion (t_1) in Equation 1.35 are replaced in Equation 2.5 with the duration of drug input (t_{in}). Although both equations represent the same basic process, Equation 1.35 is

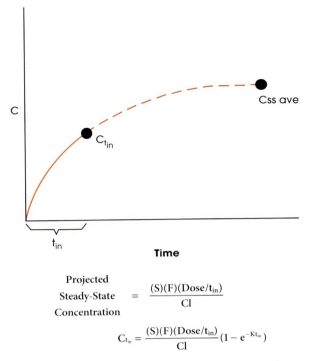

$$\text{Projected Steady-State Concentration} = \frac{(S)(F)(Dose/t_{in})}{Cl}$$

$$Ct_{in} = \frac{(S)(F)(Dose/t_{in})}{Cl}(1 - e^{-Kt_{in}})$$

FIGURE 2.3 Graphic representation of a short infusion. The plasma concentration at the end of a short infusion $(1 - e^{-Kt_{in}})$ can be calculated by multiplying the "projected steady-state concentration" (*dotted line*) by the fraction of steady state achieved $(1 - e^{-Kt_{in}})$ during the infusion period (t_{in}).

most commonly used when a continuous infusion (e.g., theophylline, lidocaine, etc.) is discontinued or sampled before steady state is achieved, and Equation 2.5 is used when a dose is to be administered over a relatively short period (e.g., aminoglycoside antibiotics). Note, in Equation 2.5, that the "function" of t_{in} in $(S)(F)(Dose/t_{in})$ is to convert the dose into a rate of drug input, and the t_{in} in $(1 - e^{-kt_{in}})$ is the duration over which the drug input occurs. While the value of t_{in} is usually the same in Equation 2.5, for example, 0.5 hour as one generally thinks of the dose being infused over 0.5 hours, the pharmacokinetic function of the two t_{in}s is different.

Once the infusion has been concluded, any subsequent drug concentration (C_2) can be calculated by multiplying the concentration at the end of the infusion $(C_{t_{in}})$ by the fraction remaining at any time interval since the end of the infusion (t_2).

$$C_2 = \frac{(S)(F)(Dose/t_{in})}{Cl}(1 - e^{-Kt_{in}})(e^{-Kt_2}) \qquad \textbf{(Eq. 2.6)}$$

The relationship between plasma concentrations predicted by the bolus dose equation (Equations 2.1 and 2.2) and the short infusion equation (Equations 2.5 and 2.6)

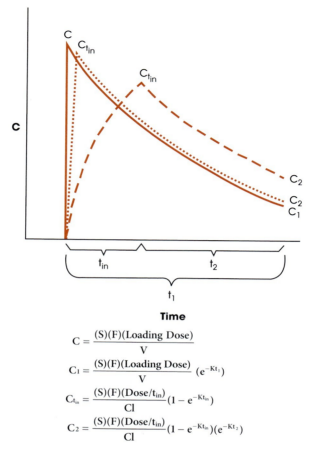

$$C = \frac{(S)(F)(\text{Loading Dose})}{V}$$

$$C_1 = \frac{(S)(F)(\text{Loading Dose})}{V}(e^{-Kt_1})$$

$$C_{t_{in}} = \frac{(S)(F)(\text{Dose}/t_{in})}{Cl}(1 - e^{-Kt_{in}})$$

$$C_2 = \frac{(S)(F)(\text{Dose}/t_{in})}{Cl}(1 - e^{-Kt_{in}})(e^{-Kt_2})$$

FIGURE 2.4   Graphic representation of a drug administered as a bolus (*solid line*) or as a short infusion (*dashed line*) and (*dotted line*). The bolus dose model assumes that drug input or absorption is instantaneous. The decay interval, t_1 (i.e., $t_{in} + t_2$), is therefore assumed to begin at the start of the infusion. In contrast, the infusion model assumes that the decay interval (t_2) begins at the conclusion of the infusion period (t_{in}). When t_{in} is $\leq 1/6$ $t\frac{1}{2}$ (*dotted line*), the concentrations are approximately the same for the short infusion and bolus dose model. When t_{in} is considerably $> 1/6$ $t\frac{1}{2}$ (*dashed line*), the concentrations calculated by the short infusion and bolus dose model are substantially different.

is depicted in Figure 2.4. Note that the bolus dose is assumed to be instantaneously absorbed at the beginning of the infusion; therefore, the initial peak concentration is higher than would be predicted by the short infusion model.

However, plasma concentrations corresponding to the conclusion of the short infusion model (t_{in} hours after starting the infusion) and all subsequent plasma levels are lower for the bolus dose model than for the infusion model. If the infusion time t_{in} is less than one-sixth of a drug's half-life, then the difference between the plasma concentrations predicted by the bolus dose and the short infusion model will be minimal. Although either equation can be used, the bolus dose model is much simpler.

LOADING DOSE FOLLOWED BY INFUSION

When a patient is given a loading dose followed by an infusion, the plasma concentration (C_1) at any time (t_1) can be calculated by summing the equations that describe the concentration produced by the loading dose at t_1 (Equation 2.2) and the concentration produced by the infusion at t_1 (Equation 1.35) (refer to C_1 in Fig. 2.1 and C_1 in Fig. 1.19).

$$C_1 = \begin{array}{c} \text{Concentration} \\ \text{Produced by the} \\ \text{Loading Dose at } t_1 \end{array} + \begin{array}{c} \text{Concentration} \\ \text{Produced by the} \\ \text{Infusion at } t_1 \end{array}$$

$$C_1 = \left[\frac{(S)(F)(\text{Loading Dose})}{V} (e^{-Kt_1}) \right] + \left[\frac{(S)(F)(\text{Dose}/\tau)}{Cl} (1 - e^{-Kt_1}) \right]$$

Note that $(S)(F)(\text{Dose}/\tau)$ in the second portion of the above equation represents the infusion rate. It is important to recall in this situation that the loading dose is eliminated according to first-order pharmacokinetics, as described in Figure 2.1, even when a maintenance infusion is initiated. This must be taken into account when predicting a plasma concentration. In other words, the maintenance infusion is accumulating, whereas the concentration resulting from the loading dose is diminishing (Fig. 2.5).

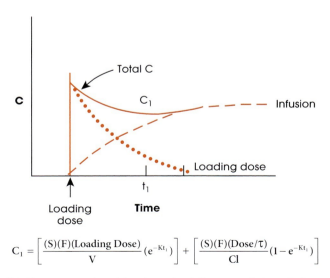

$$C_1 = \left[\frac{(S)(F)(\text{Loading Dose})}{V} (e^{-Kt_1}) \right] + \left[\frac{(S)(F)(\text{Dose}/\tau)}{Cl} (1 - e^{-Kt_1}) \right]$$

FIGURE 2.5 Graphic representation of the plasma level–time curve that results from a loading dose followed by a maintenance infusion. The curve (*solid line*) represents a summation of a loading dose curve (*dotted line*) and an infusion curve (*dashed line*). C_1 is the concentration any time (t_1) after the loading dose has been administered and after the maintenance infusion has been initiated.

INTERMITTENT ADMINISTRATION AT REGULAR INTERVALS TO STEADY STATE

When a drug is administered intermittently at regular dosing intervals until steady state is achieved (at least three to five half-lives), the average steady-state concentration can be calculated using Equation 1.33.

$$\text{Css ave} = \frac{(S)(F)(\text{Dose}/\tau)}{Cl}$$

Assuming absorption is rapid relative to $t\frac{1}{2}$, the steady-state maximum and minimum concentrations can be approximated using Equations 1.41 and 1.45, respectively.

$$\text{Css max} = \frac{\dfrac{(S)(F)(\text{Dose})}{V}}{1 - e^{-K\tau}}$$

$$\text{Css min} = \frac{\dfrac{(S)(F)(\text{Dose})}{V}}{1 - e^{-Kt}} e^{-K\tau}$$

Prediction of a plasma concentration at any time (t_1) following the peak can be accomplished using Equation 1.46. Figure 2.6 depicts the plasma concentration versus time curve that occurs with this type of dosing regimen (also see Maximum and Minimum Plasma Concentrations in Chapter 1).

$$\text{Css}_1 = \frac{\dfrac{(S)(F)(\text{Dose})}{V}}{1 - e^{-K\tau}} e^{-Kt_1}$$

SERIES OF INDIVIDUAL DOSES

When a series of individual doses is administered and a concentration before steady state must be calculated, there are several approaches that can be taken. One approach is to sum the contributions of each individual dose. This is done by decaying the peak concentration of each dose to the time at which the plasma concentration needs to be predicted. Figure 2.7 represents a series of three doses whose individual contributions were calculated and then summed to estimate the total plasma concentration existing at some time point after the third dose. Note that this is simply the sum of three individual doses, as modeled by Equation 2.2. This approach is most practical when the interval between doses or the amount of drug administered with each dose varies. Note that depending on where the brackets are placed, the summation equation may predict the concentration from one dose to the next or the contribution of each dose to the final concentration or C_{sum}. The approach of calculating the concentration from dose to dose is most useful when the pattern of drug accumulation and the potential of drug effect at each point in time are of interest. However, if the intent is to see how much each of the individual doses contribute or if an iterative solution for revision of a pharmacokinetic

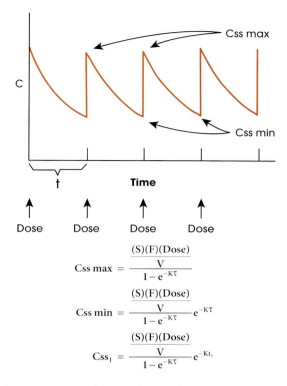

$$Css\ max = \frac{\dfrac{(S)(F)(Dose)}{V}}{1-e^{-K\tau}}$$

$$Css\ min = \frac{\dfrac{(S)(F)(Dose)}{V}}{1-e^{-K\tau}}e^{-K\tau}$$

$$Css_1 = \frac{\dfrac{(S)(F)(Dose)}{V}}{1-e^{-K\tau}}e^{-Kt_1}$$

FIGURE 2.6 Graphic representation of the steady-state plasma concentration versus time curve that occurs when drugs are given intermittently at regular dosing intervals. Any maximum concentration (Css max) is interchangeable with any other maximum concentration, and any minimum concentration (Css min) is interchangeable with any other minimum concentration. In addition, any concentration (Css₁) at time t₁ within a dosing interval is interchangeable with a corresponding concentration at the same t₁ within any other interval.

parameter is to be performed, then the approach that allows one to see how much each dose is contributing to the final solution is preferred.

If each dose and the intervals between doses are the same, it may be simpler to multiply Css max or the peak concentration that would be achieved at steady state (Equation 1.41)

$$Css\ max = \frac{\dfrac{(S)(F)(Dose)}{V}}{1-e^{-K\tau}}$$

by the fraction of steady state achieved after N doses.

$$\text{Fraction of Steady State}\atop\text{Achieved after (N) Doses} = (1-e^{-K(N)\tau}) \qquad \textbf{(Eq. 2.7)}$$

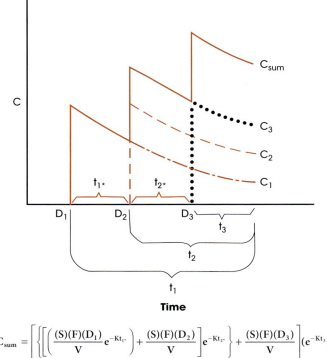

$$C_{sum} = \left[\left\{ \left[\left(\frac{(S)(F)(D_1)}{V} e^{-Kt_{1*}} \right) + \frac{(S)(F)(D_2)}{V} \right] e^{-Kt_{2*}} \right\} + \frac{(S)(F)(D_3)}{V} \right] (e^{-Kt_3})$$

$$C_{sum} = \left[\frac{(S)(F)(D_1)}{V} (e^{-Kt_1}) \right] + \left[\frac{(S)(F)(D_2)}{V} (e^{-Kt_2}) \right] + \left[\frac{(S)(F)(D_3)}{V} (e^{-Kt_3}) \right]$$

FIGURE 2.7   Graphic representation of non–steady-state summation of individual doses. The solid line represents the top summation equation and a plasma concentration because each dose is administered (D_1, D_2, D_3) as they accumulate. t_{1*} is the time from D_1 to D_2, t_{2*} is the time from D_2 to D_3, and t_3 is the time from D_3 to the time at which the plasma concentration (C_{sum}) is to be calculated. The *dashed and dotted lines* represent the bottom summation equation and the contribution of each of the individual doses to the total concentration or C_{sum}. The t_1, t_2, and t_3 represent the time from each administered dose to the time at which the plasma concentration (C_{sum}) is to be calculated.

In Equation 2.7, τ is the interval between each dose, and N represents the number of doses that have been administered. The peak concentration following N doses can be calculated by combining Equations 1.41 and 2.7. Any concentration (C_2) following the Nth dose can be calculated by multiplying the peak concentration following N doses by e^{-Kt_2}), where t_2 is the number of hours since the last dose.

$$Css_2 = \frac{\dfrac{(S)(F)(Dose)}{V}}{1 - e^{-K\tau}} (1 - e^{-K(N)\tau})(e^{-Kt_2}) \qquad \textbf{(Eq. 2.8)}$$

Note that if the doses and dosing intervals were the same in Figure 2.7, the concentration (C_{sum}) could be calculated using Equation 2.8 where N would be 3 and t_2 would be the number of hours after the third dose. Equation 2.8 is most useful when a number of doses have been administered with a consistent τ, but steady state has not yet been achieved. Equation 2.8 represents the concentration of drug produced by a series of consistently administered bolus doses that have not yet achieved steady state. This equation can be further expanded to represent a series of doses that are absorbed over a significant fraction of the drug's half-life (i.e., $t_{in} > \frac{1}{6} t\frac{1}{2}$).

$$Css_2 = \frac{\dfrac{(S)(F)(Dose / t_{in})}{Cl}(1 - e^{-Kt_{in}})}{(1 - e^{-K\tau})}(1 - e^{-K(N)\tau})(e^{-Kt_2}) \qquad \textbf{(Eq. 2.9)}$$

Equation 2.9 is similar to Equation 2.8 except that the bolus dose input model is now replaced with the short infusion input model. Equation 2.9 is seldom used in clinical practice. This is because the half-life of the drug, which requires the use of a short infusion input model, is likely to be sufficiently brief such that steady state will be achieved after two to three doses have been administered.

SUSTAINED-RELEASE DOSAGE FORMS

Most sustained-release dosage forms are designed to produce concentrations that fluctuate little within the dosage interval. Therefore, in most cases, concentrations produced by sustained-release products can be estimated by use of the equation that describes the average steady-state concentration (Equation 1.33):

$$Css\ ave = \frac{(S)(F)(Dose/\tau)}{Cl}$$

As illustrated in the following equation, the use of the Css ave formula for sustained-release products is based on the assumption that the time required for absorption (t_{in}) is approximately equal to the dosing interval (τ).

$$Css_2 = \frac{\dfrac{(S)(F)(Dose / t_{in})}{Cl}(1 - e^{-Kt_{in}})}{(1 - e^{-K\tau})}(e^{-Kt_2}) \qquad \textbf{(Eq. 2.10)}$$

$$Css_2 = \frac{\dfrac{(S)(F)(Dose/\tau)}{Cl}\left(1 - e^{-K\tau}\right)}{\left(1 - e^{-K\tau}\right)}\left(e^{-Kt_2}\right)$$

In the above equation, the $1 - e^{-K\tau}$ in the numerator and denominator cancel, and assuming t_2 is 0, we have Equation 1.33.

$$Css\ ave = \frac{(S)(F)(Dose/\tau)}{Cl}$$

If the t_{in} is exactly equal to τ, the input from one dose stops at the same time the next dose begins its infusion process. As a result, an average steady-state concentration with no rise or fall within the dosing interval is achieved. This would be exactly the same as changing an IV bag for a constant infusion without interrupting the infusion process. In practice, absorption times are not exactly equal to the dosing interval, but for most sustained-release drug products, they are reasonably close and, therefore, plasma concentrations can be considered as an average steady-state value. It should be emphasized, however, that the use of Equation 1.33 is not universal and depends on not only the absorption of the drug product but also the dosing interval selected and half-life of the drug in the specific patient. As a general rule, absorption times that exceed the dosing interval are not a problem. However, if the duration of absorption (t_{in}) is substantially less than the dosing interval, then there will be some fluctuation of the plasma concentrations. A useful approach is to consider the duration over which the plasma concentrations will decay following the end of absorption. This can be approximated by subtracting the absorption time from the dosing interval.

$$\tau - t_{in} = \text{Time within the Dosing}$$
$$\text{Interval with No Drug Absorption} \qquad \textbf{(Eq. 2.11)}$$

If this time within the dosing interval when there is no drug input is short compared to the drug's half-life, it suggests that there will be little fluctuation of the plasma concentration within the dosing interval. As a clinical guideline, if $\tau - t_{in}$ is $\leq \frac{1}{3}\ t\frac{1}{2}$, the average steady-state equation (Equation 1.33) can be used. Note that this guideline is very similar to the guidelines used for substituting the average steady-state equation (Equation 1.33) for the intermittent bolus dose equation (Equation 1.46) (see Fig. 2.11 and Interpretation of Plasma Drug Concentrations: Choosing a Model to Revise or Estimate a Patient's Clearance at Steady State). Note, however, in Figure 2.11, that the time of decay is considered to be the entire dosing interval, because the absorption is assumed to be instantaneous and t_{in} is 0.

ALGORITHM FOR CHOOSING THE APPROPRIATE EQUATION

Selecting the appropriate equation to use in a specific clinical situation can be a complex process. The algorithm in Figure 2.8 offers a stepwise approach to this process. The rules follow those outlined in the text. First, one must consider whether steady state has been achieved; then, the appropriate model is chosen to predict or calculate drug concentrations.

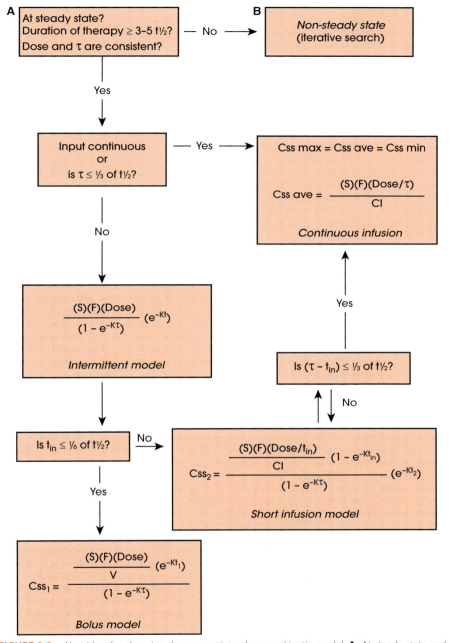

FIGURE 2.8   Algorithm for choosing the appropriate pharmacokinetic model. **A.** At steady state and **B.** Non-steady state. (*continued*)

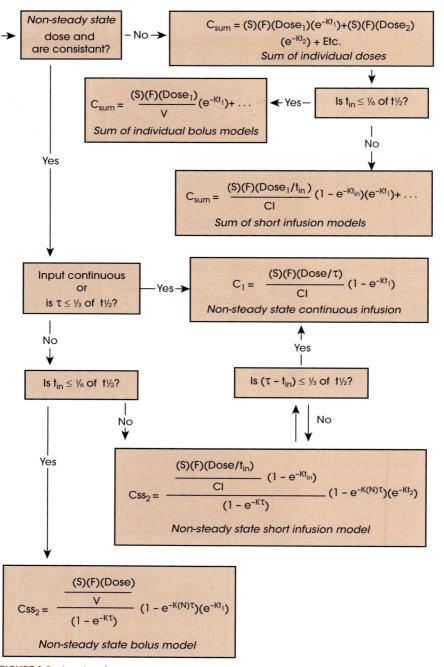

FIGURE 2.8   *(continued)*

Interpretation of Plasma Drug Concentrations

Plasma drug concentrations are measured in the clinical setting to determine whether a potentially therapeutic or toxic concentration has been produced by a given dosage regimen. This process is based on the assumption that plasma drug concentrations reflect drug concentrations at the receptor and, therefore, can be correlated with pharmacologic response. This assumption is not always valid. When plasma samples are obtained at inappropriate times or when other factors (such as delayed absorption or altered plasma binding) confound the usual pharmacokinetic behavior of a drug, the interpretation of serum drug concentrations can lead to erroneous pharmacokinetic and pharmacodynamic conclusions and ultimately inappropriate patient care decisions. These factors are discussed in the subsequent sections.

PLASMA SAMPLING TIME

To properly interpret a plasma concentration, it is essential to know when a plasma sample was obtained in relation to the last dose administered and when the drug regimen was initiated. If a plasma sample is obtained before distribution of the drug into tissue is complete (e.g., digoxin), the plasma concentration will be higher than predicted based on the dose and response. Peak (Css max) plasma levels are helpful in evaluating the dose of antibiotics used to treat severe, life-threatening infections. Although serum concentrations for many drugs peak 1 to 2 hours after an oral dose is administered, factors such as slow or delayed absorption can significantly delay the time at which peak serum concentrations are attained. Large errors in the estimation of Css max can occur if the plasma sample is obtained at the wrong time (Fig. 2.9). Therefore, with few exceptions, plasma samples should be drawn as trough or just before the next dose (Css

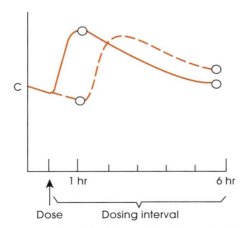

FIGURE 2.9   Schematic representation of the effect of delayed absorption (*dashed line*) on plasma-level measurements (*solid line*). Note the magnitude of error at 1 hour (theoretical time to reach Css max) as compared to 6 hours (Css min).

min) when determining routine drug concentrations in plasma. These trough levels are less likely to be influenced by absorption and distribution problems.

When the full therapeutic response of a given drug dosage regimen is to be assessed, plasma samples should not be obtained until steady-state concentrations of the drug have been achieved. If drug doses are increased or decreased based on the drug concentrations that have been measured while the drug is still accumulating, disastrous consequences can occur. Nevertheless, in some clinical situations, it is appropriate to measure drug levels before steady state has been achieved. For example, pharmacokinetic parameters for a drug administered to a severely ill patient may change so rapidly that extrapolations from a reported plasma concentration may not be valid from one day to the next. Similarly, if there is reason to suspect that the pharmacokinetic parameters in a given patient are likely to differ substantially from those reported in the literature (e.g., lidocaine in a patient with congestive heart failure),[1] or the accumulation process is prolonged because of a long t½ (e.g., phenobarbital),[2,3] it may be reasonable to obtain plasma samples before steady state to avoid excessive accumulation or unnecessarily prolonged subtherapeutic concentrations from the current dose. If possible, plasma samples should be drawn after a minimum of two half-lives because clearance values calculated from drug levels obtained less than one half-life after a regimen has been initiated are very sensitive to small differences in the volume of distribution and minor assay errors (Fig. 2.10).

REVISING PHARMACOKINETIC PARAMETERS

The process of using a patient's plasma drug concentrations and dosing history to determine patient-specific pharmacokinetic parameters can be complex and difficult. If the relationship between pharmacokinetic equations, the specific parameters, and the resultant plasma levels is understood, however, this process can be simplified. A single plasma sample obtained at the appropriate time can yield information to revise only one parameter, either the volume of distribution or clearance, but not both. Drug concentrations measured from poorly timed samples may prove to be useless in estimating a patient's V or Cl values. Thus, the goal is to obtain plasma samples at times that are likely to yield data that can be used with confidence to estimate pharmacokinetic parameters. In addition, it is important to evaluate available plasma concentration data to determine whether they can be used to estimate, with some degree of confidence, V and/or Cl. Which pharmacokinetic parameter is revised has much to do with the timing of the sample and the drug's pharmacokinetic profile. The goal in pharmacokinetic revisions is not only to recognize which pharmacokinetic parameter can be revised but also the accuracy or confidence one has in the revised or patient-specific pharmacokinetic parameter. In the clinical setting, based on the way drugs are dosed and the recommended time to sample, bioavailability is almost never revised, volume of distribution is sometimes revised, and most often clearance is the pharmacokinetic parameter that can be revised to determine a patient-specific value.

Volume of distribution

A plasma concentration that has been obtained soon after administration of an initial bolus is primarily determined by the dose administered and the volume of distribution.

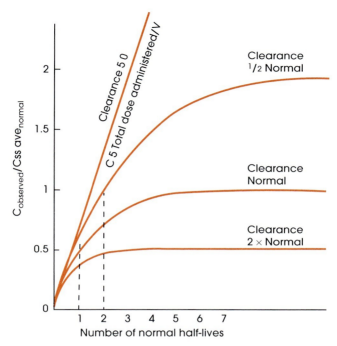

FIGURE 2.10   Relationship between observed plasma concentrations ($C_{observed}$) and the normal steady-state concentration (Css ave$_{normal}$) following initiation of a maintenance regimen at various clearance values. At steady state, the plasma concentrations are inversely proportional to clearance. Plasma concentrations obtained at or before one normal half-life are all very similar regardless of clearance. After two half-lives, alterations in a patient's clearance and ultimately steady-state concentrations can be detected by unexpectedly high or low plasma drug concentrations. After three half-lives, more confident predictions of steady-state concentrations can be made.

This assumes that both the absorption and distribution phases have been avoided. This is illustrated by Equation 2.2 (also see Figs. 2.1 and 2.12):

$$C_1 = \frac{(S)(F)(\textbf{Loading Dose})}{V}(e^{-Kt_1})$$

When e^{-Kt_1} approaches 1 (i.e., when t_1 is much less than $t\frac{1}{2}$), the plasma concentration (C_1) is primarily a function of the administered dose and the apparent volume of distribution. At this point, very little drug has been eliminated from the body. As a clinical guideline, a patient's volume of distribution can usually be estimated if the absorption and distribution phase are avoided and t_1, or the interval between the administration and sampling time, is less than or equal to one-third of the drug's half-life. Because t_1 exceeds one-third of a half-life, the measured concentration is increasingly influenced by clearance. Because more of the drug is eliminated (i.e., t_1 increases), it is difficult to estimate the patient's V with any certainty. The specific application of this clinical guideline depends on the confidence with which one knows clearance. If clearance is extremely variable and uncertain, a time interval of less than one-third of a half-life would be necessary to revise volume of distribution. On the other hand, if a patient-specific value for clearance has already been determined, then t_1 could exceed one-third of a half-life, and a reasonably accurate estimate of volume of distribution could be obtained. It is important to recognize that the pharmacokinetic parameter that most influences the drug concentration is not determined by the model chosen to represent the drug level. For example, even if the dose is modeled as a short infusion (Equation 2.6), the volume of distribution can still be the important parameter controlling the plasma concentration. V is not clearly defined in the equation; nevertheless, it is incorporated into the elimination rate constant (K).

$$C_2 = \frac{(S)(F)(\text{Dose}/t_{in})}{Cl}(1 - e^{-Kt_{in}})(e^{-Kt_2})$$

Although one would not usually select Equation 2.6 to demonstrate that the drug concentration is primarily a function of volume of distribution, it is important to recognize that the relationship between the observed drug concentration and volume is not altered as long as the total elapsed time $(t_{in} + t_2)$ does not exceed one-third of a half-life.

Our assumption in evaluating the volume of distribution is that although we have not sampled beyond one-third of a $t\frac{1}{2}$, we have waited until the drug absorption and distribution process is complete.

Clearance

A plasma drug concentration that has been obtained at steady state from a patient who is receiving a constant drug infusion is determined by clearance. This is illustrated by Equation 1.33:

$$\text{Css ave} = \frac{(S)(F)(\text{Dose}/\tau)}{Cl}$$

Note that the average steady-state plasma concentration is not influenced by volume of distribution. Therefore, plasma concentrations that represent the average steady-state level can be used to estimate a patient's clearance value, but they cannot be used to estimate a patient's volume of distribution. As illustrated in Figure 2.11, all steady-state plasma concentrations within a dosing interval that is short relative to a drug's half-life ($\tau \leq \frac{1}{3} t\frac{1}{2}$) approximate the average concentration. Therefore, these concentrations are also primarily a function of clearance and only minimally influenced by V. If the average drug concentration is assumed to occur approximately in the middle of the dosing interval, the trough concentration will have decayed from the average for only half of the dosing interval or by one-sixth of a drug half-life (assuming the dosing interval is one-third of a half-life or less). Under these conditions, the trough concentration is approximately 90% of the average drug level, an error that is usually acceptable in clinical practice. Thus, in this circumstance, the equation for Css ave (Equation 1.33) or the equation that represents a steady-state plasma concentration

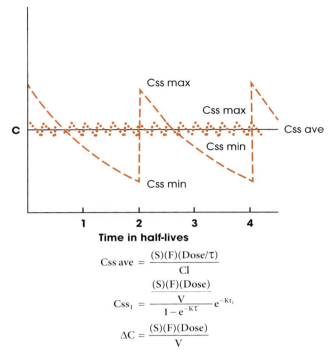

$$Css\ ave = \frac{(S)(F)(Dose/\tau)}{Cl}$$

$$Css_1 = \frac{\dfrac{(S)(F)(Dose)}{V}}{1 - e^{-K\tau}}e^{-Kt_1}$$

$$\Delta C = \frac{(S)(F)(Dose)}{V}$$

FIGURE 2.11   Plasma concentrations relative to Css ave (*solid line*) when τ is much less than (*dotted line*) and greater than (*dashed line*) the half-life. When τ is much less than t½ (*dotted line*), all plasma concentrations approximate the average concentration (Css ave) and are, therefore, primarily a function of clearance. When τ is much greater than t½ (*dashed line*), the plasma concentrations fluctuate significantly. The degree to which plasma concentrations are determined by clearance and/or volume of distribution is a function of when the plasma level is obtained within the dosing interval. Also, note that with the bolus model, the difference between Css max and Css min (ΔC) is a function of the dose and volume of distribution.

sampled any time within the dosing interval (Equation 1.46) can be used to estimate a patient-specific clearance.

$$Css_1 = \frac{\dfrac{(S)(F)(Dose)}{V}}{1 - e^{-K\tau}}e^{-Kt_1}$$

If Equation 1.46 is used, the expected volume of distribution should be retained, and the elimination rate constant should be adjusted such that Css_1 at t_1 equals the observed drug plasma concentration. Clearance could then be calculated using Equation 1.31:

$$Cl = (K)(V)$$

Sensitivity analysis

Whether a measured drug concentration is a function of clearance or volume of distribution is not always apparent. When this is difficult to ascertain, one can examine the sensitivity or responsiveness of the predicted plasma concentration to a parameter by changing one parameter while holding the other constant. For example, Equation 1.35 represents a plasma concentration (C_1) at some time interval (t_1) after a maintenance infusion has been started.

$$C_1 = \frac{(S)(F)(Dose/\tau)}{Cl}(1 - e^{-Kt_1})$$

When the fraction of steady state that has been reached ($1 - e^{-Kt_1}$) is small, large changes in clearance are frequently required to adjust a predicted plasma concentration to the appropriate value. If a large percentage change in the clearance value results in a disproportionately small change in the predicted drug level, then something other than clearance is controlling (responsible for) the drug concentration. In this case, the volume of distribution and the amount of drug administered are the primary determinants of the observed concentration. In addition, in cases where the drug concentration is very low, it might be assay error or sensitivity that is the predominant factor in determining the drug concentration, thereby making the ability to revise for any pharmacokinetic parameter limited if not impossible. This concept is illustrated graphically in Figure 2.10. Note that plasma concentrations within the first two half-lives are all very similar, whereas the steady-state concentrations are quite different. Within the first two half-lives of initiating a maintenance regimen, very large changes in clearance are required to account for small changes in plasma levels.

This type of sensitivity analysis is useful to reinforce the concept that the most reliable revisions in pharmacokinetic parameters are made when the predicted drug concentration changes by approximately the same percentage as the pharmacokinetic parameter undergoing revision. To illustrate this principle, let us examine the relationship between a theophylline drug concentration obtained 6.93 hours after starting a theophylline infusion of 30 mg/hr in a patient with the following expected parameters for theophylline: Cl 3 L/hr, V 30 L, K 0.1 hr^{-1}, t½ 6.93 hour. Because the drug being administered is theophylline, S and F are assumed to be 1.0. Using Equation 1.35, the expected plasma concentration (C_1) is calculated to be 5 mg/L.

$$\begin{aligned}
C_1 &= \frac{(S)(F)(Dose/\tau)}{Cl}(1 - e^{-Kt_1}) \\
&= \frac{(1)(1)(30 \text{ mg/hr})}{3 \text{ L/hr}}(1 - e^{-(0.1 \text{ hr}^{-1})(6.93 \text{ hr})}) \\
&= 10 \text{ mg/L}(1 - 0.5) \\
&= 5 \text{ mg/L}
\end{aligned}$$

As can be seen from the calculations, the expected steady-state concentration is 10 mg/L, and the fraction of steady state achieved ($1 - e^{-Kt_1}$) is 0.5 because the time of sampling is at one drug half-life and 50% of the steady-state plasma concentration has been achieved. If the observed plasma concentration was 6 mg/L, only slightly higher than the calculated or expected value of 5 mg/L, one might expect the patient's clearance on revision to be only slightly less than the expected 3 L/hr. This relationship, however, is deceiving because, in order to calculate a plasma concentration of 6 mg/L at 6.93 hours with a volume of 30 L, a clearance of approximately 1.32 L/hr with a corresponding K and t½ of 0.044 hr^{-1} and 15.7 hours, respectively, is required.

$$
\begin{aligned}
C_1 &= \frac{(S)(F)(Dose/\tau)}{Cl}(1-e^{-Kt_1}) \\
&= \frac{(1)(1)(30\ mg/hr)}{1.32\,L/hr}(1-e^{-(0.044\ hr^{-1})(6.93\ hr)}) \\
&= 22.7\ mg/L\,(1-0.737) \\
&= 22.7\ mg/L\,(0.263) \\
&= 5.97\ mg/L
\end{aligned}
$$

As can be seen from this illustration, the clearance value of 3 L/hr had to be reduced by more than one-half (i.e., from 3 to 1.32 L/hr) to increase the predicted drug concentration by ≈20%. This poor response of the calculated drug concentration to a change in clearance suggests that clearance is not the primary pharmacokinetic parameter responsible for the drug concentration. Therefore, any estimates of clearance and future dosing regimen based on these calculations would be tenuous at best. While knowing that the patient's theophylline concentration is 6 mg/L may be a useful clinical information, it is important to recognize that very little additional pharmacokinetic information can be obtained from this drug level. Therefore, while it may be that the patient's theophylline clearance is approximately as predicted, it is also possible that it is quite different, and additional drug levels later in the accumulation process would be necessary to determine what the final steady-state theophylline concentration would be (see Fig. 2.10).

When a predicted drug concentration changes in direct proportion, or inverse proportion to an alteration in only one of the pharmacokinetic parameters, it is likely that a measured drug concentration can be used to estimate that patient-specific parameter. When both clearance and volume of distribution have a significant influence on the prediction of a measured drug concentration, revision of a patient's pharmacokinetic parameters will be less certain because there is an infinite number of combinations for clearance and volume of distribution values that could be used to predict the observed drug concentration. When this occurs, the patient-specific pharmacokinetic characteristics can be estimated by adjusting one or both of the pharmacokinetic parameters. Nevertheless, in most cases such as this, additional plasma-level sampling will be needed to accurately predict the patient's clearance or volume of distribution so that subsequent dosing regimens can be adjusted.

If a plasma drug concentration calculated from a specific equation is similar to the reported value, the pharmacokinetic parameters used in that equation may not necessarily be the most important determinants of the drug concentration. Equation 1.46 and Figure 2.11 can be used to demonstrate this principle.

$$
Css_1 = \frac{\dfrac{(S)(F)(Dose)}{V}}{1-e^{-K\tau}}e^{-Kt_1}
$$

When the dosing interval is much shorter than the drug's half-life, the changes in concentration within a dosing interval are relatively small, and any drug concentration obtained within a dosing interval can be used as an approximation of the average steady-state concentration. Even though Equations 1.41 and 1.45

$$\text{Css max} = \frac{\dfrac{(S)(F)(Dose)}{V}}{1 - e^{-K\tau}}$$

$$\text{Css min} = \frac{\dfrac{(S)(F)(Dose)}{V}}{1 - e^{-K\tau}} e^{-K\tau}$$

could be used to predict peak and trough concentrations, a reasonable approximation could also be achieved by using Equation 1.33 for Css ave:

$$\text{Css ave} = \frac{(S)(F)(Dose/\tau)}{Cl}$$

This suggests that even though Equations 1.41 and 1.45 do not contain the parameter clearance per se, the elimination rate constant functions in such a way that the clearance derived from Equations 1.41 or 1.45 and 1.33 would all essentially be the same.

In the situation in which the dosing interval is greater than one-third of a half-life, the use of Equations 1.41 and 1.45 are appropriate, because not all drug concentrations within the dosing interval can be considered as the Css ave. However, as long as the dosing interval has not been extended beyond one half-life, clearance is still the primary pharmacokinetic parameter that is responsible for the drug concentrations within the dosing interval. Although the elimination rate constant and volume of distribution might be manipulated in Equations 1.41 and 1.45, it is only the product of those two numbers (i.e., clearance) that can be known with any certainty:

$$Cl = (K)(V)$$

If a drug is administered at a dosing interval that is much longer than the apparent half-life (see Fig. 2.11), peak concentrations may be primarily a function of volume of distribution. Because most of the dose is eliminated within a dosing interval, each dose can be thought of as something approaching a new loading dose. Of course, for steady-state conditions, at some point within the dosing interval, the plasma concentration (Css ave) will be determined by clearance. Trough plasma concentrations in this situation are a function of both clearance and volume of distribution. Because clearance and volume of distribution are critical to the prediction of peak and trough concentrations when the dosing interval is much longer than the drug t½, a minimum of two plasma concentrations is needed to accurately establish patient-specific pharmacokinetic parameters and a dosing regimen that will achieve desired peak and trough concentrations. Aminoglycoside antibiotics are examples of drugs that are administered at dosing intervals that greatly exceed their apparent half-life; therefore, if it is important to achieve targeted peak and trough concentrations, at least two plasma concentrations would be needed (see Chapter 6).

When an observed drug concentration correlates with the level that was predicted based on pharmacokinetic parameters from the literature, the particular pharmacokinetic parameter that is the primary determinant of the observed drug concentration should be determined before making future predictions. For example, successful prediction of an appropriate loading dose to achieve a specific plasma level does not guarantee that the maintenance dose is correct. Therefore, critical evaluation of the parameters affecting a patient's measured drug concentration will minimize incorrect assumptions about the applicability of literature-based pharmacokinetic parameters to a specific patient's situation or about the predictability of future plasma concentrations.

CHOOSING A MODEL TO REVISE OR ESTIMATE A PATIENT'S CLEARANCE AT STEADY STATE

As previously discussed, a drug's half-life often determines the pharmacokinetic equation that should be used to make a revised or patient-specific estimate of a pharmacokinetic parameter. A common problem encountered clinically, however, is that the half-life observed in the patient often differs from the expected value. Because a change in either clearance or volume of distribution or both may account for this unexpected value, the pharmacokinetic model is often unclear. One way to approach this dilemma is to first calculate the expected change in plasma drug concentration associated with each dose:

$$\Delta C = \frac{(S)(F)(Dose)}{V} \qquad \text{(Eq. 2.12)}$$

where ΔC is the change in concentration following the administration of each dose [(S)(F)(Dose)] into the patient's volume of distribution (V). This change in concentration can then be compared to the steady-state trough concentration measured in the patient.

$$\frac{(S)(F)(Dose)}{V} \quad \text{versus Css min}$$

or

$$\Delta C \quad \text{versus Css min}$$

Note, in Figure 2.11, that when the dosing interval (τ) is much less than the drug half-life, ΔC will be small when compared to Css min. As the dosing interval increases relative to τ, ΔC will increase relative to Css min. Therefore, a comparison of ΔC or (S)(F)(Dose)/V to Css min can serve as a guide to estimating the drug t½ and the most appropriate pharmacokinetic model or technique to use for revision. With few exceptions, drugs that have plasma-level monitoring are most often dosed at intervals less than or equal to their half-lives. Therefore, clearance is the pharmacokinetic parameter most often revised or calculated for the patient in question. The following guidelines can be used to select the pharmacokinetic model that is the least complex and, therefore, the most appropriate to estimate a patient-specific pharmacokinetic parameter.

Condition 1

When

$$\frac{(S)(F)(Dose)}{V} \leq \tfrac{1}{4}\, Css\ min$$

then,

$$\tau \leq \tfrac{1}{3}\, t\tfrac{1}{2}$$

Under these conditions,

$$Css\ min \approx Css\ ave$$

and Cl can be estimated by Equation 1.15:

$$Cl = \frac{(S)(F)(Dose/\tau)}{Css\ ave}$$

Rules/Conditions: must be at steady state.

Condition 2

When

$$\frac{(S)(F)(Dose)}{V} \leq Css\ min$$

then,

$$\tau \leq t\tfrac{1}{2}$$

Under these conditions,

$$Css\ min + (\tfrac{1}{2})\frac{(S)(F)(Dose)}{V} \approx Css\ ave \qquad \textbf{(Eq. 2.13)}$$

and Cl can be estimated by Equation 1.15:

$$Cl = \frac{(S)(F)(Dose/\tau)}{Css\ ave}$$

Rules/Conditions: must be at steady state C is Css min.
   Bolus model for absorption is acceptable.
   That is, dosage form is not sustained release.
   Short infusion model is not required, that is, $t_{in} \leq \frac{1}{6} t\frac{1}{2}$.

Condition 3

When

$$\frac{(S)(F)(Dose)}{V} > Css\ min$$

then,

$$\tau > t\frac{1}{2}$$

Under these conditions,

$$Css\ min + \frac{(S)(F)(Dose)}{V} = Css\ max \qquad \textbf{(Eq. 2.14)}$$

where V is an assumed value from the literature.
K is revised ($K_{revised}$):

$$K_{revised} = \frac{ln\left(\dfrac{Css\ min + \dfrac{(S)(F)(Dose)}{V}}{Css\ min}\right)}{\tau} = \frac{ln\left(\dfrac{Css\ max}{Css\ min}\right)}{\tau} \qquad \textbf{(Eq. 2.15)}$$

Clearance is revised ($Cl_{revised}$) using $K_{revised}$ in Equation 1.31: $Cl_{revised} = (K_{revised})(V)$
Rules/Conditions: must be at steady state C is Css min.
   Bolus model for absorption is acceptable.
   That is, dosage form is not sustained release.
   Short infusion model is not required, that is, $t_{in} \leq \frac{1}{6} t\frac{1}{2}$

   Note that the approaches used become more complex as the dosing interval increases relative to the drug half-life. If a drug is administered at a dosing interval less than or equal to one-third of its half-life and the technique in Condition 3 is used to revise clearance, the revised clearance would be correct. The calculation is not wrong, just unnecessarily complex. However, if a drug is administered at a dosing interval that exceeds one half-life and the technique in Condition 1 is used to revise clearance, the revised clearance value would be inaccurate because Css min cannot be assumed to be approximately equal to Css ave. While it could be argued that the technique used in Condition 3 would suffice for all the previous conditions, it is more cumbersome and tends to focus on the intermediate parameters, K and V, rather than Cl. One should also be aware that as the dosing interval increases relative to the drug's half-life, the confidence in a revised clearance diminishes because the volume of distribution, which is an assumed value from the literature, begins to influence the revised clearance to a greater degree. As a general rule, the confidence in Cl is usually good when the dosing interval is <t½, steady state has been achieved, and drug concentrations are obtained properly.

NON–STEADY-STATE REVISION OF CLEARANCE (ITERATIVE SEARCH)

The techniques described in the previous section allow one to calculate a revised clearance directly. However, there are a number of situations in which revision of the clearance value is possible, but there are no explicit solutions. These situations require an iterative search technique. The first situation is when the parameter being revised appears in both the exponential and the nonexponential portions of the equations, as illustrated by Equation 1.35.

$$C_1 = \frac{(S)(F)(Dose/\tau)}{Cl}(1 - e^{-Kt_1})$$

Although it may not be obvious that clearance appears in both the exponential and nonexponential portions of the equation, the elimination rate constant consists of both clearance and V.

$$C_1 = \frac{(S)(F)(Dose/\tau)}{Cl}\left(1 - e^{-\left(\frac{Cl}{V}\right)t_1}\right)$$

Therefore, if V is held constant, the revision process would be associated with a changing clearance (and the corresponding elimination rate constant) to match the observed plasma concentration (C_1). The clearance that "fits" or calculates a value for C_1 that is the same as the assayed concentration would be the revised clearance. As stated earlier, there is no direct solution, and the clearance value (which when placed in Equation 1.35 calculates the specific C_1) can only be found by trial and error. The second situation that requires an iterative search is any time there are multiple exponential terms (e^{-Kt}) where t differs. This might occur when there are multiple bolus doses being administered, and the plasma concentration is the sum of the residual of each of these doses (see Fig. 2.7). Another example is the short infusion model at steady state or Equation 2.10.

$$Css_2 = \frac{\dfrac{(S)(F)(Dose/t_{in})}{Cl}(1 - e^{-Kt_{in}})}{(1 - e^{-K\tau})}(e^{-Kt_2})$$

In Equation 2.10, clearance is expressed in both the exponential (i.e., $K = Cl/V$) and the nonexponential portions. In addition, each of the exponential terms has a different value for t, which in itself is a condition that would require an iterative search to find a unique solution for Cl.

Although an iterative search process can be cumbersome, in most cases, approximate values for the revised clearance can be arrived at within one to three attempts. One technique is to adjust the Cl by the ratio that the predicted C_1 and the assayed drug concentration are different. If, for example, the predicted drug concentration is 10 mg/L and the assayed drug concentration is 12 mg/L, the Cl in Equation 2.10 would be decreased by about 20% in the hope that a 20% decrease in Cl would increase the calculated C_1 by 20%. However, this may not be the case because, in Equation 2.10, the relationship between Cl and C_1 is not proportional. If the required change in Cl is significantly out of proportion to the ratio of C_1 to the assayed drug concentration, it is a strong indication that Cl is not the only pharmacokinetic parameter responsible for C_1. Therefore, any estimates of Cl under conditions where a large change in Cl is required to make small changes in C_1 would be tenuous at best. Many pharmacokineticists use programmed calculators or computers to facilitate these repetitive trial and error calculations. While use of computers is to be encouraged as a labor-saving device, the user must understand the fundamental process and the limits of the method (see Interpretation of Plasma Drug Concentrations: Revising Pharmacokinetic Parameters: Sensitivity Analysis: Interpretation of Plasma Drug Concentrations: Bayesian Analysis).

NON–STEADY-STATE REVISION OF CLEARANCE (MASS BALANCE)

The mass balance technique has been suggested as a more direct alternative to the iterative approach.[4,5] The mass balance technique is relatively simple and can be best visualized by examining the relationship between the rate of drug administration and the rate of drug elimination. At steady state, the rate of drug elimination (R_E) is equal to the rate of administration (R_A) and the change in the amount of the drug in the body with time is 0.

$$R_A - R_E = \text{Change in the Amount of Drug in the Body with Time} = 0$$

Under non–steady-state conditions, however, there will be a change in the amount of drug in the body with time. This change can be estimated by multiplying the difference in the plasma concentration (ΔC) by the volume of distribution and dividing by the time interval between the two drug concentrations.

$$R_A - R_E = \frac{(\Delta C)(V)}{t} \qquad \text{(Eq. 2.16)}$$

By substituting the appropriate values in the above equation, an estimate of clearance can be derived as follows:

$$R_A - R_E = \frac{(\Delta C)(V)}{t}$$

$$(S)(F)(Dose/\tau) - R_E = \frac{(C_2 - C_1)(V)}{t}$$

$$(S)(F)(Dose/\tau) - \frac{(C_2 - C_1)(V)}{t} = R_E$$

$$(S)(F)(Dose/\tau) - \frac{(C_2 - C_1)(V)}{t} = (Cl)(C\ ave)$$

$$\frac{(S)(F)(Dose/\tau) - \frac{(C_2 - C_1)(V)}{t}}{C\ ave} = Cl \qquad \text{(Eq. 2.17)}$$

Note that the average plasma concentration (C ave) is generally assumed to be the average of C_1 and C_2.

$$C\ ave = \frac{C_1 + C_2}{2} \qquad \text{(Eq. 2.18)}$$

Although this C ave is not the steady-state average, it is assumed to be the average concentration that results in the elimination of drug as the concentration proceeds toward steady state. Equation 2.17 is an accurate method for estimating clearance if the following conditions are met:

1. t, or time interval between C_1 and C_2, should be equal to at least one but no longer than two of the revised drug half-lives. This rule helps to ensure that the time interval is not so short as to be unable to detect any change in concentration and yet not so long that the second concentration (C_2) is at steady state.
2. The plasma concentration values should be reasonably close to one another. If the drug concentrations are increasing, C_2 should be less than two times C_1; if the plasma concentrations are declining, C_2 should be more than one-half of C_1 (i.e., $0.5 < C_2/C_1 < 2.0$). This rule limits the change in concentration so that the assumed value for V will not be a major determinant for the value of Cl calculated from Equation 2.17.
3. The rate of drug administration $[(S)(F)(Dose/\tau)]$ should be regular and consistent. This rule helps to ensure a reasonably smooth progression from C_1 to C_2 such that the value of C ave $[(C_1 + C_2)/2]$ is approximately equal to the true average drug concentration between C_1 and C_2.

The mass balance approach is a useful technique if the above conditions are met. It is relatively simple and allows for the calculation of clearance under non–steady-state conditions by a direct solution process. There are certain situations in which the above conditions are not met but the mass balance technique still works relatively well. For example, if the time interval between C_1 and C_2 is substantially greater than two half-lives but the value of C_2 is very close to C_1, then Equation 2.17 approximates Equation 1.15 because the average plasma concentration approximates the average steady-state value.

$$\frac{(S)(F)(Dose/\tau) - \dfrac{(C_2 - C_1)(V)}{t}}{C\ ave} = Cl$$

$$\frac{(S)(F)(Dose/\tau) - (\approx 0)}{C\ ave} = Cl$$

$$\frac{(S)(F)(Dose/\tau)}{C\ ave} = Cl$$

The mass balance approach is most commonly applicable for drugs that are given as a continuous IV infusion, as a sustained-release product, or at a dosing interval that is much less than the half-life.

As an example, let's look at a patient who has a phenobarbital level of 10 mg/L on day 1 and is given 100 mg daily for 10 days. At the end of day 10, the phenobarbital level is reported to be 18 mg/L. Given that the usual $t\frac{1}{2}$ of phenobarbital is approximately 4 or 5 days, it seems unlikely that the phenobarbital level of 18 mg/L represents steady state (i.e., less than three to five $t\frac{1}{2}$s on this regimen). One of several approaches could be taken to resolve this problem. One approach would be to write an equation that was the sum of the initial concentration decayed to the time of the second sample plus each of the 10 doses decayed individually to the time of the second sample. To solve the equation, values of S, F, and V would have to be assumed and then in an iterative fashion values of K would be substituted until the equation equaled the observed phenobarbital level of 18 mg/L.

$$C_{sum} = C(e^{-Kt}) + \left[\frac{(S)(F)(D_1)}{V}\left(e^{-Kt_1}\right)\right] + \left[\frac{(S)(F)(D_2)}{V}\left(e^{-Kt_2}\right)\right] + \cdots$$

The K value could then be used in combination with the assumed V in Equation 1.31 to calculate a clearance value.

$$Cl = (K)(V)$$

A second approach might be to again start with the initial concentration decayed to the time of the second sample and add to that concentration the contribution of a continuous infusion model that was accumulating toward steady state. The continuous infusion model could be used because the interval of 1 day between the phenobarbital doses is sufficiently short compared to the $t\frac{1}{2}$ so that the accumulation is a relatively smooth process (see Chapter 13 and Fig. 13.1).

$$C_1 = \left[C(e^{-Kt_1})\right] + \left[\frac{(S)(F)(Dose/\tau)}{Cl}(1 - e^{-Kt_1})\right]$$

In the above equation, Cl/V would be substituted for K or (K)(V) for Cl so there is only one unknown to be resolved in the equation.

Lastly, the mass balance approach could be used.

$$\frac{(S)(F)(Dose/\tau) - \dfrac{(C_2 - C_1)(V)}{t}}{C\ ave} = Cl$$

where t would be the 10-day interval between the initial phenobarbital level and the second level. This last approach using mass balance is a direct solution and does not require an iterative search. The solution for clearance should be reasonably good as long as the three rules previously mentioned are met. If there are concerns that the value of Cl is incorrect, this value of Cl could be used in one of the previous equations to see whether the more complex equation will predict the observed second phenobarbital concentration. A word of caution: If the clearance value predicts the phenobarbital concentration well (calculated value is close to the observed value), it does not necessarily mean the clearance is correct—only that regardless of which equation is used, you will calculate the same answer.

SINGLE-POINT DETERMINATION OF CLEARANCE

A drug concentration obtained approximately 1.44 half-lives after a single bolus dose is primarily a function of clearance and is also referred to as the mean residence time. This concept is represented in Figure 2.12. The ability to predict clearance using this

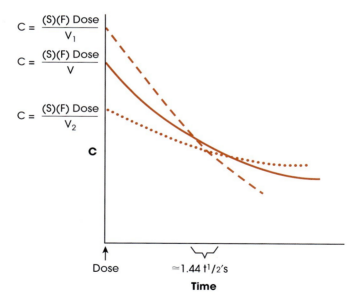

FIGURE 2.12   Single-point determination of clearance. The plasma concentrations following a single bolus dose when clearance is held constant and volume of distribution is altered tend to pivot around a single point that occurs at approximately 1.44 half-lives after the dose. When the volume of distribution is smaller (*dashed line* V_1), the concentrations before 1.44 half-life points are elevated, relative to the concentrations found in patients with larger volumes of distribution (*dotted line* V_2). The opposite is true after the 1.44 half-life point.

principle is based on a complex relationship between volume of distribution, clearance, and half-life. As can be seen from Equation 2.1 for C and Equation 1.30 for $t^{1/2}$:

$$C = \frac{(S)(F)(\text{Loading Dose})}{V} \qquad t\tfrac{1}{2} = \frac{(0.693)(V)}{Cl}$$

if clearance is held constant, and volume of distribution is decreased, the initial plasma levels will be higher and the elimination half-life will be decreased. However, if volume of distribution is increased, the initial plasma concentrations will be lower and the elimination half-life will be longer.

By examining Figure 2.12, it can be seen that over a range of volume of distribution values, there is a locus or point about which the decaying plasma concentration versus time curves appear to pivot. This pivot point is at 1.44 half-lives. For this reason, a single plasma concentration obtained at 1.44 half-lives following an initial bolus dose can be used to estimate a clearance.[6–8] This approach is essentially a rearrangement of Equation 1.28:

$$K = \frac{\ln\left(\dfrac{C_1}{C_2}\right)}{t}$$

where $(S)(F)(\text{Dose})/V$ is substituted for C_1, and C_2 the measured plasma concentration at time t after the loading dose.

$$K = \frac{\ln\left(\dfrac{(S)(F)(\text{Loading Dose})/V}{C_2}\right)}{t} \qquad \textbf{(Eq. 2.19)}$$

Equation 1.31 can then be used with the assumed value for V to calculate the patient's clearance.

$$Cl = (K)(V)$$

It is important to recognize that if the patient's clearance or volume of distribution values differ substantially from those assumed, a sampling time based on a literature-derived half-life may not represent 1.44 half-lives for the patient. In this instance, accurate patient-specific clearance would not be derived from this method outlined using Equations 2.19 and 1.31. For example, if a patient has a very low clearance and a longer-than-expected elimination half-life, plasma samples obtained at 1.44 times the drug's reported half-life will represent a sampling time that is sooner than 1.44 times the patient's actual half-life. Plasma samples obtained at this time are primarily a function of volume of distribution and would be influenced much less by clearance. Conversely, if the patient's clearance is much greater than the literature value, a sample obtained at 1.44 of the usual $t^{1/2}$ may represent several of the patient's true half-lives. Under these conditions, the observed plasma concentration is influenced to a large degree by both volume of distribution and clearance. As a result, the ability to extract (with any level of confidence) revised values for clearance or volume of distribution is extremely limited. As can be seen from the above discussion, the single-point determination of clearance only works when patient's t½ is approximately as predicted. When the patient is much different from predicted, clearance cannot be accurately determined from a single sample.

It is often difficult to accurately plan a sampling time that can be used for the single-point method. However, if sensitivity testing reveals that clearance is the primary determinant of a concentration obtained approximately 1.44 half-lives after a bolus dose, this concentration may be used to ascertain a patient-specific clearance.

BAYESIAN ANALYSIS

As previously discussed, the usual approach when using pharmacokinetics in the clinical setting is to solve our kinetic problem by using simple manipulations of an equation and then solving the equation by revising or changing one or sometimes two variables, usually volume of distribution and/or clearance. This technique works well if the clinician has a good understanding of pharmacokinetics and good clinical judgment. One of the potential dangers is that a clinical decision might be made using pharmacokinetic data that have a very low level of reliability. To help guard against this type of error, many pharmacokinetic computer programs use Bayesian analysis.

The mathematics in this approach is complicated and requires significant computational capacity. However, the concept is relatively simple. The basic approach used in this analysis technique is to adjust each element in the equation to the degree that it helps solve the equation and to the degree that it is likely that the initial estimates are wrong. Depending on the way the program is designed, everything from adherence to bioavailability, concentration measurement variability, and our usual parameters of clearance and volume of distribution can be considered in the revision process. There are three key issues with the Bayesian approach. One is that the average population value is a good and a reasonable estimate for the patient. Second is that the uncertainty or variability in the individual parameters is known. Third is that the pharmacokinetic model is appropriate.

As an example, we can consider Equation 2.2:

$$C_1 = \frac{(S)(F)(\text{Loading Dose})}{V}\left(e^{-Kt_1}\right)$$

If we take a situation in which we obtain two drug samples relatively soon after a loading dose of 100 mg is administered, both of the drug concentrations would have information about V but very little information about clearance. In this problem, we start by assuming that S and F are 1, V is 10 L, Cl is 1 L/hr, K = 0.1 hr^{-1} (t½ = 6.93 hours), and the two sampling times are at 0.5 and 1 hour after the dose.

$$C_1 = \frac{(S)(F)(\text{Loading Dose})}{V}\left(e^{-(K)(t_1)}\right)$$

$$= \frac{(1)(1)(100 \text{ mg})}{10\,\text{L}}\left(e^{-(0.1\,\text{hr}^{-1})(0.5\,\text{hr})}\right)$$

$$= 10 \text{ mg/L}\,(0.951)$$

$$= 9.51 \text{ mg/L}$$

And the second concentration would be:

$$= \frac{(1)(1)(100 \text{ mg})}{10 \text{ L}} (e^{-(0.1 \text{ hr}^{-1})(1 \text{ hr})})$$

$$= 10 \text{ mg/L} (0.905)$$

$$= 9.05 \text{ mg/L}$$

If the laboratory reported the drug concentration at 0.5 and 1 hour to be 9.8 and 8.7 mg/L, respectively, we would, from a clinical point of view, simply look at the expected values of 9.51 and 9.05 and consider the predictions to be excellent. We would assume that the less than 10% differences in the predicted and observed drug concentrations were owing to assay error. Knowing that the two drug levels were obtained very soon after the initial loading dose suggests that our volume of distribution is approximately correct. However, very little information about clearance is "contained" in the two drug samples. This would mean that our maintenance dosing regimen should be based on our original estimate of 1 L/hr for clearance. We would use the expected clearance value not because we know it is correct, but rather because we do not have any additional information that would suggest changing our original expectation.

There are computer programs (and clinicians with calculators) that would use what is commonly thought of as an "exact fit" method of analysis. This method tries to make everything fit the drug concentrations as closely as possible. In our example, S, F, t_1, and C_1 would be assumed to be exact values, and any differences between the observed values in C and the expected value are because of differences in our expected V and Cl. Following this line of reasoning, Equation 1.28 and the two drug concentrations can be used to calculate a new elimination rate constant of 0.238 hr^{-1}

$$K = \frac{\ln\left(\dfrac{C_1}{C_2}\right)}{t}$$

where C_1 is 9.8 mg/L, C_2 8.7 mg/L, and t the 0.5-hour time interval between the first and second sample. (Note that these two samples were obtained less than one t½ apart, indicating that the calculated K will be suspect.)

$$K = \frac{\ln\left(\dfrac{9.8 \text{ mg/L}}{8.7 \text{ mg/L}}\right)}{0.5 \text{ hr}}$$

$$= 0.238 \text{ hr}^{-1}$$

Now using Equation 1.26 and rearranging to solve for C_1, just after the bolus dose or 0.5 hour before the first sample, we calculate a drug level of 11.04 mg/L.

$$C_2 = C_1(e^{-(K)(t)})$$

$$9.8 \text{ mg/L} = C_1 (e^{-(0.238 \text{ hr}^{-1})(0.5 \text{ hr})})$$

$$9.8 \text{ mg/L} = C_1(0.888)$$

$$\frac{9.8 \text{ mg/L}}{(0.888)} = C_1$$

$$11.04 \text{ mg/L} = C_1$$

Now using this concentration of 11.04 mg/L that would correspond to the C in Equation 2.1, we can calculate a revised volume of distribution of 9.1 L.

$$C = \frac{(S)(F)(\text{Loading Dose})}{V}$$

$$11.04 \text{ mg/L} = \frac{(1)(1)(100 \text{ mg})}{V}$$

$$V = \frac{(1)(1)(100 \text{ mg})}{11.04 \text{ mg/L}}$$

$$V = 9.1 \text{ L}$$

Note that the revised V of 9.1 L is reasonably close to the initial estimate of 10 L. This is because we would expect considering that the timing of the samples is close to the loading dose.

However, if we use the revised K of 0.238 hr^{-1} and V of 9.1 L in Equation 1.31 to calculate a revised value for Cl, we would obtain 2.17 L/hr.

$$Cl = (K)(V)$$

$$Cl = (0.238 \text{ hr}^{-1})(9.1 \text{ L})$$

$$Cl = (2.17 \text{ L/hr})$$

This revised clearance is more than twice our initial estimate of 1 L/hr and would have a major impact on the maintenance regimen.

This revision is an example of making too much out of too little information. A Bayesian pharmacokinetics program would try to balance the change in the calculated drug concentrations as a result of a change in clearance, and attempt to come up with a reasonable estimate or compromise considering that there is an expected assay error as well as some error in V and Cl. The end result would probably be a slightly higher clearance, a slightly smaller volume of distribution, and some slight differences in the observed and predicted drug concentrations. This approach would help to avoid the huge change in clearance that occurred using the "exact fit" type of analysis. The Bayesian analysis would be similar to our initial conclusion that the observed and predicted drug concentrations are a close fit and confirm V but do not contain much information on Cl.

When drug levels are obtained at an "optimal" time, and the appropriate pharmacokinetic parameter is being analyzed, both the "exact fit" and Bayesian approaches usually give essentially the same answer. It should also be pointed out that although the Bayesian approach will help prevent the error of making too much of too little, it cannot correct or account for large real errors. Bayesian computer programs cannot adjust for gross errors. For example, errors in dose (200 mg administered vs. 100 mg recorded as given), sample labeling (sample labeled with incorrect patient name or peak labeled as a trough), model (linear vs. nonlinear elimination), and so on cannot be successfully corrected by Bayesian or any other type of computer program. Another potential problem with Bayesian programs occurs when the patient is truly different from the expected patient population. In this situation, the computer will tend to place less emphasis on the drug concentrations from the patient and try to revise toward parameters that are more like the average patient. This problem should be taken in the context that in most clinical situations, data that are very unusual are often the result of an error. Regardless of what type of approach is taken, it is important for the clinician to evaluate the drug concentration in the context of the patient and use rational judgment as to how pharmacokinetics is used in designing drug regimens.

ASSAY SPECIFICITY

The accuracy and specificity of assays used by the clinical laboratory to measure serum drug concentrations is critical. Historically, laboratories developed their assay procedures using a variety of analytical methods ranging from radioimmunoassays to high-performance liquid chromatography assay procedures. Currently, however, the vast majority of drug assays performed in the clinical setting are some variant of commercially available immunobinding assay procedures. The most commonly used procedures are variants of the fluorescence polarization immunoassay and enzyme immunoassay (enzyme-multiplied immunoassay technique and enzyme-linked immunosorbent assay).[9,10]

These assays are generally specific; however, in isolated instances, metabolites or other drug-like substances are also recognized by the antibody.[11–15] Most assay interferences are the result of cross-reactivity with the drug's metabolites, but, in some cases, endogenous compounds or drugs with similar structures can cross-react, resulting in either a falsely elevated or a decreased assayed drug concentration.[14–19]

Pharmacokinetic parameters derived from nonspecific assays or plasma concentrations that are in error may influence clinicians to make decisions that are not optimal for patient care.[16–19] Whereas the current literature is usually associated with relatively specific drug assays, caution should always be exercised when using serum drug concentrations as part of the clinical decision-making process.[20,21] This is especially true when the older literature is used because pharmacokinetic parameters that have been derived from assays with differing specificities are not interchangeable. The usual therapeutic range will also be altered when more specific assays are used.

For assays that measure the parent compound only, it is important to determine the pharmacologic activity and pharmacokinetic behavior of the metabolites. Many drugs have active metabolites that may affect a patient's pharmacologic response (Table 2.1); the pharmacokinetic behavior of these metabolites cannot be predicted by assaying only the parent compound.[22]

Whenever possible, one should evaluate the patient's clinical response directly. If drug levels and clinical response do not correlate as predicted, it may be owing to a laboratory error. Similarly, factors unique to the patient, such as concurrent disease states or antagonist drug therapy, may alter one's interpretation of the plasma drug concentration. For example, it is a common clinical observation that higher-than-usual plasma concentrations of digoxin are required to achieve a clinical response in patients with atrial fibrillation. Furthermore, for drugs that have high plasma protein binding, the same therapeutic effect will be achieved with a lower plasma concentration when plasma protein binding is decreased. This is because, for most clinical assays, the total plasma concentration (bound + free) is reported. As discussed earlier, decreased binding

TABLE 2.1   Examples of Drugs with Active Metabolites[2,22]

Amitriptyline
Carbamazepine
Chlordiazepoxide
Chlorpromazine
Chlorpropamide
Diazepam
Lidocaine
Meperidine
Metronidazole
Primidone
Propranolol
Warfarin

lowers the bound concentration but not the free, pharmacologically active concentration (see Desired Plasma Concentration [C]). The formation of aberrant metabolites and tachyphylaxis are other reasons why plasma drug concentrations fail to correlate with an expected therapeutic response.

REFERENCES

1. Zeisler JA, Skovseth JR, Anderson JR. Lidocaine therapy: time for re-evaluation. *Clin Pharm*. 1993;12: 527–528.
2. Thummel KE, Shen DD. Appendix II: design and optimization of dosage regimens: pharmacokinetic data. In: Hardman JG, ed. *Goodman and Gilman's The Pharmacologic Basis of Therapeutics*. 10th ed. New York, NY: McGraw-Hill; 2001:1917–2023.
3. Wilensky AJ, Friel PN, Levy RH, et al. Kinetics of phenobarbital in normal subjects and epileptic patients. *Eur J Clin Pharmacol*. 1982;23:87–92.
4. Chiou WL, Gadalla MA, Peng GW. Method for rapid estimation of the total body drug clearance and adjustment of dosing regimen in patients during a constant-rate intravenous infusion. *J Pharmacokinet Biopharm*. 1978;6:135–151.
5. Vozeh S, Kewitz G, Wenk M, et al. Rapid prediction of steady-state serum theophylline concentration in patients treated with intravenous aminophylline. *Eur J Clin Pharmacol*. 1980;18:473–477.
6. Slattery JT, Gibaldi M, Koup JR. Prediction of maintenance dose required to attain a desired drug concentration at steady state from a single determination of concentration after an initial dose. *Clin Pharmacokinet*. 1980;5:377.
7. Koup JR. Single-point prediction methods: a critical review. *Drug Intell Clin Pharm*. 1982;16:855.
8. Unadkat JD, Rowland M. Further considerations of the "single-point, single-dose" method to estimate individual maintenance dosage requirements. *Ther Drug Monit*. 1982;4:201.
9. Glazko AJ. Phenytoin: chemistry and methods of determination. In: Levy RH, Mattson RH, Meldrum BS, et al, eds. *Antiepileptic Drugs*. 3rd ed. New York, NY: Raven Press; 1989:159–176.
10. Steijns LS, Bouw J, van der Weide J. Evaluation of fluorescence polarization assays for measuring valproic acid, phenytoin, carbamazepine and phenobarbital in serum. *Ther Drug Monit*. 2002;24:432–435.
11. Patel JA, Clayton LT, LeBel CP, et al. Abnormal theophylline levels in plasma by fluorescence polarization immunoassay in patients with renal disease. *Ther Drug Monit*. 1984;6:458–460.

12. Hicks JM, Brett EM. Falsely increased digoxin concentrations in samples from neonates and infants. *Ther Drug Monit*. 1984;6:461–464.

13. Flachs H, Rasmussen JM. Renal disease may increase apparent phenytoin in serum as measured by enzyme-multiplied immunoassay [letter]. *Clin Chem*. 1980;26:361.

14. Frank EL, Schwarz EL, Juenke J, et al. Performance characteristics of four immunoassays for antiepileptic drugs on the IMMULITE 2000 automated analyzer. *Am J Clin Pathol*. 2002;1:124–131.

15. Dasgupta A. Digoxin-like immunoreactive substances in elderly people. Impact on therapeutic drug monitoring of digoxin and digitoxin concentrations. *Am J Clin Pathol*. 2002;118;4:600–604.

16. Steimer W, Muller C, Eber B. Digoxin assays: frequent, substantial and potentially dangerous interference by spironolactone, canrenone, and other steroids. *Clin Chem*. 2002;48:507–516.

17. Somerville AL, Wright DH, Rotschafer JC. Implications of vancomycin degradation products on therapeutic drug monitoring in patients with end-stage renal disease. *Pharmacotherapy*. 1999;19:702–707.

18. Sym D, Smith C, Meenan G, et al. Fluorescence polarization immunoassay: can it result in an overestimation of vancomycin in patients not suffering from renal failure? *Ther Drug Monit*. 2001;23:441–444.

19. Kingery JR, Sowinski KM, Kraus MA, et al. Vancomycin assay performance in patients with end-stage renal disease receiving hemodialysis. *Pharmacotherapy*. 2000;20:653–656.

20. Rainey PM, Rogers KE, Roberts WL. Metabolite and matrix interference in phenytoin immunoassays. *Clin Chem*. 1996;42:1645–1653.

21. Roberts WL, Annesley TM, De BK, et al. Performance characteristics of four free phenytoin Immunoassays. *Ther Drug Monit*. 2001;23:148–154.

22. Drayer E. Pharmacologically active metabolites, therapeutic and toxic activities, plasma and urine data in man, accumulation in renal failure. *Clin Pharmacokinet*. 1976;1:426.

3

DRUG DOSING IN KIDNEY DISEASE AND DIALYSIS

Thomas C. Dowling

Learning Objectives

By the end of the drug dosing in kidney disease and dialysis chapter, the learner shall be able to:

Renal Drug Clearance and Creatinine Clearance (Cl$_{Cr}$)

1. Describe the key drug clearance mechanisms in the kidney, and estimate creatinine clearance in various patient populations including CKD, acute kidney disease, pediatrics, obesity and elderly.
2. Describe the key drug clearance mechanisms in the kidney, with respect to passive and active drug transport and renal drug–drug interactions.
3. Describe the production of creatinine, and the inverse relationship between serum creatinine and creatinine clearance.
4. Know the usual creatinine clearance for a young adult with normal renal function.
5. Calculate, using Cockcroft and Gault equation, a patient's estimated creatinine clearance.
6. Estimate lean body weight and recognize/identify when a patient is considered "obese," using BMI as an indicator.
7. Estimate creatinine clearance for children in mL/min/1.73 m^2.
8. Convert creatinine clearance in mL/min/1.73 m^2 to creatinine clearance in mL/min for a child using either body surface area or weight per 70 kg raised to the power 0.7.
9. Estimate creatinine clearance from two non–steady-state serum creatinine values.
10. Identify at least one reason why a rising serum creatinine makes estimates of renal function difficult.
11. Calculate a patient's creatinine clearance, given a 24-hour urine collection.

12. Compare the creatinine production (mg/kg/day) with the expected production of creatinine for the patient; and if the two values differ significantly, list the possible reasons.
13. Compare the estimated creatinine clearance as calculated by the Cockcroft and Gault equation with the value calculated from a 24-hour collection and if the two values differ significantly, list the possible reasons.
14. Compare and contrast the MDRD, CKD-EPI, and Cockcroft and Gault equations with regard to appropriate use, units of measure, and patient size.
15. Explain why, unless specific information is available, eGFR equations should NOT be used to estimate kidney function for the purpose of adjusting doses of drugs that are cleared by kidney mechanisms.

Dialysis of Drugs

1. Obtain an appreciation for the types of dialysis (intermittent, continuous, and peritoneal) and to know how each is likely to affect drug elimination and dosing strategies.
2. Choose the appropriate model for postdialysis replacement dosing, given the patient's residual drug clearance and the estimated dialysis clearance.
3. Calculate the expected pre- and postdialysis drug concentrations, given a patient's steady-state peak drug concentration.
4. Explain why in most cases immediate postdialysis sampling of drugs is not recommended.
5. Explain why it is the unbound volume of distribution that determines whether or not a drug will be significantly removed by hemodialysis.
6. Know the unbound volume of distribution above which it is unlikely that a drug will be significantly removed by hemodialysis.
7. Know the usual limit for drug clearance by hemodialysis and the usual residual patient clearance above which it is unlikely that hemodialysis will remove significant additional drug.
8. Know the molecular weight (molecular mass) cutoff for low- and high-flux hemodialysis, above which it is unlikely that dialysis will be able to remove a significant amount of drug.
9. Describe the difference in molecular weight cutoff between low- and high-flux hemodialysis.
10. List at least one drug that is significantly removed by high- but not low-flux hemodialysis.
11. Describe the usual total CRRT flow rate (ultrafiltration and dialysis) and the relationship of the flow to the fraction unbound (fu) and CRRT clearance.
12. Given a target drug concentration and the CRRT flow rate, given a patient's residual drug clearance, volume of distribution, and fu:
    a. Determine whether a continuous input and Css ave model or an intermittent bolus model can be used to calculate a dosing regimen.
    b. Calculate a maintenance dose, using the appropriate model.
13. Describe the typical peritoneal volume exchange and duration or dwell time.
14. Calculate the expected Cl_{CAPD}, given a drug's fu and the peritoneal dialysate exchange rate.

TABLE 3.1 Factors Affecting Renal Drug Elimination

Glomerular filtration
  Molecular weight
  Plasma Protein binding
  Glomerular capillary pressure

Tubular secretion
  Membrane transporters (organic anion transporter [OAT], P-glycoprotein [PgP], multidrug resistant protein [MRP])
  Drug-transporter interactions
  Renal blood flow

Tubular reabsorption
  Drug pKa
  Urine pH
  Urine flow rate
  Drug transporters (PEPT2, OATP1A2)

Because many drugs are partially or totally eliminated by the kidney, it is important to understand the impact of changing kidney function on drug pharmacokinetics. Drugs can be eliminated or cleared as unchanged drug through the kidney (renal clearance) and liver (including biliary secretion and metabolic biotransformation). These two routes of clearance are assumed to be independent of one another and additive.[1,2]

$$Cl_t = Cl_m + Cl_r$$

where Cl_t is total clearance, Cl_m the metabolic clearance or the fraction cleared by metabolism, and Cl_r the renal clearance or the fraction cleared by the renal route.

The primary mechanisms within the kidney that contribute to drug clearance are glomerular filtration, tubular secretion and tubular reabsorption (Table 3.1). In patients with chronic kidney disease (CKD), the capacity of these renal mechanisms to eliminate drugs is reduced, leading to an overall reduction in total drug clearance. Because the volume of distribution for most drugs remains largely unchanged until severe renal impairment (CKD Stage 5), the reduced elimination rate constant leads to a proportional increase in t½. If dose adjustments are not made, then excessive accumulation may occur leading to toxicity and unwanted pharmacologic side effects.

Creatinine clearance is the primary clinical biomarker of glomerular filtration rate (GFR) and overall kidney function. Estimating creatinine clearance is typically the first step in designing a drug dosage regimen that is appropriate, given a patient's kidney function.

Creatinine Clearance (Cl$_{Cr}$)

Estimating kidney function is an important component in the application of pharmacokinetics to designing drug therapy regimens. Creatinine clearance as determined by a urine collection and corresponding plasma sample is considered by many clinicians to be the most accurate test of renal function. In the clinical setting, the time delay and the difficulty in obtaining the 24-hour creatinine collection limit the utility of the 24-hour urine collection. In addition, all too often, the urine collection is inaccurate because a portion is accidentally discarded or the time of collection is shorter or longer than requested.[3,4] Perhaps, the most common error is an incomplete collection, which will result in an underestimation of renal function. Because decisions with regard to drug dosing must often be made quickly, several authors have suggested a variety of methods by which Cl_{Cr} can be estimated using a serum creatinine value. The most accurate of these equations include serum creatinine, body weight or size, age, and gender.[4,5]

CREATININE PHARMACOKINETICS

The pharmacokinetics of creatinine is presented in far more detail elsewhere,[3,6–9] but a brief overview is necessary. Creatinine is a metabolic by-product of muscle, and its rate of formation (R_A) is primarily determined by an individual's muscle mass or lean body weight (LBW). It varies, therefore, with age (lower in the elderly) and gender (lower in females).[10–12] For any given individual, the rate of creatinine production is assumed to be constant. Once creatinine is released from muscle into plasma, it is eliminated largely by glomerular filtration. A smaller component is eliminated by tubular secretion via drug transporters such as the organic cationic transporter-2 (OCT2) and the multi drug and toxin extrusion protein (MATE1). Thus, observed elevations in serum creatinine because of drug-creatinine interactions must be evaluated in a given patient. For example, elevated serum creatinine values have been observed during administration of cobicistat, a CYP3A-inhibitor used as a booster with HIV integrase inhibitors, without a reduction in measured GFR. The mechanism has been identified as inhibition of OCT2 and MATE1-mediated tubular secretion of creatinine.[13] Any decrease in the GFR ultimately results in a rise in the serum creatinine level until a new steady state is reached and the amount of creatinine cleared per day equals the rate of production. In other words, at steady state, the rate in must equal the rate out. Because the rate of creatinine production remains constant even when renal clearance diminishes, the serum creatinine must rise until the product of the clearance and the serum creatinine again equals the rate of production. This concept is represented by Equation 3.1 and has been discussed earlier in "Creatine Clearance" section.

$$\leftrightarrow R_A = \left(\downarrow Cl\right)\left(\uparrow Css\ ave\right) \tag{Eq 3.1}$$

where $\leftrightarrow R_A$ is a constant rate of creatinine production, $\downarrow Cl$ the decreased creatinine clearance, and $\uparrow$ Css ave the increased steady-state serum creatinine level or SCr_{ss}, such that when steady state is achieved the product of ($\downarrow Cl$)($\uparrow$ Css ave) will be equal to the R_A or production rate of creatinine.

ESTIMATING CREATININE CLEARANCE FROM STEADY-STATE SERUM CREATININE CONCENTRATIONS (STABLE KIDNEY FUNCTION)

The degree to which a steady-state serum creatinine rises is inversely proportional to the decrease in creatinine clearance. Therefore, the new creatinine clearance can be estimated by multiplying a normal Cl_{Cr} value by the fractional change in the serum creatinine: normal SCr/patient's SCr_{ss}. For a man weighing 70 kg, it can be assumed that the normal SCr is 1.0 mg/dL and that the corresponding Cl_{Cr} is 120 mL/min.

$$\text{New } Cl_{Cr} = (120 \text{ mL/min}) \left[\frac{1 \text{ mg/dL}}{SCr_{ss}} \right] \qquad \textbf{(Eq 3.2)}$$

Based on this concept, one can see that each time the serum creatinine doubles, the creatinine clearance falls by half and that small changes in the serum creatinine at low concentrations are of much greater consequence than equal changes in the serum creatinine at high concentrations. To illustrate, if a patient with a normal serum creatinine of 1.0 mg/dL is reported to have a new steady-state serum creatinine of 2.0 mg/dL, the estimated creatinine clearance has decreased from 120 to 60 mL/min. However, if a patient with CKD has a baseline serum creatinine of 4.0 mg/dL ($Cl_{Cr} = 30$ mL/min), a similar 1.0 mg/dL increase in the serum creatinine to 5.0 mg/dL would result in a small drop in the Cl_{Cr} (6 mL/min) and a new clearance value of 24 mL/min. However, at some point even small changes in Cl_{Cr} can be physiologically significant to the patient. As an example, for a patient with a creatinine clearance of 100 mL/min, a 10 mL/min (or 10%) reduction in kidney function is of very little clinical consequence. However, for a patient with a creatinine clearance of 20 mL/min, a 10 mL/min decrease (or 67%) would likely change their clinical status from CKD Stage 4 to CKD Stage 5 requiring dialysis.

The estimation of Cl_{Cr} from SCr_{ss} alone is reasonably satisfactory as long as the patient's daily creatinine production is average (i.e., 20 mg/kg/day); the patient weighs approximately 70 kg and the serum creatinine is at steady state (i.e., either rising or falling). These conditions are usually present in the young healthy adult, but young healthy adults are not the typical patients for whom pharmacokinetic manipulations are most useful.

Adjusting to body size: weight or body surface area

To account for any changes in creatinine production and clearance that may result from a difference in body size, Equation 3.2 can be modified to compensate for any deviation in body surface area (BSA) from the typical 70-kg patient (1.73 m^2):

The patient's BSA can be obtained from a nomogram (see Appendix II), estimated from Equation 1.17:

$$\text{BSA in m}^2 = \left(\frac{\text{Patient's Weight in kg}}{70 \text{ kg}} \right)^{0.7} (1.73 \text{ m}^2)$$

or calculated from the following equation[14]:

$$BSA \text{ in } m^2 = (W^{0.425})(H^{0.725})0.007184 \qquad \textbf{(Eq. 3.3)}$$

where the BSA is in meters squared (m^2), W is weight in kilograms, and H is the patient's height in centimeters.

A disadvantage of using only weight or BSA is that the elderly or emaciated patients who have a reduced muscle mass may not have a typical steady-state serum creatinine value of 1.0 mg/dL. For this reason, it may be erroneous to assume that an SCr of 1.0 mg/dL is "normal" and indicative of a creatinine clearance of 120 mL/min in these individuals.

On average, as patients age, their muscle mass represents a smaller proportion of their total weight and creatinine production is decreased (Table 3.2). There are a number of equations that consider age, gender, body size, and serum creatinine when calculating or estimating creatinine clearance for adults.[11,15,16] Although all these methods are similar and equivalent in clinical practice, the most common method used by clinicians is probably the one proposed by Cockcroft and Gault.[15]

$$Cl_{Cr} \text{ for Males } (mL/min) = \frac{(140 - Age)(Weight)}{(72)(SCr_{ss})} \qquad \textbf{(Eq. 3.4)}$$

$$Cl_{Cr} \text{ for Females } (mL/min) = (0.85)\frac{(140 - Age)(Weight)}{(72)(SCr_{ss})} \qquad \textbf{(Eq. 3.5)}$$

TABLE 3.2   Expected Daily Creatinine Production for Males[12]

AGE (yr)	DAILY CREATININE PRODUCTION (mg/kg/day)
20–29	24[a]
30–39	22
40–49	20
50–59	19
60–69	17
70–79	14
80–89	12
90–99	9

[a]Daily creatinine production for females would be expected to be 85% of the above values.

where age is in years, weight is in kg, and serum creatinine is in mg/dL. Equations 3.4 and 3.5 calculate creatinine clearance as mL/min for the patient's characteristics entered into the equation.

The two most critical factors to consider when using the above equations are the assumptions that the serum creatinine is at steady state and the weight, age, and gender of the individual reflect normal muscle mass. In patients with obesity, most commonly defined by the World Health Organization as having a body mass index (BMI) of $\geq 30\ kg/m^2$ (obese) and BMI $\geq 40\ kg/m^2$ (morbidly obese), weight adjustments for estimating creatinine clearance are recommended. Here, BMI is calculated using Equation 3.6 as:

$$BMI = \frac{Weight\ (kg)}{Height^2\ (m)} \qquad \text{(Eq. 3.6)}$$

It is well-known that use of total body weight (TBW) can lead to significant over-estimation of creatinine clearance in obesity. To adjust for this extra non-LBW when estimating creatinine clearance in obesity, alternative measures of weight such as ideal body weight (IBW), adjusted body weight (AdjBW) and LBW have been proposed. Here, IBW is calculated as:

$$\begin{array}{l}\text{Ideal Body Weight}\\ \text{for Males in kg}\end{array} = 50 + (2.3)(Height\ in\ inches > 60) \qquad \text{(Eq. 3.7)}$$

$$\begin{array}{l}\text{Ideal Body Weight}\\ \text{for Females in kg}\end{array} = 45 + (2.3)(Height\ in\ inches > 60) \qquad \text{(Eq. 3.8)}$$

AdjBW is calculated as:

$$\text{Adjusted Body Weight} = IBW + 0.4(TBW - IBW) \qquad \text{(Eq. 3.9)}$$

LBW[17] is calculated as

$$LBW_{Male}: (9{,}270 \times TBW)/(6{,}680 + 216 \times BMI) \qquad \text{(Eq. 3.10)}$$

$$LBW_{Female}: (9{,}270 \times TBW)/(8{,}780 + 244 \times BMI) \qquad \text{(Eq. 3.11)}$$

To address the question "what weight do I use when estimating creatinine clearance in obesity"?, one study was conducted by the *Food and Drug Administration* based on a review of new drug applications that included renal pharmacokinetic studies. The results showed that for patients with BMI > 30 (obese), it is generally acceptable to use either TBW or AdjBW in the Cockcroft and Gault equation to estimate creatinine clearance. In patients with BMI ≥ 40 (morbidly obese), it is recommended that the LBW equation be used.[18]

There are other factors not considered in these equations that could account for additional weight in patients with BMI > 30. Here, the best approach will be to use clinical judgment and to recognize the limitation of creatinine-based equations to estimate kidney function. As an example, in patients with extensive third spacing of fluid (i.e., edema or ascites), the liters (kilograms) of excess third-space fluid should probably not be included in the patient's estimate of TBW. As an example, consider a 5-foot 4-inch male patient weighing 75 kg and having an estimated 15 kg of edema and ascitic fluid. To avoid assumptions associated with using weight-based indices such as IBW or LBW in this patient, it is recommended to conduct an accurately timed and measured 24-hour creatinine clearance for the purpose of renal drug dose adjustment.

In terms of drug dose individualization in this population, it is known that significant third-space fluid does contribute to the apparent volume of distribution for some drugs (see Chapter 6), but is unlikely to be an important contributor to volume of distribution if the apparent volume of distribution is large (e.g., digoxin) or if there is significant plasma protein binding (e.g., phenytoin, cyclosporine, lidocaine).

Third-space fluid weight is unlikely to contribute to and should not be used when initial estimates of clearance are made. However, although not directly influencing clearance, it is possible that the presence of ascites or edema may indicate the presence of a hepatobiliary disease process that is known to alter drug clearance.

Patients with very low BMI who are emaciated also require special consideration when estimating kidney function. While it may seem counterintuitive, a creatinine clearance calculated for an emaciated subject using the patient's weight tends to overpredict the patient's creatinine clearance. This is because patients who are emaciated tend to have a disproportionally greater loss in muscle mass than TBW, often accompanied by low values of serum creatinine. Consequently, serum creatinine in the denominator of Equations 3.4 and 3.5 may decrease more than the weight in the numerator, resulting in an overestimate of creatinine clearance. In such cases, it has been suggested that when serum creatinine values are very low (<1.0 mg/dL), an upward adjustment of creatinine to an arbitrary value may help to downwardly "correct" the creatinine clearance. This suggestion is based on the assumption that low serum creatinine values are related to small muscle mass and a decreased creatinine production rather than to an unusually large creatinine clearance. However, the practice of using "corrected" or arbitrary values for serum creatinine is not supported by scientific literature, and in fact there is data indicating that correction of low serum creatinine values up to 1.0 mg/dL falsely lowers creatinine clearance in elderly[19]. Because of the inherent difficulty in estimating creatinine clearance accurately in some populations, it is important to use clinical judgment in evaluating the risk versus the benefit of drug therapy. Here, the most reliable approach, that is least susceptible to assumptions related to body weight and serum creatinine, would be to conduct an accurately timed 24-hour measured creatinine clearance.

Pediatric patients

Estimation of kidney function in children is inherently difficult. There are several approaches,[20–22] and the fact that muscle mass and kidney function continue to mature for the first year of life makes the infant especially challenging. One of the more commonly used equations to estimate GFR for children from 1 to 18 years of ages is as follows:[20,23]

$$GFR \text{ (mL/min/1.73 m}^2) = \frac{(K)(Height \text{ in cm})}{SCr_{ss}} \qquad \text{(Eq. 3.12)}$$

where the K value is based on the infant's/child's age.

AGE	K
Preterm infants up to 1 yr	0.33
Full-term infants up to 1 yr	0.45
1–12 yr	0.55
13–21 yr female	0.55
13–21 yr male	0.70

A newer version of this equation was developed from a population of children with mild-to-moderate CKD enrolled in the Chronic Kidney Disease in Children study.[24] This simplified equation is commonly referred to as the Schwartz "Bedside" equation:

$$GFR \text{ (mL/min/1.73 m}^2) = \frac{(0.41)(Height \text{ in cm})}{SCr_{ss}} \qquad \text{(Eq. 3.13)}$$

It has been reported that this equation performs better than the original Schwartz equation for patients with mild-to-moderate CKD, although the accuracy in subpopulations is yet to be fully determined.

The above equations estimate GFR, not creatinine clearance, in children based on standardization to 1.73 m². Although these equations do not calculate the creatinine clearance for the child, it is useful as a guide to the child's relative renal function; values near 100 mL/min/1.73 m² would be considered relatively normal, and many dosing guides express creatinine clearance in this way.

The principles and cautions to be exercised when estimating GFR and creatinine clearance in children are the same as in adults. The serum creatinine should be at steady state, and the muscle mass should be reasonably close to average for the child's age and size. In cases where extremes in body weight are expected, a measured 24-hour creatinine clearance should be employed.

ESTIMATING TIME TO REACH STEADY-STATE SERUM CREATININE

All the above methods for estimating Cl_{Cr} require a steady-state serum creatinine concentration. When a patient's renal function suddenly changes, some period of time will be required to achieve a new steady-state serum creatinine concentration. In this situation, it is important to be able to estimate how long it will take for the SCr to reach steady state. If a rising serum creatinine is used in any of the previous equations, the patient's creatinine clearance will be overestimated.

As presented earlier, half-life is a function of both the volume of distribution and the clearance. If the volume of distribution of creatinine (0.5 to 0.7 L/kg)[25,26] is assumed to remain constant, the time required to reach 90% of steady state in patients with normal renal function is less than 1 day.[25,27] As an example, the average 70-kg patient with a creatinine clearance of 120 mL/min (7.2 L/hr) with a volume of distribution for creatinine of 45.5 L (0.65 L/kg) would be expected to have a creatinine t½ of 4.4 hours as calculated by Equation 3.14:

$$t\,{\textstyle\frac{1}{2}} = \frac{0.693\,(V)}{Cl}$$

$$= \frac{0.693\,(45.5\,\text{L})}{7.2\,\text{L/hr}} \qquad \textbf{(Eq. 3.14)}$$

$$= 4.4\,\text{hr}$$

Under these conditions, 90% of steady state should be achieved in approximately 15 hours (3.3 t½s). However, if the same patient had a creatinine clearance of 10 mL/min (0.6 L/hr), the creatinine t½ would be 52.5 hours and more than a week would be required to ensure that steady state had been achieved. One useful approach, that helps clinicians to make relatively rapid assessments of SCr, is to remember that because a drug (in this case creatinine) concentration is accumulating toward steady state, half of the total change will occur in the first half-life. Therefore, two serum creatinine concentrations obtained several hours apart (8 to 12 hours) that appear to be similar (i.e., not increasing or declining significantly) and that represent reasonably normal renal function probably represent steady-state conditions. As renal function declines, proportionately longer intervals between creatinine measurements are required to assure that steady-state conditions exist.

In clinical practice, patients occasionally have a slowly increasing serum creatinine. As an example, a patient might have the following serum creatinine concentrations on 4 consecutive days: 1, 1.2, 1.6, and 1.8 mg/dL. First, it should be recognized that the increase in serum creatinine from day 1 to day 2 could be caused by assay error alone because the absolute error for most creatinine assays is ±0.1 to 0.2 mg/dL. In addition, given that the t½ of creatinine at concentrations in the range of 1 to 2 mg/dL is approximately 4 to 8 hours, steady state should have been achieved on the first day. Therefore, the continued increase in serum creatinine probably reflects ongoing changes in creatinine clearance over the 4 days. The difficult clinical issue is not what the creatinine clearance is on each of the 4 days, but rather what it will be tomorrow, what is the cause, and how to prevent or minimize the ongoing renal damage.

ESTIMATING CREAINING CLEARANCE FROM NON-STEADY-STATE SERUM CREATININE

Using non–steady-state serum creatinine values to estimate creatinine clearance is difficult, and a number of approaches have been proposed.[6,7] The author uses

Equation 3.15 to estimate creatinine clearance when steady-state conditions have not been achieved.

$$\text{Cl}_{\text{Cr}} \text{ mL/min} = \frac{\left(\dfrac{\text{Production of Creatinine}}{\text{in mg/day}}\right) - \left[\left(\dfrac{(\text{SCr}_2 - \text{SCr}_1)(\text{V}_{\text{Cr}})}{t}\right)(10 \text{ dL/L})\right]}{(\text{SCr}_2)(10 \text{ dL/L})}$$

$$\times \left(\frac{1{,}000 \text{ mL/L}}{1{,}440 \text{ min/day}}\right)$$

(Eq. 3.15)

The daily production of creatinine in milligram is calculated by multiplying the daily production value in mg/kg/day from Table 3.2 by the patient's weight in kilogram. The serum creatinine values in Equation 3.15 are expressed in units of mg/dL; t is the number (or fraction) of days between the first serum creatinine measurement (SCr_1) and the second serum creatine measurement (SCr_2). The volume of distribution for creatinine (V_{Cr}) is calculated by multiplying the patient's weight in kilogram times 0.65 L/kg. Equation 3.15 is essentially a modification of the mass balance Equation 3.16.

$$\text{Cl} = \frac{(\text{S})(\text{F})(\text{Dose}/\tau) - \dfrac{(C_2 - C_1)(V)}{t}}{\text{Css ave}}$$

(Eq. 3.16)

where the daily production of creatinine in milligram has replaced the infusion rate of the drug and the second serum creatinine value replaced Css ave. The second serum creatinine is used primarily because Equation 3.15 is most commonly applied when creatinine clearance is decreasing (serum creatinine rising), and using the higher of the two serum creatinine values results in a lower, more conservative estimate of renal function. Some have suggested that the iterative search process, as represented by the Equation 3.17, be used:

$$C_2 = (C)\left(e^{-\text{Kt}}\right) + \frac{(\text{S})(\text{F})(\text{Dose}/\tau)}{\text{Cl}}\left(1 - e^{-\text{Kt}_1}\right)$$

(Eq. 3.17)

where C_2 represents SCr_2, and C represents SCr_1. (S)(F)(Dose/τ) represents the daily production of creatinine, and t represents the time interval between the first and second serum creatinine concentrations. Cl represents the creatinine clearance with the corresponding elimination rate constant K being Cl/V or the creatinine clearance divided by the creatinine volume of distribution. As discussed previously (see Interpretation of Plasma Drug Concentrations: Non–Steady-State Revision of Clearance [Iterative Search] in Chapter 2), the solution would require an iterative search, and the inherent errors in the calculation process probably do not warrant this type of calculation.

The use of Equation 3.15 can be illustrated by considering a 45-year-old, 70-kg man who has a serum creatinine concentration of 1.0 mg/dL on day 1 and a concentration of 2.0 mg/dL 24 hours later on day 2. Using Table 3.2, the expected daily production of creatinine for this patient would be 1,400 mg/day (20 mg/kg/day $\times$ 70 kg). The volume of distribution for creatinine is 45.5 L (0.65 L/kg $\times$ 70 kg), and the time between samples (t) is 1 day. Using these values, Equation 3.15 estimates a creatinine clearance of 32.8 mL/min.

$$Cl_{Cr} \text{ mL/min} = \frac{\left(\begin{array}{c} \text{Production of} \\ \text{Creatinine in mg/day} \end{array}\right) - \left[\left(\dfrac{(SCr_2 - SCr_1)(V_{Cr})}{t}\right)(10\,\text{dL/L})\right]}{(SCr_2)(10\,\text{dL/L})} \left(\dfrac{1,000\,\text{mL/L}}{1,440\,\text{min/day}}\right)$$

$$= \frac{(1,400\,\text{mg/day}) - \left[\left(\dfrac{(2\,\text{mg/dL} - 1\,\text{mg/dL})(45.5\,\text{L})}{1\,\text{day}}\right)(10\,\text{dL/L})\right]}{(2\,\text{mg/dL})(10\,\text{dL/L})} \left(\dfrac{1,000\,\text{mL/L}}{1,440\,\text{min/day}}\right)$$

$$= \frac{(1,400\,\text{mg/day}) - (455\,\text{mg/day})}{(2\,\text{mg/L})(10)} \left(0.694\,\dfrac{\text{mL/L}}{\text{min/day}}\right)$$

$$= 47.25\,\text{L/day}\left(0.694\,\dfrac{\text{mL/L}}{\text{min/day}}\right)$$

$$= 32.8\,\text{mL/min}$$

Although Equation 3.15 can be used to estimate a patient's creatinine clearance when a patient's serum creatinine is rising or falling, there are potential problems associated with this and all other approaches using non–steady-state serum creatinine values. First, a rising serum creatinine concentration may represent a continually declining renal function. To help compensate for the latter possibility, the second creatinine (SCr$_2$) rather than the average is used in the denominator of Equation 3.15. Furthermore, there are nonrenal routes of creatinine elimination that become significant in patients with significantly diminished renal function.[25] Because as much as 30% of a patient's daily creatinine excretion is the result of dietary intake, the ability to predict a patient's daily creatinine production in the clinical setting is limited.[27] One should also consider the potential errors in estimating creatinine production for the critically ill patient, the errors in serum creatinine measurements, and the uncertainty in the volume of distribution estimate for creatinine. Estimating creatinine clearance in a patient with a rising or falling serum creatinine should be viewed as a best guess under difficult conditions, and ongoing reassessment of the patient's renal function is warranted.

MEASURING CREATININE CLEARANCE: URINE COLLECTIONS

As noted earlier, in cases where the underlying assumptions of estimating creatinine clearance cannot be met, it may be most appropriate to conduct a measured creatinine clearance. In fact, pharmacokinetic studies conducted during new drug development often utilize 24-hour measured creatinine as the primary index for stratifying patients into renal function categories. The accuracy of a measured creatinine clearance highly depends on the complete and accurate measurement of creatinine concentration and urine volume over a specified time period. Errors in the collection process should always be considered, especially when collections are made in the ambulatory or nonobserved setting.

As a way to check the completeness of a timed (24-hour) urine collection, the predicted amount of creatinine produced or excreted for the patient (considering age, gender, weight, and body stature) should be compared with the amount of creatinine actually collected in the urine sample. At steady state, rate in (creatinine production) equals rate out (creatinine excretion). If the amount collected differs significantly from the patient's predicted production, the reported creatinine clearance is likely to be inaccurate. The patient's age, gender, and muscle mass should be considered when estimating the amount of creatinine produced. Increasing age and smaller muscle mass will reduce the expected amount of creatinine produced (see Table 3.2).

This principle will be illustrated using the following example. The following data were reported for a 55-year-old, 50-kg male patient for whom a 24-hour urine collection for Cl_{Cr} was ordered.

Total collection time	24 hr
Urine volume	1,200 mL
Urine creatinine concentration	42 mg/dL
Serum creatinine	1.5 mg/dL
Creatinine clearance	23 mL/min (uncorrected)
	30 mL/min (corrected)

The creatinine clearance of 23 mL/min (uncorrected) represents the patient's creatinine clearance as calculated from the urine collection. The creatinine clearance of 30 mL/min (corrected) represents what the patient's creatinine clearance would have been if the patient were 70 kg or 1.73 m². This "corrected" value is most useful as a relative estimate of renal function when the patient is substantially smaller or larger than our average 70 kg, 1.73 m² patient.

The uncorrected Cl_{Cr} was calculated using the following equation:

$$Cl_{Cr} = \frac{(U)(V)}{P}$$

(Eq. 3.18)

where U is the urine creatinine concentration in mg/dL, V the volume of urine per time of collection in mL/min, and P the plasma creatinine concentration in mg/dL. Equation 3.18 results in a Cl_{Cr} in the units of mL/min.

$$Cl_{Cr} = \frac{(U)(V)}{P}$$

$$= \frac{(42\ mg/dL)(1,200\ mL/1,440\ min)}{1.5\ mg/dL}$$

$$= 23\ mL/\ min$$

The laboratory computer performs these calculations of the uncorrected or corrected creatinine clearance. By performing the above calculation, all we have checked is the math skill of the computer and not the validity of the collection.

To determine whether the collection was complete, the total amount of creatinine collected in the 24-hour period should be calculated.

Because the patient weighs 50 kg, the apparent creatinine production per day can be calculated using the urine collection data and the appropriate conversion factors as follows:

$$\begin{array}{l}\text{Apparent Rate of} \\ \text{Creatinine Production} \\ \text{mg/kg/day}\end{array} = \frac{\begin{array}{c}\text{Amount of Creatinine} \\ \text{Extracted per Day in mg}\end{array}}{\text{Patient's Weight in kg}} = \frac{(U)(V)}{\text{Patient's Weight in kg}} \qquad \textbf{(Eq. 3.19)}$$

$$= \frac{(42\ mg/dL)(1,200\ mL/day)(1\ dL/100\ mL)}{50\ kg}$$

$$= 10.08\ mg/kg/day$$

This apparent production rate of creatinine of 10 mg/kg/day is considerably less than the normal production rate of 19 mg/kg/day as estimated from Table 3.2 for a 55-year-old man. Therefore, one possibility is that the urine collection was incomplete, and the reported value for creatinine clearance is much less than the patient's actual Cl_{Cr}. However, if the patient has a smaller than average muscle mass, the urine collection may be considered adequate and the reported creatinine clearance of 23 mL/min is the best estimate of the patient's renal function. In clinical practice, it is important to evaluate the patient for their "body composition." Patients who have a muscle mass that is less than average usually appear emaciated or very thin and/or have been physically inactive for a prolonged period (e.g., patients who are bedridden secondary to chronic illness or a spinal cord injury). Whether to accept the 24-hour urine collection as complete would depend on our assessment of the patient's physical stature.

An alternative approach to evaluating the 24-hour urine collection could be to compare the Cl_{Cr} as calculated from Cockcroft and Gault, Equation 3.4, to the uncorrected creatinine clearance from the 24-hour urine collection.

$$\begin{aligned}
\text{Cl}_{\text{Cr}} \text{ for Males (mL/min)} &= \frac{(140 - \text{Age})(\text{Weight})}{(72)(\text{SCr}_{\text{ss}})} \\
&= \frac{(140 - 55)(50)}{(72)(1.5 \text{ mg/dL})} \\
&= 39.4 \text{ mL/min}
\end{aligned}$$

In this case, Equation 3.4 calculated a Cl_{Cr} of approximately 40 mL/min and the 24-hour urine collection as a value of 23 mL/min. Clearly they both cannot be correct. Because both Equation 3.4 and the 24-hour collection used the SCr of 1.5 mg/dL, the difference must be the rate of creatinine production. Equation 3.4 assumes that the average creatinine production for a 55-year-old man is about 19 mg/kg/day (see Table 3.2). This is in contrast to the creatinine in the 24-hour collection, suggesting a production rate of about 10 mg/kg/day. Which is correct? As previously stated, if the patient has an unusually small muscle mass for their size, age, and gender, one might conclude that Equation 3.4 overestimated the production rate and the creatinine clearance. If this were the case, the 24-hour urine collection would be the most reasonable estimate of the patient's creatinine clearance. However, if the patient appears to have a normal amount of muscle mass (i.e., average physical stature for a 55-year-old man), then one might conclude that the 24-hour collection was inadequate and has underestimated the patient's creatinine production rate and, therefore, the creatinine clearance. If this were the case, the creatinine clearance of 40 mL/min from Equation 3.4 might be considered the better estimate of the patient's renal function. It is always important when determining renal function, either by use of an equation or by collecting urine that the results be evaluated in the context of the patient's muscle mass.

ESTIMATING GLOMERULAR FILTRATION RATE (eGFR)

Another method to estimate kidney function is to use eGFR equations that were developed by public health researchers for the purpose of categorizing or staging CKD. This approach is recommended by international kidney disease organizations, such as the National Kidney Foundation and the Kidney Disease Improving Global Outcomes, as a critical biomarker to evaluate and monitor patients with CKD.

The eGFR equation was originally derived from the Modification of Diet in Renal Disease (MDRD) study, with a four-variable version that has been validated to estimate GFR in patients with a GFR of <60 mL/min/1.73 m². However, at higher eGFR values, it was found that this equation loses its accuracy and could lead to over-estimation of GFR in some patients. It is for this reason that eGFR values over 60 mL/min/1.73 m² are not reported, and may appear in the electronic medical record (EMR) as "eGFR >60 mL/min/1.73 m²."

$$\text{eGFR(mL/min/1.73 m}^2) = 175 \times (\text{SCr})^{-1.154} \times (\text{Age})^{-0.203} \qquad \textbf{(Eq. 3.20)}$$
$$\times (0.742 \text{ if Female}) \times (1.21 \text{ if Black})$$

where SCr is in mg/dL and age in years.

In 2012, a newer eGFR equation was developed, based on further analysis of the MDRD study along with other pooled clinical trial data. This equation is called the Chronic Kidney Disease Epidemiology Study equation, or CKD-EPI.[28]
CKD-EPI:

$$\text{GFR (mL/min/1.73 m}^2) = 141 \times \min (SCr/\kappa, 1)^{\alpha}$$
$$\times \max(SCr/\kappa, 1)^{-1.209} \times 0.993^{Age} \times 1.018 \text{ [if female]} \times 1.159 \text{ [if African American]}$$

where: SCr is serum creatinine in mg/dL, κ is 0.7 for females and 0.9 for males, α is −0.329 for females and −0.411 for males, min indicates the minimum of SCr/κ or 1, and max indicates the maximum of SCr/κ or 1.

While both eGFR equations (MDRD and CKD-EPI) are meant to be used for staging CKD patients, to date these equations have not been shown to be superior to the Cockcroft and Gault equation for dosing drugs that are renally cleared. Because of the large body of evidence and experience with Cockcroft and Gault, it is recommended that these eGFR equations not be used for dosing of drugs until studies are preformed to document the accuracy of MDRD for dose adjustment of renally cleared drugs.[29,30] This is an important issue because many hospitals and health care systems automatically calculate and display an eGFR that is calculated from the MDRD equation (see Equation 3.20). Although use of the CKD-EPI equation for automated reporting of eGFR is recommended, it is considered optional and has not been widely implemented at this time. Because eGFR values reported in the EMR are based on the MDRD equation, a patient with a calculated eGFR of 72 mL/min/1.73 m^2 will have an EMR reported value of ">60 mL/min/1.73 m^2."

When estimating creatinine clearance for dosing of renally cleared drugs, it is recommended that the Cockcroft and Gault equation be used. When comparing the results of estimated creatinine clearance and eGFR, in most cases, the estimates will be similar, especially for patients with BSA close to 1.73 m^2. The reason for this is that the units of the MDRD equation are in mL/min/1.73 m^2. Thus, back-calculation of the eGFR value to obtain the unit of mL/min is required for direct comparison with Cl_{Cr}.

$$\frac{\text{eGFR for Patient}}{\text{mL/min}} = \frac{\text{eGFR}}{\text{mL/min/1.73 m}^2} \left(\frac{\text{BSA}}{1.73 \text{ m}^2} \right) \qquad \textbf{(Eq. 3.21)}$$

or the ratio of weight/70 kg to the power 0.7

$$\frac{\text{eGFR for Patient}}{\text{mL/min}} = \frac{\text{eGFR}}{\text{mL/min/1.73 m}^2} \left(\frac{\text{Weight in kg}}{70 \text{ kg}} \right)^{0.7} \qquad \textbf{(Eq. 3.22)}$$

In a few cases, even when the renal function has been adjusted for the patient's size, the difference in estimated renal function can be significant. As an example, a 76-year-old, 52.3-kg black male with an SCr of 1 mg/dL would have the following estimates of renal function.

Using Cockcroft and Gault Equation 3.4:

$$Cl_{Cr} \text{ for Males (mL/min)} = \frac{(140 - Age)(Weight)}{72 \times SCr_{ss}}$$

$$= \frac{(140 - 76)52.3}{72 \times 1}$$

$$= 46.5 \text{ mL/min}$$

Using the MDRD Equation 3.20:

$$eGFR \text{ (mL/min/1.73 m}^2) = 175 \times (SCr)^{-1.154} \times (Age)^{-0.203}$$
$$\times \left[0.742 \text{ if Female}\right] \times \left[1.21 \text{ if Black}\right]$$

Again substituting 1 for 0.742 if female:

$$= 175 \times (1)^{-1.154} \times (76)^{-0.203} \times 1$$
$$\times \left[1.21 \text{ if Black}\right]$$
$$= 87.9 \text{ mL/min/1.73 m}^2$$

Adjusting for the patient's size using Equation 3.22:

$$\frac{eGFR \text{ for Patient}}{mL/min} = \frac{eGFR}{mL/min/1.73 \text{ m}^2}\left(\frac{Weight \text{ in kg}}{70 \text{ kg}}\right)^{0.7}$$

$$= \frac{87.9}{mL/min/1.73 \text{ m}^2}\left(\frac{52.3 \text{ kg}}{70 \text{ kg}}\right)^{0.7}$$

$$= \frac{87.9}{mL/min/1.73 \text{ m}^2}(0.815)$$

$$= 71.6 \text{ mL/min}$$

Again the most common error in comparing Cockcroft and Gault to MDRD is failing to adjust for the patient's size, that is, mL/min versus mL/min/1.73 m². However, with our example even with adjustment for the patient's size, the estimates of renal function are considerably different depending on which equation is used, and the results from the MDRD equation would seem to be much higher than expected for this 52.3-kg, 76-year-old man. This cautionary example illustrates the necessity of calculating creatinine clearance using the Cockcroft and Gault equation, even in cases where the laboratory computer indicates that eGFR is >60 mL/min/1.73 m². Again, until specific information is known about the utility of MDRD (or CKD-EPI), it is recommended that Cockcroft and Gault, Equations 3.4 and 3.5 for adults or Schwartz, and Equation 3.13 for pediatrics be used when calculating dosing regimens for renally cleared drugs.

Adjusting drug dose based on kidney function

In cases where clinical pharmacokinetic studies and renal dosing recommendations may not be readily available, calculation of dose adjustment factors based on kidney function may be needed. Because the kidneys and liver function independently, it is assumed that a change in one does not affect the other. Thus, Cl_t can be estimated in the presence of renal or hepatic failure or both. Because metabolic function is difficult to quantitate, Cl_t is most commonly adjusted when there is decreased renal function:

$$\text{Cl Adjusted} = (Cl_m) + \left[(Cl_r) \left(\frac{\text{Fraction of Normal Renal}}{\text{Function Remaining}} \right) \right] \qquad \textbf{(Eq. 3.23)}$$

A clearance that has been adjusted for kidney function can be used to estimate the maintenance dose for a patient with stable CKD (see Equation 1.16). This adjusted clearance equation, however, is only valid if the drug's metabolites are inactive and if the metabolic clearance is indeed unaffected by kidney disease as assumed. A decrease in the function of an organ of elimination is most significant when that organ serves as the primary route of drug elimination. However, as the major elimination pathway becomes increasingly compromised, the "minor" pathway becomes more significant because it assumes a greater proportion of the total clearance. For example, a drug that is usually 67% eliminated by the renal route and 33% by the hepatic route will be 100% metabolized in the event of complete renal failure; the total clearance, however, will only be one-third of the normal value.

As an alternative to adjusting Cl_t to calculate dosing rate, one can substitute fraction of the total clearance that is metabolic and renal for Cl_m and Cl_r. Using this technique, the following equation can be derived.

$$\text{Dosing Rate Adjustment Factor} =$$
$$\left(\begin{array}{c} \text{Fraction Eliminated} \\ \text{Metabolically} \end{array} \right) + \left[\left(\begin{array}{c} \text{Fraction Eliminated} \\ \text{Renally} \end{array} \right) \left(\begin{array}{c} \text{Fraction of Normal Renal} \\ \text{Function Remaining} \end{array} \right) \right]$$
$$\textbf{(Eq. 3.24)}$$

The dosing ate adjustment factor can be used to adjust the maintenance dose for a patient with altered renal function.

As an example, take a drug that is 25% metabolized and 75% renally cleared and normally administered as 100 mg every 12 hours. If this drug were to be given to a patient who has only 33% of normal renal function, the dosing rate adjustment factor would be 0.5.

$$\text{Dosing Rate Adjustment Factor} =$$

$$\left(\begin{array}{c}\text{Fraction Eliminated}\\ \text{Metabolically}\end{array}\right) + \left[\left(\begin{array}{c}\text{Fraction Eliminated}\\ \text{Renally}\end{array}\right)\left(\begin{array}{c}\text{Fraction of Normal Renal}\\ \text{Function Remaining}\end{array}\right)\right]$$

$$= (0.25) + [(0.75)(0.33)]$$
$$= (0.25) + [0.25]$$
$$= 0.5$$

The dosing rate adjustment factor of 0.5 suggests that the drug should be administered at half the usual rate. This could be accomplished by decreasing the dose and maintaining the same interval (e.g., 50 mg every 12 hours) or by maintaining the same dose and increasing the interval (e.g., 100 mg every 24 hours). Depending on the situation and therapeutic intent, either method (or a combination of dose and dosing interval adjustment) might be appropriate.

Dialysis of Drugs

PHARMACOKINETIC MODELING: HEMODIALYSIS

The pharmacokinetic model for drugs in patients undergoing intermittent hemodialysis generally follows one of two patterns. In Figure 3.1, a maintenance drug dose produces plasma concentrations that are relatively constant between dialysis periods. This plasma concentration of drug represents the steady-state condition with very little fluctuation of the drug concentration between doses. This pattern occurs when the input is continuous (intravenous [IV] or oral sustained release) or the dosing interval is much less than the drug half-life (i.e., $\tau < \frac{1}{3}\ t\frac{1}{2}$). The rapid decline in the drug concentration corresponds to periods of hemodialysis when drug is being rapidly removed, and the rapid return of the plasma drug concentration to steady state reflects the administration of a post-dialysis replacement dose. This pattern can be represented by the following equations:

$$Cl_{pat} = Cl_m + Cl_r \tag{Eq. 3.25}$$

$$Css\ ave = \frac{(S)(F)(Dose/\tau)}{Cl_{pat}} \tag{Eq. 3.26}$$

$$Dose = \frac{(Css\ ave)(Cl_{pat})(\tau)}{(S)(F)} \tag{Eq. 3.27}$$

where Cl_{pat} is the patient's drug clearance during nondialysis periods and is the sum of the patient's metabolic clearance (Cl_m) and any residual renal clearance (Cl_r). S and F

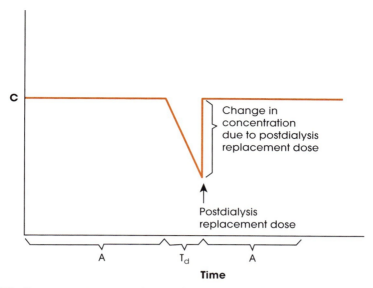

FIGURE 3.1   Plasma concentration curve between dialysis procedures. This figure represents a plasma concentration curve for a patient receiving a maintenance dose of a drug between dialysis procedures at intervals that result in small fluctuations in plasma concentration. The dosing interval during the interdialysis period (A) is arbitrary but should be less than the half-life of the drug. During the intradialysis period (T_d), the drug is rapidly removed by the dialysis procedure. The subsequent increase in the plasma concentration of drug is because of the postdialysis replacement dose. This model assumes that the drug is significantly removed during dialysis and does not include the distribution phase following the postdialysis replacement dose.

are the salt form and bioavailability of the drug, respectively and τ is the dosing interval. Equation 3.26 may be used to predict the average steady-state plasma concentration, and Equation 3.27 may be used to calculate the maintenance dose based on the estimated Cl_{pat} and the desired Css ave. In addition to the maintenance dose, the patient may also require additional doses following dialysis to replace the drug lost during the dialysis period.

$$\begin{array}{c} \text{Postdialysis} \\ \text{Replacement} \\ \text{Dose} \end{array} = \begin{bmatrix} \text{Amount of Drug} \\ \text{in the Body} \\ \text{Prior to Dialysis} \end{bmatrix} \begin{bmatrix} \text{Fraction of Drug} \\ \text{Lost during Dialysis} \end{bmatrix}$$

$$\begin{array}{c} \text{Postdialysis} \\ \text{Replacement} \\ \text{Dose} \end{array} = (V)(Css\ ave)\left(1 - e^{-\left(\frac{Cl_{pat} + Cl_{dial}}{V}\right)(T_d)}\right) \qquad \textbf{(Eq. 3.28)}$$

$$\begin{array}{c} \text{Postdialysis} \\ \text{Replacement} \\ \text{Dose} \end{array} = (V)(Css\ ave)(1 - e^{-K_{dial}(T_d)}) \qquad \textbf{(Eq. 3.29)}$$

In the above equations, (V)(Css ave) is the amount of drug in the body at the beginning of dialysis, and the elimination rate constant during the dialysis (K_{dial}) represents the sum of the patient's clearance and the clearance by dialysis divided by the volume of distribution $[(Cl_{pat} + Cl_{dial})/V]$. T_d is the duration of dialysis. If the patient's maintenance dose is given in divided daily doses or once daily, the patient's dose would be calculated using Equation 3.27 on nondialysis days. On dialysis days, the patient would receive, in addition to the maintenance dose, a postdialysis replacement dose as calculated by Equation 3.28 or 3.29.

The second pharmacokinetic model for drug dosing in patients undergoing hemodialysis is depicted in Figure 3.2. In this model, a single dose is given at the conclusion of each dialysis period. Significant amounts of drug are lost between dialysis periods, and additional drug is lost during dialysis. In this model, the dose administered at the end of dialysis replaces all of the drug lost by the patient's own clearance, as well as by dialysis clearance, and returns the drug level to a targeted "peak" concentration. This replacement dose can be calculated by use of Equation 3.30 or 3.31:

$$\text{Postdialysis Replacement Dose} = (V)(\text{Css peak})\left(1 - \left[\left(e^{-\left(\frac{Cl_{pat}}{V}\right)(t_1)}\right)\left(e^{-\left(\frac{Cl_{pat} + Cl_{dial}}{V}\right)(T_d)}\right)\right]\right) \qquad \textbf{(Eq. 3.30)}$$

$$\text{Postdialysis Replacement Dose} = (V)(\text{Css peak})\left(1 - \left[\left(e^{-(K_{pat})(t_1)}\right)\left(e^{-(K_{dial})(T_d)}\right)\right]\right) \qquad \textbf{(Eq. 3.31)}$$

where t_1 is the interdialysis period or the period from the peak concentration to the beginning of dialysis, and T_d the dialysis period or the time interval from the beginning to the end of the dialysis procedure. K_{pat} is the elimination rate constant during the interdialysis period where drug loss is caused by Cl_{pat} alone and K_{dial} is the elimination rate constant during the dialysis period where drug loss is the result of both Cl_{pat} and Cl_{dail}.

In some cases it may be appropriate to calculate the drug concentrations at the beginning and end of the dialysis period. This can be accomplished using Equations 3.32 and 3.33.

$$\text{Predialysis Concentration} = (\text{Css peak})\left(e^{-\left(\frac{Cl_{pat}}{V}\right)(t_1)}\right) \qquad \textbf{(Eq. 3.32)}$$

$$\text{Postdialysis Concentration} = \left(\text{Predialysis Concentration}\right)\left(e^{-\left(\frac{Cl_{pat} + Cl_{dial}}{V}\right)(T_d)}\right) \qquad \textbf{(Eq. 3.33)}$$

These equations are used when there are specifically targeted peak and/or trough concentrations or when transient declines in the plasma concentrations might result in

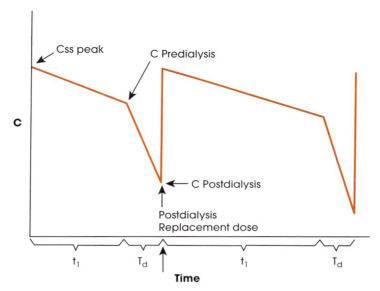

FIGURE 3.2   Plasma profile for a drug administered only at the postdialysis period for a patient receiving intermittent hemodialysis. The interdialysis period (t_1) represents the time from the steady-state peak concentration to the beginning of dialysis and may vary according to the number of days between each hemodialysis period. The intradialysis period is represented by T_d. The postdialysis dose represents the amount of drug that is lost from the body because of the patient's clearance during the interdialysis period and the dialysis clearance during the intradialysis period.

therapeutic failures, as with antiarrhythmics or anticonvulsant agents. Depending on the therapeutic intent, the specific drug concentrations may be of more or less interest. As an example, in the case of aminoglycoside antibiotics, the predialysis and not the postdialysis concentration should be thought of as the "trough" in assessing the risk of aminoglycoside toxicity. This is because the pattern of decay is more rapid during the intradialysis period and as a result, the postdialysis aminoglycoside "trough" concentration is transient and does not easily translate into drug exposure and risk of toxicity (see Fig. 3.2). Given that the interval between dialysis runs is often about 48 hours, it is not possible to dose aminoglycosides in a way that will achieve the usually targeted high peak and low trough concentrations in the dialysis patient. For these patients the usual gentamicin/tobramycin steady-state peak and predialysis trough concentration are approximately 5 and 2 mg/L. Because of this, the risk of aminoglycoside toxicity may be greater in dialysis patients.

ESTIMATING DRUG DIALYZABILITY

To calculate dosing requirements for patients undergoing intermittent hemodialysis, the dialysis clearance must be known. Although a number of general references are available,[8,9,31–38] it is frequently difficult to find information on specific drugs, especially for drugs that are poorly dialyzable. To determine the dialyzability of a drug, the apparent volume of distribution, plasma protein binding, the patient's clearance, and the drug's half-life should be considered as follows:

1. Divide the volume of distribution by fu or the usual free fraction to calculate the apparent unbound volume of distribution. It is only the unbound drug that can pass through the dialysis membrane, and therefore, it is the unbound volume of distribution against which the drug will be dialyzed. If the unbound volume of distribution exceeds 3.5 L/kg or approximately 250 L/70 kg, it is unlikely that a significant amount of drug will be removed by dialysis.

$$\text{Unbound Volume}\atop\text{of Distribution} = \frac{V}{fu} \qquad \text{(Eq. 3.34)}$$

2. Estimate the patient's clearance (Cl_m + residual Cl_r). If this value is >10 mL/min/kg or 700 mL/min/70 kg, it is unlikely that hemodialysis will add significantly to the patient's intrinsic drug elimination process. This is because most drugs have a hemodialysis clearance less than 150 mL/min.
3. If the usual dosing interval is much greater than the drug's t½ in patients with end-stage renal failure, it is unlikely that hemodialysis will significantly alter the dosing regimen. The key here is to schedule the drug administration shortly after rather than shortly before dialysis, so that even if the drug is dialyzable, very little remains to be removed by dialysis.
4. Drugs with a low molecular weight are more likely to be removed significantly by dialysis. Drugs with a molecular weight >1,000 Da are unlikely to be removed by low-flux hemodialysis. Highflux hemodialysis can remove molecules with molecular weight 1,000 Da (see Low-versus High-Flux Hemodialysis).

For almost all drugs, if any one of the above criteria is met, it is unlikely that the drug in question will be significantly removed by hemodialysis. However, if a drug has an unbound volume <3.5 L/kg, a clearance of <10 mL/min/kg, a τ that is not significantly greater than the drug's t½, and a molecular weight <1,000 Da if low-flux or <5,000 Da if high-flux, it is possible, but not a certainty, that hemodialysis will significantly alter the drug elimination pattern. In these cases it is necessary to review the literature to establish whether the drug is significantly removed by hemodialysis. If Cl_{dial} adds significantly to the patient's clearance, then additional drug replacement following hemodialysis may be appropriate.

As an additional check, the drug half-life during the dialysis period can be calculated:

$$t\tfrac{1}{2}\text{ during Hemodialysis} = \frac{(0.693)(V)}{\left(Cl_{pat} + Cl_{dial}\right)} \qquad \text{(Eq. 3.35)}$$

If the t½ during hemodialysis greatly exceeds the duration of dialysis, very little drug will be removed during any individual period of dialysis.

Whereas the techniques outlined previously can be used to estimate the dialyzability of drugs and thereby model their pharmacokinetic behavior during dialysis, there are a number of potential limitations. For many drugs, relatively little is known about either the activity or dialyzability of their metabolites. In addition, these guidelines must be used cautiously in acute overdose situations because saturation of plasma and tissue binding as well as possible alterations in the pathways for elimination may occur when drug concentrations are very high. Considerable differences in dialysis equipment, the types of membranes used in hemodialysis, and the duration of dialysis can result in data that may not be applicable to all dialysis situations.[39]

Although it would be ideal to have data derived from the specific dialysis equipment used for the patient in question, this will not be the case in most instances. Instead, one must rely on the data in the literature to estimate the average amount of drug that most likely would be removed during the patient's hemodialysis.

Dialysis procedures also vary in duration and effectiveness, but most patients receive hemodialysis three times a week, with each dialysis period being approximately 3 to 4 hours. The duration of dialysis can usually be found on the hemodialysis record sheets and should be checked to be certain that the initial plans for dialysis were successfully completed. In some cases because of hypotension, lack of venous access, or equipment malfunction, dialysis is not completed as planned, either in duration of the dialysis or the ability to maintain the patient's blood flow through the artificial kidney (dialysis membrane) during the dialysis period. As stated earlier, the usual duration of dialysis is 3 hours, and the usual blood flow through the artificial kidney is 200 to 350 mL/min. If the usual dialysis parameters are not met, the estimated drug loss during dialysis is probably less than expected.

The uncertainties and potential problems associated with predictions of drug levels during hemodialysis suggest that plasma drug concentrations guide the approach to therapy when possible. When plasma samples are obtained, the distribution phase associated with IV drug administration, as well as the transient period of disequilibrium between the plasma and tissue compartments associated with the hemodialysis process, should be avoided. The disequilibrium between plasma and tissue occurs to varying degrees with most drugs because as the drug is removed from the plasma by dialysis, additional time is required for the drug in the tissue to re-equilibrate with the decreased plasma concentration. Although the time required to re-establish equilibrium between the tissue and plasma is not documented for most drugs, it would seem reasonable to wait at least 60 minutes following the end of hemodialysis if postdialysis plasma samples are to be obtained.

LOW-VERSUS HIGH-FLUX HEMODIALYSIS

High-flux or high-efficiency hemodialysis refers to a dialysis process that utilizes a dialysis membrane that has larger pores through which both solvent (water) and solute (electrolytes, drugs, etc.) can pass.[9,10] Because the pore size is larger, high-flux hemodialysis is more efficient in removing smaller compounds and can remove some larger compounds that low-flux hemodialysis cannot remove. High-flux dialysis is more efficient than low-flux dialysis, thereby making the earlier techniques to estimate dialyzability less reliable as a predictor but not invalid. To illustrate, vancomycin with its large molecular weight (approximately 1,450 Da) is relatively unaffected by low-flux hemodialysis. This is because the pore size associated with the lowflux hemodialysis membranes only allows the passage of compounds with a molecular weight of less than 1,000 Da and has a limited ability to remove drugs with a molecular weight between 500 and 1,000 Da. However, when a high-flux dialysis membrane is used, the large pore size allows compounds of greater than 1,000 Da to pass through and be eliminated. As a result, during a usual 3-hour high-flux hemodialysis run, there is a rapid drop in the vancomycin drug concentrations followed by a postdialysis rebound in concentration, indicating that approximately 17% of the body stores of vancomycin is removed.[39-42]

For those compounds that are eliminated to a significant extent during low-flux dialysis, more drug is eliminated during high-flux hemodialysis. However, the differences in elimination are usually one of degree and not in most cases as significant as seen with vancomycin.

CONTINUOUS RENAL REPLACEMENT THERAPY

Continuous renal replacement therapy (CRRT) utilizes an ultrafiltration process with a large pore membrane similar to those in high-flux hemodialysis to filter free water and solute, including unbound drug. The rate of plasma filtration is commonly 1 L/hr but ranges from 0.5 to 2 L/hr. Of course, patients could not tolerate this rate of fluid removal unless the vast majority of fluid being removed was continuously being replaced. Dialysate is sometimes added to the ultrafiltration process, which can further increase solute and drug elimination through a passive diffusion process. Total CRRT output (ultrafiltration + dialysate) is usually in the range of 1 to 2 L/hr. The advantage of CRRT is that it is more hemodynamically forgiving than hemodialysis and is used in critically ill patients who cannot tolerate intermittent hemodialysis, usually because of hypotension.[8,9,43-45]

CRRT is also referred to as continuous arteriovenous hemofiltration or continuous venovenous hemofiltration; when dialysate is added to the process, it is referred to as continuous arteriovenous hemodiafiltration (CAVHD) or continuous venovenous hemodiafiltration (CVVHD). CRRT with or without dialysate is well documented to remove vancomycin and other drugs.[46-50] Although the absolute clearance of CRRT is not high, it is continuous and can add significantly to the elimination of some drugs.

One approach to identifying which drugs might be significantly influenced by CRRT is to calculate the maximum CRRT dialysis clearance (Cl_{CRRT}). Because the CRRT membranes, like low- and high-flux membranes, do not allow plasma proteins to pass through, only the unbound drug (Cu) can be removed by CRRT. One method of estimating the maximum Cl_{CRRT} is to multiply the total CRRT flow rate (volume of ultrafiltrate + volume of dialysate per interval of time) by the fraction of unbound drug in plasma (fu). This process assumes that the ultrafiltrate and the dialysate will be at equilibrium with plasma and have a concentration of drug that is equal to the concentration of unbound drug in plasma. This assumption is probably true because most drugs have a molecular weight that is less than 2,000 Da. While the molecular weight "cut off" for CRRT membranes is in the range of 30,000 Da, large molecules are not likely to be able to pass through the membrane and be cleared. However, molecules with a molecular weight of <5,000 and almost certainly <2,000 Da should be able to be efficiently filtered and come to equilibrium.

$$\text{Cl}_{\text{CRRT}} \text{ Maximum} = (\text{fu})(\text{CRRT Flow Rate}) \qquad \textbf{(Eq. 3.36)}$$

In Equation 3.36, fu is the fraction of drug unbound in plasma, and CRRT flow rate is the average volume output of ultrafiltration + dialysate per unit of time. Units for CRRT flow rate are usually expressed as mL/min or L/hr depending on the preference of the clinician. If the Cl_{CRRT} maximum is ≤25% of the patient's residual clearance (Cl_{pat}), then CRRT does not add significantly to the patient's drug elimination process, and no dose adjustment would be necessary relative to the presence or absence of CRRT. If Cl_{CRRT} maximum adds significantly to the patient's clearance, then the literature will have to be reviewed to identify either Cl_{CRRT} values or recommended replacement doses for patients undergoing CRRT.[45,47–53]

Dose calculations are similar to the usual methods because the CRRT process is intended to be continuous. In many cases, the t½ is extended, even when the patient is receiving CRRT, and doses can be calculated using Equation 3.37:

$$\text{Maintenance Dose} = \frac{(\text{Cl}_{\text{pat}} + \text{Cl}_{\text{CRRT}})(\text{Css ave})(\tau)}{(\text{S})(\text{F})} \qquad \textbf{(Eq. 3.37)}$$

where Css ave is the average targeted steady-state concentration, Cl_{pat} the metabolic clearance (Cl_{m}) plus an estimate of the patient's residual renal clearance (Cl_{r}), and Cl_{CRRT} an estimate of the CRRT clearance from one of the literature sources or Equation 3.36 above. When there is likely to be significant fluctuation in drug concentration between doses (i.e., $\tau > ⅓ \text{ t½}$), the following equation can be used:

$$\text{Dose} = \frac{(\text{Css}_1)(\text{V})(1 - e^{-\text{K}_{\text{CRRT}}\tau})}{(\text{S})(\text{F})(e^{-\text{K}_{\text{CRRT}}t_1})} \qquad \textbf{(Eq. 3.38)}$$

where Css_1 is the desired drug concentration, usually Css max or Css min, t_1 the time interval from the dose to Css_1, and K_{CRRT} represents the elimination rate constant consisting of Cl_{pat} ($\text{Cl}_{\text{m}} + \text{Cl}_{\text{r}}$) plus Cl_{CRRT} divided by the drug's volume of distribution.

As with hemodialysis, patients undergoing CRRT need to be monitored to ensure that the CRRT process is proceeding as planned. Because patients receiving CRRT are critically ill and the process is complex, CRRT is often adjusted on an hour-by-hour and day-by-day basis. The two most important issues to consider are whether the CRRT process has been interrupted and/or whether the CRRT flow rate has been significantly altered. Small changes in CRRT flow rates are normal, but if the patient's CRRT vascular access fails or for some other reason the process is discontinued or the flow rates changed, then many of the drug dosing recommendations will also have to be altered.

PERITONEAL DIALYSIS

Peritoneal dialysis, and especially continuous ambulatory peritoneal dialysis (CAPD), is occasionally used as an alternative to intermittent hemodialysis. This technique takes advantage of the large semipermeable surface area of the intraperitoneal space and is performed by instilling dialysate fluid via a catheter into the peritoneal space. The dialysate is allowed to equilibrate with the surrounding tissue vasculature and then is removed. This creates a clearance mechanism for solutes including body waste products and drugs. The usual volume instilled into the peritoneal space for an adult is ≈ 2 L, although this can vary somewhat depending on the size of the patient and the intent of dialysis. The efficiency of peritoneal dialysis in removing both drugs and body waste products depends on a number of factors. Assuming that the solute in plasma comes to equilibrium with the dialysate fluid, one would expect the concentration of drug in the dialysate to equal the unbound plasma drug concentration. Therefore, the maximum expected CAPD clearance (Cl_{CAPD}) would be approximately equal to the following:

$$Cl_{CAPD} \text{ Maximum} = (fu)\left(\frac{\text{Volume of Dialysate}}{T_D}\right) \qquad \textbf{(Eq. 3.39)}$$

where fu is the fraction of unbound drug in plasma, volume of dialysate is the peritoneal exchange volume, and T_D the dwell time or the time the dialysate is allowed to remain in the peritoneal space before removal.

Using the usual volume of dialysate instilled into the peritoneal space of $\approx 2,000$ mL, the usual exchange or dwell time (T_D) of ≈ 6 hours and if fu is assumed to be 1 (no plasma binding), the expected Cl_{CAPD} maximum for solute and drugs would be approximately 5.5 mL/min.

$$Cl_{CAPD} \text{ Maximum} = (fu)\left(\frac{\text{Volume of Dialysate}}{T_D}\right)$$
$$= (1)(2 \text{ L}/6 \text{ hr})$$
$$= 0.333 \text{ L/hr}$$

or

$$= (0.333 \text{ L/hr})(1,000 \text{ mL/L})(1 \text{ hr}/60 \text{ min})$$
$$= 5.5 \text{ mL/min}$$

Drugs with a residual Cl_{pat} substantially greater than 5.5 mL/min or 0.333 L/hr will not be significantly influenced by peritoneal dialysis. As a general guideline, if the Cl_{CAPD} maximum is <25% of the patient's residual clearance (Cl_{pat}), one would not anticipate a need to adjust a drug's dose if peritoneal dialysis is initiated or discontinued.

One of the assumptions in Equation 3.39 is that equilibrium is achieved between the unbound plasma drug concentration (Cu) and the dialysate fluid. This assumption is probably true for drugs of relatively low molecular weight (i.e., <500 Da). Larger compounds may not come to equilibrium within the usual 6-hour dwell time, and very large molecules (e.g., proteins) cannot diffuse across the peritoneal cell walls. Some of the plasma proteins do cross into the peritoneal space and while it can be an issue with regard to protein loss it is not significant in regard to drug elimination.

In theory, the Cl_{CAPD} for larger compounds could be calculated by taking into account the fraction of steady-state equilibrium achieved in the dialysate dwell time as follows:

$$Cl_{CAPD} \approx (fu)\left(\frac{\text{Volume of Dialysate}}{T_D}\right)(1 - e^{-(K_{eq})(T_D)}) \qquad \textbf{(Eq. 3.40)}$$

where, fu is the free fraction in plasma of the compound or drug in question, T_D the dwell time of the dialysate, K_{eq} the equilibrium rate constant for the equilibrium between the unbound drug in plasma and the dialysate, and $1 - e^{(-K_{eq})(T_D)}$ the fraction of equilibrium achieved during the dialysate dwell time (T_D). Whereas the fu is available for many drugs, it should be recognized that in renal disease the fu is often increased. Also, the equilibrium rate constant (K_{eq}) is not generally available for most drugs. The fraction of equilibrium achieved can be estimated, however, based on the molecular weight of a drug. For example, urea and creatinine, with molecular weights of approximately 60 and 113 Da, respectively, appear to come to equilibrium relatively rapidly. The average equilibrium half-time for urea and creatinine appears to be approximately 0.66 and 2 hours, respectively.

Therefore, in the usual 6-hour exchange, urea has essentially reached equilibrium and creatinine approximately 85% of equilibrium.[8,54] Interestingly, the aminoglycoside antibiotics with fu ≈ 1 and molecular weight ≈ 500 Da have a CAPD clearance that approaches the dialysis exchange rate when the dwell time (T_D) is ≈ 6 hours.[54–56] If equilibrium is approached in 6 hours, this suggests that the equilibrium half-time is probably in the range of 2 hours. Vancomycin, on the other hand, has a peritoneal dialysis clearance of only 1 to 3 mL/min. Given that vancomycin has a fu approaching 1,[46,57,58] this low Cl_{CAPD} suggests that equilibrium between plasma and dialysate is not achieved within the usual 6-hour dwell time. This observation is consistent with the fact that vancomycin is a large molecule with a molecular weight of $\approx 1,450$ Da.

The significance of high plasma protein binding on drug clearance is fairly obvious. Compounds that are extensively bound to plasma proteins and have low free concentrations are not likely to be significantly cleared by peritoneal dialysis unless their residual clearance is exceedingly low. The influence of molecular weight and time to reach equilibrium on a drug's dialyzability is less well understood because relatively few data are available. However, the clearance of compounds that appear to come to equilibrium rapidly is likely to be altered if the dwell time is changed. For example, if a patient is taking a drug that has low molecular weight, more drug will be removed if the peritoneal dialysate fluid is exchanged more frequently as predicted by Equation 3.39.

As a result, replacement doses of a drug that is necessitated by dialysis are likely to be influenced by the dialysate exchange rate. In contrast, replacement doses of drugs with high molecular weights are not likely to be significantly influenced by the exchange rate. This is because an increase in the exchange rate is offset by the decrease in dwell time and the fraction of equilibrium achieved. Consequently, the total calculated clearance by Equation 3.39 would tend to overestimate Cl_{CAPD} and, if possible, Equation 3.40 should be used for these larger, more slowly equilibrating compounds.

Because the surface area of the peritoneal membrane is large and peritoneal infections are frequent, it has become a common practice to administer antibiotics directly into the peritoneal space.[59-63] When administered by the peritoneal route, the drug does not remain in the peritoneal space but diffuses from the high concentration in the dialysate fluid to the plasma and the systemic circulation. The most common antibiotics administered intraperitoneally are the cephalosporins, aminoglycosides, and vancomycin. Techniques used to administer these drugs vary from intermittently adding large doses of drug to a single dialysate exchange on a daily or weekly basis, to the addition of smaller amounts of drug in each individual exchange. When drugs are placed in the peritoneal dialysate fluid either intermittently or with each exchange, the ability to achieve peak and trough concentrations is limited (for usual dosing recommendations see Chapters 6 and 16).

REFERENCES

1. Rowland M. Drug administration and regimens. In: Melmon K, Morelli H, eds. *Clinical Pharmacology and Therapeutics*. 2nd ed. New York, NY: Macmillan; 1978:25–70.
2. Rowland M, Tozer TN. *Clinical Pharmacokinetics: Concepts and Applications*. 2nd ed. Philadelphia, PA: Lea & Febiger; 1989.
3. Kassirer JP. Clinical evaluation of kidney-glomerular function. *N Engl J Med*. 1971;285:385.
4. Toto RD. Conventional measurement of renal function utilizing serum creatinine, creatinine clearance, inulin and para-aminohippuric acid clearance. *Curr Opin Nephrol Hypertens*. 1995;4:505–509.
5. Manjunath G, Sarnak MJ, Levey AS. Estimating the glomerular filtration rate. Dos and don'ts for assessing kidney function. *Postgrad Med*. 2001;110:55–62.
6. Lott RS, Hayton WL. Estimation of creatinine clearance from serum creatinine concentration: a review. *Drug Intell Clin Pharm*. 1978;12:140.
7. Bjornsson TD. Use of serum creatinine concentrations to determine renal function. *Clin Pharmacokinet*. 1979;4:200.
8. Daugirdas JT, Blake PG, Ing TS. *Handbook of Dialysis*. New York, NY: Lippincott Williams & Wilkins; 2001.
9. Henrich W. *Principles and Practice of Dialysis*. Philadelphia, PA: Lippincott Williams & Wilkins; 1998.
10. Goldman R. Creatinine excretion in renal failure. *Proc Soc Biol Med*. 1954;85:446.
11. Jelliffe RW. Creatinine clearance: bedside estimate. *Ann Intern Med*. 1973;79:604.
12. Siersbaek-Nielson K, Hansen JM, Kampmann J, et al. Rapid evaluation of creatinine clearance [letter]. *Lancet*. 1971;1:1133.
13. Lepist EL, Zhang X, Hao J, et al. Contribution of the organic anion transporter OAT2 to the renal active tubular secretion of creatinine and mechanism for serum creatinine elevations caused by cobicistat. *Kidney Int*. 2014;86(2):350–357.
14. Lentner C, Lentner C, Wink A, eds. *Geigy Scientific Tables. Body Surface of Children/Adults*. West Caldwell, NJ: Ciba-Geigy; 1981:226–227.
15. Cockcroft DW, Gault MH. Prediction of creatinine clearance from serum creatinine. *Nephron*. 1976;16:31

16. Hernandez de Acevedo L, Johnson CE. Estimation of creatinine clearance in children: comparison of six methods. *Clin Pharm.* 1982;1:158.

17. Janmahasatian S, Duffull SB, Ash S, et al. Quantification of lean bodyweight. *Clin Pharmacokinet.* 2005;44:1051–1065.

18. Park EJ, Pai MP, Dong T, et al. The influence of body size descriptors on the estimation of kidney function in normal weight, overweight, obese, and morbidly obese adults. *Ann Pharmacother.* 2012;46:317–328.

19. Dowling TC, Wang ES, Ferrucci L, et al. Glomerular filtration rate equations overestimate creatinine clearance in older individuals enrolled in the Baltimore longitudinal study on aging: impact on renal drug dosing. *Pharmacotherapy.* 2013;33(9):912–921.

20. Schwartz GJ, Brion LP, Spitzer A. The use of plasma creatinine concentration for estimating glomerular filtration rate in infants, children and adolescents. *Pediatr Clin North Am.* 1987;34:571–590.

21. Schwartz GJ, Haycock GB, Edelmann CM Jr, et al. A simple estimate of glomerular filtration rate in children derived from body length and plasma creatinine. *Pediatrics.* 1976:104;259–263.

22. Schwartz GJ, Feld LG, Langford DJ. A simple estimate of glomerular filtration rate in full-term infants during the first year of life. *J Pediatr.* 1984;104:849–854.

23. Schwartz GJ, Gauthier B. A simple estimate of glomerular filtration rate in adolescent boys. *J Pediatr.* 1985;106:522–526.

24. Schwartz GJ, Muñoz A, Schneider MF, et al. New equations to estimate GFR in children with CKD. *J Am Soc Nephrol.* 2009;20(3):629–637.

25. Mitch WE, Collier VU, Walser M. Creatinine metabolism in chronic renal failure. *Clin Sci.* 1980;58:327.

26. Chow MS, Schweitzer R. Estimation of renal creatinine clearance in patients with unstable serum creatinine concentrations: comparisons of multiple methods. *Drug Intell Clin Pharm.* 1985;19:385–390.

27. Bleiler RE, Schedl HP. Creatinine excretion: variability and relationships to diet and body size. *J Lab Clin Med.* 1962;59:945.

28. Levey AS, Stevens LA, Schmid CH, et al. A new equation to estimate glomerular filtration rate. *Ann Intern Med.* 2009;150:604–612.

29. NKDEP National Disease Education Program. Laboratory Professionals Creatinine Standardization Program. Recommendations for Pharmacists and Authorized Drug Prescribers; July 2006. http://www.nkdep.nih.gov/labprofessionals/Pharmacists_and_Authorized_Drug_Prescribers.htm. Accessed June 28, 2008.

30. Melloni C, Peterson, ED, Chen AY, et al. Cockcroft-Gault versus modification of diet in renal disease. *J Am Coll Cardiol.* 2008;51:991–996.

31. Aweeka FT. Appendix: drug reference table. In: Schrier RW, Gambertoglio JG, eds. *Handbook of Drug Therapy in Liver and Kidney Disease.* Boston, MA: Little, Brown and Co.; 1991.

32. Takki S, Gambertoglio JG, Honda DH. Pharmacokinetic evaluation of hemodialysis in acute drug overdose. *J Pharmacokinet Biopharm.* 1978;6:427.

33. Lee CC, Marbury TC. Drug therapy in patients undergoing haemodialysis. Clinical pharmacokinetic considerations. *Clin Pharmacokinet.* 1984;9:42.

34. Maher JF. Pharmacokinetics in patients with renal failure. *Clin Nephrol.* 1984;21:39–46.

35. Gokal R, Hutchison A. Dialysis therapies for end-stage renal disease. *Semin Dial.* 2002;14:220–226.

36. Pallotta KE, Manley HJ. Vancomycin use in patients requiring hemodialysis: a literature review. *Semin Dial.* 2008;21:63–70.

37. Israni RK, Kasbekar N, Haynes K, et al. Use of antiepileptic drugs in patients with kidney disease. *Semin Dial.* 2006;19:408–416.

38. Renal Pharmacy Consultants, LLC. Dialysis of Drugs 2016 by Mason and Bailie. http://renalpharmacy consultants.com. Accessed August 02, 2017.

39. Decker BS, Mueller BA, Sowinski KM. Drug dosing considerations in alternative hemodialysis. *Adv Chronic Kidney Dis.* 2007;14:e17–e26.

40. Lanese DM, Alfrey PS, Molitoris BA, et al. Markedly increased clearance of vancomycin during hemodialysis using polysulfone dialyzers. *Kidney Int.* 1989;35:1409–1412.

41. Pollard TA, Lampasona V, Akkerman S, et al. Vancomycin redistribution: dosing recommendations following highflux hemodialysis. *Kidney Int.* 1994;45:232–237.

42. Zoer J, Schrander-van der Meer AM, van Dorp WT. Dosage recommendation of vancomycin during haemodialysis with highly permeable membranes. *Pharm World Sci.* 1997;19:191–196.

43. Gloper TA. Continuous arteriovenous hemofiltration in acute renal failure. *Am J Kidney Dis.* 1985;6:373–386.

44. Pattison ME, Lee SM, Ogden DA. Continuous arteriovenous hemodiafiltration: an aggressive approach to the management of acute renal failure. *Am J Kidney Dis.* 1988;11:43–47.

45. Pea F, Viale P, Furlanut M. Pharmacokinetic considerations for antimicrobial therapy in patients receiving renal replacement therapy. *Clin Pharmacokinet.* 2007;46:997–1038.

46. Bickley SK. Drug dosing during continuous arteriovenous hemofiltration. *Clin Pharm.* 1988;7:198–206.

47. Davies JG, Kingswood JC, Sharpstone P, et al. Drug removal in continuous haemofiltration and haemodialysis. *Br J Hosp Med.* 1995;12:524–528.

48. Bugge JF. Pharmacokinetics and drug dosing adjustments during continuous venovenous hemofiltration or hemodiafiltration in critically ill patients. *Acta Anaesthesiol Scand.* 2001;45:929–934.

49. Bohler J, Donauer J, Keller F. Pharmacokinetic principles during continuous renal replacement therapy: drugs and dosage. *Kidney Int Suppl.* 1999;72:S24–S28.

50. Reetze-Bonorden P, Bohler J, Keller E. Drug dosage in patients during continuous renal replacement therapy: pharmacokinetic and therapeutic considerations. *Clin Pharmacokinet.* 1993;24:362–379.

51. Golper TA, Marx MA. Drug dosing adjustments during continuous renal replacement therapies. *Kidney Int Suppl.* 1998;66:S165–S168.

52. Domoto DT, Brown WW, Bruggensmith P. Removal of toxic levels of N-acetyl procainamide with continuous arteriovenous hemofiltration or continuous arteriovenous hemodiafiltration. *Ann Intern Med.* 1987;106:550–552.

53. Fissell WH. Antimicrobial dosing in acute renal replacement. *Adv Chronic Kidney Dis.* 2013;20(1):85–93.

54. Lamier N, Bogaert M. Peritoneal pharmacokinetics and pharmacological manipulation of peritoneal transport. In: Gokal R, ed. *Continuous Ambulatory Peritoneal Dialysis.* New York: Churchill Livingstone; 1986:56–93.

55. Matzke GR, Millikin SP. Influence of renal function and dialysis on drug disposition. In: Evans WE, Schentag JJ, Jusko WJ, eds. *Applied Pharmacokinetics: Principles of Therapeutic Drug Monitoring.* 3rd ed. Vancouver, WA: Applied Therapeutics; 1992.

56. Mars RL, Moles K, Pope K, et al. Use of bolus intraperitoneal aminoglycosides for treating peritonitis in end-stage renal disease patients receiving continuous ambulatory peritoneal dialysis and continuous cycling peritoneal dialysis. *Adv Perit Dial.* 2000;16:280–284.

57. Thummel KE, Shen DD. Appendix II: design and optimization of dosage regimens: pharmacokinetic data. In: Hardman JG, ed. *Goodman and Gilman's The Pharmacologic Basis of Therapeutics.* 10th ed. New York: McGraw-Hill; 2001:1917–2023.

58. Matzke GR. Vancomycin. In: Evans WE, Schentag JJ, Jusko WJ, eds. *Applied Pharmacokinetics: Principles of Therapeutic Drug Monitoring.* 3rd ed. Vancouver, WA: Applied Therapeutics; 1992.

59. O'Brien MA, Mason NA. Systemic absorption of intra-peritoneal antimicrobials in continuous ambulatory peritoneal dialysis. *Clin Pharm.* 1992;11:256.

60. Voinescu CG, Khanna R. Peritonitis in peritoneal dialysis. *Int J Artif Organs.* 2002;25:249–260.

61. Keller E, Reetze P, Schollmeyer P. Drug therapy in patients undergoing continuous ambulatory peritoneal dialysis. Clinical and pharmacokinetic considerations. *Clin Pharmacokinet.* 1990;18:104–117.

62. Keane WF, Everett ED, Golper TA, et al. Peritoneal dialysis-related peritonitis treatment recommendations 1993 update. *Perit Dial Int.* 1993;13:14–28.

63. Wiggins KJ, Craig JC, Johnson DW, et al. Treatment for peritoneal dialysis associated peritonitis. *Cochrane Database Syst Rev.* 2008;23:CD005284.

4

PEDIATRICS

Irving Steinberg

Learning Objectives

By the end of the pediatrics chapter, the learner shall be able to:

1. Provide overarching perspective on the needs for specific pediatric pharmacokinetic studies and clinical application concepts, and differences between children and adults.
2. Describe physiologic and pathophysiologic factors affecting absorption of drugs from various routes of administration in different age groupings, including transporter maturation and genetic expression, and provide examples of specific drugs affected.
3. Detail the influence of size maturation, fluid compartment developmental changes, physicochemical properties, and protein binding variations on volume of distribution of drugs in children, and described population pharmacokinetic models for this parameter.
4. Specify differences in protein binding affinity and capacity in children versus adults that affects serum and tissue binding, and drug distribution.
5. Delineate the ontogeny of phase 1 and phase 2 metabolism and hepatic clearance, and provide specific examples of drugs where age-dependent clearance and pharmacogenetic expression impact the dosing and effect of therapeutic agents throughout childhood, and in contrast to adults.
6. Explain the developmental and pathophysiologic aspects of renal drug clearance through early postnatal life, and the impact on dosage regimen design through infancy and childhood.
7. Comprehend the need for and application of proper size scaling of pharmacokinetic parameters and resultant dosing in infants, children, and adolescents, and how scaling is incorporated into pediatric population pharmacokinetic modeling.

8. Provide examples where weight-based dosing or body surface area (BSA) dosing is preferred.
9. Illustrate the incorporation of size, maturation, organ function, disease, genetics, and other components into population models for initiation/modification of dosage regimens to target goal concentrations or systemic exposure in children, and demonstrate calculation competency in applying such modeled pharmacokinetic parameters.
10. Note selected differences in pharmacodynamics between children and adults, the consideration of pharmacokinetically guided dosing in treating pediatric disease states.

The days of describing pediatric patients as "therapeutic orphans," and when insufficient study of pediatric drug therapy was common, are effectively ending, if not already over. As of this writing, pediatric studies represent 21% of the total number, and 12% of the pharmacokinetic trials, listed on ClinicalTrials.gov.[1] The Best Pharmaceuticals for Children Act and Pediatric Research Equity Act, and other research and practice initiatives in the area of pediatric clinical pharmacology, have provided the incentive, funding, and practical information needed to escalate the rate of discovery and optimized usage of medications specific to the needs of children.[2,3] Within that framework is the constant need to "get the dose right" for children, and the requirement for study designs to address this need.[4,5]

Adverse drug effects may often be linked to pharmacokinetic and pharmacodynamic issues unique to the pediatric patient. Immaturity of glucuronidation pathways resulted in fatal chloramphenicol toxicity when adult dosages were being used in neonates. This led to initiatives of size and maturation adjustments in dosing, and initial therapeutic drug monitoring efforts to individualize the dose to reach safe therapeutic target concentrations.[6]

Pharmacokinetic inference via descriptive and population pharmacokinetic data and modeling has added to the sophistication of translational efforts to optimize dosing strategies for drugs to treat children with acute and chronic diseases effectively and safely. Furthermore, correlative studies of pharmacokinetic behavior linked to the pharmacodynamics and pharmacogenetics of the drug,[7] the disease state, and the patient, creates further specificity of the dose to obtain the desired therapeutic outcomes. While the same is held true for adults, in children, the complexities of maturation or organ function, changes in size and body habitus, varying manifestation of disease states, and receptor avidity and sensitivity are among features that impose six or seven overlapping pharmacokinetic and therapeutic populations, from the preterm neonate to the older adolescent, with organ dysfunction and clinical and laboratory parameters accounting for additional sources of variability in drug disposition.[8] Efforts to model these group differences, and the continuum of ontogeny in kinetic behavior of drugs, add pharmacometric precision toward managing the most vulnerable of patients through their illness, and assist regulatory agencies to approve drugs and biologic agents for pediatric use with translational data applied to practice.[9,10]

DRUG DISPOSITION AND ELIMINATION IN PEDIATRICS

Absorption

Developmental aspects of pharmacokinetics create impact and change throughout childhood. Absorption rate and/or extent of drugs from all extravascular administration modes tend to vary depending on gestational and postnatal age, and physiologic and anatomic maturation.[12–14]

At birth, newborns have a more neutral to alkaline gastric pH (pH 6 to 8) because of residual amniotic fluid in the stomach and inability of the stomach to express acid (achlorhydria). Gastric acid production increases over the next 24 to 48 hours to achieve adult pH levels, but then declines quickly, and acidity remains relatively low in the first months of life. Slow maturation of gastric acid secretion progresses through infancy until adult production is reached at around 2 years of age. Therefore, penicillins will have greater stomach epithelial permeation and decreased decomposition and, consequently, higher concentration in preterm and term neonates compared to older children. In contrast, decreased oral bioavailability of weak acids (e.g., phenobarbital, phenytoin) and weak bases with low pKa (e.g., itraconazole) is observed. Slower rates of absorption may be accounted for by delayed biphasic gastric emptying, with adult values reached at about 6 to 8 months of age, by irregular peristalsis, or by outlet obstructions such as pyloric stenosis. Gastric emptying time is slower for preterm compared with term infants, and is more than halved from postconceptional ages (PCAs) of 28 to 36 weeks until 42 to 54 weeks.[15] Therefore, prolonged drug action within a dosing interval may result from a longer time to maximum concentration. Additionally, shorter bowel length than adults can diminish the capability to fully absorb sustained-release medications.

Reduced exocrine function occurs in newborns with low lipase production, and despite increased circulating bile acids, there is immature transporter-mediated secretion resulting in low biliary canalicular transport and intestine luminal bile acid concentrations, which can limit oral absorption of fat-soluble drugs such as oral corticosteroids. Additionally, pediatric diseases of exocrine function (e.g., cystic fibrosis) or biliary disruption (e.g., biliary atresia) are conditions where fat malabsorption of nutrients (e.g., vitamins A, D, E, and K) and lipid-soluble drugs is expected.

Other transporter maturation and intestinal metabolic and functional status influences absorption and disposition. The iron transporter DMT1 increases linearly with age in children, with the percent of iron absorbed being the lowest in those less than 6 months old.[16] Immaturity of gastrointestinal MDR1 efflux leads to higher zidovudine bioavailability in the first 14 days of life (89%) compared to those >14 days to 12 years old (61%).[17] Intestinal activity of CYP1A1 and CYP3A appears to increase with age, with less presystemic intestinal clearance in young children. Intestinal glutathione conjugation is at its highest in 1- to 3-year olds, as observed in distal duodenal biopsies of measured glutathione conjugates of the antineoplastic agent, busulfan.[18] Intestinal p-glycoprotein expression is reduced in infants, allowing more oral bioavailability.

In contrast, OATP2B1 expression is increased in young infants, with greater bioavailability for substrates such as oral methotrexate.[19] Additionally, degradation by intestinal flora, as for digoxin, is already evident in infancy and is age dependent. Sepsis, short-gut syndrome, and administration via jejunostomy tube are additional situations where oral bioavailability may be compromised for some drugs. Intramuscular absorption may be variable and ineffective in neonates because of autonomic and vasomotor instability, with relative regional blood flow changes, and inefficient muscular contractions. However, in infants, drugs such as epinephrine, cephalosporins and aminoglycosides can achieve adequate peak concentrations when given intramuscularly, relying on the 25% to 50% increase in capillary density. Rectal uptake of drugs in neonates and infants is reliable in providing systemic concentrations adequate for clinical effect (e.g., acetaminophen, diazepam). Skin penetration of many topically administered drugs is often better than it is for adults, with the hydration of the skin and thinness of the stratum corneum as fundamental to allowing more diffusion through the skin barrier compared with older children and adults.[13] Methemoglobinemia seen more frequently with EMLA (topical prilocaine and lidocaine eutectic mixture), adverse systemic effects of topical antihistamines and corticosteroids, and topical anesthetic toxicity are examples of the greater risk seen in young infants because of enhanced percutaneous absorption.

Distribution and protein binding

Generally, drugs have a wider range of weight-normalized distribution volumes in pediatric patients than in adults. One of the major differentiating factors among pediatric and adult patients across the age span is the continual changes in body habitus, especially body fluid compartments and the influence this creates on the distribution volume of medications (Fig. 4.1).[11–14] Additional alterations from pathophysiologic states that augment fluid and tissue compartments; electrolyte and extracellular fluid protein content; and inflammation and capillary integrity, can be observed to alter pharmacokinetic disposition of drugs in similar fashion, if not magnitude, as in adults.

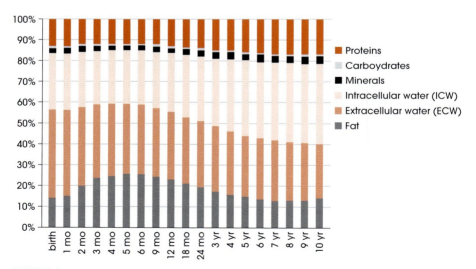

FIGURE 4.1   Changes in body composition over time during childhood. (From Jong G. Pediatric development: physiology. Enzymes, rug metabolism, pharmacokinetics and pharmacodynamics. In: Bar-Shalom D, Rose K, eds. *Pediatric Formulations: A Roadmap, AAPS Advances in the Pharmaceutical Sciences Series* 11;2014:9–23.)

Premature neonates have the highest body water to total body weight ratio, and the same is true for their extracellular fluid to weight relationship. The former has implication for drugs that distribute to a space commensurate with total body water (e.g., phenytoin, 1 to 1.5 L/kg in neonates), and the latter to those distributing to extracellular fluid spaces (e.g., aminoglycosides, 0.4 to 0.5 L/kg). The progressive decreases in the weight ratio of these fluid compartments with age will translate to linear or exponential decreases in the volume of distribution normalized to body weight of these drugs as the child matures to adolescence. Therefore, incremental doses standardized to body weight for drugs such as gentamicin (e.g., 4 to 5 mg/kg) and vancomycin (e.g., 15 to 20 mg/kg) will be higher in the neonate and infant in order to reach similar peak concentrations as those obtained at lower per kg doses in adolescents and adults (gentamicin dose = 1.5 to 2.5 mg/kg; vancomycin dose = 8 to 15 mg/kg).

Serum protein binding differences may also play a role in the differences seen in V_d, with more unbound drug available to leave the intravascular space and bind with receptor and nonreceptor tissue. In neonates, reduced albumin binding capacity results from lower quantity (e.g., 2 to 3 g/dL) and retained fetal albumin, which has less affinity for binding than normal albumin. Cefazolin has twice the average unbound fraction in neonates compared to adults,[20] and saturability of albumin binding is seen for this drug in neonates, but not typical of adults.[21] Disease states occurring predominantly in pediatric patients such as nephrotic syndrome, protein-losing enteropathy, and Kawasaki disease demonstrate significant hypoalbuminemia and diminished drug protein binding, potentially altering the kinetics and dynamics of drugs such as furosemide, mycophenolic acid, and aspirin.

Likewise, lower concentration of α_1-acid glycoprotein (AAG) in infancy is responsible for reduced protein binding of basic drugs (e.g., meperidine, fentanyl, propranolol, and lidocaine).[22] This allows for more free drug to interact with receptors and increases the potency of effect for any given weight-based dose when compared with older children and adults. This must be factored into assessing dosage needs to meet therapeutic endpoints. Some drugs, such as clindamycin, show impact of reductions in both albumin and AAG quantity, and resultant reduced protein binding, on the volume of distribution (V_d) in infants.[23] In children with sickle cell disease, increases in AAG as a result of pain crises can yield less analgesic effect of meperidine at customary doses, because the higher binding will produce less unbound meperidine.[24] Yet, the need for higher doses is met with higher repository of bound meperidine for conversion to the neurotoxic normeperidine metabolite that can cause seizures (particularly in those patients with renal compromise who accumulate normeperidine while on patient-controlled analgesia).[25]

Other binding capacity differences may comparatively reduce serum protein binding in pediatric patients. Vancomycin was shown to have lower serum binding than three groups of adults with critical care, orthopedic, and hematologic diseases.[26] Unbound fractions averaged 81% in the pediatric group versus 56% to 62% among the adults groups. Multivariate modeling revealed total vancomycin and albumin concentrations as expected predictors of unbound concentration in all four groups, but immunoglobulin A (IgA) concentration was a significant variable only for the adult patient groups, where the IgA concentrations were 3- to 7.5-fold higher than in the pediatric patients. Lower trough level targets of 7 to 10 mg/L are seen as beneficial in achieving pharmacodynamics endpoints (e.g., area under the curve to minimum inhibitory concentration [AUC/MIC] ratio $\geq$ 400) in children when compared to those suggested for adults. The higher unbound fraction may contribute to the clinical and microbiologic success of vancomycin therapy at these serum concentration and systemic exposure measures. Binding interactions of particular concern in pediatrics include the disruption of the albumin binding of high concentrations of bilirubin (and the potential risk of kernicterus) in the young infant by highly bound drugs, such as sulfisoxazole, ceftriaxone, salicylates, and others.[27]

Tissue binding differences can also translate into altered pharmacodynamic response. Infants have threefold greater number of erythrocyte (and by association, myocardial) receptors for digoxin, and a two times higher dissociation constant, leading to relative insensitivity compared with older children and adults.[28] Additionally, greater tissue binding leads to a volume of distribution of digoxin averaging 12.8 L/kg in patients 2 to 3 months old, and 16.2 L/kg in 1.3- to 5–year-old (compared with a typical 7 L/kg in adults).[29] Therefore, doses of digoxin to treat cardiac arrhythmias or heart failure in young infants are 8 to 15 mcg/kg/day, as compared with 2 to 4 mcg/kg/day for adults.[30]

Metabolism and excretion

Maturation of phase 1 and phase 2 metabolic pathways occurs at differing rates in neonates, infants, and children until adult rates are achieved or, for some pathways, surpassed.[12-14,31-33] Evidence of primordial drug metabolic enzymes and activity exists in the fetus. CYP3A7 is present at 50 to 60 days PCA, peaks within 1-week postnatal age, and then diminishes rapidly to be replaced with developing levels of the similar-acting CYP3A4. This creates a shift in the dominant metabolite of male hormones before and after birth.[34] Whereas CYP2E1, CYP2C19, and CYP2D6 show activity within hours to days, CYP2C9, CYP3A4, and CYP1A2 are delayed in onset of activity and maturation (see Fig. 4.2).[32] Note that the capacity for CYP3A4, CYP3A5, CYP2C9, CYP2C19, and CYP1A2 reach 150% to 200% of adult values in early childhood.[32] Probe drugs such as theophylline provide example to the development of drug metabolism. With CYP2E1 functional early in postnatal life, the major metabolite of theophylline is 1,3-dimethyluric acid, with more primitive pathways such a methylation represented (producing the active metabolite, caffeine early in postnatal life), along with reliance of unchanged drug elimination via the kidney (Table 4.1).[35] With maturation, these latter pathways reduce or disappear, and the enhancement of 1,3-dimethyluric acid is observed with the contributions of the later-developing CYP1A2 and CYP3A4 pathways; the former isoenzyme also contributing to 1-methyluric acid and 3-methylxanthine metabolite production, and less unchanged drug being renally excreted.[35] Similarly, phenobarbital metabolism is slow in the neonate and young infant because of immaturity of CYP2C9 and CYP2C19 oxidation pathways, with elimination half-lives in the range of 100 to 140 hours, and diminishing an average of 4.6 hr/day to a half-life of 60 to 70 hours by 4 weeks' postnatal age.[36]

Dextromethorphan is another probe drug to examine the ontogeny of metabolism. Because CYP2D6 matures faster than CYP3A4, the O-demethylation of dextromethor-phan exceeds that of N-demethylation derived from CYP3A4 metabolism during the

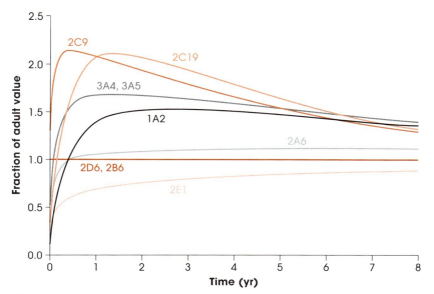

FIGURE 4.2   Maturations rates of noted cytochrome p450 enzymes as a percentage of adult activity. Data represents meta-analysis of in vivo determinations from multiple sources. (From Upreti VV, Wahlstrom JL. Meta-analysis of hepatic cytochrome P450 ontogeny to underwrite the prediction of pediatric pharmacokinetics using physiologically based pharmacokinetic modeling. *J Clin Pharmacol.* 2016;56(3):266–283.)

first 2 to 3 months of infancy. These pathways produce these metabolites equivalently after 4 months, and by 1 year the CYP3A4 products exceed those of CYP2D6.[37] Although CYP3A4 becomes a more dominant pathway in the maturing child for substrate drugs such as midazolam, critical illness may temporally negatively affect this metabolic potential.[32]

Even anatomy may define differing clearance values. Liver weight to body weight ratio is higher in children than in adults, peaking at 2 to 3 years of age. Therefore, it is not surprising that with a full complement of liver microsomal enzymes and wild-type genetic expression, that the metabolic clearance of many drugs when standardized to body weight is higher in ages 2-year to pre-adolescence than in adults. Warfarin clearance

TABLE 4.1   Molar Mean % Recovery of Theophylline and Its Metabolites in Urine, and Clearance Values, after Multiple Doses Given to Infants[35]

POSTCONCEPTIONAL AGE (wk)	THEO	3-MX	1-MU	1,3-diMU	CAFFEINE	CLEARANCE (mL/hr/kg)
30–40	55.2	1.4	8.2	24.0	8.5	21.5
40–50	32.6	5.0	11.1	42.3	3.3	30.3
>50	17.9	12.8	22.0	43.7	0.8	60.7

3-MX, 3-methyxanthine; 1-MU, 1-methyluric acid; 1,3-diMU, 1, 3 dimethyluric acid.

is a good example of this, where prepubertal children are observed to have higher weight-standardized clearances than adults, but when standardized to liver weight, as assessed by ultrasonography, these clearances were not significantly different.[38] Other hepatically cleared drugs have also shown no relationship between liver weight-normalized clearance and age.[39] This provides partial reasoning for allometric scaling of body weight as a preferable size function to quantitatively relate to clearance (see further discussion).

Phase 2 metabolism is mostly subject to maturation influences. Sulfation and acetylation capacity are present very early in life. The balance of predominant sulfation to mostly glucuronidation of acetaminophen shifts during childhood. Modeling of metabolites formation clearances in neonates of varying gestational ages demonstrated at an average of 1-week postnatal age a clearance by sulfation of 0.21 L/hr, by glucuronidation of 0.049 L/hr, and by oxidation of 0.058 L/hr. The fraction by oxidation increased by less than 15% through the restricted PCA range studied.[40] The efficiency of metabolism in young children is noted by the comparative lack of toxicity of acetaminophen acute overdose because of the protection of higher conjugation capacity (sulfation and glucuronidation), but greater risk of severe toxicity from chronic supratherapeutic dosing in this age group owing to higher p450 enzyme metabolism to the toxic intermediate, combined with less conjugation if the child is continually ill and not ingesting adequate food substrate.[41] Moreover, serum concentrations of acetaminophen dose of 160 mg recommended by the manufacturer for ages 2 to 3 (11 to 16 kg) were simulated using a population pharmacokinetic model and found to be inadequate at achieving therapeutic levels, and, therefore, weight-based dosing of 10 to 15 mg/kg/dose is preferred.[42] In contrast, the cardiotonic agent amrinone's clearance was shown to be age independent in children 1 to 24 months of age, which is unusual for the great majority of drugs where age- or size-dependent elimination is observed.[43] The early presence of acetylation of amrinone produces a metabolite that causes thrombocytopenia even in the youngest infants. Therefore, the particular metabolic pathway, its efficiency, and the production of active versus inactive metabolites must be evaluated for the individual drug and assessed for age and maturation.

UGT 1A1 matures fairly early; bilirubin conjugation is only 1% of adult values at gestational ages of 30 to 40 weeks (hence the risk of unconjugated hyperbilirubinemia and kernicterus in that age group early after birth), which then accelerates rapidly to adult values obtained at 2 to 4 months.[44] Slightly more delayed are UGT 1A6 and UGT 2B7, which mature with half-maximal adult values at 50.1 and 54.6 weeks' postmenstrual age.[45,46] UGT 2B7-mediated glucuronidation of the antiretroviral zidovudine increasing rapidly after 40 weeks' PCA, with adult clearance values of around 20 mL/min/kg reached at 46 to 52 weeks' PCA,[47] whereas others describe full maturation values occurring through the first 2 years of life.[44,47] Slower maturation rates are seen in premature infants.[48] Additionally, the expression of transporters that allow incorporating of drugs into or pumping out of organs of elimination or receptor sites, such as OCT1, OATP1B3, and p-glycoprotein, is low in neonates and steadily increases during childhood, gaining near-adult values during adolescence.[19,49,50] This, combined with immaturity in pathways expression, may diminish metabolism and conversion to active and inactive metabolites.

As an example, morphine clearances ranges from 1.7 mL/min/kg in premature neonates 24 weeks' PCA weighing 0.5 kg, to 2.5 mL/min/kg in a 1 kg neonate at 28 weeks'

PCA, to 3.5 mL/min/kg in a 2 kg infant at 32 weeks' PCA.[51] Morphine is metabolized to morphine 6-glucuronide (M6G) through the action of UGT, and its developmental immaturity yields lower production in young infants.[52] Because M6G is three to five times more potent as an analgesic but the production is less, more of the analgesic effect must come from the parent drug, and, therefore, despite an immature blood–brain barrier, the morphine EC50 is (paradoxically) higher in neonates than in older children and adults.[52] However, with continued therapy, immature renal function begins to play a larger role, and any formation of M6G is inadequately cleared, accumulates, and begins to contribute to the overall pharmacodynamic effect. Moreover, immature p-glycoprotein expression and diminished blood–brain barrier protection enhance brain sensitivity to morphine.[19] Therefore, morphine dosing later in therapy may need to be reduced if accumulation of M6G creates a toxicity risk.

Additionally, lower OCT1 activity (responsible for drug transport into the liver cell) would predict decreased incorporation into the liver for glucuronidation,[49,50,53] further limiting M6G production.[52] This is true not only for young infants but exists with the pharmacogenetic differences observed between African-American and Caucasian children. Decreased function OCT1 alleles are more common in Caucasian children,[54] and with the demonstrated comparative diminished clearance, the potential for more adverse reactions in Caucasian children could be anticipated. This may account for African-American children needing significantly more analgesic interventions, and having higher maximum pain scores and opioid requirements than Caucasian children in a large study of post-tonsillectomy pain study.[55] Despite lower opioid doses, the Caucasian children had greater opioid-related adverse effects. The pharmacogenetic factors can be mathematically incorporated into pediatric population models, as has been performed for warfarin, tacrolimus, and voriconazole,[56–58] with varying genetic penetrance, clearance influence, and clinical implementation.[7]

Concerns over the balance of pharmacogenetically endowed CYP2D6 and UGT2B7 activity with codeine use, especially in ultrafast metabolizers, has resulted in diminished use[59] and a recent call for the restriction of its use in pediatric patients,[60] especially those with respiratory problems or in breastfeeding infants exposed via mothers using codeine, particularly with use for a longer number of days.[61] Ultrafast CYP2D6 metabolizers of codeine can more quickly convert codeine into the more potent morphine.[62] This has resulted in deaths reported in breastfeeding infants of mothers with alleles for ultrafast conversion and augmented p-glycoprotein activity,[63] and for children with these alleles exposed to codeine after tonsillectomy and adenoidectomy,[64] when the child's airway is more vulnerable to respiratory depression. Little ability to determine at-risk children is available beyond use pattern and pharmacogenetic testing.[61,62]

Renal elimination begins in utero with the development of renal structures and urine production as early as at 9 weeks. Full nephrogenesis occurs at 34 to 36 weeks, and those born prematurely will need to complete development ex utero.[65–67] Perinatal sepsis or hypoxia can stunt this maturation and further delay renal elimination of drugs. Postnatal glomerular filtration rate (GFR) development has a flatter upward trajectory in lower birthweight preterm neonates than those with higher birthweight, and steeper still in full-term newborns. Small-for-gestational-age neonates have a reduced GFR and renal drug clearance compared to normal weight neonates of comparable gestational age.[67,68] Three- to fourfold increases in GFR (from 15 to 20 increases to 60 mL/min/1.73 m^2)

are seen in full-term normally developed neonates during the first month of life,[65,66] because increases in cardiac output and renal blood flow, and diminished renovascular resistance, lead to more peripheral glomerular perfusion to the more abundant cortical nephrons. As with the liver, kidney weight to body weight ratio also peaks at 2 to 3 years of age.[67] Models to describe the nonlinear increases in GFR during the first months of life have been developed.[69] The postmenstrual age at which GFR reaches 50% of adult values is estimated at 47.7 weeks (or about 8 weeks' postnatal age in a full-term infant), with continued increases during infancy, achieving maximum values for body surface area (BSA)–normalized GFR at 2 to 6 years of age. Consequently, the elimination half-life of the renally cleared drug acyclovir falls from approximately 13 hours in infants of 26 weeks' postmenstrual age to 4 hours at 40 weeks' postmenstrual age.[70] As with the liver, the kidney weight to body weight ratio also peaks at 2 to 3 years of age,[67] forecasting that the fastest half-lives of drugs such as cephalosporins, aminoglycosides, vancomycin, levetiracetam, and acyclovir are observed in early childhood. Renal impairment will predictably slow elimination as in adults, and doses should be tailored to estimated or measured creatinine clearance.[8] There are a large number of equations used to calculate creatinine clearance in children, from linear to power function to quadratic formulae, with widely varying precision, and used in first approximations of GFR and renal drug clearance.[71] Although higher in output quantity, tubular secretion maturation rate initially lags behind that of GFR maturation, but equals or exceeds it after 2 to 3 months' postnatal age, and until adult values are reaches at 1 year of age.[67] Tubular secretion can also be induced when young infants are exposed to drugs using the carboxylic acid secretion pathway for clearance (e.g., penicillin, furosemide).[72]

Gestational age, postnatal age, weight, and serum creatinine all can have individual or collective influence on the ability of infants and children to eliminate drugs renally (thought the maternal contribution of creatinine during the first couple of days of postnatal life may create a falsely low drug clearance to creatinine clearance relationship).[8] As an example, fluconazole population modeling in infants 23 to 40 weeks' gestation and less than 120 days' postnatal age revealed that all four of the above factors were statistically significant in a population pharmacokinetic model of fluconazole in infants.[73] Many such population models exist for commonly used drugs in pediatric patients, and further construction and applications of these models will be discussed below.

Other factors that impact on renal elimination of drugs (via glomerular filtration, renal blood flow, or tubular secretion) in children are similar to those in adults. Combining these factors with those of maturation gives a more comprehensive evaluation of clearance. As seen in Figure 4.3, the aminoglycoside antibiotic amikacin clearance develops through renal maturation both on a gestational or an antenatal development basis, and on a postnatal maturation basis.[74] If ibuprofen is given to the infant for the indication of patent ductus arteriosis, this can reduce renal blood flow and blunt the magnitude increase in clearance within each developmental time period. Predictive pharmacokinetic modeling of one renally cleared drug can also help to predict the clearance development of other such drugs in the target population.[75] Furthermore, augmented renal clearance has been recently demonstrated in children, as seen with more rapid clearance of vancomycin in neurotrauma and pediatric cancer patients, and amoxicillin-clavulanic acid in critically ill children.[76–78] This requires increases in dosage or more frequent administration to meet target concentrations or exposure.

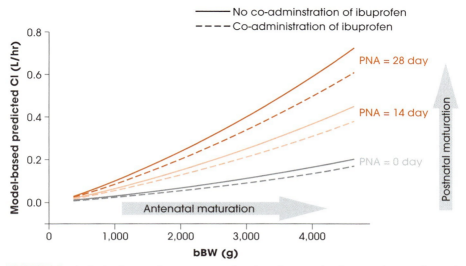

FIGURE 4.3   Amikacin clearance in neonates as a function of antenatal and postnatal maturation, and influence of ibuprofen on renal elimination.[8,74] PNA, postnatal age.

PEDIATRIC DOSING: PHARMACOKINETIC SCALING AND MODELING

It is obvious that some method of downsizing doses from adults to children is necessary to provide systemic exposure that will at least equate to those of adults in attempting to achieve similar pharmacologic effect (presuming little differences in pharmacodynamic response).[79,80] Yet, old rules such as Clark's rule for downsizing doses do not mathematically account properly for variables such as weight, BSA, age, organ function, disease, and genetics of the child, nor the physicochemical properties of the drug in assigning the proper dose to be administered.[81] These variables, their expression and maturation over time, and their manifold changes during the composite of childhood, must be assessed for their linear and nonlinear properties in relation to pharmacokinetic parameters such as clearance and volume of distribution (Table 4.2). This will allow for better a priori estimation of these parameters, and improved empiric dosing, to meet therapeutic, laboratory, or other measured targets of efficacy while avoiding toxicity. Unique pharmacodynamics in children may further pose differences between adult and pediatric dose scaling.[82]

Weight-based dosing (e.g., mg/kg) is a logical step toward downsizing, but still needs to be related in many cases to maturation, organ function, and other variables in order to more precisely assign the dose needed.[83] The Joint Commission requires weight-based dosing drug protocols in all accredited hospitals treating children.[84] However, as shown earlier for theophylline, digoxin, and aminoglycosides, weight-normalized clearance values vary by age, and selection of a weight-based daily dose often needs to be grouped by ages sharing similar average clearance values (e.g., mL/min/kg). Nonstandardized drug clearances (e.g., mL/min) are generally not linear with weight or age, and the efficiency of metabolism and renal elimination of many drugs chronologically matures, peaks,

TABLE 4.2   Pharmacokinetic Alterations in Childhood

PHYSIOLOGIC SYSTEM	TRENDS RELATED TO AGE	PHARMACOKINETIC IMPLICATION	CLINICAL IMPLICATIONS
GI tract	Neonates and young infants: reduced and irregular peristalsis followed by slow gastric emptying Neonates: increased gastric pH (>4) in relation to infants Infants: increased motility of lower GI	Slower absorption of the drug (e.g., elevated Tmax) • Faster absorption of acid labile drugs (e.g., penicillin G, erythromycin) • Reduced absorption of weak-acid drugs (e.g., phenobarbital, phenytoin) • Decreased retention of suppositories	Possible sustained action after oral administration of the drug Possible altered bioavailability ↓ rectal bioavailability
Skin	Neonates and young infants: a thinner stratum corneum (neonates), increased skin perfusion, increased water content and higher BSA to weight ratio	• ↑ Rate and extent of absorption through the skin during infancy • Higher systemic exposure to drugs for topical use in relation to adults (e.g., corticosteroids)	Increased bioavailability and potential toxicity of drugs applied topically; need for a reduced amount of the drug applied to the skin and care in application
Muscle tissue	Neonates: reduction in muscle perfusion, decreased muscle contractility Infants: higher density of capillaries in skeletal muscles	Neonates: poor perfusion limits the absorption, unpredictable PK Infants: ↑ absorption	Neonates: avoid IM administration of drugs Infants: effectiveness of drugs applied IM is higher (e.g., epinephrine)
Spatial compartments	Neonates and infants: lower proportion of adipose tissue (10%), ↓ muscle mass, ↑ amount of water related to the body weight (80%), and ↑ proportion of the extracellular fluid (45%) as compared to the intracellular fluid	Neonates: ↑ V_d for water-soluble drugs (e.g., gentamicin), and a reduced V_d of drugs that bind to muscles and adipose tissue (e.g., morphine, propofol)	Necessary to adjust the loading/maintenance dosing (mg/kg) to achieve therapeutic concentrations of drug in plasma

TABLE 4.2 Pharmacokinetic Alterations in Childhood (*continued*)

PHYSIOLOGIC SYSTEM	TRENDS RELATED TO AGE	PHARMACOKINETIC IMPLICATION	CLINICAL IMPLICATIONS
Plasma protein binding	Neonates: reduced concentrations of albumin and α_1-acid glycoprotein, with a decreased drug protein binding affinity relative to children and adults; residual fetal albumin in early neonatal period less capable of binding drugs	Increased plasma concentration of unbound drug, with increased V_d and the possibility of occurrence of toxic effects; lower total plasma concentration for low-extraction ratio drugs in children with efficient intrinsic metabolism	For drugs with high binding affinity for proteins (e.g., >80%), it is necessary to adjust the dose to maintain the drug levels in the plasma close to the lower limit of the recommended therapeutic range
Drug metabolism	Neonates and young infants: immature isoform of cytochrome P450 and phase 2 enzymes with harsh developmental expression	Neonates and young infants: reduced hepatic drug metabolism, with increase in half-life	Neonates and young infants: increase dosage interval of drug and/or reduce maintenance dose
	Children aged 1–6 yr: apparent increased activity of certain enzymes over the normal values for adults	Children aged 1–6 yr: enhanced drug clearance (e.g., decrease in half-life) for the specific pharmacologic substrates	Children aged 1–6 yr: for certain drugs is necessary to increase the dose and/or reduce the dosage interval compared to recommended adult dose
Renal drug excretion	Neonates and young infants: decreased GFR (first 6 mo) and active tubular secretion (first 12 mo). Adult values are achieved by the 24th month of life	Neonates and young infants: accumulation of drugs that are secreted via the kidneys and/or the active metabolite; ↓ plasma clearance and ↑ half-life during early infancy	Neonates and young infants: ↑ dosage interval and/or reduce maintenance dose during early infancy

Modified from Samardzic J, Allegaert K, Bajcetic M. Developmental pharmacology: a moving target. *Int J Pharm*. 2015;15;492(1–2):335–337. Copyright 2015, with permisson from Elsevier.
GI, gastrointestinal; BSA, body surface area; PK, pharmacokinetic; IM, intramuscular; GFR, glomerular filtration rate.

and deceases across the pediatric and adolescent age spectrum (see Fig. 4.4). Alternate expressions of size attempt to encompass more patients across pediatrics age groups.

BSA dosing in children has been used successfully for more fat-soluble drugs with wide distribution volumes and hepatic metabolism, and is traditionally applied to numerous antineoplastic agents.[85,86] Use of BSA for PK parameterization follows similar standardization of physiologic parameters such as cardiac output and GFR, and attempts to reduce age-related differences in clearance values.[87] For some agents, such

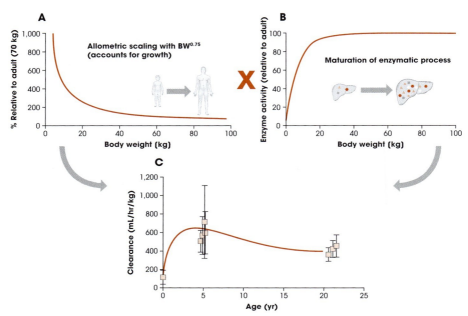

FIGURE 4.4 Influence of scaling of size and maturation of elimination pathways create typical pattern of drug clearance manifested throughout childhood. Pharmacogenetic expression may be more significant than maturation in determining transporter, metabolic, and elimination pathway efficiencies than maturation as the child develops. (From Samant TS, Mangal N, Lukacova V, et al. Quantitative clinical pharmacology for size and age scaling in pediatric drug development: a systematic review. *J Clin Pharmacol.* 2015;55(11):1207–1217, with permission.)

as the antiarrhythmic sotalol, the volume of distribution and clearance both correlate best with BSA,[88] and dosing per BSA can be used throughout childhood and adolescence for those greater than 0.33 m², providing the same AUC as seen in adults.[89] Use of BSA may, however, provide for imprecise dosing in morbidly obese patients where drugs may only have fractional penetration into adipose tissue,[90,91] reduced enzymatic clearances impacted by in nonalcoholic fatty liver disease,[92] or alterations in clearance of active metabolites, as is seen for with a 30% reduced clearance in obese children of doxorubicinol, a cardiotoxic metabolite of doxorubicin.[93] Adjustments of antineoplastic drug dosing from BSA to weight based is recommended for children less than 3 years of age to avoid hepatoxicity and vaso-occlusive disease.[94] Higher incidence of vincristine neurotoxicity is exhibited when dosing in infants is based on BSA, with additional contribution of reduced vincristine CYP35A clearance in this age group.[95] Additionally, prednisone doses calculated using BSA administered to children with nephrotic syndrome are not equivalent to per kg doses for those who weigh less than 30 kg, with children who weigh 10 kg and receiving a standard dose of 60 mg/m²/day achieving a 3.5 mg/kg/day dosage, well above the recommended 2 mg/kg/day for achieving remission.[96] A randomized trial of children with nephrotic syndrome comparing daily doses of 60 mg/m² with 2 mg/kg found no significant differences in time to remission, but more hypertension was observed in the BSA-adjusted dose group,[97] and advocacy for the weight-based dose was posited.[98]

More difficulty exists for polar drugs with restricted volumes of distribution when BSA dosing is utilized, particularly in children less than 2 years. In these younger children, the BSA to volume ratio increases with decreased age, and the relationship of weight to BSA shifts with age.[87] Bias is highest and precision is least when BSA is used to scale adult doses to infants for water-soluble, renally-cleared drugs.[99] This can prove dangerous for drugs like acyclovir. As an example, if BSA is calculated from the 50th percentile weights and heights for age in boys, handbook-suggested doses of 1,500 mg/m^2/day would yield acyclovir doses of 89.5, 84.2, and 81.1 mg/kg/day in 1-, 2-, and 3-month-old infants, respectively, well above the 60 mg/kg/day dose established in clinical studies in young infants as safe and effective.[100] Doses in excess of 60 mg/kg/day or 1,500 mg/m^2/day have been associated with increased evidence of acute kidney injury.[101]

Better attempts to scale size in pediatric patients and bridge to pharmacokinetic parameter estimates in pediatric age groups and extrapolate to adults are through use of allometric scaling, in analogy to interspecies scaling performed to assign initial drug doses in human trials based on physiologic and pharmacokinetic animal study.[102,103] The general expression for this using clearance as the parameter as a power model:

$$Cl = a \cdot (Wt)^b$$

where "a" is the coefficient and b the exponent that relate size (in this case weight) to clearance. This can be expanded and related to adults as:

$$Cl_{child} = Cl_{adult} \, (Wt_{child}/Wt_{adult})^{0.75}$$

Although 0.75 is commonly used and validated as a workable exponent,[99,102,103] this applies best when relating a child's clearance to that of an adult for more renally cleared drugs and in children $\geq$1 years old. For hepatically eliminated agents, 0.75 consistently provided little prediction error when used in children aged 2 years and older.[104] As simulations and compiled data reveal, the exponent for clearance can deviate moderately or greatly away from 0.75 for certain drugs, and approaches 1 to 1.2 in infants and neonates.[105] Serum protein binding and alterations in hepatic enzyme and drug transporter performance can further modify this exponent relationship.[104] Therefore, deriving the specific exponent for clearance of each drug may ultimately be more useful for empiric and Bayesian dosing of that drug in individual patients. An exponent of approximately 1 is often acceptable for most drugs for volume of distribution (i.e., a linear function of weight).

The selection and application of allometric exponents, or other size descriptors, can be used more effectively when other maturation and organ function variables are added to the model.[106] Maturation parameters can be added to size descriptors to produce useful models for infants.

Example—maturation model

A 4.5-month-old 7-kg infant with a normal-for-age serum creatinine of 0.35 mg/dL, born at 8 months' gestation, is given vancomycin attempting to target an AUC$_{24hr}$ of

400 mg · hr/L to provide effective therapy of staphylococcal bacteremia. What dose would you empirically start?

$$Cl_{child} = Cl_{adult} \times \left(\frac{Wt}{70}\right)^{0.75} \times \frac{(PCA)^{\Theta}}{(PCA)^{\Theta} + (TM_{50})^{\Theta}} \qquad \textbf{(Eq. 4.1)}$$

Vancomycin maturation parameters[107]:

Cl adult = 93.5 mL/min/70 kg
PCA = Postconceptional age (gestational + postnatal ages)
TM50 = PCA at which Cl is 50% of adult values = 9.5 months
Θ = Hill coefficient $\approx$ 3.4

$$Cl_{child} = 93.5 \times \left(\frac{7}{70}\right)^{0.75} \times \frac{(12.5)^{3.4}}{(12.5)^{3.4} + (9.5)^{3.4}}$$

$$= 93.5 \times 0.1778 \times 0.7177$$

$$= 11.93 \text{ mL/min}$$

$$= 0.716 \text{ L/hr}$$

The dose can then be calculated using Equation 4.2 to achieve the targeted AUC.

$$\text{Dose (mg)} = Cl(\text{L/hr})(\text{Target AUC}_{24hr} \text{ in mg} \cdot \text{h/L}) \qquad \textbf{(Eq. 4.2)}$$

$$= 0.716 \text{ L/hr} \times 400 \text{ mg} \cdot \text{h/L}$$

$$= 286.3 \text{ mg/day}$$

$$= 40.9 \text{ mg/kg/day}$$

Likewise, the mathematical description of the function of the organs of elimination provides numeric input for calculating drug clearance and the dose needed to reach target exposure. For example, valganciclovir for cytomegalovirus prophylaxis in solid organ transplant patients was one of the first examples of a package insert containing a population pharmacokinetic model to calculate the dose of a drug for a pediatric patient[108]:

$$\text{Pediatric Dose (mg)} = 7 \times \text{BSA} \times Cl_{Cr} \text{ (in mL/min/1.73 m}^2\text{)}.$$

The essence of pharmacokinetic modeling is to find statistically associated variables that best explain the kinetic parameters and their variability in a group or population, and mathematically quantify these relationships.[109] In pediatrics, because of the clinical and ethical limits on drawing blood, having validated population pharmacokinetic models that can be used in a Bayesian framework, without and then with serum concentration feedback, can provide for more assured initial and adjusted dosing of drugs in children, particularly where a narrow therapeutic range and therapeutic drug monitoring applies.[110,111] Microdosing (ultra-low dose, radiolabeled medication)[112] and microsampling (utilizing dried blood spots)[113] are techniques that have been applied to infants and children to model kinetic parameters while sparing potentially toxic exposure and multiple blood draws.[114]

Taking into account the features of size, maturation and organ function provides for a general approach to modeling clearance in infants and children that can be linked to the adult or standard clearance, but with function parameterization analyzed and itemized to the data (expressed as linear, exponential, power, hyperbolic, etc.), and with additional factors (disease, pharmacogenetics, etc.) incorporated[3,115]:

$$Cl_{child} = Cl_{adult} \cdot (f_{size}) \cdot (f_{maturation}) \cdot (f_{organ\ function}) \cdot (f_{genetic\ typing}) \cdot (f_{disease\ severity/intervention})$$

Examples of disease states or interventions that may markedly alter the pharmacokinetics in children of various drugs include therapeutic hypothermia,[116] extracorporeal membrane oxygenation,[117] HIV infection,[118] burns,[119] and other critical care conditions.[120]

We can use the above infant data calculating vancomycin dosing using this modeling approach, with a published pediatric model derived from a one-compartment data fit.[121]

Example—population pharmacokinetic model

$$Cl\ (L/hr) = 0.248 \times Weight^{0.75} \times (0.48/SCr)^{0.361} \times [\ln(Age)/7.8]^{0.995} \qquad \textbf{(Eq. 4.3)}$$

where weight is in kg, SCr is the serum creatinine in mg/dL, and postnatal age in days (4.5 months = 135 days).

$$= 0.248 \times 4.304 \times 1.1208 \times 0.6303$$

$$= 0.7541\ L/hr$$

$$= 1.8\ mL/min/kg$$

The dose can then be calculated using Equation 4.2.

$$Dose = Cl \times Target\ AUC_{24hr}$$

$$= 0.7541\ L/hr \times 400\ mg \cdot h/L$$

$$= 301.64\ mg/day$$

$$= 42.9\ mg/kg/day$$

Note that this model gives a similar calculated daily dose as the maturation model used previously.

While no model is perfect in construction or application,[122] the advances in population modeling in pediatrics, with extension to pharmacodynamic linkage,[123,124] allows further refinement of dose and effect prediction, and advises on study design and the potential for extrapolation from adults to children.

PHARMACODYNAMICS AND PHARMACOKINETICALLY DIRECTED DOSING

For most drugs, the extrapolation of effect and a pharmacokinetic search of the correct dose in children and adolescents to provide that effect can initially be derived from studies and experiences in adults.[79,125] An antihypertensive medication in adults is expected to have similar blood pressure reducing effects in children, but finding the dose (total and weight-adjusted) to provide a similar percentage decrease in systolic and diastolic pressures may take further pharmacokinetic and pharmacodynamic investigation. Precise efficacy and adverse effect profiles may differ in children in relationship to dose depending on the comorbidities and indication circumstances.[82] Unique pharmacodynamic effects exist for some immunosuppressive agents with qualitative and quantitative differences between children and adults in cellular and humoral immune systems. Age-varying vitamin K-dependent clotting factor concentrations impact the amount of warfarin needed for therapeutic anticoagulation. And sotalol has different QTc prolongation potential relative to the serum concentration, with greater sensitivity seen in neonates than infants, and in infants more than in children and adolescents, because of immaturity of potassium channels in the former age groups.[126]

Finding the proper pediatric dosing can often be challenging depending on the target response sought. While with antimicrobials, the target response is generally set to adult microbiologic and clinical endpoints (e.g., AUC to MIC ratio, peak concentration to MIC ratio, time above the MIC, quantitative pathogen eradication, etc.), the target may move with time and organism resistance. Fluoroquinolones are secondary agents in the management of community-acquired pneumonia (CAP) owing to adverse effects that may be more worrisome in children.[127] Dosing calculations derived from a pediatric population model for levofloxacin based on a goal of unbound serum concentration AUC to MIC ratio of 33.7 mg · h/L (published breakpoint for success against *Streptococcus pneumoniae*) challenge current pediatric CAP guidelines.[128] Clearance (mL/min/kg) was determined to be equal to:

$$\alpha \cdot \left(\text{Weight}\right)^{\beta} \cdot \frac{\text{Age}}{\text{Age} + A_{50}}$$

where $\alpha = 1.5 \pm 0.06$, mL/min/kg, $\beta = 0.43 \pm 0.06$, and $A_{50} = 0.32 \pm 0.18$ years.

The volume of distribution was 1.4 to 1.6 L/kg for the five evaluated age groups. Projected AUCs using these parameter estimates revealed that the doses suggested by the current pediatric CAP guidelines would provide low target responses of 50% to 60% of 5-to <10-year olds, and 76% to 81% among 10- to 16-year olds.[128] In order to assure a greater than 90% success, the doses would need to be raised to 12 mg/kg every 12 hours in those 6 months to <5-year olds, and 8 mg/kg every 12 hours in 5- to <14-year olds, which are higher than the current guideline doses of 10 mg/kg every 12 hours for patients 6 months to <5-year olds, and 10 mg/kg every 24 hours for 5- to 16-year olds.[129] Similarly, based on construction of a population pharmacokinetic model, more aggressive doses than the currently recommended 50 mg/kg every 8 or 12 hours for cefepime may be necessary in pediatric patients when simulating the effect against a gram-negative rod with

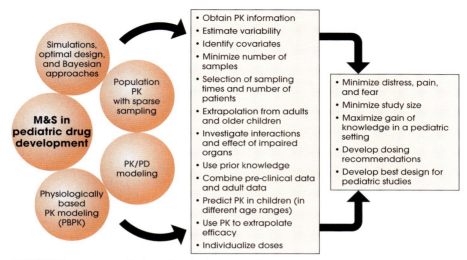

FIGURE 4.5   Design, methods, and goals of pharmacokinetic and pharmacodynamic investigation in children. (From Zisowsky J, Krause A, Dingemanse J. Drug development for pediatric populations: regulatory aspects. *Pharmaceutics*. 2010;2(4):364–388.)

an MIC is 8 mg/L.[130] Likewise, using a population kinetic model in children with HIV infection, reduction of the Food and Drug Administration–recommended zidovudine doses in the 20 to 40 kg weight category from 9 to 8 mg/kg twice daily is projected to reduce the serum concentration exposure that promotes a higher incidence of anemia.[131]

More investigation of pharmacodynamic differences between children and adults, and guidance of dosing using population pharmacokinetics with Bayesian adjustment based on individual parameter estimates subsequently modified by concentration feedback should assist both the practical application to individualize dosing for optimal response, and the development and approval of new drug entities with optimized doses for the targeted age group of children and adolescents (see Fig. 4.5).[5,111]

REFERENCES

1.   https://clinicaltrials.gov/. Accessed July 26, 2017.

2.   Committee on Pediatric Studies Conducted Under the Best Pharmaceuticals for Children Act (BPCA) and the Pediatric Research Equity Act (PREA); Board on Health Sciences Policy; Institute of Medicine; Field MJ, Boat TF, eds. *Safe and Effective Medicines for Children: Pediatric Studies Conducted Under the Best Pharmaceuticals for Children Act and the Pediatric Research Equity Act*. Washington, DC: National Academies Press (US); 2012.

3.   Vinks AA, Emoto C, Fukuda T. Modeling and simulation in pediatric drug therapy: application of pharmacometrics to define the right dose for children. *Clin Pharmacol Ther*. 2015;98(3):298–308.

4.   Vermeulen E, van den Anker JN, Della Pasqua O, et al; Global Research in Paediatrics (GRiP). How to optimise drug study design: pharmacokinetics and pharmacodynamics studies introduced to paediatricians. *J Pharm Pharmacol*. 2017;69(4):439–447.

5.   Rieder M, Hawcutt D. Design and conduct of early phase drug studies in children: challenges and opportunities. *Br J Clin Pharmacol*. 2016;82(5):1308–1314.

6. Momper JD, Wagner JA. Therapeutic drug monitoring as a component of personalized medicine: applications in pediatric drug development. *Clin Pharmacol Ther.* 2014;95(2):138–140.

7. Maagdenberg H, Vijverberg SJ, Bierings MB, et al. Pharmacogenomics in pediatric patients: towards personalized medicine. *Paediatr Drugs.* 2016;18(4):251–260.

8. Rodieux F, Wilbaux M, van den Anker JN, et al. Effect of kidney function on drug kinetics and dosing in neonates, infants, and children. *Clin Pharmacokinet.* 2015;54(12):1183–1204.

9. Standing JF. Understanding and applying pharmacometric modelling and simulation in clinical practice and research. *Br J Clin Pharmacol.* 2017;83(2):247–254.

10. Wilbaux M, Fuchs A, Samardzic J, et al. Pharmacometric approaches to personalize use of primarily renally eliminated antibiotics in preterm and term neonates. *J Clin Pharmacol.* 2016;56(8): 909–935.

11. Jong G. Pediatric development: physiology. Enzymes, drug metabolism, pharmacokinetics and pharmacodynamics. In: Bar-Shalom D, Rose K, eds. *Pediatric Formulations: A Roadmap, AAPS Advances in the Pharmaceutical Sciences Series 11*;2014: 9–23.

12. Batchelor HK, Marriott JF. Paediatric pharmacokinetics: key considerations. *Br J Clin Pharmacol.* 2015;79(3):395–404.

13. Samardzic J, Allegaert K, Bajcetic M. Developmental pharmacology: a moving target. *Int J Pharm.* 2015;15;492(1–2):335–337.

14. Lu H, Rosenbaum S. Developmental pharmacokinetics in pediatric populations. *J Pediatr Pharmacol Ther.* 2014;19(4):262–276.

15. Kearns GL, Robinson PK, Wilson JT, et al; Pediatric Pharmacology Research Unit Network. Cisapride disposition in neonates and infants: in vivo reflection of cytochrome P450 3A4 ontogeny. *Clin Pharmacol Ther.* 2003;74(4):312–325.

16. Garrick MD. Human iron transporters. *Genes Nutr.* 2011;6(1):45–54.

17. Mirochnick M, Capparelli E, Connor J. Pharmacokinetics of zidovudine in infants: a population analysis across studies. *Clin Pharmacol Ther.* 1999;66(1):16–24.

18. Gibbs JP, Liacouras CA, Baldassano RN, et al. Up-regulation of glutathione S-transferase activity in enterocytes of young children. *Drug Metab Dispos.* 1999;27(12):1466–1469.

19. Rodieux F, Gotta V, Pfister M, et al. Causes and consequences of variability in drug transporter activity n pediatric drug therapy. *J Clin Pharmacol.* 2016;56(suppl 7):S173–S192.

20. Smits A, Roberts JA, Vella-Brincat JW, et al. Cefazolin plasma protein binding in different human populations: more than cefazolin-albumin interaction. *Int J Antimicrob Agents.* 2014;43(2):199–200.

21. De Cock RF, Smits A, Allegaert K, et al. Population pharmacokinetic modelling of total and unbound cefazolin plasma concentrations as a guide for dosing in preterm and term neonates. *J Antimicrob Chemother.* 2014;69(5):1330–1338.

22. McNamara PJ, Alcorn J. Protein binding predictions in infants. *AAPS PharmSci.* 2002;4(1):E4.

23. Gonzalez D, Delmore P, Bloom BT, et al. Clindamycin pharmacokinetics and safety in preterm and term infants. *Antimicrob Agents Chemother.* 2016;60(5):2888–2894.

24. Perlman KM, Myers-Phariss S, Rhodes JC. A shift from demerol (meperidine) to dilaudid (hydromorphone) improves pain control and decreases admissions for patients in sickle cell crisis. *J Emerg Nurs.* 2004;30(5):439–446.

25. Hagmeyer KO, Mauro LS, Mauro VF. Meperidine-related seizures associated with patient-controlled analgesia pumps. *Ann Pharmacother.* 1993;27(1):29–32.

26. Oyaert M, Spriet I, Allegaert K, et al. Factors impacting unbound vancomycin concentrations in different patient populations. *Antimicrob Agents Chemother.* 2015;59(11):7073–7079.

27. Bhutani VK, Wong RJ. Bilirubin neurotoxicity in preterm infants: risk and prevention. *J Clin Neonatol.* 2013;2(02):61–69.

28. Kearin M, Kelly JG, O'Malley K. Digoxin "receptors" in neonates: an explanation of less sensitivity to digoxin than in adults. *Clin Pharmacol Ther.* 1980;28 (3):346–349.

29. Gong Y, Chen Y, Li Q, et al. Population pharmacokinetic analysis of digoxin in Chinese neonates and infants. *J Pharmacol Sci.* 2014;125(2):142–149.

30. Bendayan R, McKenzie MW. Digoxin pharmacokinetics and dosage requirements in pediatric patients. *Clin Pharm*. 1983;2(3):224–235.

31. de Wildt SN, Tibboel D, Leeder JS. Drug metabolism for the paediatrician. *Arch Dis Child*. 2014;99(12):1137–1142.

32. Upreti VV, Wahlstrom JL. Meta-analysis of hepatic cytochrome P450 ontogeny to underwrite the prediction of pediatric pharmacokinetics using physiologically based pharmacokinetic modeling. *J Clin Pharmacol*. 2016;56(3):266–283.

33. Sadler NC, Nandhikonda P, Webb-Robertson BJ, et al. Hepatic cytochrome p450 activity, abundance, and expression throughout human development. *Drug Metab Dispos*. 2016;44(7):984–991.

34. Lacroix D, Sonnier M, Moncion A, et al. Expression of CYP3A in the human liver—evidence that the shift between CYP3A7 and CYP3A4 occurs immediately after birth. *Eur J Biochem*. 1997;247(2):625–634.

35. Kraus DM, Fischer JH, Reitz SJ, et al. Alterations in theophylline metabolism during the first year of life. *Clin Pharmacol Ther*. 1993;54(4):351–359.

36. Pacifici GM. Clinical pharmacology of phenobarbital in neonates: effects, metabolism and pharmacokinetics. *Curr Pediatr Rev*. 2016;12(1):48–54.

37. Blake MJ, Gaedigk A, Pearce RE, et al. Ontogeny of dextromethorphan O- and N-demethylation in the first year of life. *Clin Pharmacol Ther*. 2007;81(4):510–516.

38. Takahashi H, Ishikawa S, Nomoto S, et al. Developmental changes in pharmacokinetics and pharmacodynamics of warfarin enantiomers in Japanese children. *Clin Pharmacol Ther*. 2000;68(5):541–555.

39. Kanamori M, Takahashi H, Echizen H. Developmental changes in the liver weight- and body weight-normalized clearance of theophylline, phenytoin and cyclosporine in children. *Int J Clin Pharmacol Ther*. 2002;40(11):485–492.

40. Cook SF, Stockmann C, Samiee-Zafarghandy S, et al. Neonatal maturation of paracetamol (acetaminophen) glucuronidation, sulfation, and oxidation based on a parent-metabolite population pharmacokinetic model. *Clin Pharmacokinet*. 2016;55(11):1395–1411.

41. Acheampong P, Thomas SHL. Determinants of hepatotoxicity after repeated supratherapeutic paracetamol ingestion: systematic review of reported cases. *Br J Clin Pharmacol*. 2016;82:923–931.

42. Abourbih DA, Gosselin S, Villeneuve E, et al. Are recommended doses of acetaminophen effective for children aged 2 to 3 years? A pharmacokinetic modeling answer. *Pediatr Emerg Care*. 2016;32(1):6–8.

43. Allen-Webb EM, Ross MP, Pappas JB, et al. Age-related amrinone pharmacokinetics in a pediatric population. *Crit Care Med*. 1994;22(6):1016–1024.

44. Krekels EH, Danhof M, Tibboel D, et al. Ontogeny of hepatic glucuronidation; methods and results. *Curr Drug Metab*. 2012;13(6):728–743.

45. Anderson BJ, Holford NH. Mechanistic basis of using body size and maturation to predict clearance in humans. *Drug Metab Pharmacokinet*. 2009;24:25–36.

46. Anderson BJ, Larsson P. A maturation model for midazolam clearance. *Paediatr Anaesth*. 2011;21(3):302–308.

47. Capparelli EV, Englund JA, Connor JD, et al. Population pharmacokinetics and pharmacodynamics of zidovudine in HIV-infected infants and children. *J Clin Pharmacol*. 2003;43(2):133–140.

48. Capparelli EV, Mirochnick M, Dankner WM, et al; Pediatric AIDS Clinical Trials Group 331 Investigators. Pharmacokinetics and tolerance of zidovudine in preterm infants. *J Pediatr*. 2003;142(1):47–52.

49. Elmorsi Y, Barber J, Rostami-Hodjegan A. Ontogeny of hepatic drug transporters and relevance to drugs used in pediatrics. *Drug Metab Dispos*. 2016;44(7):992–998.

50. Prasad B, Gaedigk A, Vrana M, et al. Ontogeny of hepatic drug transporters as quantified by LC-MS/MS proteomics. *Clin Pharmacol Ther*. 2016;100(4):362–370.

51. Anand KJ, Anderson BJ, Holford NH, et al; NEOPAIN Trial Investigators Group. Morphine pharmacokinetics and pharmacodynamics in preterm and term neonates: secondary results from the NEOPAIN trial. *Br J Anaesth*. 2008;101(5):680–689.

52. Pacifici GM. Metabolism and pharmacokinetics of morphine in neonates: a review. *Clinics (Sao Paulo)*. 2016;71(8):474–480.

53. Hahn D, Emoto C, Vinks AA, et al. Developmental changes in hepatic OCT1 protein expression from neonates to children. *Drug Metab Dispos*. 2017;45(1):23–26.

54. Fukuda T, Chidambaran V, Mizuno T, et al. OCT1 genetic variants influence the pharmacokinetics of morphine in children. *Pharmacogenomics*. 2013;14(10):1141–1151.

55. Sadhasivam S, Chidambaran V, Ngamprasertwong P, et al. Race and unequal burden of perioperative pain and opioid related adverse effects in children. *Pediatrics*. 2012;129(5):832–838.

56. Marek E, Momper JD, Hines RN, et al. Prediction of warfarin dose in pediatric patients: an evaluation of the predictive performance of several models. *J Pediatr Pharmacol Ther*. 2016;21(3):224–232.

57. Jacobo-Cabral CO, García-Roca P, Romero-Tejeda EM, et al. Population pharmacokinetic analysis of tacrolimus in Mexican paediatric renal transplant patients: role of CYP3A5 genotype and formulation. *Br J Clin Pharmacol*. 2015;80(4):630–641.

58. Teusink A, Vinks A, Zhang K, et al. Genotype-directed dosing leads to optimized voriconazole levels in pediatric patients receiving hematopoietic stem cell transplantation. *Biol Blood Marrow Transplant*. 2016;22(3):482–486.

59. Livingstone MJ, Groenewald CB, Rabbitts JA, et al. Codeine use among children in the United States: a nationally representative study from 1996 to 2013. *Paediatr Anaesth*. 2017;27(1):19–27.

60. Tobias JD, Green TP, Coté CJ; Section on Anesthesiology And Pain Medicine; Committee On Drugs. Codeine: time to say "No". *Pediatrics*. 2016;138(4):pii: e20162396.

61. Kelly LE, Chaudhry SA, Rieder MJ, et al. A clinical tool for reducing central nervous system depression among neonates exposed to codeine through breast milk. *PLoS One*. 2013;8(7):e70073.

62. Crews KR, Gaedigk A, Dunnenberger HM, et al; Clinical Pharmacogenetics Implementation Consortium. Clinical Pharmacogenetics Implementation Consortium guidelines for cytochrome P450 2D6 genotype and codeine therapy: 2014 update. *Clin Pharmacol Ther*. 2014;95 (4):376–382.

63. Sistonen J, Madadi P, Ross CJ, et al. Prediction of codeine toxicity in infants and their mothers using a novel combination of maternal genetic markers. *Clin Pharmacol Ther*. 2012;91 (4):692–699.

64. Prows CA, Zhang X, Huth MM, et al. Codeine-related adverse drug reactions in children following tonsillectomy: a prospective study. *Laryngoscope*. 2014;124(5):1242–1250.

65. Chen N, Aleksa K, Woodland C, et al. Ontogeny of drug elimination by the human kidney. *Pediatr Nephrol*. 2006;21(2):160–168.

66. Alcorn J, McNamara PJ. Ontogeny of hepatic and renal systemic clearance pathways in infants: part I. *Clin Pharmacokinet*. 2002;41(12):959–998.

67. Goldman J, Becker ML, Jones B, et al. Development of biomarkers to optimize pediatric patient management: what makes children different? *Biomark Med*. 2011;5(6):781–794.

68. Allegaert K, Anderson BJ, van den Anker JN, et al. Renal drug clearance in preterm neonates: relation to prenatal growth. *Ther Drug Monit*. 2007;29(3):284–291.

69. Rhodin MM, Anderson BJ, Peters AM, et al. Human renal function maturation: a quantitative description using weight and postmenstrual age. *Pediatr Nephrol*. 2009;24(1):67–76.

70. Sampson MR, Bloom BT, Lenfestey RW, et al; Best Pharmaceuticals for Children Act–Pediatric Trials Network. Population pharmacokinetics of intravenous acyclovir in preterm and term infants. *Pediatr Infect Dis J*. 2014;33(1):42–49.

71. Pottel H. Measuring and estimating glomerular filtration rate in children. *Pediatr Nephrol*. 2017;32(2):249–263.

72. Baum M. Renal tubular development. In: Avner ED, Harmon WE, Niaudet P, eds. *Pediatric Nephrology*. 7th ed. Berlin, Heidelberg: Springer; 2016:61–96.

73. Wade KC, Wu D, Kaufman DA, et al; National Institute of Child Health and Development Pediatric Pharmacology Research Unit Network. Population pharmacokinetics of fluconazole in young infants. *Antimicrob Agents Chemother*. 2008;52(11):4043–4049.

74. De Cock RF, Allegaert K, Schreuder MF, et al. Maturation of the glomerular filtration rate in neonates, as reflected by amikacin clearance. *Clin Pharmacokinet*. 2012;51(2):105–117.

75. De Cock RF, Allegaert K, Sherwin CM, et al. A neonatal amikacin covariate model can be used to predict ontogeny of other drugs eliminated through glomerular filtration in neonates. *Pharm Res*. 2014;31(3):754–767.

76. Kim AJ, Lee JY, Choi SA, et al. Comparison of the pharmacokinetics of vancomycin in neurosurgical and non-neurosurgical patients. *Int J Antimicrob Agents*. 2016;48(4):381–387.

77. Hirai K, Ihara S, Kinae A, et al. Augmented renal clearance in pediatric patients with febrile neutropenia associated with vancomycin clearance. *Ther Drug Monit*. 2016;38(3):393–397.

78. De Cock PA, Standing JF, Barker CI, et al Augmented renal clearance implies a need for increased amoxicillin-clavulanic acid dosing in critically ill children. *Antimicrob Agents Chemother*. 2015;59(11): 7027–7035.

79. Mulugeta Y, Barrett JS, Nelson R, et al. Exposure matching for extrapolation of efficacy in pediatric drug development. *J Clin Pharmacol*. 2016;56(11):1326–1334.

80. Zimmerman K, Putera M, Hornik CP, et al. Exposure matching of pediatric anti-infective drugs: review of drugs submitted to the Food and Drug Administration for pediatric approval. *Clin Ther*. 2016;38(9):1995–2005.

81. Mahmood I. Dosing in children: a critical review of the pharmacokinetic allometric scaling and modelling approaches in paediatric drug development and clinical settings. *Clin Pharmacokinet*. 2014;53(4):327–346.

82. Mulla H. Understanding developmental pharmacodynamics: importance for drug development and clinical practice. *Paediatr Drugs*. 2010;12(4):223–233.

83. Pan SD, Zhu LL, Chen M, et al. Weight-based dosing in medication use: what should we know? *Patient Prefer Adherence*. 2016;10:549–560.

84. Joint Commission Resources. *Joint Commission International Accreditation Standards for Hospitals*. 5th ed. Oak Brook, IL: Joint Commission Resources; 2013.

85. Chatelut E, Puisset F. The scientific basis of body surface area-based dosing. *Clin Pharmacol Ther*. 2014;95(4):359–361.

86. Bins S, Ratain MJ, Mathijssen RH. Conventional dosing of anticancer agents: precisely wrong or just inaccurate? *Clin Pharmacol Ther*. 2014;95(4):361–364.

87. Johnson TN, Rostami-Hodjegan A, Tucker GT. Prediction of the clearance of eleven drugs and associated variability in neonates, infants and children. *Clin Pharmacokinet*. 2006;45(9):931–956.

88. Saul JP, Schaffer MS, Karpawich PP, et al. Single-dose pharmacokinetics of sotalol in a pediatric population with supraventricular and/or ventricular tachyarrhythmia. *J Clin Pharmacol*. 2001;41(1):35–43.

89. Saul JP, Ross B, Schaffer MS, et al; Pediatric Sotalol Investigators. Pharmacokinetics and pharmacodynamics of sotalol in a pediatric population with supraventricular and ventricular tachyarrhythmia. *Clin Pharmacol Ther*. 2001;69(3):145–157.

90. Kendrick JG, Carr RR, Ensom MH. Pediatric obesity: pharmacokinetics and implications for drug dosing. *Clin Ther*. 2015;37(9):1897–1923.

91. Harskamp-van Ginkel MW, Hill KD, Becker KC, et al; Best Pharmaceuticals for Children Act–Pediatric Trials Network Administrative Core Committee. Drug dosing and pharmacokinetics in children with obesity: a systematic review. *JAMA Pediatr*. 2015;169(7):678–685.

92. Merrell MD, Cherrington NJ. Drug metabolism alterations in nonalcoholic fatty liver disease. *Drug Metab Rev*. 2011;43(3):317–334.

93. Thompson PA, Rosner GL, Matthay KK, et al. Impact of body composition on pharmacokinetics of doxorubicin in children: a Glaser Pediatric Research Network study. *Cancer Chemother Pharmacol*. 2009;64(2):243–251.

94. Arndt C, Hawkins D, Anderson JR, et al. Age is a risk factor for chemotherapy-induced hepatopathy with vincristine, dactinomycin, and cyclophosphamide. *J Clin Oncol*. 2004;22:1894–1901.

95. Woods WG, O'Leary M, Nesbit ME. Life-threatening neuropathy and hepatotoxicity in infants during induction therapy for acute lymphoblastic leukemia. *J Pediatr*. 1981;98:642–645.

96. Feber J, Al-Matrafi J, Farhadi E, et al. Prednisone dosing per body weight or body surface area in children with nephrotic syndrome: is it equivalent? *Pediatr Nephrol*. 2009;24(5):1027–1031.

97. Raman V, Krishnamurthy S, Harichandrakumar KT. Body weight-based prednisolone versus body surface area-based prednisolone regimen for induction of remission in children with nephrotic syndrome: a randomized, open-label, equivalence clinical trial. *Pediatr Nephrol*. 2016;31(4):595–604.

98. Filler G, Robinson LA. Should we stop dosing steroids per body surface area for nephrotics? *Pediatr Nephrol*. 2016;31(4):519–522.

99. Johnson TN. The problems in scaling adult drug doses to children. *Arch Dis Child*. 2008;93(3):207–211.

100. Steinberg I, Kimberlin DW. Acyclovir dosing and acute kidney injury: deviations and direction. *J Pediatr*. 2015;166(6):1341–1344.

101. Rao S, Abzug M, Carosone-Link P, et al. Intravenous acyclovir and renal dysfunction in children: a matched case control study. *J Pediatr*. 2015;166(6):1462–1468.

102. Holford N, Heo YA, Anderson B. A pharmacokinetic standard for babies and adults. *J Pharm Sci*. 2013;102(9):2941–2952.

103. Liu T, Ghafoori P, Gobburu JV. Allometry is a reasonable choice in pediatric drug development. *J Clin Pharmacol*. 2017;57(4):469–475.

104. Calvier EA, Krekels EH, Välitalo PA, et al. Allometric scaling of clearance in paediatric patients: when does the Magic of 0.75 Fade? *Clin Pharmacokinet*. 2017;56(3):273–285.

105. Mahmood I. Prediction of drug clearance in premature and mature neonates, infants, and children ≤2 years of age: a comparison of the predictive performance of 4 allometric models. *J Clin Pharmacol*. 2016;56(6):733–739.

106. Anderson BJ, Holford NH. Understanding dosing: children are small adults, neonates are immature children. *Arch Dis Child*. 2013;98(9):737–744.

107. Lu H, Rosenbaum S. A model for maturation of renal function in pediatric population developed from the clearance of vancomycin and gentamicin. Abstract M-045. *J Pharmacokinet Pharmacodyn*. 2013;40:S51.

108. Valcyte® [prescribing information]. South San Francisco: Genentech, Inc; April 2015.

109. Chaturvedula A. Population pharmacokinetics. In: Jann MW, Penzak SR, Cohen LJ, eds. *Applied Clinical Pharmacokinetics and Pharmacodynamics of Psychopharmacological Agents*. Switzerland: Springer International Publishing; 2016:71–90.

110. Altamimi MI, Choonara I, Sammons H. Invasiveness of pharmacokinetic studies in children: a systematic review. *BMJ Open*. 2016;6(7):e010484.

111. Zisowsky J, Krause A, Dingemanse J. Drug development for pediatric populations: regulatory aspects. *Pharmaceutics*. 2010;2(4):364–388.

112. Roth-Cline M, Nelson RM. Microdosing studies in children: a US Regulatory Perspective. *Clin Pharmacol Ther*. 2015;98(3):232–233.

113. Dorofaeff T, Bandini RM, Lipman J, et al. Uncertainty in antibiotic dosing in critically ill neonate and pediatric patients: can microsampling provide the answers? *Clin Ther*. 2016;38(9):1961–1975.

114. Cohen-Wolkowiez M, Ouellet D, Smith PB, et al. Population pharmacokinetics of metronidazole evaluated using scavenged samples from preterm infants. *Antimicrob Agents Chemother*. 2012;56(4):1828–1837.

115. Samant TS, Mangal N, Lukacova V, et al. Quantitative clinical pharmacology for size and age scaling in pediatric drug development: a systematic review. *J Clin Pharmacol*. 2015;55(11):1207–1217.

116. Empey PE, Velez de Mendizabal N, Bell MJ, et al; Pediatric TBI Consortium: Hypothermia Investigators. Therapeutic hypothermia decreases phenytoin elimination in children with traumatic brain injury. *Crit Care Med*. 2013;41(10):2379–2387.

117. Himebauch AS, Kilbaugh TJ, Zuppa AF. Pharmacotherapy during pediatric extracorporeal membrane oxygenation: a review. *Expert Opin Drug Metab Toxicol*. 2016;12(10):1133–1142.

118. Antwi S, Yang H, Enimil A, et al. Pharmacokinetics of the first-line antituberculosis drugs in Ghanaian children with tuberculosis with and without HIV coinfection. *Antimicrob Agents Chemother*. 2017;61(2):pii: e01701–e017016.

119. Sherwin CM, Wead S, Stockmann C, et al. Amikacin population pharmacokinetics among paediatric burn patients. *Burns*. 2014;40(2):311–318.

120. Thakkar N, Salerno S, Hornik CP, et al. Clinical pharmacology studies in critically ill children. *Pharm Res*. 2017;34(1):7–24.

121. Le J, Bradley JS, Murray W, et al. Improved vancomycin dosing in children using area under the curve exposure. *Pediatr Infect Dis J*. 2013;32(4):e155–e163.

122. Germovsek E, Barker C, Sharland M, et al. Scaling clearance in paediatric pharmacokinetics: all models are wrong, which are useful? *Br J Clin Pharmacol*. 2017;83(4):777–790.

123. Huurneman LJ, Neely M, Veringa A, et al. Pharmacodynamics of voriconazole in children: further steps along the path to true individualized therapy. *Antimicrob Agents Chemother*. 2016;60(4):2336–2342.

124. Brussee JM, Calvier EA, Krekels EH, et al. Children in clinical trials: towards evidence-based pediatric pharmacotherapy using pharmacokinetic-pharmacodynamic modeling. *Expert Rev Clin Pharmacol*. 2016;9(9):1235–1244.

125. Momper JD, Mulugeta Y, Green DJ, et al. Adolescent dosing and labeling since the Food and Drug Administration Amendments Act of 2007. *JAMA Pediatr*. 2013;167(10):926–932.

126. Läer S, Elshoff JP, Meibohm B, et al. Development of a safe and effective pediatric dosing regimen for sotalol based on population pharmacokinetics and pharmacodynamics in children with supraventricular tachycardia. *J Am Coll Cardiol*. 2005;46(7):1322–1330.

127. Patel K, Goldman JL. Safety concerns surrounding quinolone use in children. *J Clin Pharmacol*. 2016;56(9):1060–1075.

128. Courter JD, Nichols KR, Kazazian C, et al. Pharmacodynamically guided levofloxacin dosing for pediatric community-acquired pneumonia. *J Pediatric Infect Dis Soc*. 2017;6(2):118–122.

129. Bradley JS, Byington CL, Shah SS, et al; Pediatric Infectious Diseases Society and the Infectious Diseases Society of America. The management of community-acquired pneumonia in infants and children older than 3 months of age: clinical practice guidelines by the Pediatric Infectious Diseases Society and the Infectious Diseases Society of America. *Clin Infect Dis*. 2011;53(7):e25–e76.

130. Shoji K, Bradley JS, Reed MD, et al. Population pharmacokinetic assessment and pharmacodynamic implications of pediatric cefepime dosing for susceptible-dose-dependent organisms. *Antimicrob Agents Chemother*. 2016;60(4):2150–2156.

131. Fauchet F, Treluyer JM, Frange P, et al. Population pharmacokinetics study of recommended zidovudine doses in HIV-1-infected children. *Antimicrob Agents Chemother*. 2013;57(10):4801–4808.

5

PHARMACOGENETICS

Reginald F. Frye

Learning Objectives

By the end of the chapter on pharmacogenetics, the learner shall be able to:

1. Understand how genetic variation in drug-disposition proteins affects therapeutic efficacy and toxicity.
2. Describe the molecular basis for a genetic variation influencing the functional activity of drug-disposition proteins.
3. Discuss relevant genetic polymorphisms of important drug-disposition proteins.
4. Evaluate potential application of pharmacogenetics to tailor drug therapy in the context of therapeutic drug management.

Variability in drug response has long been recognized. Inherent differences in pharmacokinetics, pharmacodynamics, or both contribute to the variability, and therapeutic drug monitoring emerged in the 1970s as a means to individualize (or personalize) therapy for a patient. In addition to patient factors, such as adherence, age, sex, and weight, the observed variability in drug response may result from genetic variation in genes that encode for drug-disposition proteins (i.e., drug-metabolizing enzymes and drug transporters) and drug-target proteins (e.g., receptors). Studies in this field have evolved from examining genetic variants within one or more candidate genes (pharmacogenetics) to studies evaluating multiple genes or the entire genome (pharmacogenomics). This chapter will review clinically relevant consequences of common genetic variation in drug-disposition proteins on drug pharmacokinetics and describe how this information provides the foundation for pharmacogenomics-informed therapeutic drug monitoring.

PHARMACOGENETICS AND DRUG DISPOSITION

Most marketed drugs are metabolized by oxidative metabolism, which is primarily mediated by enzymes in the cytochrome P450 (CYP) family.[1] The expression and metabolic activity of these enzymes are modulated by many nongenetic factors including age, concomitant drugs or dietary supplements, sex, disease states (e.g., liver disease or inflammatory conditions), and environmental influences (e.g., smoking).[1] Additionally, genetic variation in genes that encode for drug-metabolizing enzymes may contribute substantially to variability in pharmacokinetics. The net effect is that CYP enzyme activity has been reported to vary substantially between individuals, yielding potentially large differences in drug clearance and corresponding steady-state drug concentrations.[2]

The standard nomenclature for individual CYP enzymes includes the root "CYP," followed by an Arabic number designating the enzyme family (based on sequence homology), a letter for the enzyme subfamily, and another number denoting the individual CYP enzyme (e.g., CYP2D6). For each enzyme, the reference or "wild type" allele is denoted as *1. Allelic variants (i.e., alleles having one or more single nucleotide polymorphisms [SNPs]) are sequentially numbered as identified (i.e., *2, *3, etc.).[3] A comprehensive listing of CYP variants is available at http://www.cypalleles.ki.se/.

SNPs, a common type of genetic variation in the human genome, may contribute significantly to variability in drug response owing to effects on the expression or function of drug-disposition proteins and corresponding effects on drug pharmacokinetics. An SNP in a gene that encodes for a drug-disposition protein, such as a CYP enzyme, may cause changes in the amino acid sequence yielding a nonsynonymous protein with altered function, that is, an enzyme with decreased (most common) or increased metabolic activity. For some enzymes, allelic variants result from SNPs that create an altered splice site, frameshift mutation, premature stop codon, or gene deletion, each of which produces a nonfunctional (or loss-of-function) allele. These variations can have a profound impact on the ability of an individual to metabolize some drugs; carriers of these alleles may be at risk for toxicities associated with high drug concentrations, particularly with narrow therapeutic index drugs that are metabolized by a single enzyme.[4] In contrast, some *CYP* genes exhibit gene duplication events, whereby an individual carries multiple functional copies of the gene. These individuals may demonstrate substantially increased drug metabolism that results in therapeutic failure due to lower-than-expected drug concentrations.

CYP ENZYMES

Genetic variation has been described for each of the major CYP enzymes that contribute to human drug metabolism.[1,4,5] The genes that encode for some CYP enzymes (e.g., *CYP1A2*, *CYP2E1*, *CYP3A4*) are fairly well conserved with few or no clinically relevant polymorphisms reported. However, other CYP-encoding genes (e.g., *CYP2A6*, *CYP2B6*, *CYP2C9*, *CYP2C19*, *CYP2D6*) are highly polymorphic, and variants having substantial functional consequences are known. The CYP enzymes that mediate the majority of drug metabolism in humans are in the subfamilies CYP2C, CYP2D, and CYP3A.

Pharmacogenetics of important CYP enzymes

CYP2D6. The gene that encodes the CYPD6 enzyme is one of the best characterized CYP genes with more than 100 known allelic variants. Early studies in large populations showed that clearance for some CYP2D6-metabolized drugs is an inherited trait.[6] For example, metabolism of the antihypertensive and CYP2D6 substrate drugs debrisoquine and sparteine was shown to be an inherited trait and most notably, absent in up to 10% of the population.[7] It is interesting to note that in drug metabolism pharmacogenetics research, the phenotype typically preceded the genotype, meaning that the phenotype (e.g., drug clearance) was used to categorize individuals into activity or "phenotype groups." Thus, individuals who lacked the ability to metabolize debrisoquine were labeled as "poor metabolizers" (PMs). It was several years later that the genetic basis for the observation of clearance as an inherited trait was linked to an SNP in the *CYP2D6* gene.[6,7]

The CYP2D6 enzyme constitutes only 2% to 4% of total CYP protein content in the human liver, but this enzyme metabolizes 25% to 30% of all clinically used drugs.[1] Substrates include antiarrhythmics, antidepressants, antipsychotics, β-blockers, and codeine.[1] About 5% to 10% of whites and 1% of Asians exhibit the PM phenotype.[2,8] The most common nonfunctional alleles are *CYP2D6*3*, *CYP2D6*4*, *CYP2D6*5*, and *CYP2D*6*. The PM phenotype results when an individual is homozygous for loss-of-function alleles, which may be the same or different alleles (e.g., *CYP2D6*4/*4* or *CYP2D6*4/*6*). There are also three common variant alleles that have been associated with decreased catalytic activity: *CYP2D6*10*, found predominantly in Asians; *CYP2D6*17*, found in blacks; and *CYP2D6*41*, found in whites and blacks. In addition to normal metabolizers (i.e., individuals having at least one functional CYP2D6 allele), some individuals (up to 5% of whites) exhibit greatly enhanced clearance, termed ultrarapid metabolizers (UMs), because they carry multiple copies of the *CYP2D6* gene (i.e., gene duplication). The nomenclature for CYP2D6 gene duplication is *CYP2D6* × N*, where "N" indicates the presence of two or more copies of the gene on the same chromosome, resulting in the UM phenotype.[8]

A broad range of substrates is metabolized by CYP2D6 and, as it is with other enzymes, the clinical consequence of CYP2D6 genetic variation depends on characteristics of the drug and the extent to which CYP2D6 metabolizes it. In general, compared with normal metabolizers, PMs will exhibit much higher plasma drug concentrations, whereas UMs will exhibit much lower plasma drug concentrations. If the parent drug is active, then a PM is at risk of an exaggerated pharmacodynamic effect and adverse effects, whereas a UM is at risk of therapeutic failure. If the drug administered is a prodrug converted to an active metabolite (e.g., codeine or clopidogrel), then a PM is at risk of therapeutic failure and a UM is at greater risk of adverse effects due to respective low and high concentrations of the active metabolite. For example, because CYP2D6 mediates the metabolism of codeine to the active moiety morphine, PMs will not experience the expected therapeutic effect. Conversely, UMs exhibit increased formation of morphine, which can result in an augmented pharmacodynamic effect and severe adverse effects.[8]

CYP2B6. The CYP2B6 enzyme constitutes 3% to 6% of total hepatic CYP content.[9] CYP2B6 plays an important role in the metabolism of cyclophosphamide, diazepam, efavirenz, and nevirapine. Nonsynonymous polymorphisms in the *CYP2B6* gene that are functionally relevant include *CYP2B6*4*, *CYP2B6*5*, *CYP2B6*6*, *CYP2B6*9*, and *CYP2B6*18*.[9,10] The nonsynonymous SNP at position 516 (G≥T) causes decreased CYP2B6 expression and activity through aberrant splicing and reduced functional mRNA; this polymorphism is part of the *CYP2B6*6*, **7*, **9*, **13*, **19*, and **20* alleles.[10]

Genetic variation in CYP2B6 contributes to clinically relevant differences in systemic exposure for efavirenz, which has a narrow therapeutic index.[11] The 516 G≥T SNP has been associated with lower efavirenz clearance and higher plasma concentrations. Indeed, homozygous 516T carriers may have two- to three-fold higher area under the curve values than 516G carriers.[10,11]

CYP2C9. The major CYP2C enzyme found in the human liver is CYP2C9, which mediates the metabolism of several clinically important drugs, including the narrow therapeutic index drugs phenytoin and warfarin.[12,13] Sixty variant alleles have been identified in the *CYP2C9* gene (http://www.cypalleles.ki.se/), many of which have clinically important racial differences in allele frequencies. SNPs within the coding region produce the variant alleles *CYP2C9*2* and *CYP2C9*3*, which are found in up to 35% of whites but are much less prevalent in blacks and Asians; the *CYP2C9*5* allele is found only in blacks.[13]

The clinical relevance of *CYP2C9* polymorphisms stems primarily from the contribution of CYP2C9 to the metabolism of the narrow therapeutic index drugs phenytoin and warfarin. The CYP2C9 variant alleles that have been identified are associated with decreased enzyme activity, though the magnitude of effect is substrate dependent. For warfarin, a strong relationship between the *CYP2C9* genotype and S-warfarin pharmacokinetics has been demonstrated. The impact of *CYP2C9* genotype on S-warfarin pharmacokinetics affects the daily dose of warfarin required to obtain a target international normalized ratio.[13]

Phenytoin is primarily metabolized by CYP2C9 and, to a lesser extent, CYP2C19. Even modest changes in CYP2C9 activity are likely to be clinically relevant with phenytoin because of its nonlinear pharmacokinetics. The dose required to achieve a therapeutic concentration is smaller in variant *CYP2C9* allele carriers compared with patients having the *CYP2C9*1/*1* genotype. Additionally, patients with one or more variant alleles appear to be more susceptible to concentration-related adverse events, particularly during therapy initiation.[12]

CYP2C19. CYP2C19 is involved in the metabolism of drugs such as citalopram, clopidogrel, diazepam, escitalopram, proton pump inhibitors (e.g., lansoprazole, omeprazole), and voriconazole.[14] Nonfunctional variants of *CYP2C19* are associated with the PM phenotype, which occurs in 1% to 3% of whites and 13% to 23% of Asians.[14] The most common allelic variants are *CYP2C19*2* and *CYP2C19*3*, which together account for about 95% of PMs. An SNP in the promoter region of the *CYP2C19* gene (*CYP2C19*17*) confers ultrarapid enzyme activity because of enhanced enzyme expression; the allele is relatively common, occurring at a frequency of up to 25% in whites.[1,5,14]

The presence of *CYP2C19* loss-of-function alleles can increase the risk of concentration-related adverse effects but may also lead to diminished response or treatment failure with drugs that require activation by CYP2C19. For example, the oral antiplatelet drug clopidogrel is a prodrug that undergoes a two-step activation process in which about 15% of the dose is converted to an active metabolite. Substantial evidence indicates that clopidogrel activation is critically dependent on CYP2C19 activity.[15]

The *CYP2C19*17* allele causes increased enzyme expression that results in rapid CYP2C19 activity. The increased expression yields higher metabolism and increased clearance, which may result in treatment failure for drugs such as voriconazole. Indeed, voriconazole exposure in *CYP2C19*17* carriers was 52% of that achieved in CYP2C19 extensive metabolizers and 15% of that achieved in CYP2C19 PMs.[14]

CYP3A4 and CYP3A5. CYP3A enzymes are the most abundantly expressed enzymes in both the liver and the intestine. CYP3A enzymes constitute 30% and 70% of the total CYP enzyme content in the human liver and intestine, respectively, and are responsible for the metabolism of almost 50% of marketed drugs. CYP3A4 is considered the most abundant and clinically significant enzyme in human drug metabolism; CYP3A5 is important for some drugs because it is polymorphically expressed.[1,5]

Several allelic variants of *CYP3A4* have been identified (http://www.cypalleles.ki.se/), but none is a loss-of-function allele; nonsynonymous polymorphisms are rare. The most common variant is *CYP3A4*1B*, which is an SNP in the promoter region that has a modest functional consequence. However, a loss-of-function allele has been identified in the gene that encodes for CYP3A5 that creates an aberrant splice site and results in a truncated, nonfunctional protein (*CYP3A5*3* allele).[16] Identification of this SNP explains some variability in CYP3A5 expression—only people who carry at least one copy of the *CYP3A5*1* allele express CYP3A5. Only 20% of whites, whereas 75% of blacks express CYP3A5.[16]

There is tremendous interindividual variability in CYP3A-mediated metabolism, with the clearance of some substrate drugs varying up to 20-fold. However, it appears that environmental influences affecting gene expression (e.g., induction), rather than genetic variation, are the most important factors contributing to variability in CYP3A4 activity. CYP3A5 may be important with respect to interindividual variability in CYP3A-mediated metabolism. It is estimated that CYP3A5 accounts for up to 50% of the total CYP3A content in people with at least one *CYP3A5*1* allele. The only drug for which *CYP3A5* genotype has consistently been shown to be clinically important is the immunosuppressant tacrolimus.[16] The dose required to achieve target therapeutic plasma concentrations in adult and pediatric transplant patients is typically 1.5- to 2-fold higher in *CYP3A5* expressers (*CYP3A5*1/*1*) compared with nonexpressers (*CYP3A5*3/*3*).[16,17]

PHARMACOGENOMICS-INFORMED THERAPEUTIC DRUG MONITORING

The goal of personalized medicine is to select, on the basis of genetic makeup, the best drug together with an individualized dosing regimen to obtain maximal efficacy and minimal toxicity, thereby avoiding therapeutic misadventures and achieving optimal therapeutic outcomes. Traditional therapeutic drug monitoring has a similar goal and accounts for nongenetic and genetic factors that contribute to pharmacokinetic and pharmacodynamic variability. However, pharmacogenomics can be used to provide information that can be used prior to the initiation of therapy to decide appropriateness and risk of drug therapy.

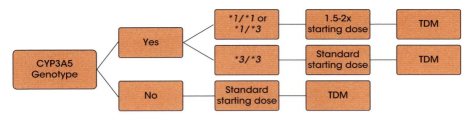

FIGURE 5.1 Pharmacogenomics-informed therapeutic drug monitoring: genotype-guided dosing for tacrolimus based on CYP3A5 genotype.

Drugs that have a narrow therapeutic index and are extensively and exclusively metabolized by a polymorphic enzyme (e.g., CYP2D6, CYP3A5) are ideal candidates for this approach. Preemptive genotyping for variants of drug-metabolizing enzymes may help guide successful treatment, such as through the development of dosing recommendations for different genetic subpopulations of patients. For example, the Clinical Pharmacogenetics Implementation Consortium (CPIC) has developed a guideline for *CYP3A5* genotype-guided dosing regimens for tacrolimus (Fig. 5.1).[16] The genotype-guided dose is intended to help achieve a therapeutic concentration earlier in therapy; traditional concentration monitoring then ensures that the target concentration is achieved or the dose is adjusted accordingly.[18] Although there is evidence to support this approach, prospective clinical studies to assess outcomes and costs are required to support the implementation of this approach in clinical practice.

CLINICAL PHARMACOGENETICS IMPLEMENTATION CONSORTIUM

The CPIC (https://cpicpgx.org/) was formed in 2009 and has a primary goal to address barriers to implementation of pharmacogenetic tests into clinical practice.[19] The consortium publishes guidelines that advise on how best to use genetic information, such as CYP3A5 genotype, in clinical practice to guide drug therapy (e.g., tacrolimus). The guidelines do not make recommendations regarding genetic testing but rather advise on how to use existing genetic information to support clinical decision-making. The guidelines are peer reviewed, published as open access, and updated regularly. The CPIC website (https://cpicpgx.org/) provides a valuable resource for additional information about specific gene–drug pairs and recommendations for drug therapy management. The guidelines have a standardized format that includes background information on genetic variability and its relevance to the drug, genotype-function translation tables, and, importantly, a summary of the levels of evidence and strength of recommendation for dosing recommendations. The CPIC guidelines are used by some institutions as the rationale and justification for implementing pharmacogenetic testing. In this text, pharmacogenomic information is included, and the CPIC guidelines are noted when relevant in the individual drug chapters—human leukocyte antigen (HLA)/carbamazepine,[20] HLA/phenytoin,[12] CYP2C9/valproic acid, CYP2C19/voriconazole,[14] and CYP3A5/tacrolimus.[16]

REFERENCES

1. Zanger UM, Schwab M. Cytochrome P450 enzymes in drug metabolism: regulation of gene expression, enzyme activities, and impact of genetic variation. *Pharmacol Ther.* 2013;138(1):103–141.

2. Sim SC, Kacevska M, Ingelman-Sundberg M. Pharmacogenomics of drug-metabolizing enzymes: a recent update on clinical implications and endogenous effects. *Pharmacogenomics J.* 2013;13(1):1–11.

3. Nelson DR, Koymans L, Kamataki T, et al. P450 superfamily: update on new sequences, gene mapping, accession numbers and nomenclature. *Pharmacogenetics.* 1996;6(1):1–42.

4. Zhang G, Nebert DW. Personalized medicine: genetic risk prediction of drug response. *Pharmacol Ther.* 2017;175:75–90.

5. Pinto N, Dolan ME. Clinically relevant genetic variations in drug metabolizing enzymes. *Curr Drug Metab.* 2011;12(5):487–497.

6. Nebert DW, Zhang G, Vesell ES. From human genetics and genomics to pharmacogenetics and pharmacogenomics: past lessons, future directions. *Drug Metab Rev.* 2008;40(2):187–224.

7. Relling MV, Evans WE. Pharmacogenomics in the clinic. *Nature.* 2015;526(7573):343–350.

8. Crews KR, Caudle KE, Dunnenberger HM, et al. Considerations for the Utility of the CPIC guideline for CYP2D6 genotype and codeine therapy. *Clin Chem.* 2015;61(5):775, 776.

9. Zanger UM, Klein K, Saussele T, et al. Polymorphic CYP2B6: molecular mechanisms and emerging clinical significance. *Pharmacogenomics.* 2007;8(7):743–759.

10. Vo TT, Varghese Gupta S. Role of cytochrome P450 2B6 pharmacogenomics in determining efavirenz-mediated central nervous system toxicity, treatment outcomes, and dosage adjustments in patients with human immunodeficiency virus infection. *Pharmacotherapy.* 2016;36(12):1245–1254.

11. Swart M, Skelton M, Ren Y, et al. High predictive value of CYP2B6 SNPs for steady-state plasma efavirenz levels in South African HIV/AIDS patients. *Pharmacogenet Genomics.* 2013;23(8):415–427.

12. Caudle KE, Rettie AE, Whirl-Carrillo M, et al. Clinical Pharmacogenetics Implementation Consortium guidelines for CYP2C9 and HLA-B genotypes and phenytoin dosing. *Clini Pharmacol Ther.* 2014;96(5):542–548.

13. Johnson JA, Gong L, Whirl-Carrillo M, et al. Clinical Pharmacogenetics Implementation Consortium guidelines for CYP2C9 and VKORC1 genotypes and warfarin dosing. *Clin Pharmacol Ther.* 2011;90(4):625–629.

14. Moriyama B, Obeng AO, Barbarino J, et al. Clinical Pharmacogenetics Implementation Consortium (CPIC) guidelines for CYP2C19 and voriconazole therapy. *Clin Pharmacol Ther.* 2016. doi:10.1002/cpt.583..

15. Scott SA, Sangkuhl K, Stein CM, et al. Clinical Pharmacogenetics Implementation Consortium guidelines for CYP2C19 genotype and clopidogrel therapy: 2013 update. *Clin Pharmacol Ther.* 2013;94(3):317–323.

16. Birdwell KA, Decker B, Barbarino JM, et al. Clinical Pharmacogenetics Implementation Consortium (CPIC) guidelines for CYP3A5 genotype and tacrolimus dosing. *Clin Pharmacol Ther.* 2015;98(1):19–24.

17. Buendia JA, Bramuglia G, Staatz CE. Effects of combinational CYP3A5 6986A≥G polymorphism in graft liver and native intestine on the pharmacokinetics of tacrolimus in liver transplant patients: a meta-analysis. *Ther Drug Monit.* 2014;36(4):442–447.

18. Lancia P, Jacqz-Aigrain E, Zhao W. Choosing the right dose of tacrolimus. *Arch Dis Child.* 2015;100(4):406–413.

19. Relling MV, Klein TE. CPIC: Clinical Pharmacogenetics Implementation Consortium of the pharmacogenomics research network. *Clin Pharmacol Ther.* 2011;89(3):464–467.

20. Leckband SG, Kelsoe JR, Dunnenberger HM, et al. Clinical Pharmacogenetics Implementation Consortium guidelines for HLA-B genotype and carbamazepine dosing. *Clin Pharmacol Ther.* 2013;94(3):324–328.

DRUG MONOGRAPHS

Below are the goals and objectives for Part II: Drug Monographs. Although we have used words to indicate that the learner should be able to independently recall and perform pharmacokinetic calculations, in many cases the learner should be able to identify the important issues and then be able to retrieve information and perform pharmacokinetic calculations. As an example, the expectations for the level of knowledge and immediate recall about digoxin versus vancomycin might be different depending on whether the learner would be dealing with cardiology or infectious disease patients. Also note that we have focused on the pharmacokinetic issues and not the pharmacodynamic issues. Depending on the level of the learner, it may be appropriate to add goals and objectives on pharmacodynamics, both therapeutic and toxic.

GOALS

The learner should be able analyze a patient history or scenario and then use that information to calculate dosing regimens using population parameters that would achieve the desired drug concentration(s). In addition, given a patient history or scenario, dosing regimen, and measured drug concentrations, the learner should be able to perform revisions of the appropriate pharmacokinetic parameter(s) and then use the revised patient-specific parameters to calculate dosing regimen that would achieve the desired drug concentration(s).

OBJECTIVES FOR EACH DRUG

After finishing each chapter in Part II, the learner shall be able to:

1. Know the therapeutic plasma concentrations, key parameters, and recommended sampling times.
2. Calculate, using the appropriate formula, a patient's expected volume of distribution, clearance, elimination rate constant, and half-life.
3. Select the appropriate equations that would be necessary to calculate an initial dose and a maintenance dosing regimen that would achieve and maintain the desired therapeutic concentrations.

4. Use the appropriate equations to calculate an initial loading (if appropriate) and maintenance dose that would achieve the desired target concentration(s).
5. Do the following if a patient history and measured plasma concentrations are given:
    a. Determine which pharmacokinetic parameter(s) can be revised.
    b. Use the appropriate equation(s) to revise the pharmacokinetic parameter(s).
    c. Use the revised pharmacokinetic parameter(s) to design a new dosing strategy to achieve the desired plasma concentrations(s).
6. Identify and know the direction of effect for the known disease and drug interactions. For the most common disease and drug interactions, the learner shall be able to adjust the appropriate pharmacokinetic parameter to account for the disease or drug interaction.
7. Defend, using pharmacokinetic principles, why a specific equation was used to design the dosing regimen—for example, why steady state versus non–steady state, a continuous versus intermittent input model, etc.

6

AMINOGLYCOSIDE ANTIBIOTICS

Emily Han and Paul M. Beringer

Learning Objectives

By the end of the aminoglycoside antibiotics chapter, the learner shall be able to:

1. Define the relationship between serum aminoglycoside concentrations and clinical/microbiological outcomes as well as risk for development of nephrotoxicity and ototoxicity.
2. List the patient factors and other drugs that are known to alter the volume of distribution or clearance of aminoglycosides.
3. State the optimal sampling times to determine therapeutic efficacy and safety of a dosing regimen.
4. Calculate an initial dosing regimen to achieve targeted serum concentrations, given patient demographics and clinical characteristics.
5. Determine the individualized pharmacokinetic parameters and develop a revised dosing regimen to achieve therapeutic drug concentrations if necessary, given measured serum concentrations.
6. Design a sampling scheme to enable dosage adjustment in a patient with changing renal function.
7. Calculate an appropriate dosage regimen for patients receiving hemodialysis, peritoneal dialysis, or continuous renal replacement therapy (CRRT).

The aminoglycosides are bactericidal antibiotics used in the treatment of serious gram-negative infections. Because absorption from the gastrointestinal tract is poor, the aminoglycosides must be administered parenterally to achieve therapeutic concentrations in the systemic circulation. In most instances, aminoglycosides are administered by intermittent intravenous (IV) infusions. The choice of an aminoglycoside dose is influenced by the specific agent (e.g., gentamicin vs. amikacin), infection (e.g., site and organism), renal function, and weight or body composition of the patient. The three most commonly monitored aminoglycoside antibiotics are gentamicin, tobramycin, and amikacin. The usual dose for gentamicin and tobramycin is 5 to 7 mg/kg/day, administered over 30 to 60 minutes as a single daily dose or in divided doses every 8 to 12 hours; the dose of amikacin is 15 to 20 mg/kg/day, administered over 30 to 60 minutes as a single daily dose or in divided doses every 8 to 12 hours. The clearance, volume of distribution, and half-life of all aminoglycosides are similar.[1] Therefore, the same pharmacokinetic model can be used for all the aminoglycosides, and the principles, which are described in this chapter for any given aminoglycoside generally, apply to the others as well. The aminoglycosides have different ranges of "therapeutic" serum concentrations and have different propensities for interaction with penicillin compounds.

PHARMACODYNAMICS OF AMINOGLYCOSIDES

Traditionally, aminoglycosides have been dosed multiple times a day. Investigations into the pharmacodynamic properties of aminoglycosides have yielded data that favor extended interval administration. Bactericidal activity of the aminoglycosides has been demonstrated to be concentration dependent (i.e., plasma concentrations that exceed 10 times the minimum inhibitory concentration [MIC] for a given bacteria are more effective than concentrations just above the MIC).[2–5] In addition to the concentration-dependent killing, there is also a post-antibiotic effect that results in depressed bacterial growth after plasma concentrations have fallen below the MIC.[2,6,7] Taken together, the pharmacodynamic properties of aminoglycosides suggest that less frequent administration of larger doses can maximize bactericidal activity. In addition, saturable uptake mechanisms within the renal cortex and inner ear indicate that extended interval dosing may also minimize the likelihood of developing nephrotoxicity and ototoxicity.[8–10] Experience from randomized controlled trials suggests that once-daily administration of aminoglycosides results in similar efficacy and perhaps a decreased risk of developing toxicities when compared with traditional dosing.[11,12]

THERAPEUTIC AND TOXIC PLASMA CONCENTRATIONS

Peak plasma concentrations for gentamicin and tobramycin using extended interval dosing (i.e., 5 to 7 mg/kg every 24 hours) are in the range of 20 to 30 mg/L. This peak concentration target is based on the pharmacodynamic goal of achieving a peak to MIC ratio of greater than 10 and the breakpoint for susceptibility of 2 mg/L.[13] Trough concentrations are below the limit of detection by design to provide a drug-free interval, which reduces the risk for development of nephrotoxicity. Peak plasma concentrations following traditional multiple daily dosing regimens are in the range of 5 to 8 mg/L.[14–16] Peak plasma concentrations <2 to 4 mg/L are likely to be ineffective,[15] and successful treatment of pneumonia may require peak concentrations of 8 mg/L or more.[14] Desirable peak concentrations for amikacin are usually 20 to 30 mg/L; trough concentrations are usually <10 mg/L.[1]

Most available data correlating aminoglycoside concentrations with ototoxicity and nephrotoxicity refer to trough plasma concentrations, although some data suggest a correlation between peak concentrations and toxicity.[17,18] Although gentamicin trough concentrations of >2 mg/L have been associated with renal toxicity, the high trough concentrations may be the result, and not the cause, of renal dysfunction. In fact, the use of elevated trough concentrations as an indication of early renal damage has been suggested by some investigators.[19,20] Fortunately, most patients who develop renal dysfunction during aminoglycoside therapy appear to regain normal renal function after the drug has been discontinued.[21]

Ototoxicity has been associated with trough plasma concentrations of gentamicin exceeding 4 mg/L for more than 10 days. When the trough concentration is multiplied by the number of days of therapy, the risk of ototoxicity is increased when the product exceeds 40 mg/day/L. Aminoglycoside ototoxicity also seems to be most prevalent in

KEY PARAMETERS: Aminoglycoside Antibiotics

THERAPEUTIC SERUM CONCENTRATIONS

Gentamicin, Tobramycin	Conventional dosing	"Once-daily" dosing
	Peak 5–8 mg/L	20 mg/L
	Trough $<$ 2 mg/L	Undetectable
Amikacin	Peak 20–30 mg/L	60 mg/L
	Trough $<$ 10 mg/L	Undetectable

V^a		
Adults, Children $>$12 yr	0.25 L/kg	
Children 5–12 yr	0.35 L/kg	

Cl		
Adults, Children $>$ 12 yr	Equal to Cl_{Cr}	
Functionally anephric patients^c	0.0043 L/kg/hr	
Surgically anephric patients^c	0.0021 L/kg/hr	
Hemodialysis^c	1.8 L/hr	
Children $\leq$ 12 yr^b	Equal to GFR	
AUC_{24}	70–100 mg · hr/L	Gentamicin and tobramycin (amikacin approximately threefold higher)

$t\frac{1}{2}$		
Normal renal function	2–3 hr	
Functionally anephric patients	30–60 hr	
fu (fraction unbound in plasma)	$>$0.95	

^{a}Volume of distribution should be adjusted for obesity and/or alterations in extracellular fluid status.
^{b}Glomerular filtration rate (GFR) calculated by modified Schwartz equation.
^{c}A functionally anephric patient is a dialysis patient with kidneys intact. A surgically anephric patient is a dialysis patient with kidneys removed. Hemodialysis clearance of 1.8 L/hr refers to low-flux hemodialysis, not high-flux or peritoneal dialysis.

patients who have existing impaired renal function or have received large doses during the course of their treatment.[17–19,22,23]

Although it is the standard practice to use aminoglycoside plasma concentrations as predictors for both efficacy and toxicity, it is controversial whether this is valid.[24] The adoption of once-daily aminoglycoside dosing at many institutions has led to less intensive monitoring of serum concentrations. The nomogram developed by Nicolau et al.[13] recommends that a single level be drawn 6 to 14 hours after the dose. The nomogram then defines in graphical form whether the dosing interval is appropriate or needs to be extended. This type of approach is much more simplified than the traditional method of determining the individualized pharmacokinetic parameters, based on measured peak and trough concentrations; however, it may not provide the same precise control of drug exposure (i.e., peak, area under the curve [AUC]) in patients who exhibit altered pharmacokinetics (i.e., third-space fluid, burns, cystic fibrosis, spinal cord injury). Alternatively, Barclay et al.[25] have defined a method of dosage individualization of extended interval aminoglycoside dosing based on a measured peak concentration and an estimation of the AUC. This dosing method is based on the assumption that the goal is to provide a similar degree of drug exposure as traditional daily dosing methods (i.e., AUC) to minimize the risk of toxicity but provide a higher peak concentration to maximize the bactericidal activity. The target AUC_{24} range for gentamicin and tobramycin is 70 to 100 mg · hr/L.

BIOAVAILABILITY (F)

The aminoglycoside antibiotics are highly water soluble and poorly lipid soluble compounds. As a result, they are poorly absorbed when administered orally and must be administered parenterally for the treatment of systemic infections.

VOLUME OF DISTRIBUTION (V)

The volume of distribution of aminoglycosides is ≈0.25 L/kg, although a relatively wide range of 0.1 to 0.5 L/kg has been reported.[26–32] Because aminoglycosides distribute very poorly into adipose tissue, lean rather than total body weight (TBW) should result in a more accurate approximation of V in obese patients.[33] The aminoglycoside volume of distribution in obese subjects also could be adjusted based on the patient's ideal body weight (IBW) plus 10% of his or her excess weight.[34,35] These adjustments in the estimation of aminoglycoside volumes of distribution in obese patients seem reasonable because aminoglycoside antibiotics appear to distribute into extracellular space, and the extracellular fluid volume of adipose tissue is approximately 10% of adipose weight versus 25%, which is an average for all the other tissues. Equation 6.1 can be used to approximate the volume of distribution (V) in obese patients:

$$\text{Aminoglycoside V (Obese Patients)} = (0.25 \text{ L/kg})(IBW) + 0.1(TBW - IBW) \qquad \textbf{(Eq. 6.1)}$$

The nonobese or IBW can be approximated using Equations 6.2 and 6.3 (see Creatinine Clearance [Cl_{Cr}] in Chapter 3).

$$\text{Ideal Body Weight for Males in kg} = 50 + (2.3)(\text{Height in inches} > 60) \qquad \textbf{(Eq. 6.2)}$$

$$\text{Ideal Body Weight for Females in kg} = 45 + (2.3)(\text{Height in inches} > 60) \qquad \textbf{(Eq. 6.3)}$$

The volume of distribution of aminoglycosides is increased in patients with ascites, edema, or other enlarged "third-space" volume.[36,37] One approach to approximating the increased volume of distribution for patients with ascites or edema is to increase the V by 1 L for each kilogram of weight gain. This approach is based on the assumption that the volume of distribution of aminoglycoside antibiotics is approximately equal to the extracellular fluid volume. This is consistent with the low plasma protein binding[1] and the fact that aminoglycosides cross membranes very poorly.

$$\text{Aminoglycoside V (L)} = \left(\begin{array}{c} 0.25\ \text{L/kg} \times \text{Nonobese,} \\ \text{Non–Excess Fluid Weight (kg)} \end{array} \right) + 0.1 \left(\begin{array}{c} \text{Excess} \\ \text{Adipose} \\ \text{Weight (kg)} \end{array} \right) + \left(\begin{array}{c} \text{Excess Third} \\ \text{Space Fluid} \\ \text{Weight (kg)} \end{array} \right)$$

$$\textbf{(Eq. 6.4)}$$

The volume of distribution of aminoglycosides can be estimated using Equation 6.4, in which the nonobese, non–excess fluid weight can usually be estimated as the IBW, and the excess adipose weight as the difference between the nonobese weight and the patient's total weight without excess third-space fluid. The excess third-space fluid weight is estimated clinically. In cases in which a rapid increase in weight has occurred over several days, this weight gain is likely to represent fluid in a third space; it is, therefore, easily estimated by taking a difference between the initial and current weights. Some patients may exhibit significant third spacing of fluids (apparent as either edema or ascites) on initial evaluation. It is most difficult to estimate an aminoglycoside V in the obese patient with significant third spacing of fluid. As Equation 6.4 illustrates, assigning excess third-space fluid to adipose weight could result in a significant underestimation of the volume of distribution. For this reason, it should be recognized that Equation 6.4 only approximates the V, and plasma concentration measurements are needed to make patient-specific adjustments.

Physiologic changes in the extracellular fluid volume occur with age in children. As the body weight increases, the percent of total body water decreases from approximately 85% in premature infants to 75% in full-term infants, to 60% in adults.[38] Accordingly, the volume of distribution of aminoglycoside continues to decline from an initial value of 0.5 L/kg to the adult value of 0.25L/kg between birth and adolescence.[39] In children younger than 5 years, the difference in V results in aminoglycoside doses that are twice that of older children or adults to achieve similar C_{max}.[32]

$$\text{Aminoglycoside} \atop \text{V(L) in Children} = \left[0.5 \text{ L/kg} - \left(\frac{\text{Age in Years}}{5} \times 0.25 \right) \right] \left(\begin{array}{c} \text{Weight} \\ \text{in kg} \end{array} \right) \qquad \textbf{(Eq. 6.5)}$$
$$\text{1 to 5 Years}$$

Because the change in volume of distribution is gradual, some clinicians have chosen to use the above algorithm to estimate the volume of distribution for patients between 1 and 5 years of age. Note that in Equation 6.5, it is assumed that the child's weight in kilogram represents a weight that is not obese and does not contain significant excess third-space fluid. Obese children have a smaller-than-average volume of distribution for their age and size, which results in lower peak concentration than children with lean body weight (LBW),[32] and children with significant third spacing of fluid should have a larger-than-average V. Pediatric patients presenting with fever and dehydration may initially have decreased V, but eventually require higher aminoglycoside doses to achieve the same target peak level to account for increase V with fluid boluses.[41] In general, the volume of distribution of 0.35 L/kg is used for patients between 5 and 12 years of age, and the adult V of 0.25 L/kg is used with older children.[40,41]

The pharmacokinetics of the aminoglycoside antibiotics has been described by a two- or three-compartment model.[42,43] However, a one-compartment model has been used widely in the clinical setting to facilitate aminoglycoside pharmacokinetic calculations. The initial distribution phase following a gentamicin IV infusion is not considered when the one-compartment model is utilized for gentamicin pharmacokinetic calculations.[43–45] For this reason, reported values for plasma samples obtained near the conclusion of an IV infusion may be higher than expected. In addition, there is some evidence that the length of the distribution phase may be dose dependent.[46] These reported values probably have no correlation with the therapeutic or toxic effects of the drug; however, they are important in terms of the optimal timing and interpretation of measured serum concentrations. A third distribution phase, or gamma phase, for gentamicin has also been identified.[42] This final volume of distribution phase for gentamicin is large, and because gentamicin clearance is decreased when plasma concentrations are low, the average half-life associated with this third compartment is in excess of 100 hours.[42,43] This large final volume of distribution and long terminal half-life may be significant when evaluating a patient's potential for aminoglycoside toxicity.[47]

Despite the existence of the three-compartment model for the aminoglycosides, pharmacokinetic calculations can be based on a one-compartment model that utilizes the second volume of distribution. The errors encountered when using a single-compartment model for aminoglycosides can be minimized if plasma drug concentrations are obtained at times that avoid the first and third distribution phases and at 24 hours after therapy has been initiated.[48] Aminoglycoside concentrations <1 mg/L should be evaluated cautiously because the influence of the large third compartment will become greater at these low concentrations.[43]

CLEARANCE (Cl)

The aminoglycoside antibiotics are eliminated almost entirely by the renal route.[1,31] Because the aminoglycoside and creatinine clearances are similar over a wide range of renal function, aminoglycoside clearance can be estimated from the formulas used to estimate creatinine clearance (Equations 6.6 and 6.7) when concentrations are within the therapeutic range.[1,26,31,43]

$$Cl_{Cr} \text{ for Males (mL/min)} = \frac{(140-Age)(Weight)}{(72)(SCr_{SS})} \qquad \textbf{(Eq. 6.6)}$$

$$Cl_{Cr} \text{ for Females (mL/min)} = (0.85)\frac{(140-Age)(Weight)}{(72)(SCr_{SS})} \qquad \textbf{(Eq. 6.7)}$$

As presented in Chapter 3, the age is in years, weight is in kg, and serum creatinine is in mg/dL. Correct estimates of creatinine clearance can only be obtained if the patient's weight represents a normal ratio of muscle mass to TBW and the serum creatinine is at steady state. For this reason, pharmacokinetic calculations for obese patients and patients who have significant third spacing of fluid should take into consideration adjustments for obesity and third spacing. Although IBW, calculated from Equation 6.2 and 6.3, is generally used to calculate creatinine clearance in obese patients, GFR has been shown to increase in proportion to the LBW, and LBW has been suggested to provide better estimation of creatinine clearance in morbidly obese patients (BMI > 40).[49] In patients who are obese (i.e., BMI, 30 to 40), creatinine clearance can be best estimated by using a weight that falls between the IBW and TBW.[50,51] For this reason, some clinicians prefer to estimate the nonobese weight by using the following equation:

$$\text{Nonobese Weight} \approx IBW + 0.4\,(TBW - IBW)$$

where IBW is estimated by Equations 6.2 and 6.3, and TBW represents the patient's TBW without the presence of excess third-space fluid. Alternately, TBW can be used to estimate creatinine clearance in patients with BMI < 40.

Predicted creatinine clearance is the most commonly employed method of estimating aminoglycoside clearance; however, this formula is known to be inaccurate at low creatinine concentrations. The Modification of Diet in Renal Disease (MDRD) equation was recently developed to provide a more accurate estimate of glomerular filtrations rate. Data correlating estimated GFRs using the MDRD equation and measured aminoglycoside clearance are currently limited.[52] More recently, the use of cystatin c concentrations has been utilized to estimate glomerular filtration. Cystatin c is an endogenous protein that is constitutively expressed from all nucleated cells and is eliminated by glomerular filtration. One advantage of cystatin c is that it is unaffected by changes in muscle mass. Several studies have demonstrated improved sensitivity in identifying early renal disease. A recent study demonstrated an improved ability to predict amikacin clearance with cystatin c clearance compared with creatinine clearance.[53] Until more definitive data are available, use of predicted creatinine clearance as a marker of aminoglycoside clearance is still recommended.

Creatinine clearance in children older than 12 years of age can be determined by using Equations 6.6 and 6.7, which are used to calculate creatinine clearance in adults.[54] However, in younger children, the ongoing maturation of the renal function and the hemodynamic and physiologic changes after birth lead to variable GFR at different stages of development.[38] Utilization of Equations 6.6 and 6.7 in these children will result in inaccurate creatinine clearance. For this reason, there are numerous methods trying to measure GFR in children, including allometric and quadratic formulas.[55,56] The most widely used equation to estimate renal clearance in pediatric population is the one utilizing the child's height and plasma creatinine concentration derived by Schwartz.[57]

$$\text{GFR (mL/min/1.73 m}^2) = 0.413 \left(\frac{\text{Height in cm}}{\text{(SCr)}} \right) \qquad \textbf{(Eq. 6.8)}$$

Because Equation 6.8 was derived from the data in children with GFR 15 to 75 mL/min/1.73 m^2, estimated GFR > 75 mL/min/1.73 m^2 should be used with caution. Equation 6.8 has been shown to overestimate GFR in those patients whose Ht/Scr ratio exceeds 251, which corresponds to GFR[58] of 103 mL/min/1.73 m^2.

Evaluation of GFR should be done with caution in neonates because the maturation of kidney depends on the birth weight and postnatal age.[56] The allometric equation using the bodyweight scaled to adults shows that the clearance is higher in neonates and young children compared with that in older children and adults,[56] which is in accordance with greater gentamicin and tobramycin clearance seen in the first weeks of life until 1 year after birth. In these young children with changing renal function, population pharmacokinetic modeling may give a better prediction of aminoglycoside clearance.

Nonrenal clearance

Another factor that should be considered when estimating the clearance of aminoglycosides is the nonrenal clearance, which is ≈0.0021 L/kg/hr (or ≈2.5 mL/min/70 kg). The nonrenal clearance of aminoglycosides is generally ignored in most patients, but it is significant in patients whose renal function is significantly diminished. In patients who are functionally anephric and receiving intermittent hemodialysis, a clearance value of ≈0.0043 L/kg/hr (5 mL/min/70 kg) represents the residual renal clearance and the nonrenal clearance. These values, however, are only approximations; serum concentrations of aminoglycosides should be monitored in patients with poor renal function.

Penicillin interaction

Aminoglycosides are often used in combination with β-lactam antibiotic for serious gram-negative infections. Carbenicillin, ticarcillin, and related extended-spectrum penicillins chemically inactivate gentamicin and tobramycin. The β-lactam ring of these penicillin compounds interacts in vivo and in vitro with one of the primary amines on both gentamicin and tobramycin to form an inactive amide.[59–61] The rate of gentamicin and tobramycin inactivation by penicillins is slow and will not be clinically significant in patient with normal clearance of these drugs.[62] In patients with severely impaired renal function, the contact time between the tobramycin or gentamicin and penicillins is increased, and the risk of inactivation is greater.[21,60,63] In these patients, the concurrent administration of carbenicillin or ticarcillin can decrease the half-life of gentamicin from approximately 46 to 22 hours. Although this interaction is usually not considered a route of aminoglycoside clearance, it does act as a mechanism for drug "elimination." This interaction is a function of the specific aminoglycoside, the penicillin compound, the concentration of the penicillin compound, and the temperature. For patients with very poor renal function who are receiving carbenicillin and ticarcillin, the additional gentamicin clearance can be approximated by multiplying the patient's apparent volume of distribution for the aminoglycoside by 0.017 hr^{-1}.

$$\begin{matrix} \text{Tobramycin, Gentamicin} \\ \text{Clearance by Carbenicillin} \\ \text{or Ticarcillin (L/hr)} \end{matrix} = (0.017 \text{ hr}^{-1}) \left(\begin{matrix} \text{Volume of Distribution} \\ \text{for Aminoglycosides} \end{matrix} \right) \qquad \textbf{(Eq. 6.9)}$$

The elimination rate constant (K) of 0.017 hr^{-1} represents the approximate in vitro elimination rate for aminoglycosides exposed to carbenicillin concentrations of 250 to 500 mg/L at a temperature of 37°C. Carbenicillin is no longer available on the market, but this equation can be used to calculate additional gentamicin clearance when ticarcillin is coadministered with gentamicin or tobramycin.

In general, tobramycin is most likely to interact with penicillins, followed by gentamicin.[59–61,63–66] Amikacin appears to be more resistant to degradation by penicillins.[59] Piperacillin/tazobactam appears to interact with gentamicin and tobramycin similarly but to a lesser extent than carbenicillin and ticarcillin.[67,68] Furthermore, the in vitro interaction between the cephalosporins (e.g., cefazolin, cefamandole, cefotaxime) and the aminoglycoside antibiotics appears to be minimal.[67–69] Because the third-generation cephalosporin antibiotics have, to a large degree, replaced the use of penicillin derivatives, the interaction between aminoglycoside antibiotics and penicillin derivatives is encountered infrequently in most clinical practices.[64,67,70] Extended infusion of β-lactam drugs (infusing each dose over 3 hours vs. 0.5 hour) is implemented at many institutions to maximize bactericidal activity by prolonging the time drug level remains above the MIC. The impact of β-lactam extended infusion in renally impaired patients also receiving aminoglycoside is unknown. The prolonged serum levels of β-lactams may increase the risk of inactivation of aminoglycosides even with those agents that showed insignificant interaction with short infusion time. Close monitoring of plasma levels of aminoglycosides is recommended in these patients.

Plasma samples for patients receiving aminoglycosides and penicillins concurrently must be obtained at a time when the in vitro interaction is minimal. Plasma samples for assay of aminoglycoside concentrations should be obtained when the penicillin is at its lowest concentration and assayed as soon as possible. If storage is required, samples should be frozen to minimize the continual in vitro effect of this interaction.

ELIMINATION HALF-LIFE

The elimination half-life of aminoglycoside antibiotics from the body is a function of the volume of distribution and clearance. Because renal function varies considerably among individuals, the half-life is also variable. For example, a 70-kg, 25-year-old man with a serum creatinine of 0.8 mg/dL might have an aminoglycoside clearance of 100 mL/min or more. If his volume of distribution is 0.25 L/kg, the corresponding elimination half-life will be approximately 2 hours. In contrast, a 75-year-old man with a similar V and a serum creatinine of 1.4 mg/dL might have an aminoglycoside clearance of $\approx$35 mL/min and a half-life of $\approx$6 hours. For this reason, the initial aminoglycoside dose and dosing interval should be selected with care. Although initial estimates of the patient's aminoglycoside pharmacokinetic parameters may be highly variable, it is hoped that pharmacokinetic adjustments will optimize the achievement of therapeutic, yet nontoxic, concentrations of aminoglycoside antibiotics.

NOMOGRAMS AND COMPUTERS

The wide availability of nomograms to dose aminoglycosides may lead one to question the necessity for pharmacokinetic calculations.[10] One nomogram that is utilized at a number of centers is the Hartford high-dose extended interval dosing nomogram.[13] The dose in this nomogram is 7 mg/kg, which targets a peak concentration of 20 to 30 mg/L that is 10 times the breakpoint for susceptibility for gentamicin and tobramycin (i.e., 2 mcg/mL). The dosing interval is adjusted based on the degree of renal function in order to maintain the target peak concentration and also achieve a drug-free interval of $\approx$6 hours to reduce accumulation within the renal cortex and inner ear.

CREATININE CLEARANCE (mL/min)	INITIAL DOSE AND INTERVAL
>60	7 mg/kg every 24 hour
40–60	7 mg/kg every 36 hour
20–40	7 mg/kg every 48 hour
<20	7 mg/kg, then follow levels to determine time of next dose (level <1 mcg/mL)

The nomogram also provides the ability to adjust the dosing interval based on a measured serum concentration obtained 6 to 14 hours after a dose. Three regions are defined in the nomogram corresponding to the appropriate dosing interval that should be chosen based on the single measured concentration. For example, if a patient was initiated on a dose of 7 mg/kg every 24 hours and had a measured concentration of 8.2 mg/L $\approx$ 9 hours after the dose, the nomogram indicates that the dosing interval should be extended to every 36 hours (see Fig. 6.1).

The limitation of these types of nomograms is that they are usually designed to achieve fixed peak and trough serum concentrations, and they do not allow the clinician to individualize the dosing regimens to account for the type of infection treated or the

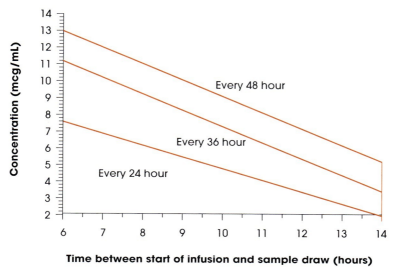

FIGURE 6.1   Gentamicin or tobramycin concentrations obtained 6 to 14 hours following a 7-mg/kg dose are plotted on the nomogram relative to the time of sampling, following the dose. Concentrations that fall within the every 24 hour quadrant indicate that the dosing interval of 24 hours should be maintained. Concentrations that fall in the every 36 hour or every 48 hour quadrant indicate that the dosing interval should be extended to 36 or 48 hours. (Adapted from Nicolau D, Freeman CD, Belliveau PP, et al. Experience with a once-daily aminoglycoside program administered to 2,184 adult patients. *Antimicrob Agents Chemother.* 1995;39:650–655, with permission from the American Society for Microbiology.)

benefit-to-risk ratio for the individual patient. Furthermore, nomograms are based on average pharmacokinetic parameters and do not provide a method for dose adjustment for unique patients (e.g., obese individuals or those who have significant third spacing of fluid). Patient-specific adjustments based on measured plasma concentrations also cannot be extrapolated from these nomograms. An understanding of the basic pharmacokinetic principles used to individualize aminoglycoside doses, coupled with a rational clinical approach, will enable the clinician to provide optimal therapy for the patient.

A number of computer programs are available to help clinicians dose aminoglycosides and other therapeutic agents. Computers tend to be more flexible than nomograms, in that the user often can select dosing intervals and peak or trough concentrations based on clinical judgment. In addition, they enable dosage determination based on data (including multiple sets of measurements) obtained under non–steady-state conditions, which is particularly important in patients with changing renal function. Bayesian analysis has been incorporated in most computerized pharmacokinetic programs and has been proven to provide very precise estimates of the pharmacokinetic parameters. One potential pitfall, however, is that the user must be familiar with the algorithms initially used to define the expected pharmacokinetic parameters and how patient-specific parameters are revised when plasma concentrations and dosing histories are supplied. In the revision process, the user must be able to recognize data that are obviously wrong and to interpret the computer output to ensure that the parameters and dosing recommendations are reasonable. The computer should be viewed as a labor-saving device, not as a substitute for a thorough understanding of the pharmacokinetic process.

TIME TO SAMPLE

Correct timing of the sample collection is important because aminoglycoside antibiotics have a relatively short half-life and a small but significant distribution phase. The most widely accepted guidelines recommend that samples for peak serum concentrations be obtained 1 hour after the maintenance dose has been initiated. This recommendation assumes that the drug is infused over about 30 minutes; an acceptable range for the infusion period is 20 to 40 minutes. If it is longer than 40 minutes, peak concentrations should be obtained ≈30 minutes after the end of the infusion to ensure that distribution is complete. Others have suggested that peak measurements should be obtained later in the dosing interval to avoid the distribution phase, particularly with extended interval dosing because of the potential dose-dependent distribution phase.[46] Trough concentrations generally should be obtained within the 0.5 hour before the administration of the next maintenance dose. In cases in which the trough concentrations are expected to be lower than the assay sensitivity (particularly with extended interval dosing), an earlier sampling time may be appropriate so that measurable trough concentrations can be obtained and patient-specific pharmacokinetic parameters derived. Ideally, the interval between the two concentration measurements should be two to four half-lives to provide more precise estimates of the half-life and reduce the potential for the later concentration to fall below the level of assay sensitivity. In all cases, the exact time of sampling and dose administration should be recorded.

When aminoglycoside plasma concentrations are sampled at a time that extends beyond the expected peak, it is possible to calculate the plasma concentration at the earlier time by simply rearranging

$$C = C_0 \ e^{-Kt} \qquad \textbf{(Eq. 6.10)}$$

where C_0 is the initial plasma concentration, C a concentration at some time t later, to

$$C_0 = \frac{C}{e^{-Kt}} \qquad \textbf{(Eq. 6.11)}$$

In the above equation, t represents the time from the measured plasma concentration (C) to the earlier plasma concentration (C_0). This equation is used to back-extrapolate a plasma concentration to the "clinical peak," which is 1 hour after the start of the infusion. The "clinical peak" concentration has generally been used as a guide to aminoglycoside efficacy.

The optimal time to sample within the first 24 hours of therapy is difficult to determine. For patients who are critically ill, a peak and subsequent trough (or midpoint for extended interval dosing) serum aminoglycoside concentration obtained after the initial loading dose allows for the most rapid evaluation of patient-specific parameters and subsequent dose adjustment, if necessary. In a large number of cases, however, this early sampling may not be necessary, particularly if the expected duration of therapy is relatively short (i.e., 3 to 5 days). The standard of practice in many institutions has been to obtain the first aminoglycoside samples after three or four doses of aminoglycoside have been administered. The majority of patients will be approaching steady state by this time; however, with the wide availability of computers and pharmacokinetic software programs, it is not absolutely necessary to wait until steady state is achieved. With extended interval dosing, there should be no significant accumulation with multiple dosing; therefore, measurements can be obtained after any dose.

Although one can estimate patient-specific pharmacokinetic parameters more accurately with three or four aminoglycoside plasma concentrations (particularly using a multicompartment model), reasonable pharmacokinetic parameters can be estimated using a one-compartment model and two plasma samples in most cases.

When aminoglycoside antibiotics are administered intramuscularly (IM), the time for absorption or drug input is less predictable; however, in most patients, plasma concentrations peak about 1 hour after the IM injection.[71] For this reason, a peak plasma concentration should be obtained 1 hour after the IM dose is administered. Because the rate of absorption is uncertain, it is difficult to know whether unusual plasma concentrations following IM administration represent delayed absorption or unusual pharmacokinetic parameters (e.g., a large volume of distribution).

Question #1   *R.W. is a 30-year-old, 70-kg, nonobese woman with a serum creatinine of 0.9 mg/dL. An initial gentamicin dose of 140 mg was infused IV over 30 minutes. Calculate the plasma concentration of gentamicin 1 hour after the infusion was started (i.e., 0.5 hour after the infusion was completed).*

A rough estimate of the peak gentamicin concentration can be calculated using Equation 6.12 by treating the 30-minute infusion as a bolus dose. The 140-mg dose would be divided by the literature value for the volume of distribution ($\approx$0.25 L/kg or 17.5 L) in this 70-kg woman.

$$C_1 = \frac{(S)(F)(\text{Loading Dose})}{V}$$

(Eq. 6.12)

$$= \frac{(1)(1)(140 \text{ mg})}{17.5}$$
$$= 8.0 \text{ mg/L}$$

The salt form (S) and bioavailability (F) were both assumed to be 1.0, and the plasma concentration of 8.0 mg/L is an approximation that assumes absorption was very rapid and that no significant drug elimination took place during the time of administration. In addition, it is assumed that the drug is distributed into a single compartment. Even though there is clearly a distribution phase associated with the IV injection of aminoglycosides, the initially high drug concentration can be ignored as long as plasma sampling is avoided during this distribution phase.[30,31,45]

A more precise calculation of the plasma concentration 1 hour after the 0.5 hour infusion has been initiated would take into account the decay of gentamicin levels from the peak concentration as calculated by Equation 6.10. In Equation 6.13 for C_1, t_1 is the time elapsed from the beginning of the IV infusion to the time of sampling at 1 hour, and the elimination rate constant (K) represents the clearance of gentamicin divided by its volume of distribution (V) (Equation 6.14).

$$C_1 = \frac{(S)(F)(\text{Loading Dose})}{V}(e^{-Kt_1}) \qquad \text{(Eq. 6.13)}$$

$$K = \frac{Cl}{V} \qquad \text{(Eq. 6.14)}$$

A creatinine clearance (and therefore gentamicin clearance) of ≈ 101 mL/min or 6.06 L/hr can be calculated for R.W., using Equation 6.7:

$$Cl_{cr} \text{ for Females (mL/min)} = (0.85)\frac{(140 - \text{Age})(\text{Weight})}{(72)(SCr_{ss})}$$

$$= (0.85)\frac{(140 - 30)(70)}{(72)(0.9)}$$

$$= 101 \text{ mL/min}$$

$$Cl_{cr} \text{ (L/hr)} = (101 \text{ mL/min})\left(\frac{60 \text{ min/hr}}{1,000 \text{ mL/L}}\right)$$

$$= 6.06 \text{ L/hr}$$

Using this clearance of ≈ 6 L/hr and the apparent volume of distribution of 17.5 L, an elimination rate constant of 0.346 hr^{-1} can be calculated using Equation 6.14. This elimination rate constant, when used in Equation 6.13 to calculate the gentamicin concentration 1.0 hour after the dose, results in a predicted concentration of 5.7 mg/L.

$$K = \frac{Cl}{V}$$

$$= \frac{6.06 \text{ L/hr}}{17.5 \text{ L}}$$

$$= 0.346 \text{ hr}^{-1}$$

$$C_1 = \frac{(S)(F)(\text{Loading Dose})}{V}(e^{-Kt_1})$$

$$= (8 \text{ mg/L})(e^{-(0.346 \text{ hr}^{-1})(1 \text{ hr})})$$

$$= (8 \text{ mg/L})(0.71)$$

$$= 5.7 \text{ mg/L}$$

To evaluate whether the IV bolus dose model is appropriate, the duration of infusion (0.5 hour) should be compared with the apparent drug half-life. When the duration of infusion or absorption is less than one-sixth of the half-life, then the bolus dose model can be used (see Chapter 2). If, however, the duration of drug input is greater than one-sixth of the half-life, then an infusion model should be used. Using Equation 6.15 and the elimination rate constant of 0.346 hr^{-1}, R.W.'s half-life is calculated to be $\approx$2 hours as follows:

$$t\,\tfrac{1}{2} = \frac{0.693}{K} \qquad \textbf{(Eq. 6.15)}$$

$$= \frac{0.693}{0.346 \text{ hr}^{-1}}$$

$$= 2.0 \text{ hr}$$

Question #2   *Using the clearance of 6.06 L/hr, the volume of distribution of 17.5 L, the elimination rate constant of 0.346 hr^{-1}, and the short infusion model, calculate the expected gentamicin concentration for R.W. 1 hour after initiating the 0.5 hour infusion of a 140-mg dose.*

Equation 6.16 represents the short infusion model and can be used to calculate the plasma concentration 1 hour after starting the 0.5 hour infusion. The duration of infusion or t_{in} would be 0.5 hour, and t_2, or the time of decay from the end of the infusion, would be 0.5 hour. Using these values, the plasma concentration 1 hour after initiation of the 0.5 hour infusion would be 6.2 mg/L.

$$C_2 = \frac{(S)(F)(Dose/t_{in})}{Cl}(1 - e^{-Kt_{in}})(e^{-Kt_2}) \qquad \textbf{(Eq. 6.16)}$$

$$= \frac{(1)(1)(140 \text{ mg}/0.5 \text{ hr})}{6.06 \text{ L/hr}}(1 - e^{-(0.346\ hr^{-1})(0.5\ hr)})(e^{-(0.346\ hr^{-1})(0.5\ hr)})$$

$$= (46.2 \text{ mg/L})(0.16)(0.84)$$

$$= (7.4 \text{ mg/L})(0.84)$$

$$= 6.2 \text{ mg/L}$$

Note that the plasma concentration of 7.4 mg/L at the end of the 0.5 hour infusion is lower than the calculated peak concentration of 8 mg/L following a bolus dose (see Question 1). This lower concentration at the end of the infusion reflects the clearance of drug during the infusion process. Also note that the plasma concentration of 6.2 mg/L at 1 hour calculated by the infusion model is greater than the comparable plasma concentration (5.7 mg/L) calculated by the bolus dose model in Question 1. Less drug remains in the body at this time when the bolus dose model is used because this model assumes that the entire dose entered the body at the beginning of the infusion.

The total dose, therefore, has been exposed to the body's clearing mechanisms for a longer time.

Question #3   *In what types of patients is it more appropriate to use the infusion equation for the prediction of aminoglycoside concentrations? When can the bolus dose model be used satisfactorily?*

Because the difference between the results obtained from these two approaches is primarily related to the amount of drug cleared from the body during the infusion period, it is reasonable to assume that in patients with decreased renal function and longer aminoglycoside half-lives, the bolus dose model could be used satisfactorily. In patients with good renal function (e.g., young adults and children), use of the infusion model is more appropriate because these patients often have very short aminoglycoside half-lives.

Question #4   *R.W., the 70-kg woman described in Question 1, was given 140 mg of gentamicin over 0.5 hour every 8 hours. Predict her peak and trough plasma concentrations at steady state.*

Again, one could treat this problem as if R.W. were receiving intermittent IV boluses or as if she were receiving 0.5 hour infusions every 8 hours. If the bolus dose model is applied, Equation 6.17 can be used to predict the peak levels, where t_1 represents the time interval between the start of the infusion and the time at which the "peak concentration" is sampled (1 hour), and τ is the interval between the doses (8 hours). Using the volume of distribution of 17.5 L and the elimination rate constant of 0.346 hr^{-1}, the calculated peak concentration would be 6.1 mg/L.

$$Css_1 = \frac{\dfrac{(S)(F)(Dose)}{V}}{(1 - e^{-K\tau})} \, e^{-Kt_1} \qquad \textbf{(Eq. 6.17)}$$

$$= \frac{\dfrac{(1)(1)(140 \text{ mg})}{17.5 \text{ L}} \left(e^{-(0.346 \text{ hr}^{-1})(1 \text{ hr})} \right)}{(1 - e^{-(0.346 \text{ hr}^{-1})(8 \text{ hr})})}$$

$$= \left(\frac{8 \text{ mg/L}}{1 - 0.063} \right)(0.71)$$

$$= \left(\frac{8 \text{ mg/L}}{0.937} \right)(0.71)$$

$$= (8.5 \text{ mg/L})(0.71)$$

$$= 6.1 \text{ mg/L}$$

The trough concentration can also be calculated using Equation 6.17, where t_1 is the time interval between the start of the infusion and the time at which trough level is sampled (8 hours). If the trough sample is obtained just before the start of the next infusion, then Equation 6.18 for Css min also can be used. Using the appropriate values for volume of distribution, elimination rate constant, and dosing interval, the calculated trough concentration would be 0.54 mg/L.

$$\text{Css min} = \frac{(S)(F)(\text{Dose})}{V}\frac{}{(1 - e^{-K\tau})}\, e^{-K\tau} \qquad \textbf{(Eq. 6.18)}$$

$$= \frac{\dfrac{(1)(1)(140\ \text{mg})}{17.5\ \text{L}}\left(e^{-(0.346\ \text{hr}^{-1})(8\ \text{hr})}\right)}{(1 - e^{-(0.346\ \text{hr}^{-1})(8\ \text{hr})})}$$

$$= \frac{8\ \text{mg/L}}{0.937}(0.063)$$

$$= 0.54\ \text{mg/L}$$

If the infusion input model,

$$C_{t_{in}} = \frac{(S)(F)(\text{Dose}/t_{in})}{Cl}(1 - e^{-K\tau_{in}}) \qquad \textbf{(Eq. 6.19)}$$

where t_{in} is the duration of the infusion, is used to replace the bolus dose model

$$\frac{(S)(F)(\text{Dose})}{V} \qquad \textbf{(Eq. 6.20)}$$

in Equations 6.17 and 6.18, then the resultant substitution results in an equation describing the intermittent infusion steady-state model (also see Chapter 2).

$$\text{Css}_2 = \frac{\dfrac{(S)(F)(\text{Dose}/t_{in})}{Cl}(1 - e^{-Kt_{in}})}{(1 - e^{-K\tau})}(e^{-Kt_2}) \qquad \textbf{(Eq. 6.21)}$$

where τ is the dosing interval and t_2 the time interval between the end of the infusion and the time at which the concentration is measured. That is, when peak concentrations are measured 1 hour after the initiation of a 0.5 hour infusion, t_2 is 0.5 hour. For trough concentrations that are sampled just before the start of a subsequent infusion (i.e., administered on an 8-hour schedule), t_2 is 7.5 hours.

Again, assuming S and F to be 1.0, the infusion time to be 0.5 hour, the dosing interval (τ) to be 8 hours, the clearance (Cl) and the elimination rate constant (K) to be 6.06 L/hr and 0.346 hr^{-1}, respectively, the "peak" concentration 1 hour after starting the 0.5 hour infusion would be calculated using Equation 6.21 as follows:

$$Css_2 = \frac{\dfrac{(S)(F)(Dose/t_{in})}{Cl}(1-e^{-Kt_{in}})}{(1-e^{-K\tau})}(e^{-Kt_2})$$

$$= \frac{\dfrac{(1)(1)(140 \text{ mg}/0.5 \text{ hr})}{6.06 \text{ L/hr}}(1-e^{-(0.346 \text{ hr}^{-1})(0.5 \text{ hr})})}{(1-e^{-(0.346 \text{ hr}^{-1})(8 \text{ hr})})}(e^{-(0.346 \text{ hr}^{-1})(0.5 \text{ hr})})$$

$$= \frac{(46.2 \text{ mg/L})(0.16)}{0.937}(0.84)$$

$$= (7.9 \text{ mg/L})(0.84)$$

$$= 6.6 \text{ mg/L}$$

Note that this steady-state "peak concentration" is not the true peak value that would occur at the end of the infusion, but a concentration that is obtained 1 hour after starting the infusion. It is this 1-hour value that is traditionally used to make the clinical correlation with aminoglycoside efficacy. Concentrations measured earlier may be considerably higher because of the two-compartment modeling associated with the IV administration of the aminoglycosides.

If the trough concentration is sampled just before the start of an infusion, a modification of Equation 6.21 can be used, where t_2 is represented by $(\tau - t_{in})$. A trough concentration of 0.59 mg/L is calculated, making the appropriate substitution of 8 hours for τ and 0.5 hour for t_{in} (Fig. 6.2).

$$Css \text{ min} = \frac{\dfrac{(S)(F)(Dose/t_{in})}{Cl}(1-e^{-Kt_{in}})}{(1-e^{-K\tau})}(e^{-K(\tau-t_{in})}) \qquad \textbf{(Eq. 6.22)}$$

$$= \frac{\dfrac{(1)(1)(140 \text{ mg}/0.5 \text{ hr})}{6.06 \text{ L/hr}}(1-e^{-(0.346 \text{ hr}^{-1})(0.5 \text{ hr})})}{(1-e^{-(0.346 \text{ hr}^{-1})(8 \text{ hr})})}(e^{-(0.346 \text{ hr}^{-1})(8 \text{ hr}-0.5 \text{ hr})})$$

$$= (7.9 \text{ mg/L})(e^{-(0.346 \text{ hr}^{-1})(7.5 \text{ hr})})$$

$$= (7.9 \text{ mg/L})(0.075)$$

$$= 0.59 \text{ mg/L}$$

Note that if the trough concentration is obtained at a time earlier than just before the next dose, Equation 6.22 should not be used. Instead, Equation 6.21 should be used where t_2 represents the time interval from the end of the infusion to the time of sampling. For example, if the trough concentration was obtained 0.5 hour before

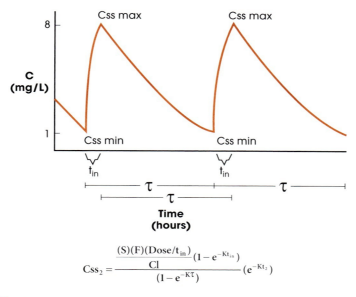

$$Css_2 = \frac{\dfrac{(S)(F)(Dose/t_{in})}{Cl}(1 - e^{-Kt_{in}})}{(1 - e^{-K\tau})}(e^{-Kt_2})$$

FIGURE 6.2 Intermittent IV infusion at steady state. The infusion is administered over t_{in} hours, and τ is the dosing interval; t_2 represents the time from the end of the infusion to the time of sampling.

the next dose, then t_2 in Equation 6.21 would be 7 hours rather than 7.5 hours in Equation 6.22.

Trough concentrations can also be calculated by multiplying the peak concentration 1 hour after the dose with the fraction of drug remaining at the time the trough level is sampled (Equation 6.10):

$$C = C_0 e^{-Kt}$$

where C_0 represents the peak concentration 1 hour after the dose, and t is the time from the peak concentration to the time of the trough sampling (7 hours if trough samples are obtained just before a dose, and 6.5 hours if trough samples are obtained 0.5 hour before a dose administered at a dosing interval of 8 hours).

Question #5 *If R.W. was given tobramycin 7 mg/kg every 24 hours, what would be the calculated steady-state peak concentration 1 hour after starting the 0.5 hour infusion? Also predict subsequent steady-state plasma concentrations 12 hours after starting the infusion and at the trough.*

Using the previously calculated gentamicin pharmacokinetic parameters of 6.06 L/hr for clearance, 17.5 L for volume, and 0.346 hr^{-1} for K, the expected steady-state peak concentration 0.5 hour after the 0.5 hour infusion would be a ≈ 21 mg/L as calculated from Equation 6.21.

$$Css_2 = \frac{\dfrac{(S)(F)(Dose/t_{in})}{Cl}(1-e^{-Kt_{in}})}{(1-e^{-K\tau})}(e^{-Kt_2})$$

$$= \frac{\dfrac{(1)(1)(480\ mg/0.5\ hr)}{6.06\ L/hr}(1-e^{-0.346(0.5)})}{(1-e^{-0.346(24)})}(e^{-0.346(0.5)})$$

$$= \frac{161.7\ mg/L(1-0.84)}{(1-0.0002)}(0.84)$$

$$= 21.6\ mg/L$$

The plasma concentrations at 12 and 24 hours can be estimated using Equation 6.10, where C_0 would be approximately 21 mg/L, and t would be 11 hours for the mid-concentration and 23 hours for the trough concentration.

$$\begin{aligned} C &= C_0 e^{-Kt} \\ &= (21\ mg/L)(e^{-(0.346)(11\ hr)}) \\ &= (21\ mg/L)(0.022) \\ &= 0.47\ mg/L \end{aligned}$$

12 hours after starting the infusion and

$$\begin{aligned} C &= (21\ mg/L)(e^{-(0.346)(23\ hr)}) \\ &= (21\ mg/L)(0.00035) \\ &= 0.007\ mg/L\ \text{at the trough} \end{aligned}$$

These calculations show that the initial plasma concentrations are well above the usual accepted therapeutic range for tobramycin, and the mid-interval and trough concentrations are very low. As previously discussed, administration of aminoglycosides as a total daily dose once every 24 hours appears in most cases to be as efficacious as the usual 8-hour divided dose and may reduce the risk of development of nephrotoxicity. Most institutions have guidelines for use of high-dose, once-daily aminoglycoside therapy. This type of regimen is usually restricted to patients who have reasonable renal function (e.g., $Cl_{Cr} > 60$ mL/min) and reasonably normal body composition (e.g., not excessively obese or having excessive third-space fluid).

One common question is whether aminoglycoside plasma concentrations should be monitored in patients receiving the drug once daily. In most cases, peak concentrations will have little meaning because they are likely to be well above the usual therapeutic range: ≈ 20 to 30 mg/L for gentamicin and tobramycin and about three times that value for amikacin. Trough plasma concentrations do not appear to be useful in that they are likely to be well below the usual detectable range and may be misinterpreted because of the tissue redistribution (gamma phase). In patients with diminished renal function, plasma level monitoring may be warranted to guard against excessive drug accumulation. One method that has been described is the peak AUC method of dosing. With this method, serum concentrations are obtained at a peak and approximately two to four half-lives later. The two levels are then used to calculate the 24-hour AUC and the extrapolated peak concentration at 1 hour into the dosing interval. The assumption with this method is that the level of drug exposure with extended interval dosing should be the same as conventional multiple daily dosing regimens (i.e., AUC_{24} 70 to 100 mg · hr/L).[25]

Question #6 *Y.B., a 70-kg, 38-year-old patient with a serum creatinine of 1.8 mg/dL, has been receiving IV tobramycin, 100 mg over 0.5 hour every 8 hours, for several days. A peak plasma concentration obtained 1 hour after the start of an infusion was 8 mg/L, and a trough concentration obtained just before the initiation of a dose was 3 mg/L. Estimate the apparent elimination rate constant (K), clearance (Cl), and volume of distribution (V) for tobramycin in Y.B.*

The two reported plasma concentrations were measured from samples obtained during the elimination phase of the plasma concentration-versus-time curve. Because the 7-hour time interval between samples exceeds the half-life of tobramycin in Y.B. (i.e., the trough concentration is less than one-half the measured peak concentration), the two concentrations can be used to estimate the elimination rate constant (see Elimination Rate Constant [K] and Half-Life [t½] in Chapter 1 and Equation 6.23).

$$K = \frac{\ln\left(\dfrac{C_1}{C_2}\right)}{t}$$

(Eq. 6.23)

$$= \ln\frac{\left(\dfrac{8.0}{3.0}\right)}{7 \text{ hr}}$$

$$= \frac{0.98}{7 \text{ hr}}$$

$$= 0.14 \text{ hr}^{-1}$$

Using the elimination rate constant of 0.14 hr^{-1}, the observed peak concentration of 8 mg/L, and the dosing regimen of 100 mg administered over 0.5 hour every 8 hours, Y.B.'s volume of distribution can be calculated by rearranging Equation 6.17

for Css_1, where τ is 8 hours and the sample is obtained 0.5 hours after the end of the 0.5 hour infusion making t_1 1 hour,

$$Css_1 = \frac{\dfrac{(S)(F)(Dose)}{V}}{(1-e^{-K\tau})}e^{-Kt_1}$$

$$V = \frac{\dfrac{(S)(F)(Dose)}{Css_1}}{(1-e^{-K\tau})}e^{-Kt_1} \qquad \textbf{(Eq. 6.24)}$$

$$V = \frac{\dfrac{(1)(1)(100\ mg)}{8\ mg/L}}{(1-e^{-(0.14\ hr^{-1})(8\ hr)})}(e^{-(0.14\ hr^{-1})(1\ hr)})$$

$$= \frac{12.5\ L}{0.67}(0.87)$$

$$= 16.2\ L$$

and the clearance can be calculated using a rearrangement of Equation 6.14

$$K = \frac{Cl}{V}$$

to solve for Cl.

$$Cl = (K)(V) \qquad \textbf{(Eq. 6.25)}$$

$$= (0.14\ hr^{-1})(16.2\ L)$$

$$= 2.3\ L/hr$$

This volume of distribution of 16.2 L corresponds to about 0.23 L/kg. The value of calculating tobramycin pharmacokinetic parameters that are specific for Y.B. is that they may now be used to calculate a dosing regimen that will produce any desired peak and trough concentrations.

Question #7   *The microbiology report reveals Pseudomonas aeruginosa with an MIC of 1 mcg/mL. Calculate a dosing regimen for Y.B. that will achieve a peak concentration of >10 mg/L (peak:MIC > 10:1) and a AUC_{24} in the range of 70 to 100 mg · hr/L.*

As before, the dose required to achieve a specific peak concentration can be calculated from Equation 6.17. To select an appropriate dosing interval, however, one should first consider Y.B.'s apparent half-life, which can be calculated using Equation 6.15 and the elimination rate constant of 0.14 hr^{-1}.

$$t\tfrac{1}{2} = \frac{0.693}{K}$$

$$= \frac{0.693}{0.14 \text{ hr}^{-1}}$$

$$= 4.9 \text{ hr}$$

As presented earlier, a dosing interval of approximately four to five half-lives is desirable to maximize the peak concentration and bactericidal activity while minimizing drug accumulation and potential nephrotoxicity and ototoxicity. Because Y.B.'s tobramycin half-life is ≈5 hours, the most convenient dosing interval is 24 hours. Using this dosing interval and the appropriate volume of distribution and elimination rate constant, Equation 6.26 (a rearrangement of Equation 6.17 to solve for dose) indicates that a dose of 200 mg administered every 24 hours should result in a peak concentration of ≈10 mg/L 1 hour after the start of a 0.5 hour infusion.

$$\text{Dose} = \frac{(Css_1)(V)(1-e^{-K\tau})}{(S)(F)(e^{-Kt_1})} \qquad \textbf{(Eq. 6.26)}$$

$$\text{Dose} = \frac{(10 \text{ mg/L})(17.5 \text{ L})(1-e^{-(0.14 \text{ hr}^{-1})(24 \text{ hr})})}{(1)(1)e^{-(0.14 \text{ hr}^{-1})(1 \text{ hr})}}$$

$$= \frac{(10 \text{ mg/L})(17.5 \text{ L})(0.97)}{(1)(1)(0.87)}$$

$$= 195.1 \text{ mg or} \approx 200 \text{ mg}$$

Equation 6.10 can be used to determine the trough concentration. A "t" of 23 hours and a C_0 of 10 mg/L should be used.

$$C = C_0 e^{-Kt}$$

$$= (10 \text{ mg/L})(e^{-(0.14 \text{ hr}^{-1})(23 \text{ hr})})$$

$$= (10 \text{ mg/L})(0.04)$$

$$= 0.4 \text{ mg/L}$$

To confirm whether the level of drug exposure is in the desirable range, Equation 6.27 can be used to calculate the AUC_{24}.

$$AUC_{24} = \frac{(\text{Dose in mg})(24 \text{ hr})/\tau \text{ in hr}}{Cl \text{ in L/hr}} \qquad \textbf{(Eq. 6.27)}$$

$$= \frac{(200 \text{ mg})(24 \text{ hr})/24 \text{ hr}}{2.3 \text{ L/hr}}$$

$$= 87 \text{ mg} \cdot \text{hr/L}$$

Question #8   *C.I. is a 50-year-old, 60-kg man with a serum creatinine of 1.5 mg/dL, who is receiving 350 mg of amikacin IV over 0.5 hour every 8 hours at midnight, 8:00 a.m., and 4:00 p.m. He had a trough concentration of 6 mg/L obtained just before the 8:00 a.m. dose and a peak concentration of 15 mg/L obtained at 9:00 a.m. Assuming these peak and trough concentrations represent steady-state levels, calculate C.I.'s elimination rate constant, clearance, and volume of distribution. Evaluate whether these parameters seem reasonable and should be used to adjust C.I.'s amikacin maintenance dose.*

The approach to calculating the revised pharmacokinetic parameters for C.I. is essentially the same as that used in the previous questions. First, the elimination rate constant of 0.13 hr^{-1} can be calculated using Equation 6.23 and the 7 hour time interval between the peak and trough concentrations (Fig. 6.3):

$$K = \frac{\ln\left(\dfrac{C_1}{C_2}\right)}{t}$$

$$= \frac{\ln\left(\dfrac{15}{6}\right)}{7 \text{ hr}}$$

$$= 0.13 \text{ hr}^{-1}$$

Next, the volume of distribution can be calculated by using Equation 6.24. A dose of 350 mg and a "τ" of 8 hours can be used. The latter t_1 represents the time from the beginning of the infusion to the "peak concentration" sampling time ($t_1 = 1$ hour).

$$V = \frac{\dfrac{(S)(F)(\text{Dose})}{Css_1}}{(1 - e^{-K\tau})}(e^{-Kt_1})$$

$$= \frac{\dfrac{(1)(1)(350 \text{ mg})}{15 \text{ mg/L}}}{(1 - e^{-(0.13 \text{ hr}^{-1})(8 \text{ hr})})}(e^{-(0.13 \text{ hr}^{-1})(1 \text{ hr})})$$

$$= \frac{(23.3 \text{ L})(0.88)}{0.65}$$

$$= 31.5 \text{ L}$$

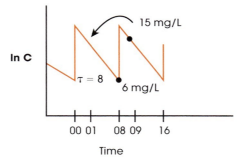

FIGURE 6.3 Calculating K by transposing Css max into the same interval as Css min. Note that steady state must have been achieved (same dose, same interval for >3 to 5 t½s). Also, the Css max is moved to the same time within the interval relative to the preceding dose (i.e., from 09:00 in one interval to 01:00 in the preceding interval). The intermittent bolus dose model has been used for the input model, and the concentrations are ln concentrations, so that the decay phase is a straight line.

Using the calculated volume of distribution of 31.5 L and the elimination rate constant of 0.13 hr^{-1}, a clearance value of 4.1 L/hr can be calculated using Equation 6.25.

$$Cl = (K)(V)$$
$$Cl = (0.13 \text{ hr}^{-1})(31.5 \text{ L})$$
$$= 4.1 \text{ L/hr}$$

Before these parameters are used to calculate an adjusted amikacin dosing regimen that will bring C.I.'s peak concentration into the range of 20 to 30 mg/L and the trough concentration below 10 mg/L, care should be taken to evaluate whether these parameters appear reasonable. The calculated clearance of 4.1 L/hr is slightly greater than the expected clearance of 3 L/hr, which would be calculated using Equation 6.6 and C.I.'s age, weight, and serum creatinine.

$$\text{Cl}_{\text{Cr}} \text{ for Males (mL/min)} = \frac{(140 - \text{Age})(\text{Weight})}{(72)(\text{SCr}_{ss})}$$
$$= \frac{(140 - 50)(60 \text{ kg})}{(72)(1.5 \text{ mg/dL})}$$
$$= 50 \text{ mL/min}$$

or

$$\text{Cl}_{\text{Cr}} (\text{L/hr}) = (50 \text{ mL/min})\left(\frac{60 \text{ min/hr}}{100 \text{ mL/L}}\right)$$
$$= 3 \text{ L/hr}$$

Although this clearance value is greater than expected, it is not so unusual as to be considered unrealistic.

The volume of distribution value of 0.53 L/kg (31.5 L/60 kg), however, is unusually large. In general, volumes of distribution >0.35 L/kg are only observed in patients who have significant third spacing of fluid (e.g., ascites or edema). If there is no evidence of any third spacing in C.I., then the volume of distribution would be unrealistically large. Therefore, the dosing history or the measured plasma concentrations are probably in error. If C.I. had received tobramycin or gentamicin, the possibility of a penicillin inter-action resulting in spuriously low plasma concentrations would have to be considered; however, amikacin does not interact with penicillins to a significant extent. Therefore, this is an unlikely explanation for the unusually large volume of distribution.

In any case, when pharmacokinetic calculations lead to parameters that are very different from those expected, there may be an error in the time of sampling, assay re-sults, or dosing history. In such cases, it may be more prudent to use the expected rather than the calculated parameters to adjust doses. In some cases, however, the patient may actually have unusual parameters. When this is suspected, the dosing history should be reevaluated and another set of plasma drug concentrations should be obtained, with special attention to precise sampling times and the dosing history.

Question #9   *D.H., a 40-year-old man, was admitted to the hospital following an automobile accident. He is 5 feet 5 inches tall and on admission weighed 85 kg. He was taken for abdominal surgery and postoperatively became hypotensive and required large volumes of fluid to maintain his blood pressure. Currently, he weighs 105 kg and has a serum creatinine of 2 mg/dL. D.H. is to receive gentamicin empirically after his abdominal surgery. Estimate his pharmacokinetic parameters and dose to achieve peak gentamicin concentrations >10 mg/L and an AUC_{24} between 70 and 100 mg · hr/L.*

To calculate D.H.'s pharmacokinetic parameters, it is first necessary to identify his nonobese, excess adipose, and excess third-space fluid weight. Using Equation 6.2, D.H.'s IBW is calculated to be ≈61.5 kg.

$$\text{Ideal Body Weight for Males in kg} = 50 + (2.3)(\text{Height in inches} > 60)$$
$$= 50 + (2.3)(\text{inches})$$
$$= 61.5 \text{ kg}$$

Assuming D.H. did not have any excess third-space fluid on admission, his excess adipose weight is ≈23.5 kg (estimated by subtracting his IBW of 61.5 kg from his admission weight of 85 kg). D.H.'s excess third-space fluid weight of 20 kg can be estimated by subtracting his initial weight of 85 kg from his current weight of 105 kg. Using these weight estimates for his body composition, Equation 6.4 can be used to estimate an aminoglycoside volume of distribution of ≈38 L:

$$\text{Aminoglycoside V(L)} = \left(\begin{array}{c} 0.25 \text{ L/kg} \times \text{Nonobese,} \\ \text{Non–Excess Fluid Weight (kg)} \end{array} \right) +$$
$$0.1 \left(\begin{array}{c} \text{Excess} \\ \text{Adipose} \\ \text{Weight (kg)} \end{array} \right) + \left(\begin{array}{c} \text{Excess Third-} \\ \text{Space Fluid} \\ \text{Weight (kg)} \end{array} \right)$$
$$= (0.25 \text{ L/kg} \times 61.5 \text{ kg}) + 0.1(23.5 \text{ kg}) + (20 \text{ kg})$$
$$= 37.7 \text{ or } 38 \text{ L}$$

To estimate D.H.'s gentamicin clearance, one would use Equation 6.6, his IBW of 61.5 kg, and his current serum creatinine of 2 mg/dL.

$$Cl_{Cr} \text{ for Males (mL/min)} = \frac{(140 - Age)(Weight)}{(72)(SCr_{ss})}$$

$$= \frac{(140 - 40 \text{ yr})(61.5 \text{ kg})}{(72)(2 \text{ mg/dL})}$$

$$= 42.7 \text{ mL/min}$$

$$= 42.7 \text{ mL/min} \times \frac{60 \text{ min/ hr}}{1000 \text{ mL/L}}$$

$$= 2.56 \text{ L/hr}$$

Using the estimated creatinine clearance of 2.56 L/hr as the gentamicin clearance and the volume of distribution of 38 L, the elimination rate constant (Equation 6.14) and half-life (Equation 6.15) are calculated to be 0.067 hr^{-1} and 10.34 hour, respectively:

$$K = \frac{Cl}{V}$$

$$= \frac{2.56 \text{ L/hr}}{38 \text{ L}}$$

$$= 0.067 \text{ hr}^{-1}$$

$$t\tfrac{1}{2} = \frac{0.693}{k}$$

$$= \frac{0.693}{0.067 \text{ hr}^{-1}}$$

$$= 10.34 \text{ hr}$$

Given D.H.'s half-life of approximately 10 hours and an infusion time of 0.5 hour, Equation 6.26, the steady-state bolus dose model, can be used to calculate his regimen.

$$Dose = \frac{(Css_1)(V)(1 - e^{-K\tau})}{(S)(F)(e^{-Kt_1})}$$

Because aminoglycoside dosing intervals are now typically greater than four to five half-lives, a dosing interval of 48 hours is reasonable given D.H.'s half-life of approximately 10 hours. Making the appropriate substitution in the rearranged equation, where Css_1 is assumed to be 10 mg/L, t_1 is 1 hour (indicating that the peak concentration is to be obtained 1 hour after the start of the infusion), a dose of $\approx$400 mg is calculated.

$$Dose = \frac{(10 \text{ mg/L})(38 \text{ L})(1 - e^{-(0.067 \text{ hr}^{-1})(48 \text{ hr})})}{(1)(1)(e^{-(0.067 \text{ hr}^{-1})(1 \text{ hr})})}$$

$$= \frac{(10 \text{ mg/L})(38 \text{ L})(1 - 0.04)}{(1)(1)(0.94)}$$

$$= 388 \text{ mg or} \approx 400 \text{ mg}$$

Although a dose of 400 mg appears to be large, this is due in part to the extensive third spacing fluid and large volume of distribution. In many cases, a somewhat lower dose might be employed; however, the peak concentration would be proportionately decreased. Also, although the dose of 400 mg seems large, D.H. is receiving this dose only every other day and based on his nonobese or IBW of 61.5 kg, this equates to ≈3.0 mg/kg/day, which is below the lower end of the usual range (5 to 7 mg/kg/day). It is also important to ensure that AUC_{24} is in the desired range (70 to 100 mg · hr/L).

$$AUC_{24} = \frac{(\text{Dose in mg})(24 \text{ hr})/\tau \text{ in hr}}{\text{Cl in L/hr}}$$

$$AUC_{24} = \frac{(400 \text{ mg})(24 \text{ hr})/48 \text{ hr}}{2.56/\text{hr}}$$

$$= 78 \text{ mg} \cdot \text{hr/L}$$

The AUC_{24} value of 78 mg · hr/L is in the lower end of the desired range (70 to 100 mg · hr/L), indicating that the dose could be increased if necessary depending on the severity of the infection. If the dosing interval remains 48 hours, an increase in dose will result in a proportional increase in AUC_{24} and peak concentration (see Equations 6.17 and 6.27). For example, a 30% increase in dose would result in an AUC_{24} of approximately 100 mg · hr/L and a peak concentration of 13 mg/L.

Question #10 *What is the significance of a changing serum creatinine in a patient receiving gentamicin?*

A rising serum creatinine level in a patient always raises the question of gentamicin-induced nephrotoxicity. In this event, the drug may be discontinued, the plasma concentration reevaluated, and/or the dose adjusted, because gentamicin may accumulate substantially when renal function is impaired. Dose modification should be based on plasma gentamicin levels rather than serum creatinine levels because serum creatinine concentrations that are not at steady state can be misleading (see Creatinine Clearance [Cl_{Cr}] in Chapter 3). The reason for this is that despite the similarity between gentamicin and creatinine clearances,[31,43] their volumes of distribution differ. Gentamicin's V of 0.25 L/kg is smaller than that of creatinine, which is 0.5 L/kg.[26,27,32,72] Because the half-life is determined by the clearance and volume of distribution (see Equation 6.28), the half-life for creatinine is approximately twice as long as that of gentamicin and the other aminoglycosides. It will, therefore, take creatinine a longer time to arrive at a new steady-state concentration after a change in renal function.

$$t\frac{1}{2} = \frac{(0.693)(V)}{Cl}$$

(Eq. 6.28)

When the serum creatinine is rising (i.e., not at steady state), the renal function is worse than that would be predicted by use of the serum creatinine, and any gentamicin dose calculated using the serum creatinine would be overestimated. Conversely, when the serum creatinine is falling, renal function may be better than that reflected by creatinine clearance, and the doses calculated on the basis of these levels would be underestimated.

Question #11   *D.W., a 20-year-old, 60-kg man, is receiving 80 mg of tobramycin infused IV over a 30-minute period every 8 hours. His serum creatinine has increased from 1 to 2 mg/dL over the past 24 hours. Because his renal function appears to be decreasing, three plasma samples were obtained to monitor serum gentamicin concentrations as follows: just before a dose, 1 hour after that same dose, and 8 hours after that dose (two troughs and one peak level). The serum gentamicin concentrations at these times were 4, 8, and 5 mg/L, respectively. Calculate the volume of distribution, elimination rate constant, and clearance of tobramycin for D.W.*

Because the second trough concentration of tobramycin is higher than the first, it is apparent that the drug is accumulating. Therefore, steady-state equations should not be used to calculate D.W.'s pharmacokinetic parameters. The first step that should be taken to resolve this dilemma is to calculate the elimination rate constant from the two plasma concentrations that were obtained during the elimination phase (8 and 5 mg/L). Equation 6.23 can be used to estimate the elimination rate constant; however, this K should only be used as an estimate because the two plasma concentrations were obtained less than one half-life apart.

$$K = \frac{\ln\left(\dfrac{C_1}{C_2}\right)}{t}$$

$$= \frac{\ln\left(\dfrac{8\ \text{mg/L}}{5\ \text{mg/L}}\right)}{7\ \text{hr}}$$

$$= 0.067\ \text{hr}^{-1}$$

This elimination rate constant of $0.067\ \text{hr}^{-1}$ was calculated by assuming that the peak concentration of 8 mg/L was obtained 1 hour after the start of the tobramycin infusion and that the trough concentration was obtained just before the next dose, resulting in a time interval of 7 hours. The elimination rate constant of $0.067\ \text{hr}^{-1}$ corresponds to a half-life of 10.3 hours (Equation 6.15):

$$t\tfrac{1}{2} = \frac{0.693}{K}$$

$$= \frac{0.693}{0.067\ \text{hr}^{-1}}$$

$$= 10.3\ \text{hr}$$

This half-life of 10.3 hours suggests that relatively little drug is lost during the infusion period; therefore, a bolus model is most appropriately used in this situation. The volume of distribution can be estimated by assuming that the bolus dose is administered instantaneously and calculating the theoretical peak concentration using Equation 6.11. C is the measured concentration of 8 mg/L, t is the 1-hour interval between the start of the infusion and the time of sampling, and C_0 is the theoretical peak concentration for an IV bolus.

$$
\begin{aligned}
C_0 &= \frac{C}{e^{-Kt}} \\
&= \frac{8 \text{ mg/L}}{e^{-(0.067 \text{ hr}^{-1})(1 \text{ hr})}} \\
&= \frac{8 \text{ mg/L}}{0.94} \\
&= 8.5 \text{ mg/L}
\end{aligned}
$$

Because the change in concentration (peak minus trough) is the result of the dose administered and the volume of distribution, the V can be calculated using Equation 6.29.

$$
V = \frac{\text{Dose}}{(C_{\text{peak}} - C_{\text{min}})}
\qquad \textbf{(Eq. 6.29)}
$$

$$
\begin{aligned}
V &= \frac{80 \text{ mg}}{(8.5 \text{ mg/L} - 4 \text{ mg/L})} \\
&= 17.8 \text{ L}
\end{aligned}
$$

This volume of distribution of 17.8 L can then be used with the elimination rate constant of 0.067 hr^{-1} in Equation 6.25 to calculate D.W.'s clearance of 1.2 L/hr or 20 mL/min:

$$
\begin{aligned}
Cl &= (K)(V) \\
&= (0.067 \text{ hr}^{-1})(17.8 \text{ L}) \\
&= 1.2 \text{ L/hr or } 20 \text{ mL/min}
\end{aligned}
$$

Question #12 *Using the pharmacokinetic parameters calculated for D.W. in Question 11, develop a dosing regimen that will produce reasonable peak and trough concentrations of tobramycin.*

Because D.W.'s tobramycin clearance is low (1.2 L/hr), it will be necessary to reduce his maintenance dose. There are two alternatives: (1) reduce the dose and maintain the same dosing interval or (2) adjust both the dose and the dosing interval such that the peak concentration and AUC_{24} will be approximately 10 mg/L and 70 to 100 mg · hr/L, respectively.

Reduce the Dose and Maintain the Same Dosing Interval. This method is not acceptable for D.W. because he has such a long half-life ($\approx$10 hours). If a dose that achieves a maximum concentration of 8 mg/L is used and the dosing interval of 8 hours is maintained, the trough level will be $\approx$4.7 mg/L.

$$Css\ min = (Css\ max)(e^{-K\tau})$$

(Eq. 6.30)

$$Css\ min = (8\ mg/L)(e^{-(0.067\ hr^{-1})(8\ hr)})$$
$$= 4.68\ mg/L$$

This level may place D.W. at risk for tobramycin toxicity.

Adjust Both the Dose and Dosing Interval to Achieve Reasonable Peak Concentration and AUC_{24} values. The only potential limitation to this approach is that most clinicians prefer to avoid prolonged periods, during which the gentamicin concentration is below the MIC of the pathogen because of the possibility of organism regrowth. Clinical experience with dosing intervals in excess of 48 hours is limited. Nevertheless, some animal data suggest that doses that result in high peak and low trough concentrations are less likely to produce renal toxicity than the same dose administered as a continuous IV infusion (i.e., the same average levels).[73] A first estimate of the dosing interval can be made by examining D.W.'s tobramycin half-life of 10 hours. If an interval of four to five half-lives is chosen, a dosing interval of 48 hours can be used. Because the half-life of tobramycin is long relative to the infusion time of 0.5 hour, the bolus dose model can be used. As previously stated, Equation 6.27 can be used to calculate a dose required to achieve a specific AUC_{24}. Using Equation 6.27 with the previously derived pharmacokinetic parameters and a dosing interval of 48 hours, a dose of $\approx$240 mg is calculated. A peak concentration that occurs 1 hour after the infusion has been initiated is also assumed (i.e., $t_1 = 1$ hour).

$$AUC_{24} = \frac{(Dose\ in\ mg)(24\ hr)/\tau\ in\ hr}{Cl\ in\ L/hr}$$

or

$$Dose\ in\ mg = \frac{(AUC_{24})(Cl\ in\ L/hr)(\tau\ in\ hr)}{24\ hr}$$
$$= \frac{(100\ mg \cdot hr/L)(1.2\ L/hr)(48\ hr)}{24\ hr}$$
$$= 240\ mg\ given\ q48h$$

The peak concentration can be calculated using the bolus dose model (Equation 6.17).

$$Css_1 = \frac{\dfrac{(S)(F)(Dose)}{V}}{(1-e^{-K\tau})}(e^{-Kt_1})$$

$$= \frac{\dfrac{(1)(1)(240\text{ mg})}{17.8\text{ L}}}{(1-e^{-(0.067\text{ hr}^{-1})(48\text{ hr})})}(e^{-(0.067\text{ hr}^{-1})(1\text{ hr})})$$

$$= \frac{13.4\text{ mg/L}}{0.96}(0.94)$$

$$= 13.96\text{ mg/L}(0.94)$$

$$= 13.1\text{ mg/L}$$

The trough concentration, 47 hours later, calculated using Equation 6.30, would be 0.6 mg/L.

$$\text{Css min} = (\text{Css max})(e^{-Kt})$$

$$\text{Css min} = (13.96\text{ mg/L})(e^{-(0.067\text{ hr}^{-1})(47\text{ hr})})$$

$$= 0.6\text{ mg/L}$$

Question #13   *M.S., a 70-kg nonobese female, undergoes 4 hours of hemodialysis every 48 hours. She is functionally (not surgically) anephric, and gentamicin is to be started. Calculate a dosing regimen that achieves a peak concentration of 6 mg/L and then maintains average levels of 3.5 mg/L.*

Because the gentamicin half-life for a patient who is functionally anephric is probably in excess of 30 hours, very little drug will be eliminated from the body over the 1-hour period following initiation of the infusion. Therefore, the loading dose may be calculated as though it were a bolus (Equation 6.31). Assuming S and F to be 1 and the volume of distribution to be 17.5 L (0.25 L/kg), a loading dose of ≈100 mg would be calculated as follows:

$$\text{Loading Dose} = \frac{(V)(C)}{(S)(F)} \qquad \textbf{(Eq. 6.31)}$$

$$= \frac{(17.5\text{ L})(6\text{ mg/L})}{(1)(1)}$$

$$= 105\text{ mg}$$

Because gentamicin elimination in M.S. will be irregular, occurring at higher rates during the dialysis, the usual maintenance dose equation cannot be used. As presented in Dialysis of Drugs in Chapter 3, there are two possible approaches to the resolution of this problem. One approach is to administer a daily dose such that average concentrations are maintained and then to calculate a replacement dose postdialysis. A second approach is to administer the drug after dialysis only. The dose used is the amount of drug lost during the interdialysis and intradialysis period. In both cases, the use of the patient's clearance (Cl_{pat}), dialysis clearance (Cl_{dial}), and the volume of distribution will be required. The reported clearance for aminoglycosides in functionally anephric patients is ≈ 0.0043 L/kg/hr,[27,74] and aminoglycoside clearance by low-flux hemodialysis is 20 to 40 mL/min, with an average value of ≈ 30 mL/min.[27,74–76]

If the approach of giving daily and postdialysis doses is taken, then the maintenance dose on non-dialysis days can be calculated using Equation 6.32, with a patient clearance of 0.3 L/hr (0.0043 L/hr/kg $\times$ 70 kg) and a dosing interval of 24 hours. In most dialysis patients, a gentamicin concentration between 3 and 4 mg/L (average: 3.5 mg/L) is set as a goal. Therefore, a dose of ≈ 25 mg would be appropriate:

$$\text{Dose} = \frac{(\text{Css ave})(Cl_{pat})(\tau)}{(S)(F)} \qquad \text{(Eq. 6.32)}$$

$$\text{Dose} = \frac{(3.5 \text{ mg/L})(0.3 \text{ L/hr})(24 \text{ hr})}{(1)(1)}$$
$$= 25.2 \text{ mg or} \approx 25 \text{ mg}$$

If the patient had been surgically anephric, the Cl_{pat} would have been approximately halved, and the corresponding maintenance dose would also have been halved or ≈ 13 mg/day. Equation 6.33 can be used to calculate the postdialysis replacement dose. Using the average C_{dial} and a dialysis time (T_d) of 4 hours, the replacement dose is calculated to be ≈ 25 mg.

$$\begin{aligned} \text{Postdialysis} \\ \text{Replacement} \\ \text{Dose} \end{aligned} = (V)(\text{Css ave})\left(1 - e^{-\left(\frac{Cl_{pat} + Cl_{dial}}{V}\right)(T_d)}\right) \qquad \text{(Eq. 6.33)}$$

$$= (17.5 \text{ L})(3.5 \text{ mg/L})\left[1 - e^{-\left(\frac{0.3 \text{ L/hr} + 1.8 \text{ L/hr}}{17.5 \text{ L}}\right)(4 \text{ hr})}\right]$$
$$= (17.5 \text{ L})(3.5 \text{ mg/L})[1 - 0.62]$$
$$= 23.3 \text{ mg or} \approx 25 \text{ mg}$$

Note that the dialysis clearance of 1.8 L/hr represents a clearance of ≈ 30 mL/min, and that this is the primary route of elimination during the intradialysis period. Also, the postdialysis dose of 25 mg can be added to the maintenance dose of ≈ 25 mg, resulting in a gentamicin dose on dialysis days of 50 mg.

If it is decided to administer the aminoglycoside only after dialysis, Equation 6.34 can be used to calculate the postdialysis replacement dose. In this situation, a steady-state peak concentration of $\approx$4 to 5 mg/L is set as a goal (peak concentrations of 6 to 8 mg/L would expose M.S. to continuously elevated concentrations of gentamicin).

Using Equation 6.34, the following are calculated: a Css peak of 5.0 mg/L, a patient clearance of 0.3 L/hr, and a t_1 of 44 hours (derived from a 48-hour interval between the dialyses and a dialysis time [T_d] of 4 hours), the postdialysis replacement dose is 62 mg.

$$\text{Postdialysis Replacement Dose} = (V)(\text{Css peak})\left(1-\left[\left(e^{-\left(\frac{Cl_{pat}}{V}\right)(t_1)}\right)\left(e^{-\left(\frac{Cl_{pat}+Cl_{dial}}{V}\right)(T_d)}\right)\right]\right) \quad \textbf{(Eq. 6.34)}$$

$$= (17.5\text{ L})(5\text{ mg/L})\left(1-\left[\left(e^{-\left(\frac{0.3\text{ L/hr}}{17.5\text{ L}}\right)(44\text{ hr})}\right)\left(e^{-\left(\frac{0.3\text{ L/hr}+1.8\text{ L/hr}}{17.5\text{ L}}\right)(4\text{ hr})}\right)\right]\right)$$

$$= (17.5\text{ L})(5\text{ mg/L})\left(1-\left[(0.47)(0.62)\right]\right)$$

$$= (17.5\text{ L})(5\text{ mg/L})\left(1-0.29\right)$$

$$= 62\text{ mg}$$

To ensure that trough concentrations just before dialysis are not excessively low, the predialysis drug concentration should be calculated using Equation 6.35.

$$\text{Predialysis Drug Concentration} = \left[\text{Css peak}\right]\left[e^{-\left(\frac{Cl_{pat}}{V}\right)(t_1)}\right] \quad \textbf{(Eq. 6.35)}$$

$$= (5\text{ mg/L})\left[e^{-\left(\frac{0.3\text{ L/hr}}{17.5\text{ L}}\right)(44\text{ hr})}\right]$$

$$= (5\text{ mg/L})(0.47)$$

$$= 2.35\text{ mg/L}$$

This predialysis concentration of $\approx$2.4 mg/L is higher than usually desired; however, because the gentamicin half-life is unusually long, it will be difficult to maintain peak levels in the range of 5 mg/L and predialysis trough concentrations of <2 mg/L. Unfortunately, the persistence of relatively high concentrations between dialysis periods will place M.S. at greater risk for ototoxicity.[77] In addition, although postdialysis concentrations can be calculated, these lower concentrations are transient and probably do not correlate well with the incidence of ototoxicity in dialysis patients. If postdialysis concentrations are to be measured, time should be allowed for equilibration between the plasma compartment (in which concentrations have been lowered during the dialysis period) and the extracellular fluid compartment.[78]

Question #14   *How would the above situation have differed if peritoneal dialysis rather than hemodialysis had been used?*

Peritoneal dialysis is much less effective in removing gentamicin; the usual clearance value is ≈ 4 mL/min/m^2, with an average value of 5 to 10 mL/min for the 70-kg patient. Nonetheless, the total amount of drug removed during dialysis may be as much as 30% or more because acute intermittent peritoneal dialysis is usually continued for ≈ 36 hours.[74,79]

Aminoglycosides can be administered either parenterally or intraperitoneally to achieve systemic plasma concentrations. When administered intraperitoneally, an initial loading dose of 2 to 3 mg/kg is added to the first peritoneal dialysis exchange. Then, 1.2 mg/kg/day is added to one exchange daily (usually the night-time exchange), or a dose that produces a dialysate concentration of ≈ 6 to 10 mg/L is added to each dialysate exchange. Both of these regimens result in steady-state plasma concentrations of ≈ 3 mg/L with relatively little fluctuation.[80] When aminoglycoside antibiotics are placed in each peritoneal exchange, many clinicians estimate the steady-state plasma concentration to be $\approx 40\%$ of the peritoneal dialysate concentration. As an example, if 16 mg were added to each 2 L peritoneal exchange volume (8 mg/L), the steady-state plasma concentration would be 3.2 mg/L, or 40% of the 8 mg/L concentration in the dialysate exchanges.[81,82]

Question #15   *T.C. is receiving tobramycin 360 mg IV over 0.5 hour every 24 hours at 9:00 a.m. Levels drawn at 11:00 a.m. and 9:00 p.m. were 15.0 and 0.9 mg/L, respectively. Calculate the peak concentration expected at 10:00 a.m., or 1 hour after starting the 9:00 a.m. tobramycin infusion, and the AUC$_{24}$ to determine the appropriateness of the current dosing regimen.*

The time interval between 11:00 a.m. and 9:00 p.m. is 10 hours, and Equation 6.23 can be used to determine the elimination rate constant for T.C.

$$K = \frac{\ln\left(\dfrac{C_1}{C_2}\right)}{t}$$

$$= \frac{\ln\left(\dfrac{15\,\text{mg/L}}{0.9\,\text{mg/L}}\right)}{10\,\text{hr}}$$

$$= \frac{2.8}{10\,\text{hr}}$$

$$= 0.28\,\text{hr}^{-1}$$

This patient-specific elimination rate constant of 0.28 hr^{-1} can be used in Equation 6.11 to calculate the expected plasma concentration at 10:00 a.m. (1 hour after the start of the infusion) or 1 hour before the observed peak of 15 mg/L.

$$C_0 = \frac{C}{e^{-Kt}}$$

$$= \frac{15\ \text{mg/L}}{e^{-(0.28\ \text{hr}^{-1})(1\ \text{hr})}}$$

$$= \frac{15\ \text{mg/L}}{0.76}$$

$$= 19.8\ \text{mg/L}$$

The steady-state infusion model (Equation 6.21)

$$Css_2 = \frac{\dfrac{(S)(F)(\text{Dose}/t_{in})}{Cl}(1 - e^{-Kt_{in}})}{(1 - e^{-K\tau})}(e^{-Kt_2})$$

can be rearranged to solve for clearance: ($t_{in} > \frac{1}{6} t\frac{1}{2}$)

$$Cl = \frac{\dfrac{(S)(F)(\text{Dose}/t_{in})}{Css_2}(1 - e^{-Kt_{in}})}{(1 - e^{-K\tau})}(e^{-Kt_2}) \qquad \textbf{(Eq. 6.36)}$$

$$Cl = \frac{\dfrac{(1)(1)\left(360\ \text{mg}/0.5\ \text{hr}\right)}{0.9\ \text{mg/L}}\left(1 - e^{(0.28\ \text{hr}^{-1})(0.5\ \text{hr})}\right)}{\left(1 - e^{-(0.28\ \text{hr}^{-1})(24\ \text{hr})}\right)}\left(e^{-(0.28\ \text{hr}^{-1})(11.5\ \text{hr})}\right)$$

$$= \frac{(800\ \text{L/hr})(0.13)}{(0.99)}(0.04)$$

$$= 4.2\ \text{L/hr}$$

The AUC$_{24}$ can then be calculated using Equation 6.27.

$$AUC_{24} = \frac{(\text{Dose in mg})(24\ \text{hr})/\tau\ \text{in hr}}{Cl\ \text{in L/hr}}$$

$$= \frac{(360\ \text{mg})(24\ \text{hr})/24\ \text{hr}}{4.2\ \text{L/hr}}$$

$$= 86\ \text{mg} \cdot \text{hr/L}$$

This peak concentration of 19.8 mg/L represents a concentration that is within the target range (peak:MIC > 10) based on the breakpoint for susceptibility (2 mcg/mL). The AUC_{24} is also in the target range (70 to 100 mg · hr/L) and suggests that T.C.'s tobramycin does not require dose adjustment.

Question #16   *E.H., an 8 year-old boy (height, 4 feet 1 inches [124 cm]; weight, 26.3 kg) with no prior medical history, is admitted for ruptured appendix. Gentamicin 60 mg IV q8h, infused over 30 minutes is started after appendectomy. His serum creatinine is 0.7 mg/dL. Calculate the predicted steady-state peak concentration of gentamicin 1 hour after the infusion was started.*

Traditionally, pediatric patients are started on gentamicin and tobramycin 2.5 mg/kg q8h and amikacin 15 mg/kg/day in 2 to 3 divided doses. However, variable Cl and V in children as they grow warrant changes in aminoglycoside dosing accordingly. In general, younger children have larger V and Cl and require higher doses, but decrease in doses is necessary as they get older and the V and Cl reach adult values. E.H.'s V can be calculated using a V of 0.35 L/kg. Cl_{cr} can be calculated by adjusting GFR from Equation 6.8 by the patient's body surface area (BSA). (See Creatinine Clearance [Cl_{Cr}] in Chapter 3.) BSA values can be obtained from the appendix.

$$V = (0.35 \text{ L/kg}) (26.3 \text{ kg})$$
$$= 9.2 \text{ L}$$

$$Cl_{Cr} \text{ for Children (mL/min/1.73 m}^2) = 0.413 \left(\frac{\text{Height in cm}}{(\text{SCr})} \right)$$

$$= 0.413 \left(\frac{124 \text{ cm}}{(0.7 \text{ mg/dL})} \right)$$

$$= 75 \text{ mL/min/1.73 m}^2$$

$$Cl_{Cr} \text{ for Children (mL/min)} = (Cl_{Cr} \text{ mL/min/1.73 m}^2) \left(\frac{\text{BSA}}{1.73 \text{ m}^2} \right) \qquad \textbf{(Eq. 6.37)}$$

$$= (75 \text{ mL/min/1.73m}^2) \left(\frac{0.95\text{m}^2}{1.73 \text{ m}^2} \right)$$

$$= 41 \text{ mL/min}$$

$$= 41 \text{ mL/min} \times \frac{60 \text{ min/hr}}{1,000 \text{ mL/L}}$$

$$= 2.46 \text{ L/hr}$$

The elimination rate can be calculated using the estimated creatinine clearance of 2.46 L/hr and V of 9.2 L (Equation 6.14). Half-life can be calculated using Equation 6.15.

$$K = \frac{Cl}{V}$$
$$= \frac{2.46 \text{ L/hr}}{9.2 \text{ L}}$$
$$= 0.27 \text{ hr}^{-1}$$

$$t_{1/2} = \frac{0.693}{K}$$
$$= \frac{0.693}{0.27 \text{ hr}^{-1}}$$
$$= 2.56 \text{ hr}$$

The steady-state peak concentration should be calculated using the short infusion model because $t_{in} > 1/6 \, t\frac{1}{2}$ (Equation 6.21)

$$Css_2 = \frac{\frac{(S)(F)(Dose/t_{in})}{Cl}\left(1 - e^{-Kt_{in}}\right)}{\left(1 - e^{-K\tau}\right)}\left(e^{-Kt_2}\right)$$

$$= \frac{\frac{(1)(1)(60 \text{ mg/0.5 hr})}{2.46 \text{ L/hr}}\left(1 - e^{-(0.27 \text{ hr}^{-1})(0.5 \text{ hr})}\right)}{\left(1 - e^{-(0.27 \text{ hr}^{-1})(8 \text{ hr})}\right)}\left(e^{-(0.27 \text{ hr}^{-1})(0.5 \text{ hr})}\right)$$

$$= \frac{(48.8 \text{ mg/L})(0.126)}{0.88}(0.87)$$
$$= 6.1 \text{ mg/L}$$

Peak level of 6 mg/L is on the lower end of therapeutic goal range, most likely because of the increased V in children. The dose can be empirically increased to target a higher peak level if needed. If the adult V of 0.25 L/kg is used without accounting for larger V in children, the actual serum peak level measured may result in a lower value than the estimated peak, subjecting patients to risk of subtherapeutic therapy.

There are many studies supporting the once-daily aminoglycoside regimen in adults, and its use, although not as prevalent, is increasing in certain populations of children. The meta-analysis of once-daily regimen demonstrated a trend for better efficacy and similar low rates of nephrotoxicity and ototoxicity in children.[83] However, lack of consensus on appropriate dosing, target population, and therapeutic drug monitoring are preventing more universal acceptance of once-daily dosing.[84] The difficulty in formulating once-daily dose that can be applied to all pediatric patients lies on the interpatient variability in pharmacokinetic differences, as well as disease states and indications for therapy. For this reason, different dosing regimens available in the literature must be reviewed for patient population before it can be applied to general population.

Many institutions initiate pediatric patients on 7 mg/kg/day regimen for gentamicin/tobramycin and 15 to 20 mg/kg/day for amikacin.[85] However, in children <8 years of age, 7 mg/kg/day dose have shown to be inadequate to produce a target peak levels of 20 to 30 mg/L.[86] In some patient populations with altered kinetics, such as critically ill patients with burn injuries or cancer, common doses used for once-daily regimen often result in less than desired C_{max} and prolonged drug-free interval. A better approach for once-daily dosing in children with cancer may be to utilize age-based dosing, followed by levels to determine patient-specific parameters.[41,87,88] The advantage of age-based dosing is that the differences in pharmacokinetics from cancer as well as from the different age group are accounted for in the regimen. Age-based dosing recommends higher doses for younger children (10 mg/kg/day in children between 6 months and 9 years of age) and gradually lowering doses in older age groups (8 mg/kg/day in children between 9 and 12 years of age, 6 mg/kg/day in children 12 years of age).[41] Burn patients exhibit significantly shorter t½, and higher Cl and V from increased blood flow to the kidney after the burn injury and fluid resuscitation. Increased amikacin doses of 12.5 to 20 mg/kg q 6 to 12 hours have been recommended for burn patients, and once daily dosing is not recommended in this population.[89]

There is no set guideline as to when to check serum levels with extended interval dosing in pediatrics. Serum level monitoring is recommended at 2 hours and 8 to 12 hours after the infusion in adult patients, but it may be prudent to check the random level earlier in children because of larger degree of interpatient variability in aminoglycoside disposition. It is suggested to obtain an initial level at 2 hours and second one at 6 to 8 hours later in children.[41,87] The random level, 6 to 8 hours after the start of infusion, is particularly important to ensure that the drug-free interval does not exceed 4 to 16 hours. The extended drug-free interval can be a challenge in those that are immunocompromised but can be overcome with dual bacterial coverage with additional antibiotics.

In neonates, checking a 22-hour post-dose level has been suggested for extended interval dosing of 5 mg/kg to establish an appropriate interval of every 24, 36 or 48 hours.[90] A 22-hour level was chosen to confirm the appropriateness of every 24 hour dosing interval before the next dose is given. Based on the 22-hour post-dose concentration, the dosing intervals can be adjusted to keep the trough level of <1 mg/L. A meta-analysis of aminoglycoside extended interval dosing in neonates reported that 8% of the peak concentrations and 6% of the trough concentrations result outside the therapeutic range.[91] Body weight of neonates change every day, and the initial aminoglycoside dose may no longer be sufficient to reach the goal C_{max} level after several days of therapy. Therefore, serum drug concentrations should be checked regularly during a prolonged aminoglycoside therapy in neonatal patients with rapidly changing body weight and renal function.

When initiating extended interval dosing in children, dosing with serum level monitoring or computer programs, such as Bayesian analysis, should be considered over nomograms because of large interpatient variability in certain disease states.[87,92]

Question #17   *J.H. is a 22-year-old female (height, 5 feet 3 inches; weight, 48 kg) with cystic fibrosis who is admitted for treatment of an acute pulmonary exacerbation. Her serum creatinine is 0.7 mg/dL. Her treatment is initiated with tobramycin 480 mg infused over 30 minutes every 24 hours. Calculate the predicted steady-state peak and trough concentrations. What is the AUC?*

The pharmacokinetics of a number of compounds, including the aminoglycoside antibiotics, has been shown to be altered in patients with cystic fibrosis. In particular, the volume of distribution appears to be larger (0.3 to 0.35 L/kg), and the clearance is faster than age-matched control subjects.[73] One potential explanation for the apparent difference in pharmacokinetic parameters is due to altered body composition. Patients with cystic fibrosis often exhibit reduced adipose mass because of malnutrition secondary to pancreatic insufficiency. When the pharmacokinetic parameters are normalized by lean body mass, the parameters are not significantly different from that of age-matched controls.[93] J.H.'s V and Cl can be calculated using a V of 0.3 L/kg, and creatinine clearance can be calculated using Equation 6.7.

$$V = (0.3 \text{ L/kg}) (48 \text{ kg})$$
$$= 14.4 \text{ L}$$

$$\text{Cl}_{\text{Cr}} \text{ for Females (mL/min)} = \frac{(140 - \text{Age})(\text{Weight in kg})}{(72)(\text{SCr})} (0.85)$$
$$= \frac{(140 - 22 \text{ yrs})(48 \text{ kg})}{(72)(0.7 \text{ mg/dL})} (0.85)$$
$$= 95.5 \text{ mL/min}$$
$$= 95 \text{ mL/min} \times \frac{60 \text{ min/hr}}{1,000 \text{ mL/L}}$$
$$= 5.7 \text{ L/hr}$$

Using the estimated creatinine clearance of 5.7 L/hr as the tobramycin clearance and the volume of distribution of 14.4 L, the elimination rate constant (Equation 6.14) and half-life (Equation 6.15) are calculated to be 0.4 hr^{-1} and 1.7 hour, respectively:

$$K = \frac{\text{Cl}}{\text{V}}$$
$$= \frac{5.7 \text{ L/hr}}{14.4 \text{ L}}$$
$$= 0.4 \text{ hr}^{-1}$$

$$t_{1/2} = \frac{0.693}{K}$$
$$= \frac{0.693}{0.27 \text{ hr}^{-1}}$$
$$= 1.7 \text{ hr}$$

The steady-state peak and trough concentrations can be calculated using the short infusion model (Equation 6.21):

$$Css_2 = \frac{\frac{(S)(F)(Dose/t_{in})}{Cl}\left(1 - e^{-Kt_{in}}\right)}{\left(1 - e^{-K\tau}\right)}\left(e^{-Kt_2}\right)$$

$$= \frac{\frac{(1)(1)(480 \text{ mg}/0.5 \text{ hr})}{5.7 \text{ L/hr}}\left(1 - e^{-(0.4 \text{ hr}^{-1})(0.5 \text{ hr})}\right)}{\left(1 - e^{-(0.4 \text{ hr}^{-1})(24 \text{ hr})}\right)}\left(e^{-(0.4 \text{ hr}^{-1})(0.5 \text{ hr})}\right)$$

$$= \frac{(168 \text{ mg/L})(0.181)}{0.99}(0.82)$$

$$= 25 \text{ mg/L}$$

The trough concentration could be calculated using the short infusion model as shown above or by decaying down the peak concentration using Equation 6.10, where "t" is the time between the two drug levels.

$$C = C_0\, e^{-Kt}$$

$$= (25 \text{ mg/L})\left(e^{-(0.4 \text{ hr}^{-1})(23 \text{ hr})}\right)$$

$$= 25 \text{ mg/L }(0.0001)$$

$$= 0.0025 \text{ mg/L}$$

$$AUC_{24} = \frac{(Dose \text{ in mg})\,(24 \text{ hr})/\tau \text{ in hr}}{Cl \text{ in L/hr}}$$

$$= \frac{(480 \text{ mg})(24 \text{ hr})/24 \text{ hr}}{5.7 \text{ L/hr}}$$

$$= 84 \text{ mg} \cdot \text{hr/L}$$

Although the dose of tobramycin appears quite high (10 mg/kg/day), the relatively rapid clearance (when expressed per TBW) results in predicted serum concentrations that are not different than the target concentrations in other patients. In the past, the use of "once-daily" aminoglycoside regimen was not as widespread in cystic fibrosis patients as in other patient populations. The relatively short elimination half-life raised concerns of bacterial resistance because of prolonged drug-free interval exceeding the duration of post-antibiotic effect. Recent systemic review demonstrated that there were no differences in efficacy between multiple daily dosing and once-daily dosing of tobramycin. No greater risk of toxicity was noted with once-daily dosing.[94] The Cystic Fibrosis Pulmonary Guideline recommends once-daily dosing of aminoglycosides over multiple daily dosing for the treatment of acute pulmonary exacerbations.[95] The recommended dose is 10 mg/kg/day because doses exceeding that has resulted in $C_{max} > 30$ mg/L and $AUC > 100$ mg · hr/L even in cystic fibrosis patients with larger V and Cl.[96] For cystic fibrosis patients, two aminoglycoside concentrations should be checked for dosage adjustment: one level 2 hour after dosing and the other 8 to 12 hours after dosing.

Question #18 *O.L., a 52-year-old man in the critical care unit with multiple organ failure, is receiving CRRT with a total output of 2 L/hr (ultrafiltration and dialysis flow rate of 1 L/hr each). His current weight is 65 kg (up from 60 kg 2 days ago), and his serum creatinine is 2.8 mg/dL. After pending cultures, he is to be started on tobramycin. What would be a reasonable starting dose for O.L.?*

There are two approaches to dosing of aminoglycosides, traditional and high-dose extended interval dosing. With traditional dosing, tobramycin would be initiated at a dose of approximately 2 mg/kg targeting peak concentrations of 6 to 8 mg/L, and a dosing interval would be chosen in order to achieve trough concentrations of less than 2 mg/L and preferably less than 1 mg/L. With high-dose extended interval dosing, a dose of 5 to 7 mg/kg would be initiated targeting peak concentrations of 20 to 30 mg/L, and a dosing interval would be chosen to target an AUC_{24} of approximately 70 to 100 mg · hr/L. To determine the tobramycin dosing regimen, we will have to estimate his residual renal function (Cl_{pat}), CRRT clearance (Cl_{CRRT}), and volume of distribution (V).

Because the patient has end-stage renal failure and is receiving CRRT, the Cockcroft and Gault equation is not a valid way to estimate renal function. Our best guess would be to use the average aminoglycoside clearance of 0.0043 L/hr/kg for functionally anephric patients. Excluding what appears to be 5 kg of excess third-space weight, the weight of 60 kg would result in a Cl_{pat} of 0.258 L/hr (0.0043 L/hr × 60 kg). Assuming that the aminoglycoside plasma binding is negligible, fu would be approximately 1 and our maximum expected Cl_{CRRT} would be 2 L/hr.

$$Cl_{CRRT} \text{ Maximum} = (fu)(CRRT \text{ Flow Rate}) \qquad \text{(Eq. 6.38)}$$

$$= (1)(2 \text{ L/hr})$$
$$= 2 \text{ L/hr}$$

Although the initial estimate of 2 L/hr is a reasonable first approach, the literature would suggest that the actual Cl_{CRRT} is approximately 0.8 of the CRRT flow rate.[97–99] Using 0.8 as the fraction of the CRRT flow that is actually cleared, we would have a Cl_{CRRT} of 1.6 L/hr (0.8 × 2 L/hr). Now combining the Cl_{CRRT} and Cl_{pat}, we estimate a total Cl of 1.86 L/hr (1.6 L/hr + 0.258 L/hr ≈ 1.86 L/hr) while the patient is receiving CRRT.

The volume of distribution would be calculated using Equation 6.4 where 60 kg represents the "Nonobese, Non–Excess Fluid Weight," 0 the "Excess Adipose Weight," and 5 kg the "Excess Third-Space Fluid Weight."

Aminoglycoside V(L) =

$$\left(\begin{array}{c} 0.25 \text{ L/kg} \times \text{Nonobese,} \\ \text{Non–Excess Fluid Weight (kg)} \end{array}\right) + 0.1 \left(\begin{array}{c} \text{Excess} \\ \text{Adipose} \\ \text{Weight (kg)} \end{array}\right) + \left(\begin{array}{c} \text{Excess Third} \\ \text{Space Fluid} \\ \text{Weight (kg)} \end{array}\right)$$

$$= 0.25 \text{ L/kg} \times 60 \text{ kg} + 0.1(0) + 1(5 \text{ kg})$$
$$= 15 \text{ L} + 0 \text{ L} + 5 \text{ L}$$
$$= 20 \text{ L}$$

Using Equations 6.14 and 6.15, we calculate a K value in hr^{-1} and a $t\frac{1}{2}$ in hr.

$$K = \frac{Cl}{V}$$

$$= \frac{1.86 \text{ L/hr}}{20 \text{ L}}$$

$$= 0.093 \text{ hr}^{-1}$$

$$t\frac{1}{2} = \frac{0.693}{K}$$

$$= \frac{0.693}{0.093 \text{ hr}^{-1}}$$

$$= 7.45 \text{ hr}$$

Considering that the usual dosing interval for "traditional" aminoglycoside dosing is three to five half-lives, our dosing interval would be somewhere between 22.4 hours (3 × 7.45 hours) and 37.3 hours (5 × 7.45 hours). Given the desire to maintain dosing intervals that are easy to calculate and adhere to an initial dosing interval of 24 hours would seem most appropriate.

To calculate the tobramycin dose, we would use Equation 6.26 where Css_1 would be our target peak concentration of 7 mg/L, V and K to be our estimates of 20 L and 0.093 hr^{-1}, respectively, and S and F would be 1. We would use 24 hours for τ and 1 hour for t_1 assuming that we want our peak concentration of 7 mg/L, 1 hour after the start of the tobramycin infusion. Inserting the above values into Equation 6.26, we calculate a tobramycin dose of 137 mg.

$$\text{Dose} = \frac{(Css_1)(V)(1 - e^{-K\tau})}{(S)(F)(e^{-Kt_1})}$$

$$= \frac{(7 \text{ mg/L})(20 \text{ L})(1 - e^{-0.093 \text{ hr}^{-1} \times 24 \text{ hr}})}{(1)(1)(e^{-0.093 \text{ hr}^{-1} \times 1 \text{ hr}})}$$

$$= \frac{(140 \text{ mg})(1 - 0.107)}{(1)(1)(0.911)}$$

$$= 137 \text{ mg}$$

The calculated dose would be rounded off to something like 135 or 140 mg given IV over 30 minutes every 24 hours. We would also want to calculate our trough concentration using Equation 6.10.

$$C = C_0 e^{-Kt}$$

where C_0 would be our steady-state peak concentration of 7 mg/L and t would be 23 hours. Note that because our steady-state peak concentration of 7 mg/L is 1 hour after starting the infusion, the time remaining in the dosing interval to the trough is 23 and not the full dosing interval of 24 hours.

$$C = C_0 e^{-Kt}$$
$$= 7 \text{ mg/L} \times e^{-0.093 \text{ hr}^{-1} \times 23 \text{ hr}}$$
$$= 7 \text{ mg/L} \times 0.118$$
$$= 0.82 \text{ mg/L}$$

Our calculated tobramycin regimen of approximately 140 mg IV every 24 hours is expected to result in a steady-state peak and trough concentration of approximately 7 and 0.8 mg/L, respectively.

With high-dose extended interval dosing, the dosing interval is approximately five half-lives in order to achieve a short drug-free interval, which is thought to reduce accumulation within the renal cortex and inner ear. Therefore, the dosing interval should be every 48 hours ($5 \times 7.45 = 37.3$ hours). Considering the in vivo post-antibiotic effect is reported to last up to 10 hours, this dosing interval would enable maximizing the peak concentration while reducing drug accumulation within the renal cortex and inner ear.

Once again, we would calculate the tobramycin dose using Equation 6.26 where Css_1 would be our target peak concentration of 20 mg/L; V and K would be our estimates of 20 L and 0.093 hr^{-1}, respectively; and S and F would be 1. We would use 48 hours for τ and 1 hour for t_1 assuming we want our peak concentration of 20 mg/L, 1 hour after the start of the tobramycin infusion. Inserting the above values into Equation 6.26, we calculate a tobramycin dose of 434 mg which would be rounded off to a dose of 440 mg.

$$\text{Dose} = \frac{(Css_1)(V)(1 - e^{-Kt})}{(S)(F)(e^{-Kt_1})}$$
$$= \frac{(20 \text{ mg/L})(20 \text{ L})(1 - e^{-0.093 \,(48 \text{ hr})})}{(1)(1)(e^{-0.093(1)})}$$
$$= \frac{(400 \text{ mg})(1 - 0.0115)}{(1)(1)(0.911)}$$
$$= 434 \text{ mg}$$

We would also want to calculate the AUC_{24} to determine the risk for toxicity using Equation 6.27.

$$AUC_{24} = \frac{(\text{Dose in mg})(24 \text{ hr})/\tau \text{ in hr}}{Cl \text{ in L/hr}}$$

Substituting $K \times V$ for clearance using the values of 0.093 hr^{-1} for K and 20 L for V:

$$= \frac{(440 \text{ mg})(24 \text{ hr})/148 \text{ hr}}{(0.093 \text{ hr}^{-1})(20 \text{ L})}$$

$$= \frac{220 \text{ mg}}{1.86 \text{ L/hr}}$$

$$= 118 \text{ mg} \cdot \text{hr/L}$$

This value of AUC_{24} exceeds our target range of approximately 70 to 100 mg · hr/L; therefore, the dose would need to be reduced. Considering the severity of O.L.'s infection, we might consider targeting an AUC_{24} of 85 to 100 mg · hr/L in order to maximize the peak concentration. This can be determined by using a simple ratio of the AUCs multiplied by the old dose to calculate a new dose.

$$\frac{AUC_{24} \text{ New}}{AUC_{24} \text{ Old}}(\text{Dose Old}) = \text{New Dose}$$

(Eq. 6.39)

$$\frac{85 \text{ mg} \cdot \text{hr/L}}{118 \text{ mg} \cdot \text{hr/L}}(440 \text{ mg}) = 316 \text{ mg}$$

or

$$\frac{100 \text{ mg} \cdot \text{hr/L}}{118 \text{ mg} \cdot \text{hr/L}}(440 \text{ mg}) = 372 \text{ mg}$$

The dose would be rounded off to a dose of 320 mg or 380 mg every 48 hours. Because the dose is significantly different than the dose we calculated earlier, we should determine the estimated peak concentration with these new doses using Equation 6.17.

$$Css_1 = \frac{\dfrac{(S)(F)(\text{Dose})}{V}}{(1 - e^{-K\tau})}(e^{-Kt_1})$$

$$= \frac{(1)(1)(320 \text{ mg})/20 \text{ L}}{1 - e^{-0.093 \, (48 \text{ hr})}} e^{-0.093(1)}$$

$$= \frac{16 \text{ mg/L}}{1 - 0.0115}(0.91)$$

$$= 14.7 \text{ mg/L}$$

Similarly, the peak concentration from a dose of 380 mg every 48 hours can be calculated to be 17.5 mg/L. Because the peak concentration is directly proportional to the dose (as long as the interval is not changed), we could also have estimated the peak concentrations based on a ratio of the dose and peak concentration already calculated. Therefore, a dose between 320 and 380 mg every 48 hours would provide a steady-state peak concentration of 14.7 to 17.5 mg/L and an AUC_{24} of 85 to 100 mg · hr/L.

We would also want to confirm our estimates with measured concentration, usually obtained around the third dose. Also as indicated in Dialysis of Drugs: Continuous Renal Replacement Therapy (CRRT) in Chapter 3, patients who are receiving CRRT are critically ill, and the CRRT procedure is often interrupted or the CRRT flow rate changed depending on the condition of the patient. For that reason, the patient should be checked frequently (minimally each day) to ensure that CRRT is progressing as initially planned.

REFERENCES

1. Pechere JC, Dugal R. Clinical pharmacokinetics of aminoglycoside antibiotics. *Clin Pharmacokinet.* 1979;4:170.

2. Craig W, Ebert SC. Killing and regrowth of bacteria in vivo: a review. *Scand J Infect Dis.* 1991;74:63–71.

3. Kapusnik JE, Hackbarth CJ, Chambers HF, et al. Single, large, daily dosing versus intermittent dosing of tobramycin for treating experimental Pseudomonas pneumonia. *J Infect Dis.* 1988;158:7–22.

4. Leggett JE, Fantin B, Ebert S, et al. Comparative antibiotic dose–effect relations at several dosing intervals in murine pneumonitis and thigh-infection models. *J Infect Dis.* 1989;159:281–292.

5. Moore RD, Lietman PS, Smith CR, et al. Clinical response to aminoglycoside therapy: importance of the ratio of peak concentration to minimal inhibitory concentration. *J Infect Dis.* 1987;155:93–99.

6. Craig WA, Vogelman B. The post-antibiotic effect. *Ann Intern Med.* 1987;106:900–902.

7. Craig WA, Redington J, Ebert SC. Pharmacodynamics of amikacin in vitro and in mouse thigh and lung infections. *J Antimicrob Chemother.* 1991;27(suppl C):29–40.

8. Powell SH, Thompson WL, Luthe MA, et al. Once-daily vs. continuous aminoglycoside dosing: efficacy and toxicity in animal and clinical studies of gentamicin, netilmicin, and tobramycin. *J Infect Dis.* 1983;5:918–932.

9. Verpooten GA, Giuliano RA, Verbist L, et al. Once-daily dosing decreases renal accumulation of gentamicin and netilmicin. *Clin Pharmacol Ther.* 1989;45:22–27.

10. Rybak MJ, Abate BJ, Kang SL, et al. Prospective evaluation of the effect of an aminoglycoside dosing regimen on rates of observed nephrotoxicity and ototoxicity. *Antimicrob Agents Chemother.* 1999;43:1549–1555.

11. Barza M, Ioannidis JP, Cappelleri JC, et al. Single or multiple daily doses of aminoglycosides: a meta-analysis. *Br Med J.* 1996;312:338–345.

12. Hatala R, Dinh T, Cook DJ. Once-daily aminoglycoside dosing in immunocompetent adults: a meta-analysis. *Ann Intern Med.* 1996;124:717–725.

13. Nicolau DP, Freeman CD, Belliveau PP, et al. Experience with a once-daily aminoglycoside program administered to 2,184 adult patients. *Antimicrob Agents Chemother.* 1995;39:650–655.

14. Noone P, Parsons TM, Pattison JR, et al. Experience in monitoring gentamicin therapy during treatment of serious gram-negative sepsis. *Br Med J.* 1979;1:477.

15. Jackson GG, Riff LJ. Pseudomonas bacteremia: pharmacologic and other basis for failure of treatment with gentamicin. *J Infect Dis.* 1971;124:185.

16. Klastersky J, Daneau D, Swings G, et al. Antibacterial activity in serum and urine as a therapeutic guide in bacterial infections. *J Infect Dis.* 1974;129:187.

17. Cox CE. Gentamicin: a new aminoglycoside antibiotic: clinical and laboratory studies in urinary tract infections. *J Infect Dis.* 1969;119:486.

18. Jackson GG, Arcieri G. Ototoxicity of gentamicin in man: a survey and controlled analysis of clinical experience in the United States. *J Infect Dis.* 1971;124:130.

19. Goodman EL, Van Gelber J, Holmes R, et al. Prospective comparative study of variable dosage and variable frequency regimens for administrations of gentamicin. *Antimicrob Agents Chemother.* 1975;8:434.

20. Schentag JJ, Cerra, FB, Plaut ME, et al. Clinical and pharmacokinetic characteristics of aminoglycoside nephrotoxicity in 201 critically ill patients. *Antimicrob Agents Chemother.* 1982;5:721.

21. Wilfret JN, Burke JP, Bloomer HA, et al. Renal insufficiency associated with gentamicin therapy. *J Infect Dis.* 1971;124(suppl):148.

22. Mawer GE, Ahmad R, Dobbs SM. Prescribing aids for gentamicin. *Br J Clin Pharmacol.* 1974;1:45.

23. Federspil P, Schätzle W, Tiesler E, et al. Pharmacokinetics and ototoxicity of gentamicin, tobramycin, and amikacin. *J Infect Dis.* 1976;134(suppl):200.

24. McCormack JP, Jewesson PJ. A critical re-evaluation of the "therapeutic range" of aminoglycosides. *Clin Infect Dis.* 1992;14:320–339.

25. Barclay ML, Duffull SB, Begg EJ, et al. Experience of once-daily aminoglycoside dosing using a target area under the concentration-time curve. *Aust N Z J Med.* 1995;25:230–235.

26. Gyselynck AM, Forrey A, Cutler R. Pharmacokinetics of gentamicin: distribution and plasma and renal clearance. *J Infect Dis.* 1971;124(suppl):70.

27. Christopher TG, Korn D, Blair AD, et al. Gentamicin pharmacokinetics during hemodialysis. *Kidney Int.* 1974;6:38.

28. Danish M, Schultz R, Jukso WJ, et al. Pharmacokinetics of gentamicin and kanamycin during hemodialysis. *Antimicrob Agents Chemother.* 1974;6:841.

29. Barza M, Brown RB, Shen D, et al. Predictability of blood levels of gentamicin in man. *J Infect Dis.* 1975;132:165.

30. Sawchuk RJ, Zaske DE. Pharmacokinetics of dosing regimens which utilize multiple intravenous infusions: gentamicin in burn patients. *J Pharmacokinet Biopharm.* 1976;4:183.

31. Regamey C, Gordon RC, Kirby WM, et al. Comparative pharmacokinetics of tobramycin and gentamicin. *Clin Pharmacol Ther.* 1973;14:396.

32. Siber GR, Echeverria P, Smith AL, et al. Pharmacokinetics of gentamicin in children and adults. *J Infect Dis.* 1975;132:637.

33. Hull J, Sarubbi FA. Gentamicin serum concentrations: pharmacokinetic predictions. *Ann Intern Med.* 1976;85:183.

34. Blouin RA, Mann HJ, Griffen WO Jr, et al. Tobramycin pharmacokinetics in morbidly obese patients. *Clin Pharmacol Ther.* 1979;26:508.

35. Bauer LA, Blouin RA, Griffen WO Jr, et al. Amikacin pharmacokinetics in morbidly obese patients. *Am J Hosp Pharm.* 1980;37:519.

36. Sampliner R, Perrier D, Powell R, et al. Influence of ascites on tobramycin pharmacokinetics. *J Clin Pharmacol.* 1984;24:43.

37. Hodgman T, Dasta JF, Armstrong DK, et al. Tobramycin disposition into ascitic fluid. *Clin Pharm.* 1984;3:203.

38. Kearns GL, Abdel SM, Blowey DL, et al. Developmental pharmacology-drug disposition, action ad therapy in infants and children. *N Engl J Med.* 2003;349:1157–1176.

39. Esheverria P, Siber GR, Paisley J, et al. Age-dependent dose response to gentamicin. *Pediatrics.* 1975;87:805.

40. Shevchuk YM, Taylor DM. Aminoglycoside volume of distribution in pediatric patients. *DICP.* 1990; 24: 273–276.

41. Dupuis LL, Sung L, Taylor T, et al. Tobramycin pharmacokinetics in children with febrile neutropenia undergoing stem cell transplantation: once-daily versus thrice-daily administration. *Pharmacotherapy.* 2004;24:564–573.

42. Schentag JJ, Jusko WJ, Plaut ME, et al. Tissue persistence of gentamicin in man. *JAMA.* 1977;238:327.

43. Schentag JJ, Jusko WJ. Renal clearance and tissue accumulation of gentamicin. *Clin Pharmacol Ther.* 1977;22:364.

44. Mendelson J, Portnoy J, Dick V, et al. Safety of bolus administration of gentamicin. *Antimicrob Agents Chemother.* 1976;9:633.

45. Lynn KL, Neale TJ, Little PJ, et al. Gentamicin by intravenous bolus injections. *N Z Med J*. 1977;80:442.

46. Demczar DJ, Nafziger AN, Bertino JS Jr. Pharmacokinetics of gentamicin at traditional versus higher doses: implications for once-daily aminoglycoside dosing. *Antimicrob Agents Chemother*. 1997;41:1115–1119.

47. Colburn WA, Schentag JJ, Jusko WJ, et al. A model for the prospective identification of the prenephro-toxic state during gentamicin therapy. *J Pharmacokinet Biopharm*. 1978;6:179.

48. Evans WE, Taylor RH, Feldman S, et al. A model for dosing gentamicin in children and adolescents that adjust for tissue accumulation with continuous dosing. *Clin Pharmacokinet*. 1980;5:295.

49. Pai MP. Estimating the glomerular filtration rate in obese adult patients for drug dosing. *Adv Chronic Kidney Dis*. 2010;17:e53–e62.

50. Dionne RE, Bauer LA, Gibson GA, et al. Estimating creatinine clearance in morbidly obese patients. *Am J Hosp Pharm*. 1981;38:841–844.

51. Bauer LA, Edwards WA, Dellinger EP, et al. Influence of weight on aminoglycoside pharmacokinetics in normal weight and morbidly obese patients. *Eur J Clin Pharmacol*. 1983;24:643–647.

52. Aronson JK. Drug therapy in kidney disease. *Br J Clin Pharmacol*. 2007;63:504–511.

53. Halacova M, Kotaska K, Kukacka J, et al. Serum cystatin c level for better assessment of glomerular filtration rate in cystic fibrosis patients treated with amikacin. *J Clin Pharm Ther*. 2008;33:409–417.

54. Bartelink IH, Rademaker CM, Schobben AF, et al. Guidelines on paediatric dosing on the basis of de-velopmental physiology and pharmacokinetic considerations. *Clin Pharamcokinet*. 2006;45:1077–1097.

55. De Cock RF, Allegaert K, Schreuder MF, et al. Maturation of the glomerular filtration rate in neonates, as reflected by amikacin clearance. *Clin Pharmacokinet*. 2012;51:105–117.

56. De Cock RF, Allegaert K, Brussee JM, et al. Simultaneous pharmacokinetic modeling of gentamicin, tobramycin and vancomycin clearance from neonates to adults: towards a semi-physiological function for maturation in glomerular filtration. *Pharm Res*. 2014;31:2643–2654.

57. Schwartz GJ, Muñoz A, Schneider MF, et al. New equations to estimate GFR in children with CKD. *J Am Soc Nephrol*. 2009;20:629–637.

58. Gao A, Cachat F, Faouzi M, et al. Comparison of the glomerular filtration rate in children by the new revised Schwartz formula and a new generalized formula. *Kidney Int*. 2013;83:524–530.

59. Holt HA, Broughall JM, McCarthy M, et al. Interactions between aminoglycoside antibiotics and carbenicillin or ticarcillin. *Infection*. 1976;4:107.

60. Ervin FR, Bullock WE Jr, Nuttall CE, et al. Inactivation of gentamicin by penicillins in patients with renal failure. *Antimicrob Agents Chemother*. 1976;9:1004.

61. Weibert RT, Keane WF. Carbenicillin-gentamicin interaction in acute renal failure. *Am J Hosp Pharm*. 1977;34:1137.

62. Lau A, Lee M, Flascha S, et al. Effect of piperacillin on tobramycin pharmacokinetics in patients with normal renal function. *Antimicrob Agents Chemother*. 1983;24:533–537.

63. Riff LJ, Jackson GG. Laboratory and clinical conditions for gentamicin inactivation by carbenicillin. *Arch Intern Med*. 1972;130:887.

64. Riff LJ, Thomason JL. Comparative aminoglycoside inactivation by beta-lactam antibiotics. Effects of a cephalosporin and six penicillins on five aminoglycosides. *J Antibiot (Tokyo)*. 1982;35:850–857.

65. Konishi H, Goto M, Nakamoto Y, et al. Tobramycin inactivation by carbenicillin, ticarcillin, and pip-eracillin. *Antimicrob Agents Chemother*. 1983;23:653.

66. Pickering LK, Gerahart P. Effect of time and concentration upon interaction between gentamicin, tobra-mycin, netilmicin, or amikacin, and carbenicillin or ticarcillin. *Antimicrob Agents Chemother*. 1979;15:592.

67. Henderson JL, Polk RE, Kline BJ. In vitro inactivation of tobramycin and netilmicin by carbenicillin, azlocillin, or mezlocillin. *Am J Hosp Pharm*. 1981;38:1167.

68. Glew RH, Pavuk RA. Stability of gentamicin, tobramycin, and amikacin in combination with four β-lactam antibiotics. *Antimicrob Agents Chemother*. 1983;24:474–477.

69. Kehoe W. Lack of effect of ceftizoxime on gentamicin serum level determinations. *Hosp Pharm*. 1986;21:340.

70. Earp CM, Barriere SL. The lack of inactivation of tobramycin by cefazolin, cefamandole, moxalactam in vitro. *Drug Intell Clin Pharm*. 1985;19:677.

71. Fischer JH, Hedrick PJ, Riff LJ, et al. Pharmacokinetics and antibacterial activity of two gentamicin products given intramuscularly. *Clin Pharm*. 1984;3:411.

72. Blieler RE, Schedl HP. Creatinine excretion: variability and relationships to diet and body size. *J Lab Clin Med*. 1962;59:945.

73. Reiner N, Bloxham DD, Thompson WL. Nephrotoxicity of gentamicin and tobramycin given once daily or continuously in dogs. *Antimicrob Agents Chemother*. 1978;4(suppl A):85.

74. Reguer L, Colding H, Jensen H, et al. Pharmacokinetics of amikacin during hemodialysis and peritoneal dialysis. *Antimicrob Agents Chemother*. 1977;11:214.

75. Christopher TG, Blair AD, Forrey AW, et al. Hemodialyzer clearance of gentamicin, kanamycin, tobramycin, amikacin, ethambutol, procainamide, and flucytosine with a technique for planning therapy. *J Pharmacokinet Biopharm*. 1976;4:427.

76. Halprin BA, Axline SG, Coplon NS, et al. Clearance of gentamicin during hemodialysis: a comparison of four artificial kidneys. *J Infect Dis*. 1976;133:627.

77. Gailiunas P Jr, Dominguez-Morenzo M, Lazarus M, et al. Vestibular toxicity of gentamicin: incidence in patients receiving long-term hemodialysis therapy. *Arch Intern Med*. 1978;138:1621.

78. Bauer LA. Rebound gentamicin levels after hemodialysis. *Ther Drug Monit*. 1982;4:99.

79. Gary NE. Peritoneal clearance and removal of gentamicin. *J Infect Dis*. 1971;124(suppl):96.

80. Lamiere N, Bogaert M, Belpaire F. Peritoneal pharmacokinetics and pharmacological manipulation of peritoneal transport. In: Gokal R, ed. *Continuous Ambulatory Peritoneal Dialysis*. New York, NY: Churchill Livingstone; 1986:56–93.

81. O'Brien MA, Mason NA. Systemic absorption of intra-peritoneal antimicrobials in continuous ambulatory peritoneal dialysis. *Clin Pharm*. 1992;11:246–254.

82. Horton MW, Deeter RG, Sherman RA. Treatment of peritonitis in patients undergoing continuous ambulatory peritoneal dialysis. *Clin Pharm*. 1990;9:102–117.

83. Contopoulos-Ioannidis DG, Giotis ND, Baliatsa DV, et al. Extended-interval aminoglycoside administration for children: a meta-analysis. *Pediatrics*. 2004;114:e111–e118.

84. Knoderer CA, Everett JA, Buss WF. Clinical issues surrounding once-daily aminoglycoside dosing in children. *Pharmacotherapy*. 2003;23:44–56.

85. Jenh AM, Tamma PD, Milstone AM. Extended-interval aminoglycoside dosing in pediatrics. *Pediatr Infect Dis J*. 2011;30:338–339.

86. McDade EJ, Wagner JL, Moffett BS, et al. Once-daily gentamicin dosing in pediatric patients without Cystic Fibrosis. *Pharmacotherapy*. 2010;30:248–253.

87. Newby B, Prevost D, Lotocka-Reysner H. Assessment of gentamicin 7 mg/kg once daily for pediatric patients with febrile neutropenia: a pilot project. *J Oncol Pharm Pract*. 2009;15:211–216.

88. Ho KK, Bryson SM, Thiessen JJ, et al. The effects of age and chemotherapy on gentamicin pharmacokinetics and dosing in pediatric oncology patients. *Pharmacotherapy*. 1995;15:754–764.

89. Yu T, Stockmann C, Healy DP, et al. Determination of optimal amikacin dosing regimens for pediatric patients with burn wound sepsis. *J Burn Care Res*. 2015;36:e244–e252.

90. Dersch-Mills D, Akierman A, Alshaikh B, et al. Performance of a dosage individualization table for extended interval gentamicin in neonates beyond the first week of life. *J Matern Fetal Neonatal Med*. 2016;29:1451–1456.

91. Nestaas E, Bangstad HJ, Sandvik L, et al. Aminoglycoside extended interval dosing in neonates is safe and effective: a meta-analysis. *Arch Dis Child Fetal Neonatal Ed*. 2005;90:F294–F300.

92. Abusham AA, Mohammed AH, Alkindi SS, et al. Sub-optimal serum gentamicin concentrations in sickle cell disease patients utilizing the Hartford protocol. *J Clin Pharm Ther*. 2012;37:212–216.

93. Hennig S, Norris R, Kirkpatrick CM. Target concentration intervention is needed for tobramycin dosing in paediatric patients with cystic fibrosis—a population pharmacokinetic study. *Br J Clin Pharmacol*. 2008;65:502–510.

94. Smyth AR, Bhatt J. Once-daily versus multiple-daily dosing with intravenous aminoglycosides for cystic fibrosis. *Cochrane Database Syst Rev*, 2014:1–27. doi:10.1002/14651858.CD002009.pub5.

95. Flume PA, Mogayzel PJ Jr, Robinson KA, et al; Clinical Practice Guidelines for Pulmonary Therapies Committee. Cystic fibrosis pulmonary guidelines: treatment of pulmonary exacerbations. *Am J Respir Crit Care Med*. 2009;180:802–808.

96. Prescott WA Jr, Nagel JL. Extended-interval once-daily dosing of aminoglycosides in adult and pediatric patients with cystic fibrosis. *Pharmacotherapy*. 2010;30:95–108.

97. Bickley SK. Drug dosing during continuous arteriovenous hemofiltration. *Clin Pharm*. 1988;7:198–206.

98. Golper TA. Continuous arteriovenous hemofiltration in acute renal failure. *Am J Kidney Dis*. 1985;6:373–386.

99. Pea F, Viale P, Furlanut M. Pharmacokinetic considerations for antimicrobial therapy in patients receiving renal replacement therapy. *Clin Pharmacokinet*. 2007;46:997–1038.

7

ANTIFUNGAL AGENTS: TRIAZOLES

Russell E. Lewis

Learning Objectives

By the end of the antifungal agents: triazoles chapter, the learner shall be able to:

1. Compare and contrast the main causes of pharmacokinetic variability among triazole antifungals that could jeopardize the efficacy and/or safety of treatment.
2. Identify specific factors for each triazole antifungal and formulation that may predispose patients to pharmacokinetic interactions.
3. Describe strategies of how triazole antifungal dosing can be optimized when inadequate drug exposures are identified by therapeutic drug monitoring.

Invasive fungal diseases are a major cause of morbidity and mortality in the immuno-compromised patients, causing an estimated 1.5 million deaths per year—a figure that surpasses the number of deaths as a result of either tuberculosis or malaria.[1] Although diagnostic advances and new antifungal agents have improved outcomes in recent years, mortality rates still approach 30% to 50% for the most commonly encountered fungal infections, or result in prolonged hospitalization or delays in life-saving treatments for malignancy or organ failure.

For over 40 years, amphotericin B-deoxycholate was the only reliable antifungal treatment for invasive yeast and mold infections. Its effectiveness, however, was compromised by frequent infusion-related reactions and high rates of nephrotoxicity that often require interruption of treatment. During the 1990s, amphotericin B was reformulated into lipid or liposomal carriers, which substantially improved the drug's tolerability profile, but did not eliminate the problem of nephrotoxicity, especially in patients with preexisting renal disease or those receiving multiple concomitant nephrotoxic therapies.

The introduction of triazole and echinocandin antifungal agents (Table 7.1) were important advances because they allowed clinicians for the first time to treat serious

TABLE 7.1   Systemic Antifungals Timeline of Introduction

SITE OF ACTION IN FUNGI	MECHANISM	DRUG (YEAR INTRODUCED)
Cell membrane	Ergosterol binding	Polyene antifungals 　Amphotericin B (1958) 　Amphotericin B lipid 　complex (1995) 　Liposomal amphotericin 　B (1996)
	Ergosterol synthesis inhibition (14α-demethylase)	Imidazoles 　Ketoconazole (1981)
		Triazoles 　Fluconazole (1990) 　Itraconazole (1992) 　Voriconazole (2002) 　Posaconazole (2006) 　Isavuconazole (2015)
Cell wall	β-Glucan synthesis inhibition (β-1,3-D-glucan synthase)	Echinocandins 　Caspofungin (2001) 　Micafungin (2005) 　Anidulafungin (2007)
Intracellular	Pyrimidine analogues/ thymidate synthase inhibitor	Flucytosine (1971)

fungal infections without serious nephrotoxicity. Triazole antifungals were also the first class of antifungals approved for use available in both oral and intravenous (IV) formulations, thus allowing patients to continue their treatment outside the hospital without a central venous catheter.

As a result, triazoles are now the most widely prescribed class of antifungal agents even though they still have many limitations. First, all triazole antifungals arrest fungal cell growth by inhibiting a key fungal cytochrome P450 enzyme (14α-demethylase) that converts lanosterol to the fungal cell membrane sterol ergosterol. This mechanism is not entirely selective for fungi, because all triazoles also inhibit, to varying degrees, human cytochrome P450 enzymes involved in the metabolism of thousands of endogenous and exogenous chemicals.[2] Consequently, treatment with triazole antifungals places patients at high risk for many pharmacokinetic (PK) drug–drug interactions.

A second limitation of triazole pharmacology is that binding affinity to 14α-demethylase largely depends on the lipophilic nature of the molecule. Chemical modifications designed to broaden the spectrum of triazole antifungals produce molecules with large volume of distribution, complex biotransformation (metabolism) profiles, and poorer bioavailability.

Collectively, these characteristics and potential for drug interactions mean that triazole PKs can be unpredictable in patients, even if dosing is standardized to body weight. In some cases, this PK variability has been shown to jeopardize the effectiveness and safety of treatment for invasive fungal diseases, suggesting that some patients could benefit from therapeutic drug monitoring (TDM).[3] This chapter focuses on the PK characteristics of triazole antifungals with particular emphasis on agents that potentially require TDM in patients at risk or documented to have invasive fungal disease.

Fluconazole

Fluconazole was the first triazole antifungal developed for clinical use. It is a relatively small (molecular weight 306 g/mol) hydrophilic molecule (log P 0.58) that is a reversible inhibitor of fungal 14α-demethylase. Consequently, fluconazole is the narrowest-spectrum triazole antifungal with activity primarily against yeast (*Candida* and *Cryptococcus* spp.), some activity against endemic (dimorphic) fungi, including *Coccidioides immitis* and *Blastomyces dermatitidis*, but no clinically useful activity against molds such as *Aspergillus* spp., *Fusarium* spp., or Mucorales. Fluconazole is frequently used for the treatment of mucocutaneous *Candida* infections, *Candida* urinary tract infections, or as a step-down (second-line) regimen for invasive candidiasis after initial echinocandin treatment if susceptibility of the isolate is known.[4] Fluconazole is also administered as prophylaxis for mucocutaneous and invasive candidiasis in some high-risk immunocompromised populations.

THERAPEUTIC RANGE OF FLUCONAZOLE

Fluconazole exhibits concentration- and time-dependent antifungal activity with a prolonged postantifungal effect. The ratio of free drug area under the concentration–time curve from 0 to 24 hours to minimum inhibitory concentration (fAUC$_{0-24hr}$/MIC) is considered the PK/pharmacodynamic (PD) index predictive of antifungal activity.[5] An AUC$_{0-24hr}$/MIC of 50 is associated with fungistatic activity, with optimal outcomes in immunocompromised or critically ill patients reported as the fAUC$_{0-24hr}$/MIC approaches 100.[6] Based on current susceptibility breakpoints for *Candida* spp., an AUC 400 mg · hr/L (roughly equivalent to a C min above 10 to 15 mg/L) is recommended. Toxicity of fluconazole has not been linked to serum fluconazole concentrations.

BIOAVAILABILITY (F)

Fluconazole is available in both IV and oral formulations (tablet and suspensions). The oral bioavailability of fluconazole is excellent (>90%) and not appreciably affected by food or gastric pH. Fluconazole achieves peak concentrations in the serum within 1 to 2 hours after oral administration.

VOLUME OF DISTRIBUTION (V)

Fluconazole is widely distributed throughout the body with a volume of distribution of approximately 0.7 L/kg and good penetration into the cerebrospinal fluid (50% to 90%

of serum levels depending on meningeal inflammation), eye, peritoneal fluid, sputum, skin, and urine.[7]

CLEARANCE (Cl)

Fluconazole is largely excreted unchanged (>80%) through the kidneys, but undergoes partial metabolism (11%) through CYP3A4 to an inactive N-oxide and glucuronide metabolites that are excreted in the urine. Fluconazole generally has predictable dose-proportional linear PKs with a nearly 1:1 relationship between the daily dose of fluconazole (in mg) and the observed serum AUC in patients with normal renal function and average body habitus. As a result, fluconazole dose/MIC is occasionally used as a surrogate to AUC/MIC in PD calculations.

The typical total body clearance rate of fluconazole in adult patients is 0.23 mL/min/kg. Fluconazole clearance in pediatric patients is more rapid (0.4 to 0.6 mL/min/kg), resulting in shorter half-life. Using the following standard PK equation (Equation 7.1), the predicted half-life is approximately 35 hours in adults and 16 to 20 hours in children.[8]

$$t\frac{1}{2} = \frac{0.693 \times V_d}{Cl} \qquad \textbf{(Eq. 7.1)}$$

Fluconazole doses are adjusted in patients with renal dysfunction. In patients with estimated glomerular filtration rate (GFR) of 50 to 80 mL/min, normal doses are recommended. If the GFR is 10 to 50 mL/min or <10 mL/min, then 50% of the daily dose is administered. The clearance of fluconazole (Equation 7.2) can be predicted in patients with renal impairment in relation to estimated (Equation 7.3) or measured (Equation 7.4) creatinine clearance using the following equations:

$$\frac{G \times (140 - Age) \times Weight\ (kg)}{Serum\ Creatinine\ (mg/dL) \times 72}\ G = 1\ (Male); 0.85\ (Female) \qquad \textbf{(Eq. 7.2)}$$

$$Cl/F\ (mL/min/kg) = 0.064 + 0.003 \\ \times\ Cockcroft\ and\ Gault\ Cl_{Cr}\ (mL/min) \qquad \textbf{(Eq. 7.3)}$$

$$Cl/F\ (mL/min/kg) = 0.129 + 0.002 \times Measured\ Cl_{Cr}\ (mL/min) \qquad \textbf{(Eq. 7.4)}$$

Fluconazole is removed by dialysis, but the dosing recommendations vary depending on the type of dialysis. In patients receiving intermitted hemodialysis, 100% of a daily dose is administered after hemodialysis or 50% of the dose is administered every 24 hours after the dialysis session. Similarly, for peritoneal dialysis, 50% of the fluconazole dose is administered daily. In patients undergoing hemofiltration, 200 to 400 mg of fluconazole is recommended once daily for patients undergoing continuous venovenous hemofiltration (CVVH). In patients undergoing continuous venovenous hemodialysis (CVVHD) or continuous venovenous hemodiafiltration (CVVHDF), 400

KEY PARAMETERS: Fluconazole[a]

THERAPEUTIC CONCENTRATIONS	C min ABOVE 10–15 mg/L
F[b]	90%
$V_d{}^c$	0.6–0.8 L/kg
Cl	0.97 L/hr
$AUC_{0-24hr}{}^d$	350 mg · hr/L
t½ in adults	35 hr
fu (fraction unbound)	89%

[a]Pharmacokinetic parameters may vary depending on patient characteristics and renal function.
[b]Bioavailability not affected by gastric pH or food.
[c]Widely distributed throughout body tissues and fluids such as the kidney, skin, saliva, sputum, nail, blister fluid, and prostate. Good Cerebrospinal fluid (CSF) penetration (50% to 94% of serum concentration attained in the CSF).
[d]400 mg daily dose.

to 800 mg/day of fluconazole is recommended; however, higher doses may be required depending on the dialysis flow rate.

Depending on the treatment indication, doses of fluconazole typically range from 400 to 800 mg daily for invasive fungal diseases. The recommended dose for patients with invasive candidiasis is a 12 mg/kg loading dose on day 1, followed by 6 mg/kg once daily. Administration of a weight-based loading and maintenance doses is recommended for bloodstream candidiasis, because the infection can progress to sepsis with marked changes in patient volume of distribution, resulting in subtherapeutic fluconazole exposures. In fact, PK point-prevalence studies in intensive care unit patients have reported that one-third of patients do not achieve therapeutic fluconazole exposures largely because fixed 200 or 400 mg daily doses are administered without loading doses, irrespective of patient weight.[9] The excellent bioavailability of the tablet and suspension formulations of fluconazole allows easy IV to oral switching when patients are clinically stable. Indeed, fluconazole is a recommended "step-down" narrowest-spectrum therapy of choice for patients who were previously receiving an echinocandin for the treatment of invasive candidiasis, provided the susceptibility of the infecting isolate to fluconazole can be confirmed.[4]

PHARMACOKINETIC DRUG INTERACTIONS

Fluconazole is a potent inhibitor of CYP2C9 and CYP2C19 and a moderate inhibitor of CYP3A4. Inhibiting effects may persist for 4 to 5 days after discontinuation owing to long half-life of fluconazole.[2] Fluconazole is also a substrate of CYP3A4. Strong inducers of CYP3A4 (i.e., rifampin) will increase the nonrenal clearance of fluconazole, possibly resulting in subtherapeutic exposures.[10] Drug–drug interactions are often dose dependent, with stronger effects observed at higher fluconazole doses.[2] Fluconazole must be used with caution when other drugs metabolized via CYP P450 enzymes are coadministered.

ADVERSE EFFECTS

Fluconazole is generally well tolerated, even at high doses. Patients occasionally develop problems of gastrointestinal (GI) intolerance or rash. Reversible alopecia has been reported in patients receiving more than 400 mg/day. Elevation of serum transaminases can also occur, and, in rare, case, hepatitis. However, in general, these toxicities are idiosyncratic and do not correlate with fluconazole serum concentrations. Similar to other triazoles, fluconazole therapy may be associated with prolongation of the QTc interval. Some experts have recommended monitoring serum levels in patients at high risk for QTc prolongation, especially in the setting the renal dysfunction.[3]

TIME TO SAMPLE

TDM is not typically recommended for patients receiving fluconazole because of the drug's relatively predictable linear PKs and excellent tolerability profile. However, special circumstances may warrant monitoring of serum drug levels, for example, patients on CVVHD with severe infections, patients infected with *Candida* spp. with a high MIC (e.g., 2 to 4 mg/L), *Candida* infections of the central nervous system (CNS), and, possibly, pediatric patients.[8] In most cases, the most practical sampling approaches to measure serum C min concentrations immediately prior to the next dose. A serum C min of 10 to 15 mg/L would be indicative of a free drug AUC/MIC >100 for *Candida* spp. with MICs up to 2 mg/L. Patients can be sampled immediately after the first maintenance dose if a loading dose is administered; otherwise, the first C min sample should be drawn between 3 and 5 days of therapy.

CLINICAL APPLICATION OF FLUCONAZOLE PHARMACOKINETICS

A relatively straightforward approach can be used to evaluate fluconazole PKs. If fluconazole C min is low, the dose (mg/day) can be increased in a proportional fashion to achieve serum concentration exposures of 10 to 15 mg/L. C min above this target range does not require dose reduction if the patient is tolerating the therapy.

Question #1   *S.V. is a 52-year-old, 68 kg female with a recent history of necrotizing pancreatitis that was complicated by sepsis, acute renal injury during sepsis, and candidemia. She was originally treated with caspofungin but has increasing transaminase levels and will be switched to IV fluconazole. There is concern about the patient having excessive fluconazole serum levels because she is receiving other medications that prolong the QTc interval. The Candida albicans isolated from the blood was found to be susceptible to fluconazole MIC (1 mg/L). Her current serum creatinine is 2.1 mg/dL. You are asked to recommend an IV dosing regimen for this patient that would ideally maintain plasma concentrations above 10 mg/L, but not produce excessive exposures that could place her at higher risk for QTc prolongation.*

The clearance of fluconazole can be estimated using an estimate of the Cl_{Cr} and Equation 7.2.

$$Cl_{Cr}(mL/min) = \frac{(0.85)(140-52)(68\text{ kg})}{(2.1\text{ mg/dL})(72)}$$

$$= 33.6\text{ mL/min}$$

Cl/F (mL/min/kg) = 0.064 + 0.003 × 34 (mL/min) or 0.17 mL/min/kg, resulting in an estimate of 11.3 mL/min or 0.68 L/hr for this patient.

The V can be estimated using the population value of 0.7 L/kg.

$$V = 0.7\text{ L/kg (68 kg)}$$

$$= 47.6\text{ L}$$

The elimination rate constant can be calculated based on the Cl and V.

$$K = \frac{Cl}{V}$$

$$= \frac{0.68\text{ L/hr}}{47.6\text{ L}}$$

$$= 0.014\text{ hr}^{-1}$$

The half-life is then calculated using Equation 7.1. In the case of this patient, the expected half-life would be $t\frac{1}{2} = (0.693 \cdot 47.6\text{ L})/0.68\text{ L/hr}$ or 48.5 hours.

The patient should be administered a standard 12 mg/kg loading dose of fluconazole (~800 mg administered as a bolus injection). Loading doses are not adjusted on the basis of renal function. An 800-mg loading dose in this patient would result in an expected C max of 16.8 mg/L, assuming a V_d of 0.7 L/kg using the following equation:

$$C\text{ max} = \frac{D}{V_d} \qquad \textbf{(Eq. 7.5)}$$

$$C\text{ max} = \frac{800\text{ mg}}{47.6\text{ L}} = 16.8\text{ mg/L}$$

The expected trough 24 hours after the loading dose in this patient can be estimated using the following equation:

$$C\text{ min} = C_0 \times e^{-K_e(\tau)} \qquad \textbf{(Eq. 7.6)}$$

$$C\text{ min} = 16.8\text{ mg/L} \times e^{-(0.014\text{ hr}^{-1})(24\text{ hr})}$$

$$= 12.0\text{ mg/L}$$

Hence, the patient has only eliminated approximately 28% of the dose after 24 hours, with 72% of the drug is remaining. The cumulative impact of slower fluconazole clearance could be estimated, for example, if the patient was administered a standard 400 mg daily maintenance dose. At day 5 of therapy, the fluconazole trough concentrations would be predicted using the non–steady-state equation:

$$C\min = \left(\frac{\frac{\text{Dose}}{V_d}}{\left(1 - e^{-K_e(\tau)}\right)} \right) \left(1 - e^{-K_e(N)(\tau)}\right)\left(e^{-K_e\tau_2}\right) \qquad \textbf{(Eq. 7.7)}$$

$$C\min = \left(\frac{\frac{400}{47.6\ \text{L}}}{\left(1 - e^{-(0.014\ \text{hr}^{-1})(24\ \text{hr})}\right)} \right) \left(1 - e^{-(0.014\ \text{hr}^{-1})(5)(24\ \text{hr})}\right)\left(e^{-(0.014\ \text{hr}^{-1})(24\ \text{hr})}\right)$$

$$= 17.1\ \text{mg/L}$$

where τ is the dosing interval of 1, N the number of doses administered,[5] and t_2 the time elapsed from the last dose until the time of the C min (1 day). The predicted C min is approximately 17 mg/L by day 5—nearly double the trough concentration that is required. Figure 7.1 shows how this accumulation would look over time. By reducing the administered dose by 50% to 200 mg every 24 hours, the patient could be maintained at therapeutic exposures of fluconazole (above 10 mg/L) while reducing excessive peak concentrations that may be a concern in the setting of this patient's risk for QTc prolongation.

$$C\min = \left(\frac{\frac{\text{Dose}}{V_d}}{\left(1 - e^{-K_e(\tau)}\right)} \right) \left(e^{-K_e\tau_2}\right) \qquad \textbf{(Eq. 7.8)}$$

$$= \left(\frac{\frac{200\ \text{mg}}{47.6\ \text{L}}}{\left(1 - e^{-(0.014\ \text{hr}^{-1})(24\ \text{hr})}\right)} \right) \left(e^{-(0.014\ \text{hr}^{-1})(24\ \text{hr})}\right)$$

$$= 14.1\ \text{mg/L}$$

Itraconazole

Itraconazole was the second triazole approved for the treatment of superficial and invasive fungal diseases. It is a larger (molecular weight 705 g/mol) more lipophilic (log P 5.48) molecule compared to fluconazole that is an irreversible inhibitor of fungal

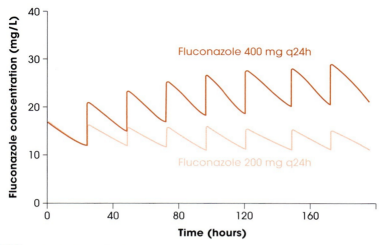

FIGURE 7.1   Predicted fluconazole serum concentrations over time in a patient with renal dysfunction.

14α-demethylase. Consequently, the spectrum of itraconazole is broader than fluco-nazole, including yeast (*Candida* and *Cryptococcus* spp.) and endemic dimorphic fungi (*C. immitis* and *B. dermatitidis*) as well as common molds such as *Aspergillus* spp. Use of itraconazole has been largely supplanted by newer, better-tolerated broad-spectrum triazoles, but it remains an important drug for the treatment of endemic mycoses, including histoplasmosis, blastomycosis, and coccidioidomycosis.

THERAPEUTIC RANGE OF ITRACONAZOLE

When corrected for protein binding, itraconazole is similar to fluconazole in that the fAUC/MIC is the PK/PD threshold associated with treatment efficacy. Several studies and a published meta-analysis of 3,957 patients have examined the relationship between itraconazole serum C min and risk for breakthrough invasive fungal diseases in patients with hematologic malignancies taking itraconazole as antifungal prophylaxis.[11–13] Breakthrough fungal infections were more common among patients with serum itraconazole C min less than 0.25 to 0.5 mg/L measured by a high-performance liquid chromatography (HPLC) assay. Therefore, a C min above 0.5 mg/L is recommended to ensure adequate protection during itraconazole prophylaxis. In a clinical study examining the use of itraconazole capsules for the treatment of invasive aspergillosis, improved outcomes were observed when itraconazole serum concentrations surpassed 8 mg/L (measured by bioassay; equivalent to >1 mg/mL measured by HPLC).[14] Therefore, C min concentrations of itraconazole >1 mg/L are advocated in patients with active fungal disease.

One study performed in patients with chronic obstructive pulmonary aspergillosis reported significantly higher rates of toxicity (GI adverse effects and fluid retention) when itraconazole serum levels measured by bioassay exceeded 17 mg/L.[15,16] This bioassay concentration is roughly equivalent to an itraconazole C min > 4 mg/L (measured by HPLC).

BIOAVAILABILITY

Itraconazole is typically administered as 200 to 400 mg daily as a divided dose. In patients with severe fungal disease, a loading dose of 200 mg three times daily for the first 3 days of therapy is recommended. Itraconazole bioavailability depends on the formulation administered (see Key Parameters: Itraconazole). The capsule formulation (100 mg) consists of drug-coated microspheres to enhance the surface area for dissolution of the drug in the stomach. In healthy volunteers with normal gastric acidity, the bioavailability of the capsules is 55% when taken with food. The time to peak serum concentrations ranges between 1 and 4 hours. However, dissolution of the drug is reduced in patients with GI dysfunction or increased gastric pH (e.g., on acid suppression therapy), resulting less absorbable drug delivered to the duodenum and significantly lower bioavailability. To overcome this problem, a cyclodextrin oral solution formulation of itraconazole was developed that can be taken without food and does not require low gastric pH. The bioavailability of the oral solution is approximately 60%, but has, for many patients, an unpalatable taste and higher rates of GI adverse effects. This is because of the fact that the cyclodextrin vehicle is not absorbed from the GI tract and acts as an osmotic agent to retain water in the intestine. An IV form of itraconazole (administered in cyclodextrin) is available in Europe and Asia, but is no longer available in the United States.

VOLUME OF DISTRIBUTION (V)

Itraconazole has a very large volume of distribution (10.7 L/kg) that includes penetration into the skin, liver, bone, adipose tissue, nail, and bronchial fluids.[7] However, high molecular weight and extensive protein binding (90% to 99%) limit its penetration into the vitreous fluid of the eye and cerebral spinal fluid (concentrations often undetectable), even though successful treatment of cerebral fungal infections and cryptococcal meningitis are reported. Little active drug is present in urine.

CLEARANCE (Cl)

Itraconazole displays a saturable, nonlinear pattern of elimination with increasing doses. The PKs are more complex than fluconazole, with serum concentrations best predicted with a two-compartment model with oral absorption described by four-transit compartments. Itraconazole is extensively metabolized in the liver by predominantly CYP3A4 to an active (hydroxyl-itraconazole) and inactive metabolites. The ratio of metabolites depends in part on the synthesis of itraconazole, which is compared of four *cis* isomers with varying affinity for CYP3A4. The active hydroxyl-itraconazole metabolite can be detected in concentrations of 1 to 1.6 times higher than the parent compound.[17] The presence of the active metabolite will influence how serum concentrations are reported; most reference laboratories will report both the metabolite and parent compound concentrations. If itraconazole concentrations are analyzed using a (microbial) bioassay methodology, the reported concentrations will be roughly fivefold higher.

Approximately 55% of the itraconazole dose is excreted via biliary elimination, and 35% excreted as active and inactive metabolites through the kidney. At steady state,

KEY PARAMETERS: Itraconazole[a]

THERAPEUTIC CONCENTRATIONS	C min 0.5–4 mg/L (MEASURED BY HPLC)
F	55% capsules (with food; solution 30% higher when administered without food)
V_d	10.7 L/kg
Cl[b]	16 L/hr
AUC_{0-24hr}[c]	15.4 mg · hr/L
t½	35 hr
fu (fraction unbound)	<5%

[a]Pharmacokinetic parameters may vary depending on patient characteristics and liver dysfunction; administered as a 200 mg dose.
[b]Mean body clearance.
[c]200 mg twice daily dose.
HPLC, high-performance liquid chromatography.

the clearance rate is approximately 3.8 mL/min/kg. Using Equation 7.1, this results in an estimated half-life of 32 hours.

Itraconazole doses do not need to be reduced in patients with renal dysfunction. However, patients with moderate-to-severe liver dysfunction are likely to have reduced rates of clearance. Patients should be carefully monitored for evidence of toxicity and consideration given to performing TDM for itraconazole.

PHARMACOKINETIC DRUG INTERACTIONS

Itraconazole is a substrate and inhibitor of CYP3A4 and P-glycoprotein (P-gp), and is associated with the potential for many drug–drug interactions. Patients should have their medication profiles carefully reviewed whenever starting or stopping itraconazole therapy. Strong inducers of CYP3A4 (i.e., rifampin, phenytoin, carbamazepine) will result in low or undetectable itraconazole concentrations and are contraindicated. Similarly, use of itraconazole with other medications metabolized through CYP3A4 pathways that increase QTc interval is contraindicated. Itraconazole will reduce the clearance of many cardiovascular, anesthesia, immunosuppressant, and chemotherapy agents. Careful dosage adjustment of the second drug or avoidance of itraconazole may be required, because some of these interactions are potentially life threatening.

In addition to CYP3A4-associated interactions, drugs that increase gastric pH (antacids, H_2 antagonists, and protein pump inhibitors) reduce the bioavailability of itraconazole capsules. Cola drinks have been shown to increase the absorption of the capsules in patients with achlorhydria or those taking H_2-receptor antagonists or other gastric acid suppressors. Grapefruit/grapefruit juice may increase itraconazole serum levels because of inhibition of intestinal P-gp.

ADVERSE EFFECTS

Although itraconazole is tolerated by many patients, it is associated with higher rates of GI intolerance and hepatic toxicity compared to fluconazole. Hypokalemia, cardiotoxicity with a negative inotropic effect, neuropathies, adrenal insufficiencies (more common with longer term, higher dose therapy), gynecomastia, leg edema, and hearing loss are also observed more frequently with itraconazole than fluconazole. Itraconazole carries a risk of QTc prolongation and interacts with many other agents that also prolong QTc. Therefore, concomitant use should be avoided.

TIME TO SAMPLE

Without a loading dose, itraconazole concentrations reach steady state after 2 weeks. If a loading dose is administered, the first C min sample can be collected on days 5 to 7 of therapy or soon thereafter. Owing to the long half-life of the drug, samples drawn for TDM in the middle of the dosing interval will not differ substantially from the actual C min concentration.

CLINICAL APPLICATION OF ITRACONAZOLE PHARMACOKINETICS

TDM is recommended for all patients receiving itraconazole to ensure adequate exposures. If the C min concentration of itraconazole is low (<0.5 mg/L) on days 5 to 7 of therapy, then the patient should be carefully assessed for factors to improve the drug bioavailability (i.e., administer with cola beverage if taking capsules, stop protein pump inhibitors), or switch to the oral solution. If the patient is going to continue taking capsules, the dose should be increased by 100 mg twice daily and recheck a serum concentration. Patients with elevated C min concentrations (>4 mg/L) can be continued on the same dose without changes if they are tolerating itraconazole, but dose reduction (100 mg twice daily) should be considered if they are experiencing adverse effects and cannot be switched to an alternative antifungal agent.

> **Question #2**   *A.J. is a 34-year-old male patient (height 5 feet 6 inches, weight 55 kg) with cystic fibrosis who is to be initiated on itraconazole 200 mg capsules orally every 12 hours for treatment of allergic bronchopulmonary aspergillosis. What is the predicted steady-state C min on this regimen?*

Because the frequency of drug administration (e.g., 12 hours) is approximately one-third of the half-life (e.g., 35 hours), the continuous infusion model (Equation 7.9) can be used to predict the average steady-state concentration.

$$Css = \frac{(S)(F)(D)}{(Cl)(\tau)} \qquad \textbf{(Eq. 7.9)}$$

$$Css = \frac{(1)(0.55)(200 \text{ mg})}{(16.7 \text{ L/hr})(12 \text{ hr})}$$
$$= 0.55 \text{ mg/L}$$

The concentration of 0.55 mg/L is within the desired therapeutic range for the trough concentration, indicating that this regimen is appropriate. A measured concentration should be obtained in 2 weeks to confirm achievement of a therapeutic concentration and to assess clinical response. Patients with cystic fibrosis typically receive acid suppressor therapy for the treatment of acid reflux or to enhance the activity of pancreatic enzymes supplements; therefore, the dose of itraconazole often needs to be increased in this population to achieve therapeutic concentrations.

Voriconazole

Voriconazole is structurally similar to fluconazole (349 g/mol) but is a more lipophilic molecule (log P 1.82) that irreversibly binds to fungal 14α-demethylase, resulting in a broader spectrum of activity compared to fluconazole that covers yeast and *Aspergillus*, some *Fusarium* spp., and black molds but not Mucorales. Along with isavuconazole, voriconazole is considered a drug of choice for the treatment of invasive aspergillosis in patients who have not received prior azole therapy.[18]

THERAPEUTIC RANGE OF VORICONAZOLE

Voriconazole exposure–response relationships have been investigated in a number of studies and are similar to other triazoles in that the fAUC/MIC best predicts outcome.[16] Specifically, serum C min concentrations are predictive of the patient AUC. A C min of >1 mg/L has been identified in several studies as a threshold voriconazole exposure associated with a higher probability of successful clinical outcome in patients with invasive aspergillosis.[19–22] In an analysis of phase 2/3 studies of voriconazole treatment for invasive aspergillosis and invasive candidiasis, C min to MIC ratios of 2 to 5 were associated with a higher probability of successful clinical outcome.[23]

Voriconazole C min greater than 5.5 to 6 mg/L are associated with a higher probability of CNS adverse effects (encephalopathy) and visual hallucinations. In one prospective study investigating voriconazole TDM, patients who were randomized to undergo routine TDM monitoring during voriconazole therapy experienced fewer adverse effects and were less likely to have treatment interruptions compared to those who did not undergo routine TDM.[24]

Although voriconazole C min is often elevated in patients with liver dysfunction, there is no evidence of a "cutoff" concentration of voriconazole that can be used to predict hepatotoxic events.[25]

BIOAVAILABILITY (F)

Voriconazole is typically administered IV as 6 mg/kg loading dose for two doses and then 4 mg/kg twice daily as a maintenance dose. An oral tablet and suspension formulations are available. Oral tablet doses are lower (fixed 200 mg dose twice daily), but many experts still recommend continued weight-based dosing (4 mg/kg twice daily) even with the tablet formulation. Time to peak serum levels is approximately 1 hour. Dosing for patients less than 40 kg is lower (100 mg twice daily), whereas pediatric patients require higher doses (discussed below). Voriconazole tablets are well absorbed without food (86% bioavailability) when taken 1 hour before or 2 hours after meals. Absorption is independent of gastric pH but is reduced by 24% if tablets are taken with food. Some population PK models in neutropenic patients have suggested that bioavailability is lower (60% to 65%) in patients with chemotherapy-associated mucositis,[19] or in pediatric patients.[26–28]

The IV formulation of voriconazole is solubilized in a sulfobutylether-cyclodextrin (SBECD) vehicle. In patients with renal dysfunction, and in animal models, accumulation of the SBCED has been associated with reversible changes in the renal and bladder epithelium, but the clinical significance of these changes in humans is unknown. The manufacturer does not recommend using the IV formulation in patients with impaired renal function (GFR < 50 mL/min), and SBECD is only moderately removed by dialysis. However, several case series have described successful use of IV voriconazole in critically ill patients with renal dysfunction or on dialysis without problems.[29–31]

VOLUME OF DISTRIBUTION (V)

Voriconazole is widely distributed in tissues, including the CNS and vitreous fluid of the eye. Cerebral spinal fluid concentrations are approximately 50% of serum concentration.[7] The volume of distribution differs between children and adults. In children, a biphasic V_d has been described with a V_d (central) compartment of 0.81 L/kg, and V_d (peripheral) compartment of 2.2 L/kg. In adults, the V_d is 4.6 L/kg. Little active drug is present in urine.

CLEARANCE

Clearance rates of voriconazole are dose dependent, saturable at higher doses, and can vary tremendously from one patient owing to a number of factors. Voriconazole is metabolized predominantly by CYP2C19, and to a lesser extent CYP2C9 and CYP3A4 to inactive metabolite (N-oxide voriconazole), which is excreted in the urine. CYP2C19 exhibits genetic polymorphism (15% to 20% Asians may be poor metabolizers of voriconazole; 3% to 5% Caucasians and African Americans may be poor metabolizers).

Pediatric patients have much higher clearance rates of voriconazole compared to adults because of a three- to fivefold greater rate of CYP2C19 metabolism and enhanced activity of flavin containing monooxygenase 3.[26–28,32] Clearance of voriconazole in adolescents (age 12 to 14 years) depends on weight with children greater than 50 kg exhibiting PK characteristics similar to adults. Currently, recommended doses for children aged 2 to 12 years less than 50 kg are an IV dose of 9 mg/kg twice daily on day 1, then 8 mg/kg twice daily thereafter. Oral dosing is 9 mg/kg twice daily and then followed by 9 mg/kg every 12 hours.[27] However, PKs are extremely variable, and TDM is often needed to guide dosing. Occasionally, infants and younger children may require every 8-hour dosing of voriconazole to achieve therapeutic concentrations.

Voriconazole clearance is not affected by renal function. However, avoidance of IV voriconazole is recommended by the manufacturer if patients have an estimated GFR < 50 mL/min owing to risk of accumulation of cyclodextrin vehicle. Lower doses of voriconazole should be considered in patients with hepatic insufficiency. For

KEY PARAMETERS: Voriconazole[a]

THERAPEUTIC CONCENTRATIONS	C min: 1–6 mg/L
F	86% capsules without food (adults)
	50%–65% (pediatrics)
V_d	4.6 L/kg
Cl^b	
$\quad Km^c$	2.07 mg/L (adults)
	5.16 mg/L (pediatrics)
$\quad Vmax^d$	1.7 mg/kg/day (pediatrics)
	0.54 mg/kg/day (adults)
$AUC_{0-12hr}{}^{e}$	17.99 mg · hr/L
$t\frac{1}{2}$	6 hr, variable and dose dependent
fu (fraction unbound)	40%

[a]Pharmacokinetic parameters may vary depending on patient characteristics and liver dysfunction; administered as a 200 mg dose.
[b]Voriconazole exhibits Michaelis-Menten (nonlinear) pharmacokinetics in some patients, meaning that dosage escalation may lead to a disproportionate increase in systemic drug exposures (AUC) because of saturable metabolism. This saturable metabolism appears to occur at lower doses (mg/kg) in adults than children owing to a greater than twofold higher concentration required to saturate metabolic capacity (Km).
[c]Km concentration in central compartment where clearance is half-maximal. Median calculated value from population pharmacokinetic studies, subject to wide interpatient variability.
[d]Vmax, maximal rate of enzymatic inactivation of voriconazole. Median calculated value from population pharmacokinetic studies, subject to wide interpatient variability.
[e]6 mg/kg loading dose, then 4 mg/kg twice daily.

mild-to-moderate hepatic insufficiency (Child-Pugh Classes A and B): 6 mg/kg every 12 hours × 2 doses (load), then 2 mg/kg IV every 12 hours with serum concentration monitoring is recommended.

PHARMACOKINETIC DRUG INTERACTIONS

Voriconazole is a substrate of CYP2C19 and a potent inhibitor of CYP3A4.[2] Patients should have their medication profiles carefully reviewed with starting or stopping voriconazole therapy. Strong inducers of CYP3A4 (i.e., rifampin, phenytoin, carbamazepine, efavirenz) generally result in low or undetectable voriconazole concentrations and are contraindicated. Similarly, use of voriconazole with other medications metabolized through CYP3A4 pathways that increase QTc interval is contraindicated. Voriconazole will reduce the clearance of many cardiovascular, anesthesia, immunosuppressant, and chemotherapy agents. Careful dosage adjustment of the second drug or avoidance of voriconazole may be required, because some of these interactions are potentially life threatening.

Medications that are inhibitors of CYP2C19 (i.e., omeprazole) have been used in some case series to "boost" voriconazole serum concentrations.[33,34]

ADVERSE EFFECTS

The most common adverse effect during voriconazole therapy is photopsia (abnormal vision described as blurriness, color changes, and enhanced vision) seen in 20.6% of patients, but fewer than <1% require treatment discontinuation. The duration of visual abnormalities usually lasts less than 30 minutes, typically starting 30 minutes after dosing. Patients may also develop increased transaminases (13%) and alkaline phosphatase with therapy discontinuation required in 4% to 8% of cases. Other less common adverse effects include rash and hallucinations.

Encephalopathy is an adverse effect of voriconazole that is associated with C min concentrations >5.5 mg/L.[19,20] Other rare adverse effects seen with long-term therapy include phototoxicity that can evolve into squamous cell carcinoma, alopecia with skin and nail changes, and periostititis and/or skeletal fluorosis.

TIME TO SAMPLE

Voriconazole concentrations reach steady state by 5 days, but a C min sample on days 2 to 5 after the loading dose is acceptable for early TDM assessment. Many experts recommend repeating a C min sample during the second week of therapy to confirm the patient is within the therapeutic range. Auto-induction of voriconazole metabolism has been reported to occur at higher-than-usual doses, resulting in decreased C min over time, which may require further dose modification to maintain therapeutic concentrations.

CLINICAL APPLICATION OF VORICONAZOLE PHARMACOKINETICS

TDM is recommended for most patients receiving voriconazole for the treatment of invasive aspergillosis, and is considered essential for effective dosing of pediatric patients.[17] Similar to other triazole antifungals, C min are reasonable predictive of AUC and are used to monitor therapy. The first C min sample for voriconazole can be drawn after 3 to 5 days (after the fifth dose, including the loading doses) to confirm serum concentrations fall between 1 and 6 mg/L.

Patients who have changes in their voriconazole dose, are switched from IV to oral therapy, or have a change in their clinical condition (e.g., suspected breakthrough infections or toxicity) should have voriconazole serum concentrations checked. TDM may also be helpful in patients who have additional medications with possible PK interactions with voriconazole started or stopped.

If the voriconazole C min is low (<1 mg/L), it is important to ensure that the voriconazole dose (including loading dose) was administered appropriately. If the patient was recently switched from IV to a fixed oral dose, the oral dose could be increased to the same weight-based (mg/kg) dose that was administered IV. If the C min is very low (<0.5 mg/L), the patient should be switched to IV if on oral, and the daily dose should be increased by 50% with follow-up monitoring 2 to 5 days later. Careful screening for clinical scenarios that alter voriconazole PKs (e.g., drug interactions, compliance) is critical.

If the predose voriconazole C min concentrations are high (>6 mg/L), the patient should be carefully screened for clinical factors that may be influencing voriconazole PKs and ensure that the C min sample was appropriately drawn. Dose reduction may not be needed if the patient is tolerating voriconazole without CNS adverse effects; however, close monitoring is recommended. In one prospective randomized study of voriconazole TDM, patients with C min >10 mg/L had the next voriconazole dose held, and subsequent doses were reduced by 50% until concentrations fell within the therapeutic range.

Question #3 *F.P. is a 9-year-old, 35 kg male who received a matched related allogeneic hematopoietic stem cell transplant for acute lymphoblastic leukemia 70 days ago that has been complicated by acute graft versus host disease. He is receiving oral trimethoprim sulfamethoxazole, valacyclovir, and fluconazole as prophylaxis. His current immunosuppression regimen is tacrolimus 0.03 mg/kg/day, and his last level was 10.2 ng/mL. His renal and liver function are within normal limits. In the last 72 hours, F.P. has developed a fever (38.5°C) that has not responded to broad-spectrum antibiotics, and a computed tomography scan of the chest reveals lesions suspicious for invasive aspergillosis. F.P. was started on IV voriconazole 250 mg (7 mg/kg) twice daily, and, on day 5 of therapy, a C min serum level is 0.5 mg/L. How should F.P.'s voriconazole dosing be managed to achieve a C min above 1.0 mg/L?*

Because F.P. is pediatric patient, he is expected to have much higher clearance of voriconazole than adults; 7 mg/kg twice daily may still not be sufficient. Although the PKs of voriconazole are complex and difficult to predict because of wide interpatient variations in metabolism, the Km value reported in most pediatric PK studies is higher than adults (see Key Parameters: Voriconazole), and surpasses average voriconazole concentrations expected in this patient. This can be demonstrated by using formula relating C min (mcg/mL) concentrations to voriconazole AUC (mcg/mL · hr) reported in pediatric population PK studies (Fig. 7.2).

$$AUC_{0-12\ hr} = 11.45 + 14.97 \times C\ min \qquad \text{(Eq. 7.10)}$$

Using this equation, a patient with a trough of 0.5 mcg/mL would have an expected AUC of 18.9 mcg/mL · hr.

$$AUC_{0-12hr} = 11.45 + 14.97 \times 0.5\ \text{mcg/mL}$$

$$= 18.9\ \text{mcg/mL} \cdot \text{hr}$$

The clearance can be calculated from the AUC using Equation 7.11 as:

$$Cl\left(L/kg \cdot hr\right) = \frac{(S)(F)(D)}{AUC} \qquad \text{(Eq. 7.11)}$$

$$= \frac{(1)(1)(7\ \text{mg/kg})}{18.9\ \text{mg/L} \cdot \text{hr}}$$

$$= 0.37\ L/kg \cdot hr$$

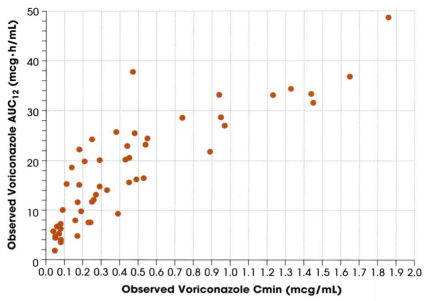

FIGURE 7.2   Observed voriconazole AUC_{0-12hr} versus C min at steady state in children receiving 7 mg/ kg IV every 12 hours and 200 mg orally every 12 hours with a C min < 2 mcg/mL. (From Driscoll TA, Yu LC, Frangoul H, et al. Comparison of pharmacokinetics and safety of voriconazole intravenous-to-oral switch in immunocompromised children and healthy adults. *Antimicrob Agents Chemother.* 2011;55(12):5770–5779.)

Using Equation 7.9, we can estimate the average steady-state concentration, Css of 1.58 mcg/mL, which is well below typical medial Km reported in population PK studies (5.16 mcg/mL).

$$Css = \frac{(S)(F)(D)}{(Cl)(\tau)}$$

$$= \frac{(1)(1)(7 \text{ mg/kg})}{(0.37 \text{L/kg} \cdot \text{hr})(12 \text{ hr})}$$

$$= 1.58 \text{ mg/L}$$

If the voriconazole dose was increased to achieve an AUC of 30 mcg/mL · h, which roughly corresponds to a Css of 2.5 mcg/mL, this value is still less than the Km.

Therefore, it would be reasonable to increase the dose by 2 mg/kg every 12 hours to 9 mg/kg every 12 hours, and recheck serum trough levels after 3 days.

Note that for an adult with a trough of 0.5 mcg/mL receiving a voriconazole 4 mg/kg maintenance dose twice daily, the predicted AUC (14.1 mcg/mL · hr) and Css (1.18) is modestly lower based on the following formula:

(Eq. 7.12)

$$AUC_{0-12hr} = 7.39 + 13.49 \times C \text{ min}$$

$$= 7.39 + 13.49 (0.5 \text{ mcg/mL})$$

$$= 14.1 \text{ mcg/mL} \cdot \text{hr}$$

However, the Css (1.18) is much closer to reported Km values (2.07 mcg/mL), suggesting adult patients will approach saturable (nonlinear) drug elimination at lower mg/kg doses. Therefore, if an adult patient has a trough of 0.5 mcg/mL, a more modest dose increase of 1 mg/kg every 12 hours to 5 mg/kg every 12 hours may be more reasonable with a recheck of the serum trough levels after 3 days.

Question #4   *How should tacrolimus dosing be changed in light of the PK drug interaction with voriconazole?*

When starting voriconazole in patients already receiving tacrolimus, it is recommended that the tacrolimus dose be reduced to one-third of the original dose and followed with frequent monitoring of the tacrolimus blood levels (therapeutic range 10 to 15 ng/mL). When voriconazole is discontinued, tacrolimus levels should be carefully monitored and the dose increased as necessary.

Posaconazole

Posaconazole is a large molecular weight (700 g/mol) highly lipophilic (log P 5.50) triazole structurally similar to itraconazole. Posaconazole is one of the two broadest-spectrum triazoles, with activity against yeast (*Candida* spp. and *Cryptococcus* spp.), molds (*Aspergillus*, *Fusarium* spp., and black molds, including Mucorales), and endemic dimorphic fungi (*C. immitis* and *B. dermatitidis*). Similar to itraconazole capsules, the solid (suspension) formulation of posaconazole requires food and low gastric pH for absorption.

THERAPEUTIC RANGE OF POSACONAZOLE

Posaconazole has similar PD characteristics as other triazoles. Exposure–response relationships for posaconazole are primarily derived from phase III studies that evaluated posaconazole prophylaxis in patients with hematologic malignancies[35] or acute graft versus host disease after allogeneic hematopoietic stem cell transplantation.[36] Additional exposure response data were also available from an open-label salvage study in patients with probable or proven invasive aspergillosis.[37] In prophylaxis studies, higher rates of breakthrough fungal infection or treatment discontinuation were observed in patients with random serum or C min less than 0.7 mg/L.[38] In the open-label salvage study of patients with invasive fungal disease, the highest response rates were observed in patients with random serum levels or Cmin > 1.25 mg/L.[37]

To date, serum concentrations of posaconazole have not been shown to be predictive of toxicity during posaconazole treatment.

BIOAVAILABILITY (F)

The bioavailability of posaconazole suspension when administered at 600 to 800 mg/day in divided doses (three to four times daily) with a high-fat meal is approximately 50%. Without food or divided doses, or in the setting of increased gastric pH, the bioavailability decreases by more than 30%. Similar to itraconazole, acidic beverages increase the bioavailability of posaconazole. The need for three to four times daily dosing with posaconazole is not related to the half-life of the drug, rather divided dosing improves the dissolution of the solid dosage form in the stomach. Doses higher than 800 mg/day of the suspension will not improve blood levels because of limited additional dissolution.

Because frequent administration of posaconazole with high-fat meals is problematic in target population who would most benefit from posaconazole prophylaxis (i.e., hematologic malignancy patients receiving chemotherapy), a delayed-release tablet formulation was introduced that releases drug in the small intestine. As a result, absorption of the tablet does not require food or low gastric pH to achieve 60% bioavailability. However, bioavailability is still further improved if the tablet is administered with food. Dosing for the delayed-release tablet differs from the suspension: 300 mg orally twice daily for 1 day 1, then 300 mg once daily.

An IV formulation of posaconazole solubilized in cyclodextrin was also introduced and is useful for patients who cannot take the gastroresistant tablet. IV dosing is similar to the tablet: 300 mg IV twice daily $\times$ 1 day, then 300 mg IV once daily.

VOLUME OF DISTRIBUTION (V)

Similar to itraconazole, posaconazole is widely distributed in tissues with a V_d of approximately 7 L/kg.[7] Posaconazole is highly protein bound (>98%) and, like itraconazole, has limited penetration into the vitreous fluid of the eye and low concentrations in the cerebral spinal fluid even though successful treatment of cerebral fungal infections has been reported.[7] The terminal elimination half-life is approximately 35 hours (steady-state attained at 7 to 10 days). Little active drug is present in urine.

CLEARANCE (Cl)

Posaconazole is primarily metabolized in the liver, where it undergoes glucuronidation, and is transformed into biologically inactive metabolites. Posaconazole is predominantly eliminated in the feces (71%). Renal clearance is a minor elimination pathway (13%).

KEY PARAMETERS: Posaconazole[a]

THERAPEUTIC CONCENTRATIONS	C min: > 0.7 mg/L
F	50% suspension with food and divided dosing; 54% tablets without food and single daily dose
V_d	7 L/kg
Cl	11 L/hr
AUC_{0-24hr}	15.9 mg · hr/L
$t\frac{1}{2}$	35 hr
fu (fraction unbound)	2%

[a]Pharmacokinetic parameters may vary depending on patient characteristics and formulation administered.

Posaconazole dosing should not be adjusted in patients with renal dysfunction. Limited data are available on dosing posaconazole in patients with liver disease; standard dosing is recommended with caution.

PHARMACOKINETIC DRUG INTERACTIONS

Posaconazole is metabolized via uridine diphosphate (UDP) glucuronidation (phase II enzymes). It is a substrate of P-gp efflux and an inhibitor of CYP3A4. As a result, the clearance of drugs metabolized although CYP3A4 will be affected by posaconazole.[2] Similar precautions are recommended as with other triazoles that inhibit CYP3A4. Posaconazole serum concentrations may be decreased with the coadministration of UDP glucuronidation or P-gp inducers.

ADVERSE EFFECTS

Posaconazole is generally well tolerated with a side effect profile similar to fluconazole. The most common adverse effects are nausea, vomiting, and abdominal pain. Increases in serum aminotransferases or hyperbilirubinemia are occasionally reported. No relationship between posaconazole serum concentrations and adverse effects has been reported.

TIME TO SAMPLE

Without a loading dose or when using the suspension formulation, posaconazole concentrations reach steady state after 7 to 10 days. Typically, the first C min sample can be collected on days 5 to 7 of therapy or soon thereafter. For tablets or IV formulation, serum levels of C min can be initially samples on days 3 to 5. Owing to the long half-life of the posaconazole, samples drawn for TDM in the middle of the dosing interval will not differ substantially from the actual C min concentration.

CLINICAL APPLICATION OF POSACONAZOLE PHARMACOKINETICS

TDM is recommended for most patients receiving posaconazole suspension, especially during the treatment of suspected or documented fungal infections. The need for routine TDM with the gastroresistant tablet or IV formulation is less well defined but could be considered in situations of suspected clinical failure or drug interactions. Typically, a C min concentration of posaconazole is checked after the first 3 to 5 days of therapy with the tablet or IV formulation to ensure that the levels are above 0.7 mg/L. A serum C min > 0.35 mg/L sample on days 2 to 3 with the suspension will likely surpass 0.7 mg/L at steady state.[18]

If predose C min concentration is low (<0.7 mg/L prophylaxis or <1 mg/L treatment), the patients should be assessed clinical scenarios affecting bioavailability and compliance. Patients receiving the suspension formulations can be switched to the gastroresistant tablet or IV formulation. If patient requires suspension formulation, the daily dose should be increased from 600 to 800 mg administered in four divided doses with food or acidic beverage, stop acid suppression therapy if feasible. C min concentrations can be rechecked after 5 to 7 days. The safety and PKs of higher maintenance doses of gastroresistant tablets of IV formulations above 300 mg/day are not well understood.

Question #5 *R.T. is a 54-year-old, 80 kg male undergoing remission-induction chemotherapy for acute myelogenous leukemia. As part of his prophylaxis regimen, he was prescribed posaconazole gastroresistant tablet (three 100 mg tablets daily); but now has difficulties swallowing as a result of mucositis and has been switched to the oral suspension formulation of posaconazole (200 mg three times daily). A trough serum level was checked after switching and returns as undetectable. How should R.T.'s posaconazole be managed to achieve a C min above 0.7 mg/L?*

Although posaconazole tablets are now the preferred formulation of posaconazole in many centers, they may be challenging to swallow in patients with poor oral intake and mucositis. Unfortunately, poor appetite or difficulty swallowing may also limit the absorption of the suspension formulation, which requires low gastric pH, food (preferably a high-fat meal), and divided dosing to maximize absorption. Strategies for maximizing the absorption of posaconazole may include increasing the dose of the suspension formulation to 800 mg/day given in four divided doses, administering each dose with Ensure or some other enteral nutrition product, or taking posaconazole suspension with an acidic cola beverage. Acid suppression therapy such as proton pump inhibitors or H_2 antagonists should be stopped if possible.

Ultimately, it may be necessary to switch the patient to IV posaconazole, recheck serum C min, to ensure that adequate concentrations are then consider switching back to oral therapy once mucositis and oral intake improves.

Question #6 *If the patient is switched to the IV formulation but not administered a loading dose, what would be the predicted trough after the first IV dose (only given 300 mg daily)*

The population estimate of the V can be used.

$$V = 7 \text{ L/kg (80 kg)}$$

$$= 560 \text{ L}$$

The elimination rate constant can be calculated based on the Cl and V.

$$K = \frac{Cl}{V}$$

$$= \frac{11 \text{ L/hr}}{560 \text{ L}}$$

$$= 0.0196 \text{ hr}^{-1}$$

Using Equation 7.5, the initial concentration after the dose is estimated as:

$$C_0 = \frac{(S)(F)(D)}{V}$$

$$= \frac{(1)(1)(300 \text{ mg})}{560 \text{ L}} = 0.54 \text{ mg/L}$$

$$= 0.54 \text{ mg/L}$$

The trough concentration can then be estimated using Equation 7.6:

$$C \min = C_0 \times e^{-K_e \tau}$$

$$= 0.54 \text{ mg/L} \times e^{-(0.0196 \text{ hr}^{-1})(24 \text{ hr})}$$

$$= 0.34 \text{ mg/L}$$

Question #7   *How long would it take for the patient to achieve a trough concentration above 0.7 mg/L*

Using the non–steady-state Equation 7.7, we can calculate the predicted troughs on days 2, 3, and 4.

$$C \min = \left(\frac{\frac{\text{Dose}}{V_d}}{(1 - e^{-K_e \cdot \tau})} \right) (1 - e^{-K_e (N)(\tau)})(e^{-K_e \tau})$$

$$C \min_{(2\text{nd dose})} = \left(\frac{\frac{300 \text{ mg}}{560 \text{ L}}}{\left(1 - e^{(-0.02 \text{ hr}^{-1}) \times 24 \text{ hr}}\right)} \right) (1 - e^{(-0.02 \text{ hr}^{-1})(2) \times (24 \text{ hr})})(e^{-0.02 \times 24 \text{ hr}})$$

With each successive dose, N is changed to 3, 4, 5, and so on.
The results are 0.55 mg/L on day 2, 0.68 mg/L on day 3, and 0.72 mg/L on day 4.

Question #8   *If the patient is administered a loading dose (300 mg twice daily on day 1), what is the predicted trough before the dose on day 2 (24 hours after loading dose started).*

Using Equation 7.7, we can calculate the predicted trough 24 hours after the loading dose was started.

$$C\,min = \left(\frac{\dfrac{Dose}{V_d}}{(1 - e^{-K_e(\tau)})}\right)(1 - e^{-K_e(N)(\tau)})(e^{-K_e\tau})$$

$$= \left(\frac{\dfrac{300\ mg}{560\ L}}{(1 - e^{(-0.02\ hr^{-1})\times(12\ hr)})}\right)(1 - e^{(-0.02^{hr^{-1}})(2)(12\ hr)})(e^{-0.02\times12hr})$$

$$= 0.75\ mg/L$$

Isavuconazole

Isavuconazole is a smaller (molecular weight 437 g/mol) lipophilic (log P 3.9) triazole with a similar spectrum of activity to posaconazole. Isavuconazole is unique, however, in that it is formulated as a water-soluble prodrug (isavuconazolium sulfate) that is rapidly cleaved by serum esterases to the active moiety (isavuconazole). As a result, both the oral tablet and IV formulation avoid the need for cyclodextrin. Isavuconazole is as effective of treatment for invasive aspergillosis as voriconazole, but is associated with fewer visual, CNS and hepatic toxicities, and less variable PKs.[39] Isavuconazole is primarily used as a first-line treatment for invasive aspergillosis,[17] but may also be an effective alternative to amphotericin B for patients with mucormycosis.[40]

THERAPEUTIC RANGE OF ISAVUCONAZOLE

Although isavuconazole exhibits similar PK/PD characteristics as other triazole antifungals, no relationship between serum drug levels and treatment outcome was reported in phase II/III clinical studies.[41] A provisional C min target of >1 mg/L has been proposed based on the isolate susceptibility of PK/PD simulations.[42] To date, serum concentrations of isavuconazole have not been shown to be predictive of toxicity during isavuconazole treatment.

BIOAVAILABILITY (F)

The typical IV or oral dose of isavuconazole is 372 mg isavuconazonium (equivalent to 200 mg isavuconazole) three times daily for the first 2 days as a loading dose and then 372 mg once daily. The loading dose is required to ensure serum drug concentrations exceed 1 mg/L in the first 24 to 48 hours of therapy.[41] Isavuconazole exhibits linear and dose-proportional PKs up to 600 mg/day. Bioavailability of oral tablets is estimated at 98%. Maximal serum concentrations are reached 2 to 3 hours after either single or multiple dosing. Absorption of isavuconazonium tablets is not markedly affected by food or gastric pH.

VOLUME OF DISTRIBUTION (V)

Isavuconazole is widely distributed into tissues with a V_d of approximately 6 to 7 L/kg at steady state. Isavuconazole is highly protein bound (99%), and achieves low concentrations in the cerebrospinal fluid, but penetrates the brain parenchyma. Little active drug is present in urine.

CLEARANCE (Cl)

Following IV administration, prodrug is not found in serum 1.25 hours after a 1-hour infusion. Isavuconazonium is rapidly hydrolyzed to isavuconazole by esterases along with some minor, inactive metabolites. Isavuconazole is a substrate of cytochrome P450 3A4 and 3A5 and undergoes extensive hepatic metabolism with fecal excretion. Renal excretion accounts for <1% of administered dose. Isavuconazole is unique among the triazoles because of the extended elimination half-life (100 hours). Clearance of isavuconazole is not impacted by renal impairment. The clearance of isavuconazole in patients with mild-to-moderate hepatic impairment (Child-Pugh Classes A and B) is reduced, but no dosage adjustment is recommended. There are no data for patients who have Child-Pugh Class C liver disease.

Isavuconazole clearance may be affected by race. Chinese subjects were found to have a lower clearance of isavuconazole (2.6 L/hr vs. 1.6 L/hr, respectively) compared to Caucasian subjects and a 50% higher AUC. However, no dosage adjustment has been recommended based on race. No PK studies of isavuconazole have been reported in children.

PHARMACOKINETIC DRUG INTERACTIONS

Isavuconazole is a substrate and a moderate inhibitor of CYP3A4. Isavuconazole is also mild inhibitor of P-gp and organic cation transporter 2. Similar to itraconazole, voriconazole, and posaconazole, concomitant use of isavuconazole is contraindicated with strong CYP3A4 inducers (e.g., rifampin). Medications that are metabolized through

---

KEY PARAMETERS: Isavuconazole[a]

THERAPEUTIC CONCENTRATIONS (PROVISIONAL)	C min: >1 mg/L
F	98%
V_d	>7 L/kg
Cl	2–3 L/hr
AUC_{0-24hr}	97.9 mg · hr/L
$t\frac{1}{2}$	100 hr
fu (fraction unbound)	1%

[a]Pharmacokinetic parameters may vary depending on patient characteristics and formulation administered.

CYP3A4 should be used with caution in combination with isavuconazole and may require dosage adjustment with careful TDM (e.g., tacrolimus, sirolimus, cyclosporine). Similar concurrent use of isavuconazole with strong CYP3A4 inducers (e.g., rifampin) should be avoided because they will result in subtherapeutic exposures of isavuconazole.

ADVERSE EFFECTS

Isavuconzole was well tolerated in clinical trials, patients who received isavuconazole experienced fewer adverse effects (visual disturbances, liver function test abnormalities) compared to voriconazole. The most common reactions are headache, GI complaints, and mild elevation in serum transaminases. Isavuconazole is uniquely associated with QTc shortening (instead of QTc prolongation observed with other triazoles) and is contraindicated in patients with familial short QTc syndrome.

TIME TO SAMPLE

Following a loading dose, steady-state concentrations of isavuconazole are achieved after 5 to 7 days. A C min sample is recommended immediately prior to the next dose after this time. Owing to the long half-life of the drug, samples drawn for TDM in the middle of the dosing interval will not differ substantially from the actual C min concentration.

CLINICAL APPLICATION OF ISAVUCONAZOLE PHARMACOKINETICS

Currently, there are limited data supporting the need for routine TDM for isavuconazole. However, TDM may be warranted in patients with suspected clinical failure or progression of the infection on treatment, infection with a resistant pathogen, or PK drug interactions. A C min concentration of >1 mg/L (but ideally 2 to 4 mg/L) would suggest adequate drug exposures. After ruling out drug interactions or other possible causes of inadequate exposures, switching to IV therapy (if on oral) or dosage escalation up to 600 mg/day could be considered in select patient with low isavuconazole blood levels.

REFERENCES

1. Brown GD, Denning DW, Gow NA, et al. Hidden killers: human fungal infections. *Sci Transl Med.* 2012;4(165):165rv13.
2. Brüggemann RJM, Alffenaar J-WC, Blijlevens NMA, et al. Clinical relevance of the pharmacokinetic interactions of azole antifungal drugs with other coadministered agents. *Clin Infect Dis.* 2009;48(10):1441–1458.
3. Ashbee HR, Barnes RA, Johnson EM, et al. Therapeutic drug monitoring (TDM) of antifungal agents: guidelines from the British Society for Medical Mycology. *J Antimicrob Chemother.* 2014;69(5):1162–1176.
4. Pappas PG, Kauffman CA, Andes DR, et al. Clinical Practice Guideline for the Management of Candidiasis: 2016 Update by the Infectious Diseases Society of America. *Clin Infect Dis.* 2016;62(4):e1–e50.
5. Nett JE, Andes DR. Antifungal agents: spectrum of activity, pharmacology, and clinical indications. *Infect Dis Clin North Am.* 2016;30(1):51–83.
6. Rodriguez-Tudela JL, Almirante B, Rodriguez-Pardo D, et al. Correlation of the MIC and dose/MIC ratio of fluconazole to the therapeutic response of patients with mucosal candidiasis and candidemia. *Antimicrob Agents Chemother.* 2007;51(10):3599–3604.

7. Felton T, Troke PF, Hope WW. Tissue penetration of antifungal agents. *Clin Microbiol Rev.* 2014;27(1):68–88.

8. van der Elst KC, Pereboom M, van den Heuvel ER, et al. Insufficient fluconazole exposure in pediatric cancer patients and the need for therapeutic drug monitoring in critically ill children. *Clin Infect Dis.* 2014;59(11):1527–1533.

9. Sinnollareddy MG, Roberts JA, Lipman J, et al. Pharmacokinetic variability and exposures of fluconazole, anidulafungin, and caspofungin in intensive care unit patients: data from multinational defining antibiotic levels in intensive care unit (DALI) patients study. *Crit Care.* 2015;19(7):33.

10. Nicolau DP, Crowe HM, Nightingale CH, et al. Rifampin-fluconazole interaction in critically ill patients. *Ann Pharmacother.* 1995;29(10):994–996.

11. Glasmacher A, Hahn C, Leutner C, et al. Breakthrough invasive fungal infections in neutropenic patients after prophylaxis with itraconazole. *Mycoses.* 1999;42(7–8):443–451.

12. Glasmacher A, Hahn C, Molitor E, et al. Itraconazole trough concentrations in antifungal prophylaxis with six different dosing regimens using hydroxypropyl-beta-cyclodextrin oral solution or coated-pellet capsules. *Mycoses.* 1999;42(11–12):591–600.

13. Glasmacher A, Prentice A, Gorschlüter M, et al. Itraconazole prevents invasive fungal infections in neutropenic patients treated for hematologic malignancies: evidence from a meta-analysis of 3,597 patients. *J Clin Oncol.* 2003;21(24):4615–4626.

14. Denning DW, Lee JY, Hostetler JS, et al. NIAID Mycoses Study Group multicenter trial of oral itraconazole therapy for invasive aspergillosis. *Am J Med.* 1994;97(2):135–144.

15. Lestner JM, Roberts SA, Moore CB, et al. Toxicodynamics of itraconazole: implications for therapeutic drug monitoring. *Clin Infect Dis.* 2009;49(6):928–930.

16. Lepak AJ, Andes DR. Antifungal pharmacokinetics and pharmacodynamics. *Cold Spring Harb Perspect Med.* 2015;5(5):a019653.

17. Wiederhold NP, Pennick GJ, Dorsey SA, et al. A reference laboratory experience of clinically achievable voriconazole, posaconazole, and itraconazole concentrations within the bloodstream and cerebral spinal fluid. *Antimicrob Agents Chemother.* 2014;58(1):424–431.

18. Patterson TF, Thompson GR III, Denning DW, et al. Practice guidelines for the diagnosis and management of aspergillosis: 2016 update by the infectious diseases society of America. *Clin Infect Dis.* 2016;63(4):e1–e60.

19. Pascual A, Csajka C, Buclin T, et al. Challenging recommended oral and intravenous voriconazole doses for improved efficacy and safety: population pharmacokinetics-based analysis of adult patients with invasive fungal infections. *Clin Infect Dis.* 2012;55(3):381–390.

20. Pascual A, Calandra T, Bolay S, et al. Voriconazole therapeutic drug monitoring in patients with invasive mycoses improves efficacy and safety outcomes. *Clin Infect Dis.* 2008;46(2):201–211.

21. Dolton MJ, McLachlan AJ. Voriconazole pharmacokinetics and exposure-response relationships: assessing the links between exposure, efficacy and toxicity. *Int J Antimicrob Agents.* 2014;44(3):183–193.

22. Dolton MJ, Ray JE, Chen SC, et al. Multicenter study of voriconazole pharmacokinetics and therapeutic drug monitoring. *Antimicrob Agents Chemother.* 2012;56(9):4793–4799.

23. Troke PF, Hockey HP, Hope WW. Observational study of the clinical efficacy of voriconazole and its relationship to plasma concentrations in patients. *Antimicrob Agents Chemother.* 2011;55(10):4782–4788.

24. Park WB, Kim NH, Kim KH, et al. The effect of therapeutic drug monitoring on safety and efficacy of voriconazole in invasive fungal infections: a randomized controlled trial. *Clin Infect Dis.* 2012;55(8):1080–1087.

25. Tan K, Brayshaw N, Tomaszewski K, et al. Investigation of the potential relationships between plasma voriconazole concentrations and visual adverse events or liver function test abnormalities. *J Clin Pharmacol.* 2006;46(2):235–243.

26. Neely M, Rushing T, Kovacs A, et al. Voriconazole pharmacokinetics and pharmacodynamics in children. *Clin Infect Dis.* 2010;50(1):27–36.

27. Groll AH, Castagnola E, Cesaro S, et al. Fourth European Conference on Infections in Leukaemia (ECIL-4): guidelines for diagnosis, prevention, and treatment of invasive fungal diseases in paediatric patients with cancer or allogeneic haemopoietic stem-cell transplantation. *Lancet Oncol.* 2014;15(8):e327–e340.

28. Friberg LE, Ravva P, Karlsson MO, et al. Integrated population pharmacokinetic analysis of voriconazole in children, adolescents, and adults. *Antimicrob Agents Chemother.* 2012;56(6):3032–3042.

29. Abel S, Allan R, Gandelman K, et al. Pharmacokinetics, safety and tolerance of voriconazole in renally impaired subjects: two prospective, multicentre, open-label, parallel-group volunteer studies. *Clin Drug Investig.* 2008;28(7):409–420.

30. Burkhardt O, Thon S, Burhenne J, et al. Sulphobutylether-beta-cyclodextrin accumulation in critically ill patients with acute kidney injury treated with intravenous voriconazole under extended daily dialysis. *Int J Antimicrob Agents.* 2010;36(1):93, 94.

31. Turner RB, Martello JL, Malhotra A. Worsening renal function in patients with baseline renal impairment treated with intravenous voriconazole: a systematic review. *Int J Antimicrob Agents.* 2015;46(4):362–366.

32. Driscoll TA, Yu LC, Frangoul H, et al. Comparison of pharmacokinetics and safety of voriconazole intravenous-to-oral switch in immunocompromised children and healthy adults. *Antimicrob Agents Chemother.* 2011;55(12):5770–5779.

33. Boyd NK, Zoellner CL, Swancutt MA, et al. Utilization of omeprazole to augment subtherapeutic voriconazole concentrations for treatment of Aspergillus infections. *Antimicrob Agents Chemother.* 2012;56(11):6001, 6002.

34. Wood N, Tan K, Purkins L, et al. Effect of omeprazole on the steady-state pharmacokinetics of voriconazole. *Br J Clin Pharmacol.* 2003;56(suppl 1):56–61.

35. Cornely OA, Maertens J, Winston DJ, et al. Posaconazole vs. fluconazole or itraconazole prophylaxis in patients with neutropenia. *N Engl J Med.* 2007;356(4):348–359.

36. Ullmann AJ, Lipton JH, Vesole DH, et al. Posaconazole or fluconazole for prophylaxis in severe graft-versus-host disease. *N Engl J Med.* 2007;356(4):335–347.

37. Walsh TJ, Raad I, Patterson TF, et al. Treatment of invasive aspergillosis with posaconazole in patients who are refractory to or intolerant of conventional therapy: an externally controlled trial. *Clin Infect Dis.* 2007;44(1):2–12.

38. Jang SH, Colangelo PM, Gobburu JV. Exposure-response of posaconazole used for prophylaxis against invasive fungal infections: evaluating the need to adjust doses based on drug concentrations in plasma. *Clin Pharmacol Ther.* 2010;88(1):115–119.

39. Maertens JA, Raad II, Marr KA, et al. Isavuconazole versus voriconazole for primary treatment of invasive mould disease caused by Aspergillus and other filamentous fungi (SECURE): a phase 3, randomised-controlled, non-inferiority trial. *Lancet.* 2016;387(10020):760–769.

40. Marty FM, Perfect JR, Cornely OA, et al. An open-label phase 3 study of isavuconazole (VITAL): focus on mucormycosis. *Risk.* 2014;8:21–26.

41. Miceli MH, Kauffman CA. Isavuconazole: a new broad-spectrum triazole antifungal agent. *Clin Infect Dis.* 2015;61(10):1558–1565.

42. Arendrup MC, Meletiadis J, Mouton JW, et al. EUCAST technical note on isavuconazole breakpoints for Aspergillus, itraconazole breakpoints for Candida and updates for the antifungal susceptibility testing method documents. *Clin Microbiol Infect.* 2016;22(6):571 e1–571 e4.

8

CARBAMAZEPINE

Laura F. Ruekert and Jeanne H. VanTyle

Learning Objectives

By the end of the carbamazepine chapter, the learner shall be able to:

1. Estimate the initial dosage for a patient on carbamazepine, including the population estimates for V_d and clearance.
2. Explain why loading doses of carbamazepine are not recommended.
3. List and perform the pharmacokinetic calculations necessary for initial adjustments in the maintenance dose of carbamazepine.
4. Describe the metabolism and clearance of carbamazepine and anticipate possible drug interactions or adverse reactions related to clearance.
5. Understand and explain the role of pharmacogenetics with pharmacokinetics and pharmacodynamics of carbamazepine and its adverse drug reaction profile.

Carbamazepine is an anticonvulsant compound that is structurally similar to the tricyclic antidepressant agents. It blocks voltage-dependent sodium channels and is the drug of choice for the treatment of trigeminal neuralgia (tic douloureux, glossopharyngeal neuralgia syndrome), and is used in the treatment of a variety of seizure disorders. It has the Food and Drug Administration (FDA) approval for generalized tonic–clonic (grand mal) and partial (psychomotor, temporal lobe) seizures, bipolar disorders, and in acute mania and mixed episodes. It is used off-label in a variety of other conditions, including pain syndromes, migraine headaches, and other neurologic disorders. Carbamazepine is most frequently prescribed for those patients who have failed to respond to other anticonvulsant therapy or for those who have developed significant side effects from other anticonvulsant agents.[1,2]

Carbamazepine is available in many dosage forms, including oral suspension, chewable tablet, oral tablet, extended-release tablets, and extended-release capsules.

KEY PARAMETERS: Carbamazepine

Therapeutic plasma concentrations	4–12 mg/L
F	80% tablets
S	1.0
V^a	1.1 L/kg
$Cl^{a,b}$	
Monotherapy	0.064 L/kg/hr
Polytherapy	0.10 L/kg/hr
Children (monotherapy)	0.11 L/kg/hr
Free fraction	0.2–0.3
$t\frac{1}{2}$	
Adult monotherapy	15 hr
Adult polytherapy[b]	10 hr

[a]The values for volume of distribution and clearance are approximations based upon oral administration data and an estimate of bioavailability.
[b]The clearance and half-life values represent adult values after induction has taken place. Polytherapy represents a patient receiving other enzyme-inducing anticonvulsants (e.g., phenobarbital, phenytoin)

High-fat meals will increase rate but not extent of absorption. The contents of the capsule cannot be altered by chewing but may be sprinkled on applesauce if required.[3] Carbamazepine is available generically from several manufacturers. It is labeled for use in children through adulthood. The most commonly used dose for children less than 6 years of age is 10 to 20 mg/kg/day initially but, at steady state, is likely to be 20 to 30 mg/kg/day orally divided twice daily. Effective doses for adults with seizure disorders are in the range of 15 to 25 mg/kg/day (or 800 to 1,200 mg/day) at steady state. Migraine prophylaxis doses are usually in the range of 10 to 20 mg/kg/day given twice daily with extended-release products.

Carbamazepine is metabolized by CYP3A4 and CYP3A5 producing a carbamazepine 10,11-epoxide, metabolite responsible for both therapeutic and adverse effects. The half-life of the 10,11-epoxide is approximately 34 hours. The carbamazepine-10,11-epoxide to carbamazepine ratios are higher in infants and preschool children. Children have been shown to have increased CYP3A4 activity as compared to adults. Less than 2% of carbamazepine is excreted unchanged in the urine. Carbamazepine is approximately 75% bound to plasma albumin and α_1-acid glycoprotein. Usual half-life of carbamazepine, 24 to 30 hours, as monotherapy would suggest achievement of steady state within a week. However, time to achieve steady state is highly variable with reports of 4 to 15 days owing to auto-induction.

THERAPEUTIC AND TOXIC PLASMA CONCENTRATIONS

The range of therapeutic serum concentrations for carbamazepine is reported to be 4 to 12 mg/L (SI: 17 to 51 μmol/L). The conversion of mass units to SI units is

1 mcg/mL = 4.23 µmol/L. Many patients will develop symptoms of toxicity, including cardiovascular toxicity, such as second- and third-degree heart block, when plasma concentrations exceed 10 mg/L. For this reason, many clinicians prefer to use a therapeutic range of approximately 4 to 8 mg/L, especially in patients on other anticonvulsants. Adverse reactions such as neuromuscular disturbances can be difficult to tolerate, and some clinicians prefer a lower therapeutic range. The clinician should be aware of conditions that can increase the formation of the 10,11-epoxide[4–6] such as simultaneous administration of quetiapine,[7] phenytoin, and valproate sodium.[8] In most patients, the carbamazepine to its major metabolite (10,11-epoxide) ratio is relatively constant,[9,10] with serum concentrations of the epoxide metabolite ranging from 15% to 40% of carbamazepine.[4,7] In some patients, such as in overdose situations when protein binding is saturated, it might be useful to monitor total carbamazepine and the 10,11-epoxide metabolite because serum concentrations will significantly increase to 50% to 80% of the carbamazepine concentration.[4,11]

ADVERSE EFFECTS

Carbamazepine is associated with numerous adverse drug reactions. The most common adverse effects associated with carbamazepine involve the central nervous system (CNS) and include dizziness, nystagmus, ataxia, blurred vision, diplopia, dry mouth, nausea, vomiting, drowsiness, and suicidality. Cardiovascular, renal, and hepatic effects vary in severity and include tachycardia, hyponatremia, hepatic porphyria, and hepatotoxicity. Idiosyncratic dermatologic and hematologic reactions associated with carbamazepine include agranulocytosis, aplastic anemia, mild maculopapular eruption and drug hypersensitivity syndrome or drug reaction with eosinophilia and systemic symptoms (DRESS), Stevens–Johnson syndrome (SJS),[12] and toxic epidermal necrolysis (TEN).[13]

The appropriateness of pharmacogenomics testing should be evaluated when considering the initiation of CBZ or when there is a diagnosis of SJS, TEN, DRESS, or other cutaneous reaction such as mild maculopapular eruption potentially secondary to CBZ, owing to the significant associated morbidity and mortality. The presence of either the HLA-A*31:01 or HLA-B*15:02 allele has been associated with the development of these cutaneous reactions, with reported odds ratios (OR) of 9 and 113 in all populations.[14,15] Clinical Pharmacogenetics Implementations Consortium guidelines and the FDA recommended patients with ancestry in at-risk populations should be screened for the presence of HLA-B*1502 allele prior to starting carbamazepine.[16–18] Studies confirm highest at-risk individuals include those of Han Chinese descent, followed by Vietnam, Cambodia, the Reunion Islands, Thailand, India, Malaysia, and Hong Kong.[14,15] Any individual with at least one copy of HLA-B15:02 allele should avoid carbamazepine unless the benefits outweighs the risks *and* the patient has taken the drug for 3 or more months without any development of cutaneous adverse reactions.[18] Whereas HLA-B*15:02 is more strongly associated with SJS/TEN particularly in Han Chinese (OR 1357),[18,19] HLA-A*31:01 is associated with all phenotypes of CBZ-induced cutaneous reactions in Japanese, Korean, European, and mixed ancestries (OR 9).[15,16,20] It is noteworthy that some patients without copies of the allele have experienced SJS/TEN, regardless of ancestry.

Carbamazepine, pregnancy class D, is teratogenic and has been associated with neural tube defects by antagonizing enzymes in folate metabolism and interfering with folate absorption.[21,22] Polymorphism in genes associated with folate metabolism, including methylenetetrahydrofolate reductase, methionine synthese reductase, and methylenetetrahydrofolate dehydrogenase, may lead to difference in the susceptibility of individuals to folate antagonists.[23] Carbamazepine and the 10,11-epoxide both pass into the breast milk, and clinicians should take into consideration the importance of the drug to the mother while balancing the risks to the nursing infant.

Many antiepileptic drugs, including carbamazepine, appear to increase the risk of suicidal thoughts or behavior. Patients should be monitored for worsening of depression, suicidal thoughts, and/or any changes in mood or behavior. In one study of 827 suicidal acts in 297,620 treatment episodes, oxcarbazepine, tiagabine, lamotrigine, valproate, and phenobarbital had rates greater than carbamazepine.[24] Unlike the risk of suicidality associated with antidepressants, the risk of suicidality associated with antiepileptics shows no relationship to age and may persist for the duration of treatment. To minimize the risk of CBZ adverse effects, a baseline comprehensive history and physical examination along with baseline and periodic complete blood count, comprehensive metabolic panel, liver function tests, drug levels, and electrocardiogram are recommended monitoring parameters.

PHARMACOKINETICS

Bioavailability (F)

Carbamazepine is a lipid-soluble compound that is slowly and variably absorbed from the gastrointestinal tract. Peak plasma concentrations following immediate-release products occur at approximately 6 hours (range 2 to 24 hours) after oral ingestion. Grapefruit juice increases the bioavailability of carbamazepine by inhibiting CYP3A4 in the gut wall and in the liver. There is evidence that CYP induction/inhibition modulates drug transporter expression of P-glycoprotein, MRP2 (multidrug resistance protein 2), and MRP3 (multidrug resistance protein 3). A high-fat meal has been shown to increase the rate of absorption and elevate the peak concentration while not changing the extent as measured by the area under the curve. Following administration of an intravenous product, bioavailability is shown to be 0.78.[25,26] Because carbamazepine is slowly absorbed, changes in gastrointestinal function, especially those associated with rapid transit, could decrease its bioavailability and result in variable plasma concentrations of carbamazepine. For clinical purposes, the authors assume the bioavailability factor (F) to be approximately 0.8 for carbamazepine when administered as the oral tablet, chewable tablet, or suspension.

Volume of distribution (V)

On average, the volume of distribution for carbamazepine is approximately 1.1 L/kg.[27] Carbamazepine, a neutral compound, is primarily bound to albumin and α_1-acid glycoprotein, and has a free fraction (α) of approximately 0.2 to 0.3. In uremic patients, increases in free carbamazepine concentrations may be seen. Although carbamazepine is bound to plasma proteins, there are very few clinical studies exploring alterations in plasma binding characteristics. This may be because carbamazepine is bound to multiple plasma proteins and, with a free fraction of 0.2 to 0.3, a fairly large change in plasma binding would be required for the change in binding to become clinically significant. Carbamazepine daily dose should be based on ideal body weight, but not on total body weight.[28] Loading doses of carbamazepine are not commonly utilized because time must be allowed for concentrations to rise to steady state, because auto-induction alters the pharmacokinetics of carbamazepine.

Clearance (Cl)

Carbamazepine is eliminated almost exclusively by metabolism, with less than 2% of an oral dose being excreted remain unchanged in the urine. Carbamazepine is metabolized in the liver by CYP3A4/5 isoenzymes and induces CYP1A2 (strong), CYP2B6 (moderate), CYP2C8/9 (strong), 2C19 (strong), and CYP 3A4 (strong) to accelerate the hepatic metabolism of other drugs (see Fig. 8.1). The average clearance value appears to be approximately 0.064 L/kg/hr in adult patients who have received the drug chronically. Data indicates gender and racial differences account for variability in carbamazepine clearance.[29] Studies indicate that absolute clearance (L/hr/kg) was significantly lower in men as compared to women (0.039 vs. 0.049, p = 0.007) and in African-Americans as compared to Caucasians (0.039 vs. 0.048, p = 0.019).[25] A majority of studies show that apparent CYP3A4 activity is higher in women (and children) than in men.[30]

In patients who are taking other enzyme-inducing antiepileptic drugs concurrently (polytherapy), the clearance is increased to approximately 0.1 L/kg/hr. Single-dose studies suggest a clearance that is one-half to one-third of the value observed in patients on chronic therapy. The increase in clearance associated with chronic therapy is apparently owing to auto-induction of its metabolic enzymes.

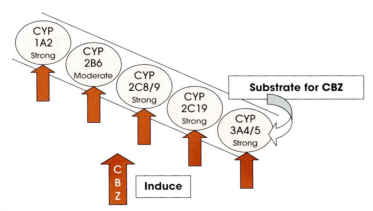

FIGURE 8.1 The metabolism of carbamazepine is via CYP3A4. Carbamazepine is capable of inducing CYP1A2, CYP2B6, CYP2C8/9, CYP2C19, and CYP3A4/5. The induction of the same system as is used for metabolism is "auto-induction." This leads to unique pharmacokinetic difficulties until steady-state conditions are reached. Carbamazepine also induces P-gp production and uses UGT1A1 and UGT2B7. CBZ, carbamazepine; P-gp, P-glycoprotein.

Drug interactions

Carbamazepine has many drug interactions resulting both from CYP inhibition and from induction that alter observed concentrations. Carbamazepine has been shown to induce the metabolism of warfarin through CYP2C9. Carbamazepine greatly reduces the serum concentrations of atorvastatin and rosuvastatin probably by inducing the metabolism.[31] Because pravastatin is not metabolized by 3A4, it is not associated with this interaction.[32] In addition, carbamazepine induces the phase II metabolism isoenzymes UGT1A9 and UGT2B7 found in the liver, kidneys, and lower gastrointestinal tract. UGT1A9 and UGT2B7 play a major role in conjugation.[33] Table 8.1 lists selected drug interactions via CYP3A4.

TABLE 8.1   Carbamazepine Drug Interactions

CYP3A4 **inhibitors** that inhibit carbamazepine metabolism and increase plasma carbamazepine include	CYP3A4 **inducers** that induce the rate of carbamazepine metabolism and decrease plasma carbamazepine include
INCREASED PLASMA CARBAMAZEPINE	**DECREASED PLASMA CARBAMAZEPINE**
Azole antifungals	Carbamazepine[b]
fluconazole, itraconazole, ketoconazole, voriconazole	Cisplatin
	Doxorubicin
Cimetidine	Felbamate
Clarithromycin[a]	Phenobarbital
Chloroquin, mefloquine	Phenytoin
Dalfopristin/Quinupristin	Primidone
Diltiazem	Rifampin
Erythromycin[a]	Theophylline
Fluoxetine	
Fluvoxamine	
Grapefruit juice	
Isoniazid	
Lithium	
Loratadine	
Loxapine	
Niacinamide	
Protease inhibitors	
indinavir, nelfinavir, ritonavir	
Quetiapine	
Quinine	
Ranolazine	
Troleandomycin	
Valproate[a]	
Verapamil	
Zileuton	

Partial list of drugs known to affect serum concentrations of carbamazepine.
[a]Inhibit epoxide-hydroxylase, resulting in increased concentrations of carbamazepine 10,11-epoxide.
[b]Auto-induction.

Carbamazepine induces its own metabolism through time- and dose-dependent auto-induction, resulting in the curvilinear relationship between the CBZ dose and the epoxide metabolite. Therefore, the use of clearance values from single-dose studies is impractical in the calculation of a maintenance dose and may lead to errors. The auto-induction of carbamazepine metabolism has many clinical implications. It is important to initiate patients on relatively low doses to avoid side effects early in therapy. The maintenance dose can be increased at 1- to 2-week intervals by 200 mg/day. The auto-induction phenomenon also limits pharmacokinetic study and manipulation of carbamazepine dosing. For example, it is uncertain whether induction is an all-or-none or a graded process that is dose related. Induction should be complete within 5 to 7 days but may take up to a few weeks. Finally, auto-induction of metabolism commonly causes changes in steady-state carbamazepine levels that are less than proportional to an increase in the maintenance dose.

As with many of the anticonvulsant agents, carbamazepine has been associated with cross-induction of other anticonvulsants. For this reason, whenever carbamazepine is added to an anticonvulsant regimen or other agents are added to a carbamazepine regimen, additional plasma level monitoring may be appropriate to ensure that the

TABLE 8.2 The Effects of Carbamazepine on Other Select Drugs

DRUG(S)	MECHANISM	EFFECT	RECOMMENDATION
Delavirdine/other NNRTIs	Induction of CYP3A4 by carbamazepine	Reduction in plasma concentration of NNRTI and loss of virologic response	Monitor carbamazepine concentrations and adjust. Consider alternative AED agent
Lithium	Pharmacodynamic effect	Neurotoxic effect and adverse effects	A reduced lithium dose may be needed
Oral contraceptives	Induction of CYP3A4 by carbamazepine	Enhanced metabolism of EE and norethindrone resulting in contraceptive failure	Backup method of contraception required; barrier or IUD
Phenytoin primidone	Hepatic metabolism induced	Combination may alter levels of both drugs; may increase CNS depression	Monitor serum concentrations of phenytoin and carbamazepine
Warfarin	Induction of CYP1A2 and CYP3A4	Decreased anticoagulant effect	Increased monitoring and change in dose may be required. Consider alternative anticoagulant

AED, antiepileptic drug; CNS, central nervous system; EE, ethinylestradiol; IUD, intrauterine device; NNRTIs, non-nucleoside reverse transcriptase inhibitors.

maintenance regimen continues to result in plasma levels that are optimal for therapeutic control. Table 8.2 provides examples of monitoring recommendations for selected drug interactions. Under certain conditions, as with valproate, erythromycin, and clarithromycin, the carbamazepine concentration is reduced, and the 10,11-epoxide concentration is increased.[33] This may explain the observation of CNS side effects in some patients with relatively low carbamazepine plasma concentrations and may warrant checking the epoxide metabolite level in addition to the CBZ drug concentration.

Patients treated with a combination of antiretroviral agents and carbamazepine are at increased risk of interactions.[34] Carbamazepine use is common in the treatment of HIV-infected patients because approximately 10% of patients have seizures secondary to neurologic manifestations of HIV and opportunistic CNS infections. Carbamazepine can reduce concentrations of antiretroviral agents and, importantly, be implicated in the loss of virologic response. In particular, the well-established efficacy of recommended first-line Integrase Strand Transfer Inhibitor regimens containing dolutegravir for HIV can be compromised and warrants dolutegravir dosing increases from once daily to twice daily when given concomitantly with CBZ.[34,35] Various protease inhibitors, nucleoside reverse transcription inhibitors (NRTIs), non-nucleoside reverse transcriptase inhibitors (NNRTIs), and their associated combination products interact with CBZ and should be carefully evaluated to optimize treatment response.

Estradiol is metabolized by CYP1A2, and CYP1A2 is induced by carbamazepine. Studies have shown lowered sex hormone levels secondary to enzyme-induced accelerated metabolism and higher sex hormone binding globulin) that reduce the free concentrations of the hormones.[36] Induced metabolism of sex steroid hormones by carbamazepine increases the risk of contraceptive failure and may result in pregnancy.[37] This is especially true for women on low-dose contraceptive hormones.[37–40]

Half-life (t½)

Single-dose studies predict a carbamazepine half-life of approximately 30 to 35 hours. However, steady-state data suggest a half-life of approximately 15 hours in adult patients receiving carbamazepine monotherapy, and approximately 10 hours in patients receiving other enzyme-inducing antiepileptic drugs (e.g., phenytoin, phenobarbital) concurrently. Children metabolize carbamazepine more rapidly than adults do with reported steady-state half-lives of 4 to 12 hours.

Time to sample

Obtaining carbamazepine plasma samples within the first few weeks of therapy may be useful to establish a relationship between carbamazepine concentration and a patient's clinical response. However, these data should be interpreted cautiously if one is attempting to predict the long-term relationship between a carbamazepine dosing regimen and plasma levels. Once steady state has been achieved, the time of sampling within a dosing interval is somewhat arbitrary given the long half-life and relatively short dosing interval for carbamazepine. It is important to establish a fixed relationship between drug intake and blood sampling. The most sensible time to take routine samples is in the early morning (trough) before the first dose of medication is administered, or later in the day, prior to the next dose. Such samples will reflect the trough concentration and are comparable from day to day. In addition, the clinician can monitor plasma drug levels without concern for artifactual errors, including the influence of diet and food intake on absorption of the drug from the gastrointestinal tract. Nevertheless, it is reasonable to obtain carbamazepine plasma samples at a consistent time within the dosing interval. As a rule, samples should be obtained just before a dose (trough) unless this is markedly inconvenient for the patient. Inconvenience is most likely to be encountered in ambulatory patients who may be taking the drug on a schedule that is not consistent with their clinic appointments.

PHARMACOGENETICS

It has been suggested that single-nucleotide polymorphisms (SNPs) within the carbamazepine pathway contribute to the variability seen with its pharmacokinetics and, thus, response or even resistance. *SCN1A* gene belongs to a family of genes that provide instructions for making sodium channels. Overall, 25 SNPs have been identified and may account for the variability in CBZ pharmacokinetics. For example, SNPs associated with CYP3A, EPHX1 (epoxide hydrolase 1), UGT2B7, and drug transporters (ABCB1 and ABCB2) may alter clearance, volume of distribution, serum drug levels, and the carbamazepine to the epoxide metabolite ratio and, subsequently, may be implicated in setting of drug interactions, adverse reactions, suboptimal treatment response.[41]

Oxcarbazepine (Trileptal)

Carbamazepine has a number of limitations, including auto-induction, many drug interactions, toxicities, and teratogenicity. Oxcarbazepine (Trileptal) was developed as chemically similar to carbamazepine with an improved safety profile. Oxcarbazepine has a chemical structure similar to carbamazepine but with different metabolism. Oxcarbazepine is a prodrug of 10-monohydroxycarbazepine (MHD), the active metabolite which is responsible for the majority of drug actions. Oxcarbazepine is completely absorbed and converted to MHD. The volume of distribution is approximately 0.7 L/kg in adults. MHD has a half-life of about 9 hours, is taken two times a day, steady state is reached in 2 to 3 days, and about 40% is protein bound primarily to albumin. Oxcarbazepine biotransformation does not involve epoxide metabolite formation. The lack of an epoxide may contribute to the better tolerability of oxcarbazepine. More than 95% appears in the urine as metabolites with <1% as unchanged drug. No dose adjustment is required for liver dysfunction, but is for creatinine clearance <30 mL/min. It is in pregnancy category C. Oxcarbazepine can inhibit CYP2C19 and induce CYP3A4/5 with potentially important effects on plasma concentrations of other drugs. The inhibition of CYP2C19 by oxcarbazepine and MHD can cause increased plasma concentrations of drugs that are substrates of CYP2C19. No auto-induction has been observed with oxcarbazepine. Coadministration of oxcarbazepine with an oral contraceptive has been shown to decrease the plasma concentrations of the two hormonal components, ethinylestradiol and levonorgestrel.[42]

Eslicarbazepine (Aptiom)

Eslicarbazepine is the newest member of this antiepileptic drug group. Eslicarbazepine is approved for both adjunctive and monotherapy of partial-onset seizures in adults and children (6 to 17 years).[43] It is used off-label for bipolar disorder and trigeminal neural-gia. It is structurally different from carbamazepine and oxcarbazepine. Eslicarbazepine has a linear pharmacokinetic profile, low binding to plasma proteins (<40%), and a half-life of 20 to 24 hours, and is mainly excreted by the kidneys in an unchanged form or as glucuronide conjugates. It has a low potential for drug interactions.[42,44,45] Like oxcarbazepine, it is not metabolized to an epoxide. A common concern of the three agents is hyponatremia that has been reported with all. The hyponatremia appears to be caused by syndrome of inappropriate antidiuretic hormone secretion and is dose related. It also induces oral contraceptives and may cause oral contraceptives to be less effective by lowering concentrations of ethinylestradiol and levonorgestrel. Oxcarbazepine and eslicarbazepine do not have black-box warnings for HLA-B*1502, aplastic anemia, or agranulocytosis.[43,45,46]

Question #1   *N.S., a 36-year-old, 60 kg female, is to be started on carbamazepine as an anticonvulsant agent. How would you initiate therapy? Explain your rationale. Estimate amount needed at steady state and then propose how to start the patient on therapy. Calculate a daily dose that will produce an average steady-state plasma concentration of approximately 6 mg/L.*

Do not give a loading dose of carbamazepine because of auto-induction. To calculate an average steady-state plasma concentration, the maintenance dose equation is used with an assumed bioavailability of 0.8 and an average clearance value of 3.84 L/hr (0.064 L/kg/hr × 60 kg). The fraction of the administered dose that is active drug (S) is 1.0.

$$Cl_{monotherapy} = 0.064 \text{ L/Kg} \times 60 \text{ kg} = 3.84 \text{ L/hr}$$

$$\text{Maintenance Dose} = \frac{(Cl)(Css \text{ ave})(\tau)}{(S)(F)} \qquad \textbf{(Eq. 8.1)}$$

$$= \frac{(3.84 \text{ L/hr})(6 \text{ mg/L})(24 \text{ hr/1 day})}{(1)(0.8)}$$

$$= 691.2 \text{ mg/day}$$

This dose (~700 mg/day) is that which would be required to achieve the steady-state level of 6 mg/L after auto-induction of carbamazepine metabolism had taken place. For this reason, N.S. should be started on a lower daily dose initially and increased at 1- to 2-week intervals based on her clinical response. The usual initial daily dose for adult patients is 200 by mouth twice daily, with increases of approximately 200 mg/day every 7 to 14 days. When discontinuing treatment, reduce the dose gradually to avoid the risk of seizure.

Question #2   *After 2 months, the carbamazepine dose of N.S. has been increased to 300 mg orally two times a day. On this regimen, she has had some reduction in seizure frequency; however, seizure control is still considered unsatisfactory. The steady-state carbamazepine level at this time is reported to be 4 mg/L. What are possible explanations for this observed plasma level? What dose would be required to achieve a new steady-state carbamazepine level of 6 mg/L?*

Using the steady-state continuous infusion equation and a clearance of 3.84 L/hr, the anticipated carbamazepine level in N.S. for a dose of 600 mg/day would be approximately 5 mg/L. One should also consider whether to use literature values or patient observations when you have patient data that allows you to calculate clearance for the patient. Using the literature information:

$$\text{Css ave} = \frac{(S)(F)(D/\tau)}{(Cl)} \qquad \text{(Eq. 8.2)}$$

$$= \frac{(1)(0.8)(300 \text{ mg}/12 \text{ hr})}{3.84 \text{ L/hr}}$$

$$= 5.2 \text{ mg/L}$$

The observed level of 4.0 mg/L is within the predicted range, considering the fact that both bioavailability and clearance values derived from average literature values may not be correct for N.S. At this point, it would be difficult to establish whether a slightly lower-than-expected bioavailability or a higher-than-average clearance was responsible for the observed level of 4.0 mg/L.

Because of carbamazepine's relatively slow absorption characteristics and long half-life, it is probable that the measured concentration of 4 mg/L represents an average steady-state value. At steady state, the average plasma concentration should be proportional to the daily dose. Therefore, to increase the plasma concentration from 4 to 6 mg/L, one would simply increase the carbamazepine dose by 50% (i.e., from 600 to 900 mg/day).

$$\text{New Maintenance Dose} = \left(\frac{\text{Css ave New}}{\text{Css ave Old}}\right) \text{Old Maintenance Dose} \qquad \text{(Eq. 8.3)}$$

$$= \left(\frac{\text{Css ave New}}{\text{Css ave Old}}\right) 600 \text{ mg/day}$$

$$= 900 \text{ mg/day}$$

Another approach might be to calculate the apparent carbamazepine clearance for patient N.S. using a rearrangement of the maintenance dose Equation 8.1, the current maintenance dose of 300 mg/12 hr, and an assumed bioavailability of 0.8. In this case, patient observations are used rather than literature clearance:

$$Cl = \frac{(S)(F)(D/\tau)}{Css\ ave} \qquad \textbf{(Eq. 8.4)}$$

$$= \frac{(1)(0.8)(300\ mg/12\ hr)}{4\ mg/L}$$

$$= 5\ L/hr$$

This clearance value could then be used in the maintenance dose equation to calculate the maintenance dose as illustrated. However, this time, the clearance value that has been derived from the patient's specific data is used rather than an average value from the literature:

$$Maintenance\ Dose = \frac{(Cl)(Css\ ave)(\tau)}{(S)(F)}$$

$$= \frac{(5\ L/hr)(6\ mg/L)(24\ hr/day)}{(1)(0.8)}$$

$$= 900\ mg/day$$

If N.S. was receiving other anticonvulsant agents, it would be appropriate to monitor their concentrations as well, because carbamazepine could induce their metabolism, thereby reducing their steady-state concentrations.

Question #3   *The decision is made to add valproic acid to attempt better control of the seizures. N.S. returns 2 weeks later to clinic. The patient complains that recently, she is sleepy and "feels funny." A carbamazepine concentration is drawn and reported to be 9 mcg/mL. What is your explanation?*

Owing to the addition of valproic acid, a CYP3A4 enzyme inhibitor, the metabolism of carbamazepine is decreased which in turn increases carbamazepine serum concentrations as well as the carbamazepine 10,11-epoxide, which also has some activity. This leads to the increased serum concentration, and because the epoxide has activity, it can cause further sedation than was seen on the lower dose of carbamazepine. After serum levels have stabilized, the body may adjust to the higher level and her sleepiness will become less of a noticeable side effect.

In addition, valproic acid can inhibit the metabolism of carbamazepine via CYP3A4 and can displace carbamazepine from protein binding sites, thus increasing the free fraction of carbamazepine. Valproic acid can increase the formation of the epoxide metabolite, which may also be picked up by the assay (about 7%) for carbamazepine.

These factors can lead to an increase in carbamazepine's serum concentration, which could result in side effects such as drowsiness.

Question #4   *A.B. is a 60-year-old male (65 kg) currently receiving the following:*

MEDICATION	STEADY-STATE CONCENTRATION (mcg/mL)
Carbamazepine 200 mg three times a day	7
Phenytoin extended 300 mg orally at bedtime	11

Despite these agents, seizures persist, and the decision is made to add valproic acid of 250 mg orally three times a day. One month following the addition of valproic acid, A.B. complains of drowsiness. Drug concentrations are drawn, and the levels obtained are carbamazepine 7.6 mcg/mL, phenytoin 8 mcg/mL, and valproic acid 50 mcg/mL. The serum albumin level reported is 4.2 g/dL. What is your explanation for the patient complaints?

Figure 8.2 depicts the effects valproic acid may have on carbamazepine and phenytoin levels. Carbamazepine level is slightly increased because of the concurrent use of valproic acid, a CYP3A4 enzyme inhibitor, which decreases the metabolism of the carbamazepine. A possibility that the increase is only modest is because of the use of phenytoin, a CYP3A4 enzyme inducer, which may also be affecting the amount of carbamazepine being metabolized. Phenytoin levels are likely decreased owing to the increased carbamazepine level with additional increase in carbamazepine epoxide levels. From these increases, an increase in CYP3A4 induction occurs, which causes an increase in phenytoin metabolism and a decrease in phenytoin serum levels. Valproic acid levels are within therapeutic range, but would potentially be higher if it was used as monotherapy, and was not being influenced by the enzyme induction of phenytoin and carbamazepine.

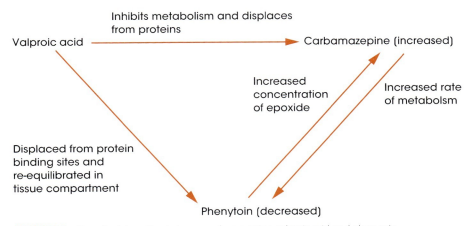

FIGURE 8.2   Complex interaction between carbamazepine, valproic acid, and phenytoin.

REFERENCES

1. Johannessen-Landmark C, Johannessen SI. Pharmacological management of epilepsy: recent advances and future prospects. *Drugs.* 2008;68:1925–1939.

2. Glauser T, Ben-Menachem E, Bourgeois B, et al. ILAE treatment guidelines: evidence-based analysis of antiepileptic drug efficacy and effectiveness as initial monotherapy for epileptic seizures and syndromes. *Epilepsia.* 2006;47:1094–1120.

3. Equetro® carbamazepine extended-release capsules [package insert]. Parsippany, NJ: Validus Pharmaceuticals; 2012.

4. Russell JL, Spiller HA, Baker DD. Markedly elevated carbamazepine-10,11-epoxide/carbamazepine ratio in a fatal carbamazepine ingestion. *Case Rep Med.* 2015;2015:369707.

5. Burianova I, Borecka K. Routine monitoring of the active metaboite of carbamazepine: is it really necessary? *Clin Biochem.* 2015;48(13–14):866–869.

6. Potter JM, Donnelly A. Carbamazepine-10,11-epoxide in therapeutic drug monitoring. *Ther Drug Monitor.* 1998;20(6):652–657.

7. Fitzgerald BJ, Okos AJ. Elevation of carbamazepine-10,11-epoxide by quetiapine. *Pharmacotherapy.* 2002;22(11):1500–1503.

8. Bernus I, Dickinson RG, Hooper WD, et al. The mechanism of the carbamazepine-valproate interaction in humans. *Br J Clin Pharmacol.* 1997;44:21–27.

9. Tutor-Crespo MJ, Hermida J, Tutor JC. Relative proportions of serum carbamazepine and its pharmacological active 10,11-epoxy derivative: effect of polytherapy and renal insufficiency. *Upsala J Med Sci.* 2008;113(2):171–180.

10. Ma CL, Jiao Z, Wu XY, et al. Association between PK/PD-involved gene polymorphisms and carbamazepine-individualized therapy. *Pharmacogenonomics.* 2015;16(13):1499–1512.

11. Sol EL, Ruggles KH, Cascino GD, et al. Seizure exacerbation and status epilepticus related to carbamazepine-10,11-epoxide. *Ann Neurol.* 1994;35(6):743–746.

12. Ferrell PB, McLeod HL. Carbamazepine, HLA-B*-1502 and the risk of Stevens-Johnson syndrome and toxic epidermal necrolysis: US FDA recommendations. *Pharmacogenomics.* 2008;9:1543–1546.

13. Anderson GD. Pharmacokinetics, pharmacodynamic, and pharmacogenetic targeted therapy of antiepileptic drugs. *Ther Drug Monitor.* 2008;30:173–180.

14. Whirl-Carrillo M, McDonagh EM, Hebert JM, et al. Pharmacogenomics knowledge for personalized medicine. *Clin Pharmacol Ther.* 2012;92(4):414–417.

15. Leckband SG, Kelsoe JR, Dunnenberger HM, et al. Clinical Pharmacogenetics Implementation Consortium (CPIC) guidelines for HLA-B genotype and carbamazepine. *Clin Pharmacol Ther.* 2013;94(3):324–328.

16. Genin E, Chen D-P, Hung S-I, et al. HLA-A*31:01 and different types of carbamazepine-induced severe cutaneous adverse reactions: an international study and meta-analysis. *Pharmacogenomics J.* 2014;14:281–288.

17. Hung S-I, Chung W-H, Jee S-H, et al. Genetic susceptibility to carbamazepine-induced cutaneous adverse drug reactions. *Pharmacogenet Genomics.* 2006;16:297–306.

18. Tangamornsuksan W, Chaiyakinapurk N, Somkrua R, et al. Relationship between the HLA-B*1502 allele and carbamazepine-induced Stevens-Johnson syndrome and toxic epidermal necrolysis. *JAMA Dermatol.* 2013;149(9):1025–1032.

19. Man CB, Kwan P, Baum L, et al. Association between HLA-B*1502 allele and antiepileptic drug-induced cutaneous reactions in Han Chinese. *Epilepsia.* 2007;48;1015–1018.

20. Amstutz U, Shear NH, Rieder MJ, et al. Recommendations for HLA-B*15:02 and HLA-A*31:01 genetic testing to reduce the risk of carbamazepine-induced hypersensitivity reactions. *Epilepsia.* 2014;55(4):496–506.

21. Tomson T, Xu WH, Battino D. Major congenital malformations in children of women with epilepsy. *Seizure.* 2015;28:46–50.

22. Arpino C, Brescianini S, Robert E, et al. Teratogenic effects of antiepileptic drugs: use of an international database on malformations and drug exposure (MADRE). *Epilepsia.* 2000;41:1436–1443.

23. van Gelder MM, van Rooij IA, Miller RK, et al. Teratogenic mechanisms of medical drugs. *Human Reprod Update.* 2010;16(4):378–394.

24. Patorno E, Bohn RL, Wahl PM, et al. Anticonvulsant medications and the risk of suicide, attempted suicide, or violent death. *JAMA*. 2010;303(14):1401–1409.

25. Marino SE, Birnbaum AK, Leppil IE, et al. Steady-state carbamazepine pharmacokinetics following oral and stable-labeled intravenous administration in epilepsy patients: effects of race and sex. *Clin Pharmacol Ther*. 2012;91(3):483–488.

26. Tolbert D, Cloyd J, Biton V, et al. Bioequivalence of oral and intravenous carbamazepine formulations in adult patients with epilepsy. *Epilepsia*. 2015;56(6):915–923.

27. Landmark CJ, Johannessen SI, Tomson T. Host factors affecting antiepileptic drug delivery-pharmacokinetic variability. *Adv Drug Deliv Rev*. 2012;64:896–910.

28. Caraco Y, Zylber-Katz E, Berry EM, et al. Carbamazepine pharmacokinetics in obese and lean subjects. *Ann Pharmacother*. 1995;29:843–847.

29. Puranik YG, Birnbaum AK, Marino SE, et al. Association of carbamazepine major metabolism and transport pathway gene polymorphisms and pharmacokinetics in patients with epilepsy. *Pharmacogenomics*. 2013;14(1):2–18.

30. Harris RZ, Benet LZ, Schwartz JB. Gender effects in pharmacokinetic and pharmacodynamics. *Drugs*. 1995;50(2):222–239.

31. Parrish RH, Pazdur DE, O'Donnell PJ. Effect of carbamazepine initiation and discontinuation on antithrombotic control in a patient receiving warfarin: case report and review of the literature. *Pharmacotherapy*. 2006;26:1650–1653.

32. Bellosta S, Paoletti R, Corsini A. Safety of statins: focus on clinical pharmacokinetics and drug interactions. *Circulation*. 2004;109(23 suppl 1):III-50–III-57.

33. Caruso A, Bellia C, Pivetti A, et al. Effects of EPHX1 and CYP3A4 polymorphisms on carbamazepine metabolism in epileptic patients. *Pharmacogenomics Pers Med*. 2014;7:117–120.

34. Günthard HF, Saag MS, Benson CA, et al. Antiretroviral drugs for treatment and prevention of HIV infection in adults. 2016 recommendations of the International Antiviral Society-USA panel. *JAMA*. 2016;316(2):191–210.

35. Song I, Weller S, Patel J, et al. Effect of carbamazepine on dolutegravir pharmacokinetics and dosing recommendation. *Eur J Clin Pharmacol*. 2016;72(6):665–670.

36. Brodie MJ, Mintzer S, Pack AM, et al. Enzyme induction with antiepileptic drugs: cause for concern? *Epilepsia*. 2013;54(1):11–27.

37. Davis AR, Westhoff CL, Stanczyk FZ. Carbamazepine coadministration with an oral contraceptive: effects on steroid pharmacokinetics, ovulation, and bleeding. *Epilepsia*. 2011;52(2):243–247.

38. Lagana AS, Triolo O, D'Amico V, et al. Management of women with epilepsy: from preconception to post-partum. *Arch Gynecol Obstet*. 2016;293(3):493–503.

39. Bhajta J, Bainbridge J, Borgelt L. Teratogenic medications and concurrent contraceptive use in women of childbearing ability with epilepsy. *Epilepsy Behav*. 2015;52(pt A):212–217.

40. Verrotti A, Mencaroni E, Castagnini M, et al. Foetal safety of old and new antiepileptic drugs. *Expert Opin Drug Saf*. 2015;14(10):1563–1571.

41. Daci A, Beretta G, Vllasaliu D, et al. Polymorphic Variants of SCN1A and EPHX1 influence plasma carbamazepine concentration, metabolism, and pharmacoresistance in a population of Kosovar Albanian Epileptic Patients. *PLoS ONE*. 2015;10(11):1–17.

42. Zaccara G, Perucca E. Interactions between antiepileptic drugs, and between antiepileptic drugs and other drugs. *Epileptic Disord*. 2014;16(4):409–432.

43. Gierbolini J, Giarratano M, Benbadis SR. Carbamazepine-related antiepileptic drugs for the treatment of epilepsy – a comparative review. *Expert Opin Pharmacother*. 2016;17(7):885–888.

44. Tambucci R, Basti C, Maresca M, et al. Update on the role of eslicarbazepine acetate in the treatment of partial-onset epilepsy. *Neuropsychiatr Dis Treat*. 2016;12:1251–1260.

45. Zelano J, Ben-Menachem E. Eslicarbazepine acetate for the treatment of partial epilepsy. *Expert Opin Pharmacother*. 2016;17(8):1165–1169.

46. Zaccara G, Giovannelli F, Cincotta M, et al. Clinical utility of eslicarbazepine: current evidence. *Drug Des Devel Ther*. 2015;9:781–789.

9

CYTOTOXIC ANTICANCER DRUGS: METHOTREXATE AND BUSULFAN

Timothy W. Synold

Learning Objectives

By the end of the cytotoxic anticancer drugs: methotrexate and busulfan chapter, the learner shall be able to:

1. Describe the methotrexate plasma concentrations and time course that would
   a. Identify patients at risk for methotrexate toxicity.
   b. Identify patients who would be most likely to have therapeutic benefit from methotrexate.
2. Convert methotrexate concentrations from mg/L to μM (10^{-6} M) and μM to mg/L.
3. Outline the usual dosing strategy for leucovorin rescue and conditions under which (concentration and time) the leucovorin rescue dose should be increased.
4. Describe the apparent two-compartment modeling of methotrexate and what would be the most appropriate volume of distribution to use when a loading dose is administered over a relatively short time period.
5. Identify patients who would be at risk for methotrexate toxicity considering the following:
   a. Renal function
   b. Significant third-spacing of fluid
   c. Receiving drugs that are known to or would be expected to decrease methotrexate clearance
6. Discuss the biphasic elimination of methotrexate and why the biphasic elimination is important to the timing of the methotrexate plasma samples and projection of when rescue will be achieved.

7. Do the following if a patient history and a methotrexate infusion dose over 36 hours are given:
   a. Calculate the patients' expected methotrexate clearance.
   b. Calculate the expected methotrexate Css ave at 36 hours.
   c. Calculate the expected methotrexate concentration 48 and 60 hours after starting the methotrexate regimen.

8. Calculate the recommended starting dose of busulfan in a patient who is:
   a. Less than 25% above their ideal body weight.
   b. More than 25% above their ideal body weight.

9. Convert busulfan concentrations from mcg/L to μM and from μM to mcg/L.

10. Convert busulfan AUC in units of μM · min to busulfan Css in units of mcg/L and Css in mcg/L to AUC in units of μM · min.

11. Describe the busulfan plasma AUC or Css that is associated with the following after hematopoietic stem cell transplant:
    a. An increased risk of developing hepatic veno-occlusive disease.
    b. An increased risk of disease relapse or failure to engraft.

12. Identify the appropriate blood sample collection schedule for determination of busulfan AUC or Css.

13. Given a set of busulfan concentration-versus-time data, determine the following:
    a. The busulfan plasma AUC using the rule of linear trapezoids.
    b. The busulfan plasma Css using the rule of linear trapezoids
    c. The busulfan AUC using the model-derived parameters obtained from a compartmental model fit of the data.
    d. The busulfan Css using the model-derived parameters.

14. Calculate the recommended adjusted dose of busulfan that will give the targeted AUC or Css.

The principle of treating patients with maximal safe doses of cytotoxic chemotherapy is reflected in the way that these drugs are developed for clinical use. During the early stages of clinical testing, doses of cytotoxic drugs are escalated in small cohorts of patients until unacceptable or dose-limiting toxicity is observed. Once toxicity is encountered, the dosage in subsequent patients is reduced to a level where an "acceptable" proportion of patients experience unacceptable toxicity (typically defined as <33%). The resulting "maximum tolerated dose" becomes the recommended starting dose for future clinical use. Moreover, cytotoxic agents typically display steep dose–response curves and narrow therapeutic windows. Optimal cytotoxic drug therapy is complicated by the contribution of both pharmacokinetic and pharmacodynamic variability. Although little is known about the causes and extent of pharmacodynamic variability, a great deal of effort has been spent determining the magnitude and potential sources of the wide patient-to-patient variations seen in the pharmacokinetics of most cytotoxic drugs. As a result of the many factors that contribute to differences in pharmacokinetics, the clearances of most of the commonly used cytotoxic drugs vary over a 3- to 10-fold range. The wide ranges in the rates of elimination result in correspondingly large variations in total drug exposures (e.g., area under the concentration–time curve [AUC] and steady-state drug concentration [Css]) in patients treated with equivalent doses. As a result, individuals given identical doses of cytotoxic agents can have up to 10-fold differences in measured drug exposures. For drugs with steep dose–response curves and narrow therapeutic windows, the implication of such pharmacokinetic variability is significant and leads to unpredictability in antitumor response and toxicity. Therefore, several methods are used in an attempt to minimize the wide inter- and intrasubject pharmacokinetic variability.[1]

DOSING BASED ON BODY SURFACE AREA

One of the earliest approaches to normalizing cytotoxic drug exposures was the use of body surface area (BSA) to correct for differences in individual patient size.[2] During the initial stages of clinical drug development, BSA is used to guide dosage escalation up to the point of a definition of the maximum tolerated dose. The recommended doses of drugs that are developed in this way are ultimately assigned on the basis of a BSA-based dosing algorithm. As a result, it has become common practice in clinical oncology to dose anticancer drugs on the basis of a patient's BSA with the aim of reducing interindividual variability in drug exposure caused by factors related to patient size.

DOSING BASED ON RENAL FUNCTION

The pharmacokinetics of anticancer agents are often associated with the functional indices of the major drug clearing organs, the liver and kidneys. Depending on the major route of elimination for a particular drug, it can be reliably predicted that significant changes in either hepatic or renal function will result in corresponding changes in drug clearance. Carboplatin is associated with an increased risk of severe toxicity in patients with creatinine clearances of less than 60 mL/min because of decreased drug clearance and greater total drug exposure.[3] Calvert and colleagues[4] first demonstrated that carboplatin AUC could be accurately predicted using an equation that takes into account the patient's pretreatment glomerular filtration rate (GFR):

$$\text{Carboplatin Dose (mg)} = \text{AUC (mg/mL} \cdot \text{min)} \times (\text{GFR} + 25)(\text{mL/min})$$

This a priori method for carboplatin dosing has led to a substantial reduction in pharmacokinetic variability, and carboplatin is one the few drugs of any class that is routinely dosed to achieve a target systemic exposure. The original Calvert formula was developed using an accurate measurement of GFR based on urinary ^{51}Cr-ethylenediaminetetraacetic acid clearance. The method of choice for current clinical practice uses either a measured or a calculated Cl_{Cr} instead of measured GFR. Although the accepted formulas for calculating Cl_{Cr} typically lead to biased estimates of GFR, they are more suited to routine clinical use. An important caveat is that since the change in the methodology for measuring serum creatinine, lower values are being reported, leading to much higher estimates of Cl_{Cr}. Therefore, the Food and Drug Administration currently recommends that when using established formulas to calculate carboplatin doses in patients with normal kidney function, the estimate of GFR should be capped at 125 mL/min to avoid overdosing.

DOSING BASED ON HEPATIC FUNCTION

The rationale for reducing the dose of cytotoxic drugs in the presence of hepatic impairment is well documented for agents such as etoposide, doxorubicin, vincristine, docetaxel, and paclitaxel. However, unlike Cl_{Cr} and kidney function, there is no single laboratory test that can be used to accurately predict pharmacokinetics. In patients with hepatic impairment, the recommended guidelines for dose adjustment are based on clinical measures of liver function such as bilirubin (e.g., doxorubicin and vincristine), serum glutamic-oxaloacetic transaminase (e.g., paclitaxel and docetaxel), alkaline phosphatase (e.g., docetaxel), or albumin (e.g., etoposide). More recently, the Childs–Pugh classification has been proposed as an alternative to single laboratory measures of hepatic capacity.

THERAPEUTIC DRUG MONITORING

Evans et al. reported the first ever large prospective randomized trial comparing individualized doses of cytotoxic chemotherapy versus standard doses.[5] In this trial, children with acute lymphoblastic leukemia were randomized to receive either conventional doses of methotrexate, cytarabine, and teniposide or individualized doses based on real-time pharmacokinetic determinations. Patients who were randomized to receive individualized chemotherapy doses had a significantly better disease-free survival than those patients who received fixed doses. Although this study established the clinical utility of therapeutic drug monitoring (TDM) of cytotoxic chemotherapy, it also illustrated the difficulty of such an approach. The ability to perform real-time pharmacokinetic monitoring of even a single cytotoxic agent requires dedicated laboratory personnel and resources typically only available at major medical centers. Therefore, despite a high degree of pharmacokinetic variability, steep dose–response relationships, and narrow therapeutic windows, there are currently only two cytotoxic agents for which TDM plays an accepted role in the management of patients.[1,6,7]

Methotrexate

Methotrexate is a folic acid antimetabolite that competitively inhibits dihydrofolate reductase, the enzyme responsible for converting folic acid to the reduced or active folate cofactors. Methotrexate is used to treat a number of neoplasms, including leukemia, osteogenic sarcoma, breast cancer, and non-Hodgkin lymphoma. Methotrexate is administered by the parenteral route when doses exceed 30 mg/m^2 because oral absorption is limited.[8] Current dosing regimens range from as low as 2.5 mg to as high as 12 g/m^2 or more. High-dose methotrexate is administered over a period as short as 3 to 6 hours to as long as 40 hours.[9,10]

Approximately 50% of methotrexate is bound to plasma proteins.[8,9] Methotrexate is primarily renally cleared. It is a weak acid with a pKa of 5.4. At low pH, the drug has limited solubility and may precipitate in the urine, causing renal damage. Therefore, a patient receiving high-dose methotrexate should receive hydration, and the urine pH should be maintained above 7. Methotrexate has some minor metabolites with weak activity, the most important of which is 7-hydroxy-methotrexate. The concentration of this metabolite may become significant with high doses of methotrexate. Although 7-hydroxy-methotrexate has only about 1/200 of the clinical activity of methotrexate, it is one-third to one-fifth as soluble. As a result, it may precipitate in the renal tubules, causing acute nephrotoxicity.[11] This solubility problem is an additional reason why patients receiving high doses of methotrexate should be adequately hydrated and have their urine alkalinized.[9,10]

UNITS

Methotrexate is generally administered in milligram or gram doses, and the plasma concentrations are reported in units of mg/L, mcg/mL, and molar or micromolar units. When methotrexate concentrations are reported in molar units, they usually range from values of 10^{-8} to 10^{-2} M. In addition, they are commonly reported in micromolar (or 10^{-6} M) units. To interpret methotrexate concentrations accurately, it is important to establish which units are being reported and how those units correspond to the generally accepted therapeutic or toxic values. Methotrexate has a molecular weight of 454 g/mol; therefore, a value of 0.454 mg/L is equal to 1×10^{-6} M or 1 µM. To convert methotrexate concentrations in units of mg/L to molar concentrations, Equation 9.1 can be used:

$$\text{Methotrexate Concentration in } 10^{-6} \text{ molar} = \frac{\text{Methotrexate Concentration in mg/L}}{0.454} \qquad \textbf{(Eq. 9.1)}$$

TOXIC PLASMA CONCENTRATIONS

The primary goal of methotrexate plasma monitoring is to ensure that patients receive adequate doses of the rescue agent to prevent serious toxicity. Because most high-dose rescue regimens are designed to "save" the average patient, the vast majority of methotrexate plasma levels that are obtained for monitoring will be routine and are unlikely to require intervention. Nevertheless, plasma concentration monitoring can be used to identify patients with unusual methotrexate disposition that could result in serious toxicity. The therapeutic and toxic effects of methotrexate are closely linked to its plasma concentrations. Plasma concentrations exceeding 1×10^{-7} M for 48 hours or more are associated with methotrexate toxicity.[12] The most common toxic effects of methotrexate include myelosuppression, oral and gastrointestinal mucositis, and acute hepatic dysfunction.[8,10,12]

Leucovorin rescue

To ensure that methotrexate toxicities do not occur in moderate- and high-dose treatment regimens, leucovorin is administered every 4 to 6 hours in doses that range from 10 to 100 mg/m². The usual course of rescue therapy is from 12 to 72 hours, or until the plasma concentration of methotrexate falls below the critical value of 1×10^{-7} M. In some rescue protocols, concentrations of 5×10^{-8} (0.05 µM) are considered to be the value indicating the rescue is complete.[9]

Methotrexate concentrations in excess of 1×10^{-6} M (1 µM) at 48 hours are associated with an increased incidence of methotrexate toxicity, even in the face of leucovorin rescue doses of 10 mg/m². When the methotrexate concentration exceeds 1×10^{-6} M at 48 hours, increasing the leucovorin rescue dose to 50 to 100 mg/m² or more reduces methotrexate toxicity.[12] Presumably, this increased dose enables leucovorin factor to compete successfully with methotrexate for intracellular transport and to thereby rescue host tissues.

Although rescue regimens vary considerably, most employ a leucovorin dosing regimen of approximately 10 mg/m² administered every 6 hours for 72 hours. If the methotrexate concentration falls below 1×10^{-7} M (0.1 µM) or 5×10^{-8} M (0.05 µM) before the completion of the 72-hour rescue period, then the rescue factor can be discontinued. If the methotrexate concentrations are still greater than 1×10^{-7} but less than 1×10^{-6} at 48 hours, then rescue with leucovorin is continued at doses of approximately 10 mg/m² every 6 hours until the methotrexate concentration falls below the rescue value of 1×10^{-7} M (0.1 µM) or 5×10^{-8} M (0.05 µM). If methotrexate concentrations are greater than 1×10^{-6} at 48 hours, leucovorin doses should be increased to 100 mg/m² intravenous (IV) every 3 hours and continued at that dose until levels are below 1×10^{-6}, at which point leucovorin can be decreased to approximately 10 mg/m² every

---

KEY PARAMETERS: Methotrexate

Therapeutic plasma concentration	Variable
Toxic concentration	
Plasma	$>1 \times 10^{-7}$ M for $>$48 hr
	$>1 \times 10^{-6}$ M at $>$48 hr requires increased leucovorin rescue doses
CNS	Continuous CNS methotrexate concentrations $>10^{-8}$ M
F	
Dose $<$ 30 mg/m²	100%
Dose $<$ 30 mg/m²	Variable
V_i (initial)	0.2 L/kg
V AUC	0.7 L/kg
Cl	$[1.6][Cl_{Cr}]$
t½	
α[a]	3 hr
β[b]	10 hr
fu (fraction unbound in plasma)	0.5

[a]t½ of 3 hours generally employed with methotrexate plasma concentrations greater than 5×10^{-7} M.
[b]t½ of 10 hours generally employed with methotrexate plasma concentrations of less than 5×10^{-7} M.
CNS, central nervous system.

6 hours until the methotrexate concentration falls below the rescue value of 1×10^{-7} M (0.1 μM) or 5×10^{-8} M (0.05 μM).

VOLUME OF DISTRIBUTION (V)

The relationship between methotrexate plasma concentrations and volume of distribution is complex. The drug displays at least a biexponential elimination curve, indicating that there is an initial plasma volume of distribution of about 0.2 L/kg and a second larger volume of distribution of 0.5 to 1 L/kg following complete distribution.[13,14] The evaluation of the apparent volume of distribution for methotrexate is further complicated by the fact that it appears to increase at higher plasma concentrations.[13] This phenomenon may reflect an active transport system that becomes saturated at high plasma concentrations and reverts to passive intracellular diffusion of methotrexate. The multi-compartmental modeling as well as the variable relationship between the plasma concentration and apparent volume of distribution of methotrexate makes calculation of methotrexate loading doses somewhat speculative. Nevertheless, when loading doses are required, a volume of distribution of 0.2 to 0.5 L/kg is usually employed.

The presence of third-space fluids such as ascites, edema, or pleural effusions can also influence the volume of distribution of methotrexate.[15] Although pleural effusions do not substantially increase the volume of distribution, the high concentrations of methotrexate that accumulate in these spaces can be important because equilibration with plasma is delayed. In patients with pleural effusions, the initial elimination half-life appears to be normal; however, the second elimination phase is prolonged.[16] Prolongation of this terminal elimination phase is significant because the time required for patients to achieve a methotrexate plasma concentration of less than 1×10^{-7} can be extended. In this situation, additional doses and/or higher doses of leucovorin rescue factor may have to be administered beyond the usual rescue period (see Fig. 9.1, Half-life [t½], and Question 2).

CLEARANCE (Cl)

The vast majority of methotrexate is eliminated by the renal route.[16] Methotrexate clearance ranges from one to as much as two times the creatinine clearance.[10,11,13] Methotrexate clearance by an active transport mechanism that may be saturable results in a renal clearance value that varies (relative to creatinine clearance) with methotrexate plasma concentrations.[11]

The renal clearance of methotrexate is also influenced by a number of compounds (e.g., probenecid and salicylates influence weak acid secretion). In addition, sulfisoxazole and other weak acids have been reported to diminish the renal transport of methotrexate.[11,17] Proton pump inhibitors such as omeprazole have also been associated with delays in methotrexate clearance and prolong methotrexate half-life.[18] Because methotrexate renal clearance may be inhibited, all drugs should be added cautiously to the regimen of a patient receiving methotrexate therapy. Although early reports attributed salicylate-induced methotrexate toxicity to plasma protein displacement of methotrexate, the most likely mechanism is an alteration in renal clearance. An alteration in plasma binding is an unlikely explanation because methotrexate is only 50% bound to plasma proteins.[11,16]

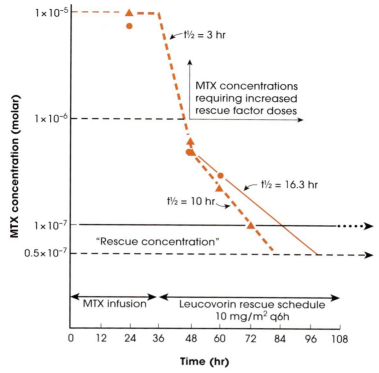

FIGURE 9.1   Methotrexate (MTX). This figure represents a semilog plot of the expected (*filled triangle*) and measured (*filled circle*) MTX plasma concentrations during and following a 36-hour infusion. Levels were obtained at 24, 48, and 60 hours after the start of the infusion. Note that leucovorin rescue should be continued as long as the MTX concentration is greater than the rescue value, represented here as either 1×10^{-7} M (0.1 µM) or 0.5×10^{-7} M (0.05 µM), and that the rescue dose should be increased for MTX levels greater than 1×10^{-6} M at 48 hours and beyond.

Changes in renal function are important when designing and monitoring methotrexate therapy. Therefore, all patients receiving moderate- and high-dose methotrexate therapy should have their plasma level of methotrexate and their renal function monitored. Although the therapeutic dose of methotrexate may range over several grams, serious toxicity and death have been attributed to doses as low as 10 mg of methotrexate when administered to a patient with inadequate renal function.[19,20]

Concomitant administration of the prostaglandin inhibitors indomethacin and ketoprofen with methotrexate has been associated with an acute decrease in renal function and a greatly prolonged exposure to high methotrexate concentrations.[21,22] This interaction presumably results from the combined renal effects of the nonsteroidal anti-inflammatory agent with methotrexate. Although this interaction has not been described for all nonsteroidal anti-inflammatory agents, these agents should be avoided in patients receiving methotrexate therapy.

A relatively small percentage of methotrexate is metabolized; nevertheless, significant amounts of methotrexate metabolites can be found in the urine when large doses are administered. This is especially true during the late phase of methotrexate elimination when the majority of the parent compound has been eliminated. The most extensively studied metabolite is the 7-hydroxy-methotrexate compound, which is considered to be potentially nephrotoxic because of its low water solubility.[11]

HALF-LIFE (t½)

The relationship between methotrexate's volume of distribution and clearance is complex. Because of the potential for capacity-limited intracellular transport and capacity-limited renal clearance, the apparent half-lives for methotrexate are determined by both a changing volume of distribution and a changing clearance. Consequently, the elimination of methotrexate is not accurately described by linear pharmacokinetic modeling. Given these problems, a relatively simple two-compartment model with an initial α half-life of 2 to 3 hours and a β or terminal half-life of approximately 10 hours appears to represent the elimination phase reasonably well.[14,16] The terminal or β half-life of approximately 10 hours often does not become apparent until plasma concentrations decline into the range of 5×10^{-7} M $(0.5 \times 10^{-6}$ or 0.5 µM). Because the terminal phase is also independent of the dose administered, it probably reflects a change in the distribution and elimination of methotrexate.

Whereas the apparent terminal half-life of methotrexate is somewhat variable, it does not appear to increase with increasing doses. Unlike most other two-compartmental drugs, significant methotrexate is eliminated during the α phase. In fact, a very large percentage of the total methotrexate dose may be eliminated during the α phase. Nevertheless, the terminal phase is also important because retention of even a very small amount of the administered dose can be potentially toxic to the patient.[14,15]

Pleural effusions or other third-space fluid collections can significantly prolong the terminal half-life of methotrexate, and leucovorin rescue regimens may need to be extended over a longer period in these situations. Some patients may unexpectedly develop acute changes in renal function or prolonged elimination characteristics that are unpredictable and independent of renal function. For this reason, continued monitoring of methotrexate is essential, even if early plasma level monitoring indicates that an adjustment of the methotrexate dose or leucovorin regimen is unnecessary.

Question #1   *P.J., a 61-year-old, 69-kg man (SCr = 1.1 mg/dL), is to receive a course of methotrexate therapy for acute lymphoblastic leukemia. His regimen will consist of a 400-mg methotrexate loading dose to be administered over 15 minutes, followed by an IV infusion of 50 mg/hr for the next 36 hours. He will then receive a 100 mg ($\approx$50 mg/m²) dose of leucovorin every 6 hours IV for the first 4 doses, followed by 8 doses orally of 20 mg ($\approx$10 mg/m²) at 6-hour intervals or until the methotrexate concentration is <0.5 × 10⁻⁷ M. The leucovorin regimen will begin immediately after the 36-hour methotrexate infusion has been discontinued and is scheduled to continue for the next 72 hours, with the last dose given 102 hours after initiation of the methotrexate therapy. Methotrexate levels are scheduled to be obtained 24 hours after the beginning of the 50-mg/hr infusion, at 48 hours (12 hours after the end of the 36-hour infusion), and at 60 hours (24 hours after the end of the methotrexate infusion). Calculate the anticipated methotrexate concentrations at the scheduled sampling times.*

Before the anticipated methotrexate concentrations can be calculated, it is first necessary to determine P.J.'s creatinine clearance, using Equation 9.2:

$$\frac{Cl_{Cr} \text{ for Males}}{(mL/\min)} = \frac{(140 - \text{Age})(\text{Weight})}{(72)(SCr_{ss})} \qquad \textbf{(Eq. 9.2)}$$

$$= \frac{(140 - 61)(69)}{(72)(1.1)}$$

$$= 68.8 \text{ mL/min}$$

The creatinine clearance of 68.8 mL/min can be converted to 4.13 L/hr:

$$\begin{aligned}
\frac{Cl_{Cr}}{(L/hr)} &= \left[\frac{Cl_{Cr}}{(mL/\min)}\right]\left[\frac{60 \text{ min/hr}}{1,000 \text{ mL/L}}\right] \\
&= [68.8 \text{ mL/min}]\left[\frac{60 \text{ min/hr}}{1,000 \text{ mL/L}}\right] \\
&= 4.13 \text{ L/hr}
\end{aligned}$$

This creatinine clearance of 4.13 L/hr can then be placed into Equation 9.3 to calculate a methotrexate clearance (Cl_{MTX}) of 6.6 L/hr.

$$Cl_{MTX} = (1.6)(Cl_{Cr}) \qquad \textbf{(Eq. 9.3)}$$

$$= [1.6][4.13 \text{ L/hr}]$$

$$= 6.6 \text{ L/hr}$$

The 24-hour concentration represents an average steady-state level. The steady-state level of methotrexate in mg/L can then be calculated by using the equation for steady-state concentration (Equation 9.4):

$$\text{Css ave} = \frac{(S)(F)(\text{Dose}/\tau)}{Cl} \qquad \textbf{(Eq. 9.4)}$$

$$= \frac{(1)(1)(50 \text{ mg}/1 \text{ hr})}{6.6 \text{ L/hr}}$$

$$= 7.6 \text{ mg/L}$$

The values of S and F were assumed to be 1, and this methotrexate concentration in mg/L can be converted to a concentration in the units of micromoles or 10^{-6} M using Equation 9.1.

$$\text{Methotrexate Concentration in } 10^{-6} \text{ molar} = \frac{\text{Methotrexate Concentration in mg/L}}{0.454}$$

$$= \frac{7.6 \text{ mg/L}}{0.454}$$

$$= 16.7 \times 10^{-6} \text{ molar or } 1.67 \times 10^{-5} \text{ molar}$$

The resultant methotrexate concentration of approximately 16.7×10^{-6} or 1.67×10^{-5} M assumes that steady state has been achieved 24 hours after the infusion rate of 50 mg/hr has been initiated. Steady state is assumed to have been achieved because the methotrexate plasma concentrations are relatively high. At concentrations greater than 10^{-7} M, a half-life of 2 to 3 hours appears to determine the elimination and accumulation of most of the methotrexate in the body. As noted earlier, this model is not consistent with the traditional view of a two-compartment model in which the terminal half-life plays an important role in the accumulation toward steady state. Although there is the possibility of some continued accumulation, this generally appears to be minor, and the use of the shorter, 2- to 3-hour, methotrexate half-life in evaluating initial methotrexate loss or accumulation is satisfactory in most cases.

Assuming the plasma concentration at the end of the 36-hour infusion is 16.7×10^{-6} M, a plasma concentration of 1.04×10^{-6} M (10.4×10^{-7} M) at 48 hours (or 12 hours after the infusion has been discontinued) can be calculated using Equation 9.5.

$$C_2 = C_1(e^{-Kt}) \qquad \textbf{(Eq. 9.5)}$$

C_1 is the methotrexate plasma concentration at the end of the infusion, and t is the 12-hour time interval spanning from the end of the 36-hour infusion to the time of sampling at 48 hours. K is the elimination rate constant calculated from a rearrangement of the equation for t½ (Equation 9.6) and using the shorter elimination half-life of 3 hours.

$$t\tfrac{1}{2} = \frac{0.693}{K} \qquad \textbf{(Eq. 9.6)}$$

$$K = \frac{0.693}{t\,\frac{1}{2}} \tag{Eq. 9.7}$$

$$K = \frac{0.693}{t\,\frac{1}{2}}$$
$$= \frac{0.693}{3\ hr}$$
$$= 0.231\ hr^{-1}$$
$$C_2 = C_1(e^{-Kt})$$
$$C_2 = (16.7 \times 10^{-6}\ molar)(e^{-(0.231\ hr^{-1})(12\ hr)})$$
$$= (16.7 \times 10^{-6}\ molar)(0.0625)$$
$$= 1.04 \times 10^{-6}\ molar\ or\ 10.4 \times 10^{-7}\ molar$$

Because this methotrexate concentration is 1×10^{-6} M 48 hours after starting the methotrexate therapy, the leucovorin rescue dose does not have to be increased. The planned leucovorin rescue schedule should be continued until the concentration falls to 0.5×10^{-7}.

Calculation of the methotrexate concentration 60 hours after the infusion has been initiated (24 hours after the infusion has been concluded) is more problematic. The half-life for methotrexate tends to increase as the methotrexate concentration approaches 0.2 to 0.7×10^{-6} M (2 to 7×10^{-7} M). Therefore, the use of a traditional two-compartment model for this drug is inappropriate because the more prolonged terminal half-life correlates more closely with a specific concentration range than with a specific time interval following discontinuation of the infusion. This unusual phenomenon may be related to a change in the active transport system that is influenced by plasma concentration.

One technique that is used to predict methotrexate concentrations several hours after the infusion has been discontinued is to decay the methotrexate concentration to a range of 0.2 to 0.7×10^{-6} M using a half-life of 3 hours. The longer or β half-life of 10 hours is then used to predict subsequent decay. If a plasma concentration of 0.5×10^{-6} is arbitrarily selected as the cutoff concentration for using a half-life of 3 hours, the time required for the initial decay can be calculated using Equation 9.8:

$$t = \frac{\ln\left(\dfrac{C_1}{C_2}\right)}{K} \tag{Eq. 9.8}$$

C_1 represents the initial plasma concentration of 16.7×10^{-6} M, C_2 the arbitrary cutoff plasma concentration of 0.5×10^{-6} M, and K the elimination rate constant corresponding to the initial half-life of 3 hours (0.231 hr^{-1}). Using Equation 9.8, the time (t) required for the methotrexate concentration to fall to 0.5×10^{-6} M would be

15.2 hours after the end of the infusion or 51.2 hours after the methotrexate regimen is begun:

$$t = \frac{\ln\left(\dfrac{16.7 \times 10^{-6} \text{ molar}}{0.5 \times 10^{-6} \text{ molar}}\right)}{0.231 \text{ hr}^{-1}}$$

$$= \frac{3.5}{0.231 \text{ hr}^{-1}}$$

$$= 15.2 \text{ hr}$$

To calculate the plasma concentration at 60 hours, the plasma level at 51.2 hours (36-hour infusion + 15.2-hour decay) would have to be decayed for an additional 8.8 hours. In this case, however, the elimination rate constant that corresponds to the terminal elimination half-life of 10 hours would be used (Equation 9.7).

$$K = \frac{0.693}{t\frac{1}{2}}$$

$$= \frac{0.693}{10 \text{ hr}}$$

$$= 0.0693 \text{ hr}^{-1}$$

Using these values and the equation for first-order elimination of a drug from the body (Equation 9.5), a methotrexate concentration of 2.7×10^{-7} M at 60 hours can be calculated.

$$C_2 = C_1(e^{-Kt})$$

$$= (0.5 \times 10^{-6} \text{ molar})(e^{-(0.0693 \text{ hr}^{-1})(8.8 \text{ hr})})$$

$$= 0.27 \times 10^{-6} \text{ molar or } 2.7 \times 10^{-7} \text{ molar}$$

These calculations suggest that an additional 24 hours will be required to decay the concentration to 0.5×10^{-7} M:

$$t = \frac{\ln\left(\dfrac{0.27 \times 10^{-6} \text{ molar}}{0.05 \times 10^{-6} \text{ molar}}\right)}{0.6931 \text{ hr}^{-1}}$$

$$= \frac{1.68}{0.0693 \text{ hr}^{-1}}$$

$$= 24 \text{ hr}$$

Because this concentration will decay to a concentration below 0.5×10^{-7} (0.05 µM) (the rescue value) in a little more than two half-lives, it would appear from our calculations that P.J. will have been rescued by leucovorin successfully.

Therefore, the rescue concentration will be achieved before leucovorin is scheduled to be discontinued. Nevertheless, these predicted concentrations are only approximations and cannot replace the measured methotrexate concentrations. A graphic representation of the expected methotrexate concentrations (filled triangle) is plotted in Figure 9.1. Unless there is a dramatic increase in the methotrexate half-life, the concentration will be well below 1×10^{-7} M long before the leucovorin is scheduled to be discontinued.

Question #2   *P.J.'s methotrexate levels were reported as 13.5×10^{-6} M at 24 hours, 0.83×10^{-6} M (8.3×10^{-7} M) at 48 hours, and 0.44×10^{-6} M (4.4×10^{-7} M) at 60 hours. How would one interpret each of these methotrexate values? What would be an appropriate course of action regarding P.J.'s rescue therapy?*

The initial plasma concentration of 13.5×10^{-6} is lower than the predicted concentration calculated in Question 1 (16.7×10^{-6} M). The lower-than-predicted concentration suggests that P.J.'s methotrexate clearance is greater than expected; however, the difference between the predicted and actual concentrations is well within the expected variation.

The plasma level of 8.3×10^{-7} M at 48 hours (12 hours after the end of the infusion) suggests that P.J. is progressing as expected during the initial elimination phase. The difference between the expected (10.4×10^{-7} M) and the observed concentrations is minimal, considering the fact that the initial plasma level was slightly lower than predicted (see Fig. 9.1). Because the observed plasma level is below 1×10^{-6} M at 48 hours, it is unnecessary to increase the leucovorin dose.

The measured methotrexate concentration of 4.4×10^{-7} M ($0.44\ \mu$M) at 60 hours is greater than the predicted concentration of 2.7×10^{-7} M ($0.27\ \mu$M). Although the differences are not remarkable, it is of some concern that P.J.'s half-life is longer than anticipated. P.J.'s elimination rate constant of $0.053\ \mathrm{hr}^{-1}$ can be calculated using these two methotrexate concentrations, the time interval between the concentrations, and rearranging Equation 9.8 to form Equation 9.9.

$$K = \frac{\ln\left(\dfrac{C_1}{C_2}\right)}{t} \qquad \textbf{(Eq. 9.9)}$$

$$t = \frac{\ln\left(\dfrac{8.3 \times 10^{-7}\ \text{molar}}{4.4 \times 10^{-7}\ \text{molar}}\right)}{12\ \text{hr}}$$

$$= \frac{0.63}{12\ \text{hr}}$$

$$= 0.053\ \mathrm{hr}^{-1}$$

P.J.'s corresponding methotrexate t½ of 13.1 hours can be calculated using the K value of 0.053 hr^{-1} and Equation 9.6.

$$t\frac{1}{2} = \frac{0.693}{K}$$
$$= \frac{0.693}{0.053\ hr^{-1}}$$
$$= 13.1\ hr$$

Although the increased methotrexate half-life appears to be substantial, the accuracy of the half-life calculation is uncertain because the plasma levels used are separated by a time interval that is less than one half-life. The increase in this terminal half-life of methotrexate could be attributed to any of the following: an assay error, accumulation of methotrexate in a pleural effusion or other third-space fluid, a drug-induced reduction in the renal clearance of methotrexate (e.g., salicylates), or a normal variance in methotrexate elimination. If this is the result of pleural effusion or third-space fluids, one would expect slower elimination, without a significant decrease in levels. Often in the case of pleural effusion, levels may fluctuate because of the redistribution of the methotrexate between the third-space fluid and intravascular circulation. One would need to continue to give leucovorin rescue and monitor levels until methotrexate levels drop below 0.05 μM. In addition, there may be times when methotrexate will cause an increase in serum creatinine. This may delay methotrexate clearance. Again, one would continue leucovorin rescue and monitor levels until methotrexate levels drop below 0.05 μM.

Regardless of the cause, it is important to determine whether P.J. will achieve a plasma concentration of less than 0.5×10^{-7} M by the time the leucovorin rescue is scheduled to be discontinued. Using the patient-specific or revised elimination rate constant of 0.053 hr^{-1} and Equation 9.8, it appears as though P.J.'s methotrexate concentration will fall to 0.5×10^{-7} M after another 41 hours (101 hours after starting the methotrexate therapy). This is just at the time scheduled for the last dose of leucovorin (102 hours after starting the methotrexate infusion).

$$t = \frac{\ln\left(\dfrac{C_1}{C_2}\right)}{K}$$
$$= \frac{\ln\left(\dfrac{4.4 \times 10^{-7}\ molar}{0.5 \times 10^{-7}\ molar}\right)}{0.053\ hr^{-1}}$$
$$= \frac{2.17}{0.053\ hr^{-1}}$$
$$= 41\ hr^{-1}$$

This calculation should not be used as the sole criterion for evaluating the success of rescue therapy because the elimination rate constant calculation is uncertain, and the methotrexate terminal half-life may become more prolonged as the plasma concentration declines. In this particular case, additional methotrexate plasma levels should be obtained to ensure that the actual plasma concentration is below the critical value of 0.5×10^{-7} before leucovorin rescue is discontinued. If this critical value has not been achieved by 102 hours, then additional doses of leucovorin will have to be administered until P.J. has achieved a plasma level below 0.5×10^{-7} M (see Fig. 9.1). Note that the observed methotrexate levels suggest that P.J. has a more prolonged terminal half-life.

Busulfan

Busulfan is a bifunctional alkylating agent that kills dividing cells by forming DNA cross-links. When the resulting DNA damage cannot be repaired, cells undergo pro-grammed cell death or apoptosis. Busulfan is especially toxic to hematopoietic cells in bone marrow and was originally introduced as a treatment for patients with chronic myelogenous leukemia.[23] Owing to its potent myelosuppressive effects, busulfan is commonly used in bone marrow ablative regimens given before hematopoietic stem cell transplantation (HSCT). Busulfan is typically used in combination with other marrow ablative agents such as radiation, cyclophosphamide, melphalan, or fludarabine. Busul-fan was originally only available as an oral tablet, and the parental formulation did not come on the market until long after its role in HSCT conditioning had been established. The dosage of busulfan most often used in adults undergoing HSCT is 0.8 mg/kg IV or 1 mg/kg orally given every 6 hours for 4 days (12 or 16 mg/kg total dose). IV busulfan is also given on a once-daily schedule at a dose of 3.2 mg/kg/day. IV administration is now the preferred route because of the high incidence of emesis that occurs with oral dosing, often requiring error prone estimation and replacement of the vomited tablets. Variability in busulfan systemic exposure and identification of a strong correlation between drug concentrations and both toxicity and therapeutic outcome in patients undergoing HSCT have led to the routine use of TDM.

UNITS

Busulfan is administered in milligram doses, and the plasma concentrations are typically reported in units of mcg/L or μM. To interpret busulfan concentrations accurately, it is critically important to know which units are being reported and how those units correspond to the therapeutic ranges being targeted. Busulfan has a molecular weight of 246 g/mol. Therefore, a value of 246 mcg/L is equal to 1×10^{-6} M or 1 μM. To con-vert busulfan concentrations in units of mcg/L to μM concentrations, the following equation can be used:

$$\text{Busulfan conc (μM)} = \text{Busulfan conc (mcg/L)/246 mcg/μmol} \qquad \textbf{(Eq. 9.10)}$$

TARGET PLASMA CONCENTRATIONS

Hepatic veno-occlusive disease (VOD) is a common life-threatening complication resulting from the chemo-ablative regimens used in HSCT, occurring in 20% to 40% of patients.[24,25] VOD results from injury to small veins and sinusoids of the liver, followed by deposition of protein aggregates that progressively block venous outflow, leading to intrahepatic hypertension. Clinically, VOD is characterized by jaundice, weight gain, ascites, and painful swelling of the liver. Mortality rates as a result of VOD range from 20% to 50%. A first dose busulfan AUC > 1,500 µmol/L · min has been linked to an increased risk of VOD.[24] Others using the average busulfan plasma concentration (C ave) as a measure of drug exposure have demonstrated that a C ave >900 mcg/L also results in an increased risk of VOD.[26] To convert the busulfan AUC to C ave, one must first convert the AUC value to units of mcg/L · hr and then divide the AUC by the dosing interval (τ) using Equation 9.11.

$$\text{Busulfan C ave (mcg/L)} = \text{Busulfan AUC (mcg/L} \cdot \text{hr)}/\tau \qquad \textbf{(Eq. 9.11)}$$

In addition to the relationship between higher exposures and toxicity, it has been demonstrated that lower busulfan exposures are associated with poorer outcomes following HSCT. Patients with busulfan AUC of <800 µmol/L · min or C ave of <600 mcg/L have a higher rate of disease relapse and engraftment failure.[26,27] Therefore, the accepted therapeutic window for busulfan when given every 6 hours for 16 doses is a first dose AUC of 900 to 1,500 µM · min or a C ave of 600 to 900 mcg/L. Although the optimal therapeutic window for once-daily busulfan has yet to be determined, most transplant centers are using an AUC range of 900 to 1,500 µM · min, which is equivalent to four times the AUC range on an every 6-hour dosing schedule.[28]

TIME TO SAMPLE

For determination of the busulfan plasma AUC, the timing for collection of samples depends on the route of administration. Following an oral dose, blood samples are collected at 15 and 30 minutes, 1, 1.5, 2, 3, 4, 5, and 6 hours following administration. Following an IV dose, samples are collected immediately before the end of the 2-hour infusion and then 15 and 30 minutes, 3, 4, 5, and 6 hours after the end of the infusion. Additional samples are required with oral dosing because of the unpredictability of oral absorption and the importance of collecting samples around the Cmax for accurate determination of the AUC. Approaches utilizing as few as two timed blood samples have been suggested for patients receiving IV busulfan; however, these limited samples strategies have not yet been validated in prospective clinical trials. Plasma is separated from whole blood, and the complete set of samples is sent to the lab for analysis. Although some transplant centers have the capability for onsite testing, many do not. There can be a 12- to 24-hour delay between the time that the samples are collected and the time the results are available. As a result, an additional two to four doses of busulfan must be given before an adjustment can be made. Because of this, some transplant centers prefer to use a test dose strategy whereby a low, subtherapeutic dose of busulfan is given before the start of the full dose regimen for prediction of busulfan pharmacokinetics.[29,30]

BUSULFAN ASSAYS

Analysis of busulfan in plasma is commonly performed using gas chromatography–mass spectrometric detection (GC–MS). GC methods require that busulfan in plasma be derivatized so that it becomes volatile enough to enter the gas phase and fly through the capillary column. Electrochemical detection is also an option but requires longer run times owing to the less selective nature of the detection method. More recently, liquid chromatography combined with tandem mass spectrometry (LC–MS/MS) has been used to measure busulfan. LC–MS/MS analysis does not require derivatization and is significantly more sensitive than GC-based methods. The major disadvantage is that LC–MS/MS instruments are significantly more expensive to purchase and maintain.

METHODS FOR ESTIMATING BUSULFAN AREA UNDER CURVE

Both noncompartmental and model-derived methods are used for the determination of busulfan AUC.[31] Noncompartmental data analysis relies on the rule of linear trapezoids and does not require special curve-fitting software. Programs that are available on almost every computer, such as Excel, can be used to calculate the AUC. Furthermore, noncompartmental analysis is the preferred approach in cases where the plasma concentration-versus-time data are erratic, for example, when the oral absorption is unpredictable. Because the target therapeutic ranges are based on the AUC extrapolated to infinity, the portion of the AUC after the last measured time point must also be calculated using the terminal elimination rate constant derived from the last two to three sample measurements. The equation (9.12) for calculating the AUC of busulfan using the trapezoidal rule is as follows:

$$AUC_{trapezoidal} = \sum_{i=0}^{n-1} \frac{(t_i + 1 - t_i)(C_i + 1 + C_i)}{2} + \frac{C_{last}}{\lambda} \qquad \textbf{(Eq. 9.12)}$$

where t_i and C_i are the times and concentrations at the ith time point. The terminal elimination rate constant for extrapolating to infinity is calculated using formula 9.13:

$$\lambda = \frac{\ln(C_{last} - 1)) - \ln(C_{last})}{t(last) - t(last - 1)} \qquad \textbf{(Eq. 9.13)}$$

Model-derived approaches depend on software packages such as ADAPT and WinNonlin. Busulfan disposition is best described by a one-compartment first-order elimination model. Figure 9.2 shows a concentration-versus-time data set from a patient receiving IV busulfan. The actual data points are depicted by the open triangles, and the smooth curve was generated using ADAPT.

BIOAVAILABILITY (F)

The availability of an IV busulfan formulation has made it possible to determine its absolute bioavailability, which has been reported to be 80%.[26,32,33] Busulfan is rapidly

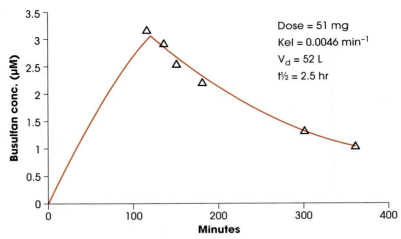

FIGURE 9.2   Busulfan. This figure is a typical busulfan plasma concentration-versus-time curve following an IV dose of 0.8 mg/kg infused over 120 minutes. The symbols (*open triangle*) indicate the measured plasma concentration at 115, 135, 150, 180, 300, and 360 minutes, and the line represents the best-fit curve generated using ADAPT software.

KEY PARAMETERS: Busulfan

Therapeutic plasma concentrations	
Q6h dosing	$AUC_{0-\infty} = 900 - 1{,}500\ \mu M \cdot min$
	or C ave $= 600 - 900$ mcg/L
Q24h dosing[a]	$AUC_{0-\infty} = 3{,}600 - 6{,}000\ \mu M \cdot min$
F	80%
V/F	
Adults and children >4 yr	0.6–1.0 L/kg
Children <4 yr	1.4–1.6 L/kg
Cl/F	
Adults and children >4 yr	2.5–4.5 mL/min/kg
Children <4 yr	6.8–8.4 mL/min/kg
t½	2.5–3.0 hr
Adults and children >4 yr	2.5–3.0 hr
Children <4 yr	1.5–2.0 hr
fu (fraction unbound in plasma)	0.6–0.7

[a]The optimal range for once-daily dosing has not yet been determined. A range of 3,600 to 6,000 µM · min has been proposed because it is equivalent to 4 times the range established for the every 6-hour dosing schedule.

absorbed with peak plasma drug concentrations occurring between 1.5 and 2.5 hours after an oral dose, with more rapid absorption after administration of crushed tablets. There are no known food–drug interactions for busulfan, although patients are advised not to eat or drink anything 1 hour before and 1 hour after each oral dose. Approximately 25% of patients experience delayed absorption or prolonged elimination of oral busulfan. In some cases, plasma concentrations can continue to increase throughout the entire 6-hour dosing interval, making it impossible to determine a terminal elimination rate constant. In such cases, the mean population terminal elimination rate constant is used to extrapolate the AUC to infinity.

VOLUME OF DISTRIBUTION

The mean volume of distribution (**V**) after administration of an IV dose of busulfan is 0.8 L/kg in adults and 1.5 L/kg in very young children.[26,32,33] There is no difference in the V_d of busulfan in older children versus adults. Age-related differences in busulfan disposition are possibly because of the larger liver volume normalized to body weight in younger children, which could explain the need for higher doses of drugs that are primarily cleared by the liver, such as busulfan, when they are dosed on a milligram per kilogram basis in very young children.

When calculating the dose of busulfan in an obese patient, it is recommended that the dose be based on an adjusted ideal body weight (IBW) calculated using the ABW25 equation[34]:

$$\text{Adjusted IBW} = \text{IBW} + (0.25 \times (\text{ABW} - \text{IBW}))\qquad \textbf{(Eq. 9.14)}$$

Approximately 30% of the drug is irreversibly bound to plasma proteins. The erythrocyte to plasma ratio of busulfan is 1.05. Busulfan freely distributes into the cerebrospinal fluid (CSF), with CSF concentrations approximating those in the plasma, accounting for why some patients experience seizures after high doses.[35]

CLEARANCE (Cl)

There are also age-related differences in busulfan Cl between very young children versus older children and adults. The Cl of busulfan in children older than 4 years and adults is in the range of 2.5 to 4.5 mL/min/kg, whereas Cl in children less than 4 years ranges from 6.8 to 8.4 mL/min/kg.[26,32,33] Cl is independent of dose up to a daily IV dose of 3.2 mg/kg. Excretion of unchanged busulfan in the urine is very low (1% to 2%), and the majority of busulfan is eliminated through hepatic metabolism via glutathione conjugation predominantly via GSTA1 with minor contributions from GSTM1 and GSTP1.[36] Children have been shown to conjugate busulfan more efficiently than adults, which likely explains the larger apparent V_d/F and faster clearance in very young children compared to older children and adults.

HALF-LIFE (t½)

The elimination half-life of busulfan in adults and older children ranges from 2.5 to 3.0 hours. In children less than 4 years, the range is between 1.5 and 2.0 hours.[26,32,33]

Question #3   *R.C., a 43-year-old, 82-kg woman (IBW = 58 kg), is receiving a course of busulfan and cyclophosphamide as her pretransplant conditioning regimen for acute myelogenous leukemia. The regimen includes 0.8 mg/kg of IV busulfan given every 6 hours for a total of 16 doses. Each busulfan dose is administered over 120 minutes, and serial blood samples are collected around the first dose for determination of the busulfan AUC. Calculate the correct starting dose for R.C.*

Because R.C. is obese, it is recommended that her starting busulfan dose be calculated on the basis of an adjusted IBW using the ABW25 Equation 9.14:

$$\text{Adjusted IBW} = \text{IBW} + (0.25 \times (\text{ABW} - \text{IBW}))$$

$$= 58 + (0.25[82 - 58 \text{ kg}])$$

$$= 64 \text{ kg}$$

According to the ABW25 equation, R.C.'s adjusted IBW is 64 kg. Therefore, the correct starting dose for R.C. would be 0.8 mg/kg × 64 kg or 51 mg.

Question #4   *The results of the analysis of her busulfan levels came back from the lab and are shown in the following table. First, calculate the busulfan AUC using the rule of linear trapezoids; then using the pharmacokinetic parameters from Figure 9.2, calculate the model-derived AUC.*

TIME (min)	BUSULFAN (μM)
115	3.18
135	2.93
150	2.56
180	2.22
300	1.34
360	1.04

The busulfan AUC can be calculated using the rule of linear trapezoids (Equation 9.12):

$$\text{AUC}_{\text{trapezoidal}} = \sum_{i=0}^{n-1} \frac{(t_i + 1 - t_i)(C_i + 1 + C_i)}{2} + \frac{C_{\text{last}}}{\lambda}$$

Based on the first term in the equation, the AUC from time zero to the time of the last busulfan measurement is 642 µM · min.

$$AUC_{0-360\ mins} = \frac{(0 + 3.18\ \mu M)(115.18\ ns)}{2} + \frac{(2.93 + 3.18\ \mu M)(1,353 + 3.18\ ns)}{2}$$

$$+ \frac{(2.56 + 2.93\ \mu M)(1,506 + 2.93\ ns)}{2} + \frac{(2.22 + 2.56\ \mu M)(1,802 + 2.56\ ns)}{2}$$

$$+ \frac{(1.34 + 2.22\ \mu M)(3,004 + 2.22\ ns)}{2} + \frac{(1.04 + 1.34\ \mu M)(3,604 + 1.34\ ns)}{2}$$

$$= (182.9 + 61.1 + 41.2 + 71.7 + 213.6 + 71.4)$$

$$= 642\ \mu M \cdot min.$$

To extrapolate the AUC to infinity, the terminal elimination rate constant is calculated according to Equation 9.13:

$$\lambda = \frac{\ln(C_{last} - 1) - \ln(C_{last})}{t(last) - t(last - 1)}$$

$$\lambda = \frac{\ln(1.34\ \mu M) - \ln(1.04\ \mu M)}{360 - 300\ min}$$

The calculated λ for R.C. is 0.0042 min^{-1}. When the last measured busulfan concentration is divided by λ and added to the first term in the trapezoidal rule, the AUC equation results in a final AUC$_{trapezoidal}$ estimate extrapolated to infinity of 890 µM · min.

$$AUC_{360-\infty} = \frac{C_{last}}{\lambda}$$

$$= \frac{1.04\ \mu M}{0.0042\ min^{-1}}$$

$$= 248\ \mu M/min$$

$$AUC_{0-\infty} = 642 + 248 = 890\ \mu M/min$$

The busulfan AUC$_{0-\infty}$ can also be calculated using the model-derived parameters provided in Figure 9.2 according to the following equations:

$$AUC_{0-\infty} = \frac{Dose}{Cl}$$

$$Cl = Vd \times \lambda$$

To be consistent with the AUC$_{trapezoidal}$, the busulfan dose of 51 mg must first be converted to units of micromoles by multiplying by 1,000 mcg/mg and dividing by the busulfan molecular weight of 246 mcg/µmol. This conversion results in a busulfan dose of 207.3 µmol.

$$\text{Busulfan Dose}\left(\mu M\right) = \frac{(\text{Dose in mg})(1,000\ \mu/\text{mg})}{246\ \mu g/\mu mol}$$

$$= \frac{(51\ \text{mg})(1,000\ \mu/\text{mg})}{246\ \mu g/\mu mol}$$

$$= 207.3\ \mu mol$$

Using the busulfan dose in µmole and substituting V × K_{el} in Figure 9.2 for Cl, the model-derived $AUC_{0-\infty}$ estimate for R.C. is 867 µM · min.

$$AUC_{0-\infty} = \frac{D\left(\mu moles\right)}{\left(K\right)\left(V\right)}$$

$$= \frac{207.3\ \mu moles}{\left(0.0046\ min^{-1}\right)\left(52\ L\right)}$$

$$= 867\ \mu M \cdot min$$

Question #5　*R.C.'s hematologist wants to target an AUC of 1,200 µM · min. What dose would you recommend? The hematologist is also considering targeting an average plasma concentration (C ave) of 750 mcg/L instead of AUC. What is R.C.'s first dose busulfan C ave, and what would be the expected Css if you were to change the dose as calculated above?*

Using the $AUC_{trapezoidal}$ of 890 µM · min measured following a dose of 51 mg, one can calculate the dose expected to result in an AUC of 1,200 µM · min by using the following equation (Equation 9.15);

$$\text{Adjusted Dose (mg)} = \text{First Dose (mg)} \times \frac{AUC\left(\text{Target}\right)}{AUC(\text{First Dose})} \qquad \textbf{(Eq. 9.15)}$$

$$= 51\ \text{mg}\left(\frac{1,200\ \mu M \cdot min}{890\ \mu M \cdot min}\right)$$

This results in a recommended adjusted busulfan dose of 69 mg.

To determine the first dose busulfan Css, one must first convert the $AUC_{trapezoidal}$ in units of $\mu M \cdot min$ to units of mcg/L $\cdot$ hr by multiplying 890 $\mu mol/L \cdot min$ by 246 mcg/μmol and dividing by 60 min/hr, which results in a $AUC_{trapezoidal}$ of 3,649 mcg/L $\cdot$ hr.

$$AUC_{trapezoidal}\ (\mu g/L \cdot hr) = \frac{AUC_{trapezoidal}\ (\mu M \cdot min)(246\ \mu g/\mu mol)}{60\ min/hr}$$

$$= \frac{(890\ \mu M \cdot min)(246\ \mu g/\mu mol)}{60\ min/hr}$$

$$= 3{,}649\ mcg/L \cdot hr$$

The Css can then be calculated using Equation 9.11, where the dosing interval τ is equal to 6 hours:

$$\textbf{Busulfan Css (mcg/L)} = \textbf{Busulfan AUC (mcg/L} \cdot \textbf{hr)}/\tau$$

$$= \frac{3{,}649\ \textbf{mcg/L} \cdot \textbf{hr}}{6\ \textbf{hr}}$$

$$= 608\ \textbf{mcg/L,}$$

resulting in a first dose busulfan Css estimate of 608 mcg/L. Increasing the busulfan dose to 69 mg, one would expect a new Css of 608 mcg/L $\times \frac{69\ mg}{51\ mg}$, or 823 mcg/L. If the hematologist truly wants to target a busulfan Css of 750 mcg/L instead of an AUC of 1,200 $\mu M \cdot min$, an adjusted busulfan dose of 51 mg $\times \frac{750\ mcg/L}{608\ mcg/L}$, or 63 mg would be more appropriate.

ACKNOWLEDGMENT

The important work of Courtney Yuen to a previous version of this chapter is acknowledged.

REFERENCES

1. Masson E, Zamboni WC. Pharmacokinetic optimisation of cancer chemotherapy: effect on outcomes. *Clin Pharmacokinet.* 1997;32:324–343.

2. Du Bois D, Du Bois EF. A formula to estimate the approximate surface area if height and weight be known. 1916. *Nutrition.* 1989;5:303–311; discussion 312–303.

3. Egorin MJ, Van Echo DA, Olman EA, et al. Prospective validation of a pharmacologically based dosing scheme for the cis-diamminedichloroplatinum(II) analogue diamminecyclobutanedicarboxylatoplatinum. *Cancer Res.* 1985;45:6502–6506.

4. Calvert AH, Newell DR, Gumbrell LA, et al. Carboplatin dosage: prospective evaluation of a simple formula based on renal function. *J Clin Oncol.* 1989;7:1748–1756.

5. Evans WE, Relling MV, Rodman JH, et al. Conventional compared with individualized chemotherapy for childhood acute lymphoblastic leukemia. *N Engl J Med.* 1998;338:499–505.

6. van den Bongard HJ, Mathot RA, Beijnen JH, et al. Pharmacokinetically guided administration of chemotherapeutic agents. *Clin Pharmacokinet.* 2000;39:345–367.

7. Paci A, Veal G, Bardin C, et al. Review of therapeutic drug monitoring of anticancer drugs part 1–cytotoxics. *Eur J Cancer.* 2014;50:2010–2019.

8. Wan SH, Huffman DH, Azarnoff DL, et al. Effect of route of administration and effusions on methotrexate pharmacokinetics. *Cancer Res.* 1974;34:3487–3491.

9. Bleyer WA. Methotrexate: clinical pharmacology, current status and therapeutic guidelines. *Cancer Treat Rev.* 1977;4:87–101.

10. Bleyer WA. The clinical pharmacology of methotrexate: new applications of an old drug. *Cancer.* 1978;41:36–51.

11. Shen DD, Azarnoff DL. Clinical pharmacokinetics of methotrexate. *Clin Pharmacokinet.* 1978;3:1–13.

12. Stoller RG, Hande KR, Jacobs SA, et al. Use of plasma pharmacokinetics to predict and prevent methotrexate toxicity. *N Engl J Med*. 1977;297:630–634.

13. Leme PR, Creaven PJ, Allen LM, et al. Kinetic model for the disposition and metabolism of moderate and high-dose methotrexate (NSC-740) in man. *Cancer Chemother Rep*. 1975;59:811–817.

14. Pratt CB, Howarth C, Ransom JL, et al. High-dose methotrexate used alone and in combination for measurable primary or metastatic osteosarcoma. *Cancer Treat Rep*. 1980;64:11–20.

15. Evans WE, Pratt CB. Effect of pleural effusion on high-dose methotrexate kinetics. *Clin Pharmacol Ther*. 1978;23:68–72.

16. Isacoff WH, Morrison PF, Aroesty J, et al. Pharmacokinetics of high-dose methotrexate with citrovorum factor rescue. *Cancer Treat Rep*. 1977;61:1665–1674.

17. Liegler DG, Henderson ES, Hahn MA, et al. The effect of organic acids on renal clearance of methotrexate in man. *Clin Pharmacol Ther*. 1969;10:849–857.

18. Beorlegui B, Aldaz A, Ortega A, et al. Potential interaction between methotrexate and omeprazole. *Ann Pharmacother*. 2000;34:1024–1027.

19. Cadman EC, Lundberg WB, Bertino JR. Systemic methotrexate toxicity: a pharmacological study of its occurrence after intrathecal administration in a patient with renal failure. *Arch Intern Med*. 1976;136:1321–1322.

20. Ahmad S, Shen FH, Bleyer WA. Methotrexate-induced renal failure and ineffectiveness of peritoneal dialysis. *Arch Intern Med*. 1978;138:1146–1147.

21. Ellison NM, Servi RJ. Acute renal failure and death following sequential intermediate-dose methotrexate and 5-FU: a possible adverse effect due to concomitant indomethacin administration. *Cancer Treat Rep*. 1985;69:342–343.

22. Thyss A, Milano G, Kubar J, et al. Clinical and pharmacokinetic evidence of a life-threatening interaction between methotrexate and ketoprofen. *Lancet*. 1986;1:256–258.

23. Jones RJ, Grochow LB. Pharmacology of bone marrow transplantation conditioning regimens. *Ann N Y Acad Sci*. 1995;770:237–241.

24. Grochow LB, Jones RJ, Brundrett RB, et al. Pharmacokinetics of busulfan: correlation with veno-occlusive disease in patients undergoing bone marrow transplantation. *Cancer Chemother Pharmacol*. 1989;25:55–61.

25. Vassal G, Koscielny S, Challine D, et al. Busulfan disposition and hepatic veno-occlusive disease in children undergoing bone marrow transplantation. *Cancer Chemother Pharmacol*. 1996;37:247–253.

26. McCune JS, Gibbs JP, Slattery JT. Plasma concentration monitoring of busulfan: does it improve clinical outcome? *Clin Pharmacokinet*. 2000;39:155–165.

27. McCune JS, Gooley T, Gibbs JP, et al. Busulfan concentration and graft rejection in pediatric patients undergoing hematopoietic stem cell transplantation. *Bone Marrow Transplant*. 2002;30:167–173.

28. Madden T, de Lima M, Thapar N, et al. Pharmacokinetics of once-daily IV busulfan as part of pretransplantation preparative regimens: a comparison with an every 6-hour dosing schedule. *Biol Blood Marrow Transplant*. 2007;13:56–64.

29. Takamatsu Y, Sasaki N, Eto T, et al. Individual dose adjustment of oral busulfan using a test dose in hematopoietic stem cell transplantation. *Int J Hematol*. 2007;86:261–268.

30. Kangarloo SB, Naveed F, Ng ES, et al. Development and validation of a test dose strategy for once-daily i.v. busulfan: importance of fixed infusion rate dosing. *Biol Blood Marrow Transplant*. 2012;18:295–301.

31. Olson MT, Lombardi L, Clarke W. Clinical consequences of analytical variance and calculation strategy in oral busulfan pharmacokinetics. *Clin Chim Acta*. 2011;412:2316–2321.

32. Hassan M, Ljungman P, Bolme P, et al. Busulfan bioavailability. *Blood*. 1994;84:2144–2150.

33. Hassan M. The role of busulfan in bone marrow transplantation. *Med Oncol*. 1999;16:166–176.

34. Bubalo J, Carpenter PA, Majhail N, et al. Conditioning chemotherapy dose adjustment in obese patients: a review and position statement by the American Society for Blood and Marrow Transplantation practice guideline committee. *Biol Blood Marrow Transplant*. 2014;20:600–616.

35. Caselli D, Rosati A, Faraci M, et al. Risk of seizures in children receiving busulphan-containing regimens for stem cell transplantation. *Biol Blood Marrow Transplant*. 2014;20:282–285.

36. Czerwinski M, Gibbs JP, Slattery JT. Busulfan conjugation by glutathione S-transferases alpha, mu, and pi. *Drug Metab Dispos*. 1996;24:1015–1019.

10

DIGOXIN

Maureen S. Boro

Learning Objectives

By the end of the digoxin chapter, the learner shall be able to:

1. State the digoxin target concentrations/therapeutic endpoint for patients with congestive heart failure versus atrial fibrillation.
2. Explain why digoxin concentrations should not be sampled soon after an intravenous dose or an oral dose, and why early digoxin plasma concentrations do not reflect the drug's potential for efficacy or toxicity.
3. List patient factors, disease states, and other drugs that alter digoxin volume of distribution and/or clearance and know how to take the factor(s) into account when determining a patient's pharmacokinetic parameters.
4. Explain the effect of renal function on the maintenance dose and loading dose of digoxin.
5. Identify in a case history, possible explanations why a patient may have an elevated or a subtherapeutic digoxin concentration.
6. Determine whether digoxin is expected to be significantly removed by dialysis, using the principles in Chapter 3: Dialysis of Drugs: Estimating Drug Dialyzability.
7. Revise the patient's digoxin clearance, and determine an appropriate revised maintenance dose, given a steady-state digoxin concentration and patient history.
8. List the three conditions necessary when using the mass balance approach for determining digoxin clearance in a patient with two non–steady-state digoxin concentrations.
9. List the criteria for when DigiFab would be indicated and, given a measured digoxin concentration, calculate the required DigiFab dose.
10. Discuss digoxin assay issues concerning the potential for drug interference, endogenous digoxin-like compound, and following the administration of digoxin.

Digoxin is an inotropic agent primarily used to treat congestive heart failure (CHF) and atrial fibrillation. It is incompletely absorbed and, once absorbed, a substantial fraction is cleared by the kidneys. In the acute care setting, historically digoxin loading doses of ≈1 mg/70 kg were administered before the initiation of the usual maintenance dose of 0.125 to 0.25 mg/day. These loading and maintenance doses were from an era when target levels were 1 to 2 mcg/L, and probably today loading doses would not be given and maintenance doses of approximately one-half would be more common in patients with heart failure (see Therapeutic Plasma Concentrations, this chapter). Because it has a relatively long elimination half-life in adults, digoxin is given once daily. Dosage adjustments can be important for patients who are being converted from parenteral to oral therapy or vice versa; patients with renal impairment, CHF, or thyroid abnormalities; or patients who take amiodarone concurrently.

THERAPEUTIC PLASMA CONCENTRATIONS

Although there is considerable variation between patients, historically plasma digoxin concentrations of ≈1 to 2 mcg/L (ng/mL) were generally considered to be within the therapeutic range.[1,2] Data now indicate that a therapeutic range of 0.5 to 0.9 mcg/L is indicated for patients with CHF.[3–6] This lower target range is based on the fact that most patients with left ventricular dysfunction do not demonstrate additional therapeutic benefits from higher digoxin concentrations and are at greater risk for toxicity with digoxin concentrations ≥1.2 mcg/L.[4,7,8] For patients on digoxin for atrial fibrillation, the goal for digoxin is rate control.[9] Rate control is achieved by atrioventricular (AV) nodal blockade and may require higher digoxin concentrations. The use of pharmacokinetics to adjust the dosing regimen can reduce the incidence of digoxin toxicity.[2,10–12] Pharmacokinetics can help guide therapy to optimize clinical response, but even simple nomograms aid clinicians to dose digoxin effectively.[13] However, it appears digoxin has declined in clinical popularity and, in time, will likely be phased out of practice.[14–17]

BIOAVAILABILITY (F)

The bioavailability of digoxin tablets ranges from 0.5 to greater than 0.9. Many clinicians use a bioavailability of 0.7 to 0.8. A bioavailability of 0.7 is used in this chapter as an estimate of the average bioavailability figures reported in the literature.[18,19] The elixir appears to have a bioavailability of approximately 0.8, and soft gelatin capsules of digoxin appear to be completely absorbed.[20,21] The intravenous (IV) route of administration is also assumed to have 100% bioavailability.

St. John wort has been reported to reduce the bioavailability of digoxin by approximately 25%. It has been postulated that the interaction is with P-glycoprotein; however, other mechanisms (such as an induction of hepatic metabolism) have also been proposed.[24–27] Similarly, various antibiotics have also been reported to alter the bioavailability of digoxin. In most cases, the antibiotics appear to increase the bioavailability, supposedly by suppressing bacteria in the gastrointestinal tract that metabolize digoxin. Other mechanisms such as metabolism or renal excretion may also play a role in how some of the antibiotics increase the plasma concentrations of digoxin. The most common class of antibiotics that have been reported to increase digoxin concentrations

KEY PARAMETERS: Digoxin

Therapeutic range[a]	
CHF	0.5–0.9 mcg/L
Non CHF	0.5–2 mcg/L for atrial fibrillation and ventricular rate control
F	
Tablets	0.7
Elixir	0.8
Soft gelatin capsule	1
S	1
V[b] (L)	(3.8)(Weight in kg) + (3.1)(Cl$_{Cr}$ in mL/min)
Cl[b] (mL/min)	
Non-CHF patients	(0.8 mL/kg/min)(Weight in kg) + (Cl$_{Cr}$ in mL/min)
Patients with CHF	(0.33 mL/kg/min)(Weight in kg) + (0.9) (Cl$_{Cr}$ in mL/min)
t½[c]	2 days
fu (fraction unbound in plasma)	0.9

[a]There are a number of studies that list the therapeutic range in patients with CHF, and all now recommend 0.5 to <1 mcg/L.[4–6,22,23] In some patients with atrial fibrillation, concentrations greater than 2 mcg/L may be required to control ventricular rate adequately.
[b]For factors that alter V and Cl for digoxin, see Table 10.1.
[c]The t½ is longer in patients with renal failure and in patients receiving amiodarone.
CHF, congestive heart failure.

are macrolides, but others such as itraconazole are not a surprise.[28–32] Coadministration of cholestyramine has been reported to decrease the bioavailability of digoxin, and both cholestyramine and charcoal have been suggested as a treatment modality in patients who are digitalis toxic.[33,34]

VOLUME OF DISTRIBUTION (V)

The average volume of distribution for digoxin is ≈7.3 L/kg.[35] This V is decreased in patients with renal disease (see Question 4).

$$V_{Digoxin}(L) = (3.8 \text{ L/kg})(\text{Weight in kg}) + (3.1)(Cl_{Cr} \text{ in mL/min}) \qquad \textbf{(Eq. 10.1)}$$

In the above equation, the factors have been selected so that when creatinine clearance is in mL/min and weight is in kilograms, the unit of the calculated volume of distribution is L.

Digoxin V is also decreased in hypothyroid patients (see Question 12) and in patients who are taking quinidine (see Question 15). The volume of distribution is increased

TABLE 10.1 Most Common Factors That Alter Digoxin Volume of Distribution and Clearance

FACTOR[a]	
Volume of distribution	
Creatinine clearance	See Equation 10.1
Obesity	IBW[b]
Quinidine	0.7
Thyroid	
Clinically hypothyroid	0.7
Clinically hyperthyroid	1.3
Clearance	
Creatinine clearance	See Equations 10.3 and 10.4
Congestive heart failure	See Equation 10.4
Obesity	IBW[b]
Amiodarone	0.5
Quinidine	0.5
Verapamil	0.75
Thyroid function	
Clinically hypothyroid	0.7
Clinically hyperthyroid	1.3

[a]Factor should be multiplied by calculated volume of distribution or clearance value. Multiple factors would increase the uncertainty of any volume or clearance prediction. Although not tested, one might anticipate the factors to be multiplicative.
[b]Ideal body weight.

in hyperthyroid patients (see Question 12). In addition, the volume of distribution for digoxin in obese subjects appears to be more closely related to the nonobese or ideal body weight (IBW) than total body weight[36] (Table 10.1).

The manner in which digoxin is distributed in the body must be considered in the interpretation of plasma levels. The plasma concentration decline of digoxin follows a two-compartment model (see in Chapter 1: Volume of Distribution: Two-Compartment Models).[37] Although the models state two compartments, the body is not two compartments but rather 100's if not 1,000's of compartments. Digoxin first distributes into a small initial volume of distribution, V_i, consisting of plasma and other rapidly equilibrating tissues, and then distributes into larger and more slowly equilibrating tissue compartments. The myocardium responds pharmacologically as though it was located in one of the larger more slowly equilibrating tissue compartments (V_t). Because plasma samples are obtained from V_i, plasma digoxin levels do not accurately reflect the drug's pharmacologic effects until the digoxin is completely distributed into large more slowly equilibrating compartments. Serum concentrations of digoxin obtained before complete distribution are often misleading. Because the initial volume of distribution (V_i) of digoxin is relatively small ($\approx 1/10 V_t$), high plasma concentrations are commonly reported immediately after a dose is administered. Because the heart behaves as though it was in one of the tissue compartments, the initial high serum concentrations that occur immediately after a dose are not reflective of either therapeutic or toxic potential of digoxin. Being able to use the plasma drug concentration requires the plasma concentration to be at equilibrium with the receptors in the myocardium. For this equilibrium to take place, several hours are required. Plasma concentrations are only meaningful when obtained after equilibration is complete (i.e., at least 4 hours after an IV dose[38] or 6 hours after an oral dose.[39] Because time is not often critical, following the package insert's sampling recommendation of no sooner than 6 hours after an IV or oral dose seems prudent.[40] The clinical effects of a dose, however, may be observed much sooner than 4 to 6 hours because the distribution half-life (α t½) is only about 35 minutes.[41] After approximately two α t½'s (i.e., 1 hour), the myocardium experiences the effects of 75% of an IV dose. However, a plasma sample taken at this time would be misleadingly high because the remaining 25% of the dose which is not yet distributed out of V_i would produce a plasma concentration that is high relative to that which would be observed once equilibrium between the compartments is complete. Figure 10.1 is a theoretical two-compartment model for digoxin illustrating that several hours are required to reach equilibrium.

CLEARANCE (CL)

Digoxin clearance varies considerably among individuals and should be estimated for each patient. Total digoxin clearance (Cl_t) is the sum of its metabolic (Cl_m) and renal (Cl_r) clearances, as illustrated by Equation 10.2:

$$Cl_t = Cl_m + Cl_r \qquad \textbf{(Eq. 10.2)}$$

In healthy individuals, the metabolic clearance of digoxin is $\approx$0.57 to 0.86 mL/kg/min, and the renal clearance is approximately equal to or a little less than creatinine clearance. CHF reduces the metabolic clearance of digoxin to about one-half its usual value and may reduce the renal clearance slightly as well[19,42–44] (see also in Chapter 1: Clearance [Cl]).

Using the data from Sheiner et al.,[42] the total digoxin clearance in mL/kg/min can be calculated in patients with and without CHF as follows:

$$\begin{aligned} &\text{Total } Cl_{\text{Digoxin}}\,(\text{mL/min}) \\ &\text{(Patients without CHF)} \end{aligned} = (0.8\ \text{mL/kg/min})(\text{Weight in kg}) + Cl_{Cr}\ \text{in mL/min} \qquad \textbf{(Eq. 10.3)}$$

$$\begin{aligned} &\text{Total } Cl_{\text{Digoxin}}\,(\text{mL/min}) \\ &\text{(Patients with CHF)} \end{aligned} = (0.33\ \text{mL/kg/min})(\text{Weight in kg}) + (0.9)(Cl_{Cr}\ \text{in mL/min}) \qquad \textbf{(Eq. 10.4)}$$

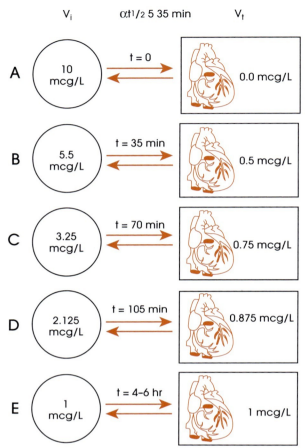

FIGURE 10.1 A theoretical two-compartment model for digoxin. The myocardium or target organ be-haves as though it was one of the compartments located somewhere in V_t and, therefore, responds to the theoretical digoxin concentration in V_t. Following complete distribution, the concentrations in V_i and V_t are assumed to be equal and the pharmacologic effect maximal. Note that the initial volume of distribution (V_i) is much smaller than the tissue volume of distribution (V_t); therefore, the digoxin concentrations are very high following an initial IV dose. **(A)** depicts digoxin concentration immediately following an IV bolus. All of the drug is in V_i and the plasma concentration is 10 mcg/L, but no digoxin is in the tissue compartments V_t; therefore, no effect is present. **(E)** depicts complete digoxin distribution. Note that the tissues in the two compartments are in equilibrium and that the digoxin concentration in both V_i and V_t is assumed to be equal (i.e., 1 mcg/L). At this point, the plasma level reflects the concentration in the tissue compartments and the potential for drug effect. **(B–D)** depict the relative digoxin concentrations in V_i and V_t after one, two, and three distribution half-lives (α t½s). After three α t½s, 87.5% of the pharmacologic effect is achieved; however, it is still much too early to obtain a digoxin level, because the concentration in V_i is more than 100% higher than the final equilibrated concentration. IV, intravenous.

Creatinine clearance can be estimated from the patient's serum creatinine using Equations 10.5 and 10.6.

$$\frac{\text{Cl}_{\text{Cr}} \text{ for Males}}{(\text{mL/min})} = \frac{(140 - \text{Age})(\text{Weight in kg})}{(72)(\text{SCr}_{\text{ss}})} \quad \textbf{(Eq. 10.5)}$$

$$\frac{\text{Cl}_{\text{Cr}} \text{ for Females}}{(\text{mL/min})} = (0.85)\frac{(140 - \text{Age})(\text{Weight in kg})}{(72)(\text{SCr}_{\text{ss}})} \quad \textbf{(Eq. 10.6)}$$

Note that, in the above equations, the units do not cancel; however, the values of 140 in the numerator and 72 in the denominator result in a creatinine clearance that has a unit value of mL/min. Also, in obese subjects, the renal clearance of digoxin is best described by IBW, therefore IBW is normally used as the weight in the creatinine clearance equation for this drug. The most common method of estimating IBW is as follows:

$$\textbf{Ideal Body Weight for Males in kg} = 50 + (2.3)(\text{Height in inches} > 60) \quad \textbf{(Eq. 10.7)}$$

$$\textbf{Ideal Body Weight for Females in kg} = 45 + (2.3)(\text{Height in inches} > 60) \quad \textbf{(Eq. 10.8)}$$

Similarly, IBW is used to estimate digoxin metabolic clearance. As presented for other drugs in this book, although the studies have not been done specifically for digoxin, it may be reasonable to consider using an adjusted body weight instead of IBW to estimate digoxin clearance in an obese patient. These and other methods for estimating digoxin clearance are illustrated in the questions later in this chapter. See Table 10.1 for common factors that alter digoxin clearance. It is the authors' opinion that $\text{Cl}_{\text{Digoxin}}$ (patients with CHF) equation is the more conservative approach and is recommended to use even in patients without a diagnosis of heart failure.

HALF-LIFE (t½)

The half-life for digoxin is approximately 2 days in patients with normal renal function. In anephric patients, the half-life increases to approximately 4 to 6 days. This increase in the digoxin half-life is less than might be expected based on the reduction in clearance because the volume of distribution is also decreased in patients with diminished renal function (see Question 4 and Equations 10.1 and 10.17). Although not unique to digoxin, a change in volume of distribution with decreased renal function is uncommon.

TIME TO SAMPLE

Plasma samples for routine digoxin level monitoring are ideally obtained 7 to 14 days after a maintenance regimen is initiated or changed. This delay in obtaining digoxin samples helps to ensure that steady state has been attained on the current dosing regimen. Samples may be obtained before steady state is achieved, but caution should be used in assessing the relationship between the current dosing regimen and the eventual steady-state concentration. In addition, in patients with end-stage renal disease, it may take 15 to 20 days to achieve steady state because of the prolonged half-life.

Plasma samples obtained within 24 hours of an initial loading dose may help confirm the relationship between the digoxin plasma concentration and pharmacologic response or establish the apparent volume of distribution. When plasma samples are obtained this early, however, they are of little value in evaluating the maintenance regimen.

Once steady state has been achieved, routine plasma samples for digoxin monitoring should be drawn just before the next dose (trough levels); however, any sampling time that avoids the distribution phase (at least 4 hours following an IV dose or 6 hours following an oral dose) is acceptable.

Patients taking digoxin who are to be given amiodarone/dronedarone are likely to require digoxin plasma level monitoring to determine the extent to which the digoxin pharmacokinetics is altered[45–48] (see Question 14). Although quinidine is rarely used, it is the classic digoxin drug–drug interaction. This interaction is especially troublesome because it results in a rapid rise in digoxin concentration (because of V) and sustained rise (because of Cl). With quinidine, there is the possibility that digoxin concentrations will fluctuate within a quinidine dosing interval. Consequently, in patients taking quinidine and digoxin, samples should be obtained at a time that corresponds to the trough of the quinidine dosing interval and that also avoids the distribution phase for digoxin. There have also been data suggesting fluctuations in digoxin concentrations with amiodarone.[49]

The time course for the expected change in digoxin concentrations will depend on whether the drug interaction alters digoxin volume of distribution or clearance or both. In addition, the time required for the interacting drug to accumulate and effect a change in digoxin pharmacokinetic parameter(s) should also be considered. When drugs are added to a patient's therapy that can alter the disposition of digoxin, the nature of the drug interaction and expected change in half-life should provide some clues as to the time course and extent of the expected change in the digoxin concentration.

Question #1   *Estimate a digoxin loading dose that will produce a plasma concentration of 1 mcg/L for a 50-year-old, 70-kg patient with a creatinine clearance of 80 mL/min being treated for CHF.*

Estimating a loading dose requires knowledge of the volume of distribution of the drug. Although one might consider using the average literature value for the V of digoxin (7.3 L/kg), a more conservative and/or logical approach would be to use patient-specific parameter estimates.[35] Taking into consideration the patient's renal function ($Cl_{Cr} = 80$ mL/min), the patient's volume can be calculated using Equation 10.1.

$$\begin{aligned}
V_{Digoxin}(L) &= (3.8\ L/kg)(\text{Weight in kg}) + (3.1)(Cl_{Cr}\ \text{in mL/min}) \\
&= (3.8\ L/kg)(70\ kg) + (3.1)(80\ mL/min) \\
&= 266\ L + 248\ L \\
&= 514\ L
\end{aligned}$$

Then, using Equation 10.9, the loading dose can be calculated as follows:

$$\text{Loading Dose} = \frac{(V)(C)}{(S)(F)} \qquad \textbf{(Eq. 10.9)}$$

$$= \frac{(514 \text{ L})(1 \text{ mcg/L})}{(1)(1)}$$

$$= 514 \text{ mcg or} \approx 500 \text{ mcg}$$

In this case, it was assumed that the loading dose was to be given IV; therefore, a bioavailability (F) of 1 was used.[18] If the loading dose was to be given orally, F would have been 0.7, and the calculated loading dose would have been 734 mcg ($\approx$750 mcg). In both cases, S is 1 because digoxin is not administered as a salt.

Loading doses of digoxin are not commonly given. In the case of rapid rate control in an acute care setting, IV digoxin might be used, but other agents are available. In treatment of CHF, it is rare to load a patient with digoxin but rather start on a maintenance dose. This example is included because if a loading dose is given, it needs to be done correctly. Even though digoxin use is declining, emergency room visits for digoxin toxicity are not emphasizing the importance of understanding dosing of digoxin.[50]

Question #2 *How should this loading dose be divided, and what would be an appropriate interval between doses?*

Loading doses of digoxin are almost always administered in divided doses so that the patient can be evaluated for toxicity and efficacy in the course of receiving the total loading dose. If the patient appears to develop toxicity or is therapeutically controlled, the remainder of the calculated loading dose is withheld. The usual procedure is to give one-half of the calculated loading dose initially, followed by two doses of one-fourth, and, in some cases, IV doses are divided into four equal parts. However, doses are based on practically, taking into consideration that oral tablets are available as 125 and 250 mcg and parenteral is 250 mcg/mL.

Historically, 6 hours is the usual interval between oral doses because it is the approximate time to ensure that the oral dose of digoxin has been absorbed and distributed into the myocardium.[39] Even following an IV injection, 2 to 4 hours are required for a single dose of digoxin to exhibit most of the effect.[38] In an emergency, when it is important to rapidly achieve pharmacologic effects, clinical decisions about efficacy/toxicity can be made 1 to 2 hours following an IV dose. This is because the majority of digoxin will have been distributed into the tissue compartment, and $\approx$75% to 90% of the pharmacologic effect can be evaluated at this time. It would still be too soon, however, to evaluate plasma concentrations because of the distribution phase (see Fig. 10.1 and in Chapter 1: Volume of Distribution [V]: Loading Dose). In this example, the loading dose of 500 mcg would be administered as 250 mcg and then two additional doses of 125 mcg each separated by 2 to 4 hours. It could also be given as two doses of 250 mcg separated by 2 to 4 hours. Again, the reason for dividing the dose is so that the patient can be evaluated for efficacy or toxicity before the next portion of the loading dose is administered.

Question #3　*R.J. is a 50-year-old, 70-kg man with CHF and has a serum creatinine of 1 mg/dL. Calculate a maintenance dose that will achieve an average plasma digoxin concentration of 0.8 mcg/L.*

Because the objective is to achieve an average digoxin concentration of 0.8 mcg/L at steady state (Css ave), Equation 10.10 can be used to calculate the maintenance dose.

$$\text{Maintenance Dose} = \frac{(Cl)(Css\ ave)(\tau)}{(S)(F)} \qquad \textbf{(Eq. 10.10)}$$

When using Equation 10.10, it is important to ensure that the units will cancel properly and are easy to use. In the case of digoxin, the concentrations are usually reported as mcg/L, and, therefore, the digoxin dose should be expressed as mcg. Given that the dosing interval (τ) is usually expressed in days, the clearance should be expressed as L/day. If the dosing interval is thought of as hours (e.g., 24 hours), then clearance would be in the units of L/hr. Therefore, assuming the dosing interval (τ) to be 1 day, the bioavailability (F) 0.7 for oral tablets, and the fraction of the dose that is digoxin (S) to be 1, the digoxin clearance (Cl) is the only remaining parameter to be calculated.

The digoxin clearance for R.J. can be determined by using Equation 10.4.

$$\frac{\text{Total } Cl_{Digoxin}\ (mL/\ min)}{(\text{Patients with CHF})} = \frac{(0.33\ mL/kg/\ min)(\text{Weight in kg})}{+ (0.9)(Cl_{Cr}\ in\ mL/\ min)}$$

Although the creatinine clearance (Cl_{Cr}) for R.J. is unknown, it can be estimated easily from his serum creatinine using Equation 10.5, assuming all the criteria for the use of this formula are met (i.e., serum creatinine is at steady state, and R.J.'s muscle mass is average for a 50-year-old man).

$$\begin{aligned}
Cl_{Cr}\ \text{for males} &= \frac{(140 - \text{Age})(\text{Weight in kg})}{(72)(SCr_{ss})} \\
&= \frac{(140 - 50\ yr)(70\ kg)}{(72)(1\ mg/dL)} \\
&= 87.5\ mL/\ min
\end{aligned}$$

This creatinine clearance can now be used in Equation 10.4 to estimate R.J.'s total digoxin clearance.

$$\begin{aligned} \text{Total Cl}_{\text{Digoxin}} \text{ (mL/min)} \\ \text{(Patients with CHF)} \end{aligned} = \begin{aligned} &(0.33 \text{ mL/kg/min})(\text{Weight in kg}) \\ &+ (0.9)(\text{Cl}_{\text{Cr}} \text{ in mL/min}) \end{aligned}$$

$$= (0.33 \text{ mL/kg/min})(70 \text{ kg})$$
$$+ (0.9)(87.5 \text{ mL/min})$$
$$= 23.1 \text{ mL/min} + 78.8 \text{ mL/min}$$
$$= 101.9 \text{ mL/min}$$

The digoxin clearance is then used to calculate the maintenance dose. Because the maintenance dose is commonly expressed in mcg/day, the clearance in mL/min can be converted to L/day by multiplying the value by the number of minutes per day (1,440 min/day) and dividing by the number of milliliters per liter (1,000 mL/L) as follows:

$$\text{Cl (L/day)} = (\text{Cl as mL/min})\left(\frac{1,440 \text{ min/day}}{1,000 \text{ mL/L}}\right) \qquad \textbf{(Eq. 10.11)}$$

$$= (101.9 \text{ mL/min})\left(\frac{1,440 \text{ min/day}}{1,000 \text{ mL/L}}\right)$$
$$= 146.7 \text{ L/day}$$

The maintenance dose can now be calculated using Equation 10.10.

$$\begin{aligned} \text{Maintenance Dose} &= \frac{(\text{Cl})(\text{Css ave})(\tau)}{(\text{S})(\text{F})} \\ &= \frac{(146.7 \text{ L/day})(0.8 \text{ mcg/L})(1 \text{ day})}{(1)(0.7)} \\ &= \frac{117.4 \text{ mg}}{0.7} \\ &= 168 \text{ mcg} \\ &= 0.168 \text{ mg} \end{aligned}$$

One could elect to give either 0.125 mg every day or 0.125 and 0.25 mg on alternate days for an average dose of 0.1875 mg/day. Given that the 0.168 mg/day dosing rate is only an estimate, most clinicians would probably give 0.125 mg/day because R.J. is being treated for CHF and a lower digoxin concentration would be desirable.

Question #4   *If the patient in Question 1 had a serum creatinine of 5 mg/dL, would the estimated loading dose have been different?*

For a number of years, it was assumed that renal function influenced only the clearance of digoxin. A number of studies have indicated, however, that patients with decreased creatinine clearance also have a decreased volume of distribution for digoxin.[35,42,51]

The relationship between volume of distribution (V), plasma concentration (C), and amount of drug in the body is described by Equation 10.12.

$$V = \frac{\text{Amount of Drug in the Body}}{C} \qquad \text{(Eq. 10.12)}$$

In uremic patients, it is assumed that digoxin is displaced from the tissue compartment. As a result, C is higher and V is smaller.

$$\downarrow V = \frac{\text{Amount of Drug in the Body}}{\uparrow C}$$

There is some controversy about the significance of this tissue displacement of digoxin. Myocardial digoxin concentrations at any given plasma digoxin level are lower relative to their nonuremic counterparts.[52] Consequently, some have suggested that no change in the loading dose is necessary.[53] Almost all clinicians today assume that the higher the digoxin concentrations, the greater the drug effect, both therapeutic and toxic. Therefore, they generally target digoxin concentrations, in renal failure patients, that are similar to or lower than the concentrations for patients with normal renal function. Many clinicians, however, do not recognize that the volume of distribution is likely to be reduced in patients with significant renal dysfunction and, therefore, do not always make the appropriate initial reduction in digoxin loading doses.

Because very little digoxin is bound to plasma proteins, only about 10%, a change in the desired therapeutic plasma concentration is unlikely to result from plasma protein displacement[54] (see in Chapter 1: Desired Plasma Concentration [C]: Protein Binding).

There are a number of ways to estimate the volume of distribution for digoxin in a patient with decreased renal function; Equation 10.1 is most commonly used. It is the authors' opinion that this equation appears to be useful over a wider range of creatinine clearance values, especially in young adults with good renal function.[55]

$$V_{\text{Digoxin}}(L) = (3.8 \text{ L/kg})(\text{Weight in kg}) + (3.1)(Cl_{Cr} \text{ in mL/min})$$

Equation 10.1 is for a specific patient; therefore, the estimated Cl_{Cr} should be expressed in mL/min for that patient. The volume of distribution for digoxin in uremic patients can vary considerably. For this reason, the values obtained from this equation and the calculated loading dose should be considered only rough estimates.

Using Equation 10.5, the patient's creatinine clearance is determined to be approximately 20 mL/min. Note that we are assuming the patient is not receiving any type of dialysis, because dialysis invalidates Equations 10.5 and 10.6.

$$\begin{aligned} Cl_{Cr} \text{ for Males} &= \frac{(140 - \text{Age})(\text{Weight in kg})}{(72)(SCr_{ss})} \\ &= \frac{(140 - 50 \text{ yr})(70 \text{ kg})}{(72)(5 \text{ mg/dL})} \\ &= 17.5 \text{ mL/min or} \approx 20 \text{ mL/min} \end{aligned}$$

Using this value in Equation 10.1, the estimated volume of distribution would be 328 L.

$$V_{Digoxin} (L) = (3.8\,L/kg)(Weight\ in\ kg) + (3.1)(Cl_{Cr}\ in\ mL/min)$$
$$= (3.8\,L/kg)(70\,kg) + (3.1)(20\,mL/min)$$
$$= (266\,L) + (62\,L)$$
$$= 328\,L$$

If the volume of distribution is assumed to be approximately 330 L (as calculated from Equation 10.1), the estimated IV loading dose using Equation 10.9 would be approximately 375 mcg if a digoxin concentration of 1 mcg/L was desired.

$$Loading\ Dose = \frac{(V)(C)}{(S)(F)}$$
$$= \frac{(330\,L)(1\,mcg/L)}{(1)(1)}$$
$$= 330\,mcg\ or \approx 375\,mcg$$

Again, as in Question 1, S and F are assumed to be 1. The total loading dose should be divided and administered as described in Question 2. Again, the loading dose is divided so that the patient's response can be evaluated between each of the partial loading doses. This is to guard against the possibility that the patient's volume of distribution is smaller than anticipated or that the patient is more sensitive to the pharmacologic effects than expected. One should also consider the possibility that the volume of distribution may be much larger than expected and additional doses may have to be administered to achieve the desired plasma concentration or pharmacologic effect.

It should be pointed out that dosing to a therapeutic endpoint is common in patients with atrial fibrillation in whom the therapeutic endpoint is increased AV nodal blockade and a decrease in ventricular rate.

Question #5 *Estimate the daily dose that would maintain the average digoxin concentration at 0.8 mcg/L in this same 70-kg, 50-year-old patient with a serum creatinine of 5 mg/dL.*

As in Question 3, Equation 10.10 would be used to estimate the maintenance dose.

$$Maintenance\ Dose = \frac{(Cl)(Css\ ave)(\tau)}{(S)(F)}$$

Using the creatinine clearance estimate of 20 mL/min (see Question 4), the digoxin clearance can be estimated using Equation 10.4 (for CHF).

$$\begin{aligned} Total\ Cl_{Diogoxin}\,(mL/min) &= (0.33\,mL/kg/min)(Weight\ in\ kg) \\ (Patients\ with\ CHF) &\quad + (0.9)(Cl_{Cr}\ in\ mL/min) \\ &= (0.33\,mL/kg/min)(70\,kg) \\ &\quad + (0.9)(20\,mL/min) \\ &= 23.1\,mL/min + 18\,mL/min \\ &= 41.1\,mL/min \end{aligned}$$

The digoxin clearance can be converted from mL/min to L/day as described in Question 3 using Equation 10.11.

$$Cl\ (L/day) = (Cl\ as\ mL/min)\left(\frac{1,440\ min/day}{1,000\ mL/L}\right)$$

$$= (41.1\ mL/min)\left(\frac{1,440\ min/day}{1,000\ mL/L}\right)$$

$$= 59.2\ L/day$$

Again, assuming S to be 1 and F to be 0.7 for digoxin tablets, the approximate daily dose (calculated using Equation 10.10) would be 68 mcg/day or 0.068 mg/day.

$$Maintenance\ Dose = \frac{(Cl)(Css\ ave)(\tau)}{(S)(F)}$$

$$= \frac{(59.2\ L/day)(0.8\ mcg/L)(1\ day)}{(1)(0.7)}$$

$$= \frac{47.4\ mcg}{0.7}$$

$$= 67.7\ mcg\ of\ digoxin\ each\ day$$

Again, this dose is not convenient, and most clinicians would probably administer either 0.125 mg every other day or one-half of a 0.125-mg tablet (0.0625 mg) every day because digoxin comes in 0.125-mg tablets, and this is a reasonable dose for patients with significantly diminished renal function.

Question #6 *Assume that the patient described above can take nothing by mouth and must be converted to daily IV doses of digoxin. Assume he was taking one-half of a 0.125-mg tablet (0.0625 mg) each day. Calculate an equivalent IV dose.*

If the bioavailability of digoxin is assumed to be 0.7, the equivalent IV dose would be 0.044 mg/day as calculated from Equations 10.13 and 10.14.

$$\begin{matrix}\text{Amount of Drug Absorbed}\\ \text{or Reaching the Systemic Circulation}\end{matrix} = (F)(Dose) \qquad \textbf{(Eq. 10.13)}$$

$$= (0.7)(0.0625\ mg)$$

$$= 0.044\ mg$$

$$\frac{\text{Dose of New}}{\text{Dosage Form}} = \frac{\text{Amount of Drug Absorbed from Current Dosage Form}}{\text{F of New Dosage Form}} \qquad \textbf{(Eq. 10.14)}$$

$$= \frac{0.044 \text{ mg}}{1}$$

$$= 0.044 \text{ mg} \quad \text{or} \quad \approx 0.05 \text{ mg}$$

If the dose is not adjusted to account for the increased bioavailability of the IV dose, higher steady-state digoxin concentrations would eventually be achieved (see in Chapter 1: Elimination Rate Constant [K] and Half-Life [t½] and Fig. 1.16). Also, note that the dose might be rounded to 0.05 mg, which would correspond to 0.2 mL of the injectable (0.25 mg/mL). The dose of 0.05 mg would be expected to achieve a Css ave of <1 mcg/L. This could be further evaluated by calculating Css ave using Equation 10.20 (see Question 9) or by comparing the ratio of the old and new doses to the old Css ave.

$$\frac{\text{Dose}_{\text{NEW}}}{\text{Dose}_{\text{OLD}}}(\text{Css ave}_{\text{OLD}}) = \text{Css ave}_{\text{NEW}} \qquad \textbf{(Eq. 10.15)}$$

$$\frac{0.05 \text{ mg}}{0.044 \text{ mg}}(0.8 \text{ mcg/L}) = 0.91 \text{ mcg/L}$$

Question #7   *B.G., a 62-year-old, 50-kg woman, with atrial fibrillation was admitted to the hospital for possible digoxin toxicity. Her serum creatinine was 3 mg/dL, and her dosing regimen at home had been 0.25 mg of digoxin daily for many months. The digoxin plasma concentration on admission was 3 mcg/L. How long will it take for the digoxin concentration to fall from 3 to 1.5 mcg/L?*

The answer to this question requires knowledge of the digoxin half-life (t½) or the elimination rate constant (K), both of which are dependent on the clearance and volume of distribution for digoxin in B.G. The relationship between these parameters is described by Equations 10.16 and 10.17.

$$K = \frac{\text{Cl}}{\text{V}} \qquad \textbf{(Eq. 10.16)}$$

$$t\frac{1}{2} = \frac{(0.693)(\text{V})}{\text{Cl}} \qquad \textbf{(Eq. 10.17)}$$

Three basic steps are required to solve this problem: (1) estimate digoxin clearance, (2) estimate the V for digoxin, and (3) calculate the half-life.

Step 1. Estimate clearance. We can estimate digoxin clearance as illustrated in previous questions by first determining B.G.'s creatinine clearance through the use of Equation 10.6 for women.

$$Cl_{Cr} \text{ for Females} = (0.85)\frac{(140 - \text{Age})(\text{Weight in kg})}{(72)(SCr_{ss})}$$

$$= (0.85)\frac{(140 - 62 \text{ yr})(50 \text{ kg})}{(72)(3 \text{ mg/dL})}$$

$$= 15.3 \text{ mL/min}$$

This estimation of Cl_{Cr} then can be used to determine the digoxin clearance using Equation 10.4 (for CHF), which is the more conservative approach.

$$\frac{\text{Total Cl}_{\text{Digoxin}} (\text{mL/min})}{(\text{Patients with CHF})} = \frac{(0.33 \text{ mL/kg/min})(\text{Weight in kg})}{+ (0.9)(Cl_{Cr} \text{ in mL/min})}$$

$$= (0.33 \text{ mL/kg/min})(50 \text{ kg}) + (0.9)(15.3 \text{ mL/min})$$

$$= 16.5 \text{ mL/min} + 13.8 \text{ mL/min}$$

$$= 30.3 \text{ mL/min}$$

Converted to L/day by Equation 10.11, the digoxin clearance would be 43.6 L/day.

$$Cl(\text{L/day}) = (\text{Cl as mL/min})\left(\frac{1,440 \text{ min/day}}{1,000 \text{ mL/L}}\right)$$

$$= (30.3 \text{ mL/min})\left(\frac{1,440 \text{ min/day}}{1,000 \text{ mL/L}}\right)$$

$$= 43.6 \text{ L/day}$$

A more patient-specific approach would be to use the patient's dosing history and the observed digoxin concentrations to derive a patient-specific digoxin clearance. If one assumes that the digoxin half-life is significantly longer than the dosing interval, the observed digoxin plasma concentration should closely reflect the average concentration at steady state; from this, the digoxin clearance can be calculated (i.e., this level is relatively independent of the volume of distribution; see Chapter 1: Elimination Rate Constant [K] and Half-Life [t½]: Clinical Application of Elimination Rate Constant [K] and Half-life [t½]: Dosing Interval [τ]). Therefore, the observed digoxin concentration can be used in Equation 10.18 to estimate B.G.'s clearance.

$$Cl = \frac{(S)(F)(\text{Dose}/\tau)}{Css \text{ ave}} \qquad \textbf{(Eq. 10.18)}$$

$$= \frac{(1)(0.7)(250 \text{ mcg/day})}{3 \text{ mcg/L}}$$

$$= \frac{175 \text{ mcg/day}}{3 \text{ mcg/L}}$$

$$= 58.3 \text{ L/day}$$

This higher-than-average digoxin clearance of 58.3 L/day calculated from B.G.'s dosing history and observed plasma level while different from population average is not unreasonable for this 50-kg, 62-year-old woman with a serum creatinine of 3 mg/dL. Given the usual uncertainty in predicting clearance, we would expect most of our patients to have an observed clearance that is between one-half to two times the predicted value. Actual clearance values outside this range should be evaluated carefully to determine whether the patient is substantially different from the assumed pharmacokinetic population. In most cases, it is more likely that we have made an error in our calculations or in our assumptions (see Question 9).

Step 2. Calculate B.G.'s digoxin volume of distribution. Because our only digoxin plasma concentration represents something approaching Css ave, we cannot derive a patient-specific volume and will have to rely on a literature estimate that we can calculate using Equation 10.1.

$$
\begin{aligned}
V_{Digoxin}\,(L) &= (3.8\text{ L/kg})(\text{Weight in kg}) + (3.1)(Cl_{Cr}\text{ in mL/ min}) \\
&= (3.8\text{ L/kg})(50\text{ kg}) + (3.1)(15.3\text{ mL/ min}) \\
&= 190\text{ L} + 47\text{ L} \\
&= 237\text{ L}
\end{aligned}
$$

Step 3. The digoxin elimination rate constant and half-life for B.G. can now be estimated from Equations 10.16 and 10.17 using our patient-specific digoxin clearance and the literature estimate of volume of digoxin.

$$
\begin{aligned}
K &= \frac{Cl}{V} \\
&= \frac{58.3\text{ L/day}}{237\text{ L}} \\
&= 0.246\text{ day}^{-1} \\
t\tfrac{1}{2} &= \frac{(0.693)(V)}{Cl} \\
&= \frac{(0.693)(237\text{ L})}{58.3\text{ L/day}} \\
&= 2.8\text{ days}
\end{aligned}
$$

We now have the data necessary to answer the original question. The time required for B.G.'s plasma concentration of digoxin to fall from 3 to 1.5 mcg/L (one-half the original level) is one half-life, or 2.8 days.

In most situations, the calculations are not this easy (i.e., one $t\tfrac{1}{2}$). When the time of decay is not obvious, the time required for the plasma concentration to fall to a predetermined level can be calculated using Equation 10.19.

$$
t = \frac{\ln\left(\dfrac{C_1}{C_2}\right)}{K}
\tag{Eq. 10.19}
$$

In the above equation, t represents the time required for C_1, the initial higher concentration, to decay to C_2, the lower concentration, for any given elimination rate constant K. Of course, the equation assumes a first-order decay process (i.e., Cl and V are constants) and that no drug is administered or absorbed between the concentrations C_1 and C_2 (see in Chapter 1: Elimination Rate Constant [K] and Half-Life [t½]: Elimination Rate Constant [K]).

$$t = \frac{\ln\left(\dfrac{C_1}{C_2}\right)}{K}$$

$$t = \frac{\ln\left(\dfrac{3\ \text{mcg/L}}{1.5\ \text{mcg/L}}\right)}{0.246\ \text{day}^{-1}}$$

$$= \frac{\ln(2)}{0.246\ \text{day}^{-1}}$$

$$= \frac{0.693}{0.246\ \text{day}^{-1}}$$

$$= 2.8\ \text{days}$$

Question #8 *Calculate a daily dose that will maintain B.G.'s average digoxin plasma concentration at 1.5 mcg/L.*

Using the clearance value of 58.3 L/day calculated from B.G.'s data, and assuming S, F, and τ to be 1, 0.7, and 1 day, respectively, the new maintenance dose can be estimated using Equation 10.10.

$$\text{Maintenance Dose} = \frac{(\text{Cl})(\text{Css ave})(\tau)}{(\text{S})(\text{F})}$$

$$= \frac{(58.3\ \text{L/day})(1.5\ \text{mcg/L})(1\ \text{day})}{(1)(0.7)}$$

$$= \frac{87.5\ \text{mcg}}{0.7}$$

$$= 125\ \text{mcg}$$

or 0.125 mg Digoxin Daily

Alternatively, the previous maintenance dose could be adjusted proportionately to the desired change in steady-state plasma level because clearance and other factors were assumed to be constant. Therefore, if the new steady-state level is to be one-half of the previous value, the new maintenance dose should be one-half the previous maintenance dose.

Question #9 *N.W., a female who has been taking the same dose of digoxin for 15 days, is seen in the clinic and is found to be doing well clinically. A digoxin plasma level drawn on the morning of her visit is 2.4 mcg/L. What are the possible explanations for this elevated serum digoxin concentration?*

Because this serum digoxin concentration theoretically represents an average steady-state concentration (Css ave), one must evaluate each of the factors that could alter steady state. The relationship of each of these factors to the average steady-state concentration may be seen by studying Equation 10.20.

$$\text{Css ave} = \frac{(S)(F)(Dose/\tau)}{Cl}$$

(Eq. 10.20)

1. *(S)(F)*. N.W. may be absorbing more than 70% (average bioavailability) from the oral dosage form. Because there are no salt forms of digoxin, S should be 1. Whereas an increase in F could account for some of the elevated digoxin concentration, F alone could only increase the digoxin by a factor of 1.4 (i.e., 1/0.7).
2. *Dose.* N.W. may be taking more than the prescribed dose, although taking less than the prescribed dose is more common.[11,56] Of course, each tablet may not contain the labeled amount. In some cases, the tablets may be larger than normal and, on physical inspection, may show that,[57] however, if the tablet is standard size but contains more drug, this would be impossible to tell. Although, given current manufacturing standards, this is not high on the list of possibilities, clinicians need to watch for US Food and Drug Administration and manufacturer alerts for this type of information.
3. τ. N.W. may be taking the proper dose more often than prescribed.
4. *Cl.* N.W.'s clearance or ability to eliminate the drug may be less than we estimated. We expect most patients to be within the range of one-half to two times the expected clearance values (i.e., two times to one-half the expected Css ave).
5. *Css ave.* The assay could be in error. Interfering substances may be present, or the plasma level may have been drawn during the distribution phase of the drug.

Plasma levels obtained during the distribution phase of digoxin are higher than anticipated because digoxin is absorbed from the gastrointestinal tract into the plasma and V_i faster than it is distributed into the tissues or V_t. Because the myocardium responds to digoxin as one of the more slowly equilibrating tissue compartments, plasma levels obtained before distribution is complete and equilibrium with the myocardium has been achieved, do not correlate with pharmacologic effects of the drug.[11,39] Digoxin plasma levels should be obtained just before the next dose is given, or at least 6 hours after the oral digoxin dose[39,40] (see the discussion on Digoxin Volume of Distribution (V) and Time to Sample, this chapter).

Question #10   *Outline a reasonable plan to determine the cause of N.W.'s higher-than-predicted digoxin level.*

1. Ask N.W. when that day's digoxin dose was taken relative to when the blood sample was obtained.

2. Determine N.W.'s adherence to the digoxin regimen. This is difficult but must be attempted through a history or pill count.
3. Determine whether any drugs interfered with the digoxin assay. Literature reports of interference by drugs having a steroid nucleus are applicable only to the antibody assay used in the particular report and to the assay techniques and may not apply to the assay used to determine N.W.'s digoxin plasma level. Therefore, the laboratory measuring the serum level would have to be contacted about the possibility of assay interference.[44,58–62] While falsely elevated digoxin concentrations are most commonly reported and should be considered in N.W.'s case, interfering substances may also result in a falsely decreased assay measurement.[61]

   Patients with poor renal function and newborn infants accumulate an endogenous digoxin-like compound that can produce a falsely elevated or false-positive digoxin assay result. The usual range of the false-positive reaction is from 0.1 to >1 mcg/L,[63–65] with an average of ≈0.1 to 0.4 mcg/L. This interference does not appear to represent a cross-reactivity with digoxin metabolites, because it has been observed in patients who have never received digoxin. The assay interference in these patients with apparent renal dysfunction is assay specific and is much more significant for some assays than for others.[64,66] Assays continue to change so clinicians need to check on which assays are used at their site and what can affect assay accuracy and specificity.[67]

4. Reschedule a second digoxin plasma level, but be certain that it is drawn at least 6 hours after a dose. Preferably, obtain the sample in the morning before the daily dose is taken.
5. Evaluating N.W.'s Cl and F is difficult and costly because such evaluation would require hospitalization. Furthermore, it would only result in the obvious conclusion that the dose should be reduced if, in fact, the dosage level was too high. This approach would only be used under the most unusual circumstances. In addition, F could only increase from the assumed 0.7 to a maximum of 1 and would not, by itself, account for the observed elevation in Css ave.

Question #11   *T.S., a female receiving digoxin 0.25 mg/day for several months, has a reported digoxin plasma concentration of 0.3 mcg/L. Her CHF is poorly controlled. What is the most probable explanation?*

The answer to this question is essentially the same as that to Question 9; the same factors should be considered. T.S. should be asked if she is receiving the same brand or dosage form of digoxin because bioavailability may vary between products, however, with today's standards, not likely an issue. Also, check if T.S. has conditions that accelerate intestinal transit time (e.g., small bowel resection), which can decrease digoxin absorption.[68] T.S. could also be one of the very rare patients who has a large metabolic and renal clearance for digoxin.[69] As indicated in Question 10, there are some drugs that result in a falsely decreased digoxin assay result and that possibility should also be considered.[61] The most likely explanation for the subtherapeutic digoxin concentrations is noncompliance with the prescribed regimen.[56]

Question #12   *In 1966, Doherty and Perkins[70] evaluated the pharmacokinetics of digoxin in hyperthyroid, hypothyroid, and euthyroid patients. Figure 10.2 is a representation of one of the graphs from this study. Using the graph, discuss the implications of thyroid disease on the loading dose, maintenance dose, and the time required to reach steady state relative to the euthyroid state. Assume that the same Css ave is desired in all patients.*

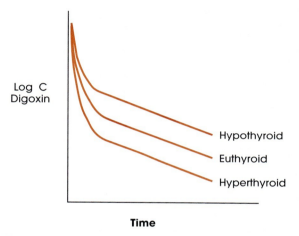

FIGURE 10.2   Digoxin and thyroid function. Note the distribution and elimination of digoxin when administered by the intravenous route to hypothyroid, hyperthyroid, and euthyroid patients.[70]

Loading Dose. Because hypothyroid patients have higher plasma levels following a single loading dose, they must have a decreased apparent volume of distribution. Therefore, a decrease in the loading dose may be appropriate. Hyperthyroid patients have lower plasma levels and would be expected to require larger loading doses because of a larger volume of distribution. In addition, atrial fibrillation is one of the common cardiac arrhythmias in hyperthyroid patients. In these patients, higher-than-average digoxin concentrations are often necessary to achieve adequate AV nodal blockade and ventricular rate control.

Time to Reach Steady State. The slope of all the decay curves is the same. Therefore, the half-lives and elimination rate constants are equal, and the time required to reach steady state will be the same for hyperthyroid, hypothyroid, and euthyroid patients receiving digoxin.

Maintenance Dose. Because K is the same in all patients, the clearance and volume of distribution must both be changed by the same proportion and in the same direction (see Equation 10.16).

$$K = \frac{Cl}{V}$$

$$K(\text{Same in All Patients Studied}) = \frac{Cl\,(\text{Variable})}{V\,(\text{Variable})}$$

Hypothyroid patients must have a decreased clearance, because the volume of distribution is decreased. This reduction in Cl would necessitate a reduction in maintenance doses. Similarly, the larger V in the hyperthyroid patients is consistent with an increased clearance; therefore, an increase in maintenance dose would be indicated if Css ave is to remain the same as that used for euthyroid patients.

It is important to reemphasize, however, that although K and V were used to estimate clearance, V is an independent variable, which, like clearance, is affected by thyroid disease. Because both Cl and V were affected in the same direction and to the same degree, the half-life (and K) did not change (see Table 10.1).

Two other studies[71,72] have examined the pharmacokinetics of digoxin in patients with thyroid disease. Both of these suggest that the changes in the digoxin clearance result from an increased glomerular filtration rate associated with hyperthyroidism. If this increased renal function is the primary factor responsible for the altered digoxin clearance observed in hyperthyroid patients, it would be possible to encounter such patients with decreased digoxin clearance if they also had intrinsic renal dysfunction.

Question #13 *Do patients receiving hemodialysis require additional digoxin following dialysis?*

One should first determine whether digoxin is expected to be significantly removed by dialysis. To evaluate digoxin's unbound volume in a dialysis patient, we need to calculate digoxin's volume. Assuming a Cl_{Cr} of 5 mL/min and a weight of 70 kg, and using Equation 10.1, the volume we would expect is 281.5 L.

$$\begin{aligned}
V_{Digoxin}\,(L) &= (3.8\,L/kg)(\text{Weight in kg}) + (3.1)(Cl_{Cr}\ \text{in mL/min}) \\
&= (3.8\,L/kg)(70\,kg) + (3.1)(5\,mL/min) \\
&= 266\,L + 15.5\,L \\
&= 281.5\,L
\end{aligned}$$

Now using Equation 10.21, we can calculate digoxin's unbound volume.

$$\text{Unbound Volume of Distribution} = \frac{V}{fu} \qquad \textbf{(Eq. 10.21)}$$

$$\begin{aligned}
&= \frac{281.5\,L}{0.9} \\
&= 313\,L
\end{aligned}$$

Based on the unbound volume of 313 L for this 70-kg patient or 4.5 L/kg, we would not expect digoxin to be significantly removed by dialysis (see in Chapter 3: Dialysis of Drugs: Estimating Drug Dialyzability).

This assessment of digoxin not being significantly removed by dialysis is further supported by the literature. Digoxin has a molecular weight of about 500 Da and will pass through the dialysis membrane; however, most of the digoxin is in the deeper, more slowly equilibrating tissue compartment and is difficult to remove by any intermittent hemofiltration process. The dialysis clearance for digoxin is only 10 mL/min using dialysis membranes having a molecular weight cutoff of about 1,000 Da. Therefore, <3% of the total amount of drug in the body is removed during hemodialysis.[73] This dialysis clearance of 10 mL/min may seem significant when compared with the metabolic clearance of 23 mL/min/70 kg for patients with CHF,[42] but the dialysis takes place for only 3 to 4 hours every few days, while the metabolic clearance is continuous. High-efficiency or high-flux membranes will have higher digoxin clearance values and be more efficient in clearing plasma digoxin, but the digoxin in the deep compartment is slowly equilibrating and unlikely to be effectively eliminated in the usual 3- or 4-hour dialysis run. Continuous renal replacement therapy may be more effective over several days in removing digoxin because it is continuous.[74] However, given the long t½ of digoxin, even with the increased clearance, changes in concentration are likely to be over several days, and any necessary dose adjustments can be made as needed.[75]

It is important to note that dialysis can induce digitalis toxicity by altering serum electrolyte concentrations and acid–base balance. For example, a decrease in serum potassium or other electrolytes may occur during dialysis and result in digoxin toxicity during or just following dialysis. If digoxin plasma samples are to be obtained around the time of dialysis, it would be wise to sample before dialysis is started or to wait at least 4 to 6 hours following the end of dialysis to ensure that the vascular and deep tissue concentrations of digoxin have had sufficient time to re-equilibrate.

Question #14 *C.B. is a patient with atrial fibrillation who was given digoxin for ventricular rate control. He is taking a maintenance dose of 0.25 mg/day of digoxin. Now, however, amiodarone will be added to C.B.'s drug regimen in an attempt to further control his ventricular response and, it is hoped, to convert him to normal sinus rhythm. What are the pharmacokinetic considerations with regard to the amiodarone–digoxin drug interaction?*

Amiodarone is well recognized to decrease both the metabolic and renal clearance of digoxin. Although estimates vary, most patients have about a 50% reduction in digoxin clearance when amiodarone is added to their regimen.[45–47,76] While the digoxin volume of distribution may also decrease slightly, the change is small.[45,46] In addition, amiodarone has a very long t½ of approximately 40 days and accumulates slowly in the body.[77] As a result, following the initiation of amiodarone, digoxin concentrations rise slowly over a 1- to 2-week period (Fig. 10.3, line C).

Given that the change in digoxin disposition is primarily a 50% reduction in clearance, we would expect to reduce the patient's digoxin maintenance dose by 50% if our goal was to maintain the same steady-state digoxin concentration after the initiation of amiodarone. Although the change in digoxin occurs slowly, most clinicians reduce the digoxin maintenance dose at the time of starting amiodarone to ensure that the change

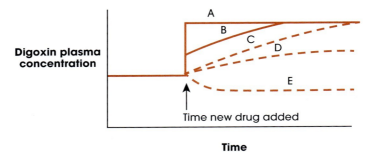

FIGURE 10.3   Digoxin. This figure represents the anticipated changes in digoxin concentration following the initiation of an interacting agent (↑). The solid line A represents the effect of a drug that changes the volume of distribution in proportion to the decrease in the digoxin clearance. Broken line B represents the effect of a drug that produces a decrease in volume of distribution that is less than proportional to the decrease in digoxin clearance (e.g., quinidine). Line C represents the effect of a drug that decreases the digoxin clearance to approximately the same extent as quinidine, but produces no apparent change in the volume of distribution (e.g., amiodarone). Line D represents the effect of a drug that decreases digoxin clearance to a lesser extent than that observed with quinidine (e.g., verapamil). Line E represents a drug that decreases bioavailability or increases clearance or both and, hence, the decline in digoxin concentrations (e.g., St. John wort).

in the digoxin regimen is not forgotten. If the digoxin steady-state concentration was very low at the time of initiating amiodarone, no change in digoxin may be necessary if the goal was to approximately double the digoxin concentration.

Although not related to the question at hand, many if not most patients with atrial fibrillation are receiving warfarin. Amiodarone also reduces the clearance of warfarin and, as a result, the International Normalized Ratio (INR) increases. If the patient's INRs are not closely monitored and the warfarin doses adjusted, the patient's INR will almost certainly increase significantly. It would not be good pharmaceutic care to prevent a digitalis intoxication only to have the patient develop a major bleeding episode.

Question #15   *What if patient C.B. above was to be given quinidine? Are the considerations the same as for amiodarone?*

Although quinidine is no longer one of the common antiarrhythmic agents, it is still used on occasion. Understanding how quinidine alters the disposition of digoxin helps to explain the differences in how the interaction is managed. Patients receiving digoxin have a rapid and sustained rise in the serum digoxin concentration following the addition of quinidine[78–80] (see Fig. 10.3, line B). This rapid rise in digoxin within the first 24 hours apparently results from the displacement of digoxin by quinidine from tissue sites. The increased digoxin concentration reflects a decrease in digoxin's volume of distribution to 70% of the original value. The initial rise in digoxin concentrations to approximately 1.5 times the original concentration is followed by a relatively slow accumulation over the next week to a steady-state digoxin concentration that is approximately double the original value.[78,81] Many patients develop signs of digitalis toxicity (primarily gastrointestinal in nature), which subside when the dose and plasma concentrations of digoxin are adjusted.[78] However, it should be recognized that although gastrointestinal side effects are the most common for digitalis, side effects do not occur in a progressive order from least to most toxic or dangerous. The first sign of digoxin toxicity could be a life-threatening cardiac arrhythmia.

The rapid and sustained changes in digoxin concentrations (see Fig. 10.3) suggest that the initial change in digoxin concentration is owing to a decline in the volume of distribution, which is slightly smaller than the decline in the clearance. This is illustrated by the initial rapid increase in serum digoxin concentration followed by a gradual increase in the serum concentration to the final steady-state value.

Given the initial rapid rise in digoxin concentration (decrease in V) and the eventual doubling of the steady-state concentration (decrease in Cl), the usual approach is to hold one daily dose of digoxin in an attempt to blunt the initial rapid rise in digoxin and then reinitiate the digoxin maintenance dose at half the previous rate.[82–86] Again, this approach assumes that the goal is to maintain the same digoxin concentration following the initiation of quinidine therapy.[87–89]

The patient's digoxin concentration at the time of adding quinidine should be considered carefully. For example, adding quinidine to a patient with a digoxin level of 0.5 mcg/L may require no digoxin dose adjustment. A patient with a level of ≈1 mcg/L may have one dose withheld and the maintenance dose halved.

In addition, digoxin concentrations may vary within a quinidine dosing interval because of the varying degrees of tissue displacement. This has been demonstrated at relatively low quinidine concentrations and should be considered when obtaining digoxin plasma levels. For this reason, it is generally advisable to obtain plasma digoxin concentrations just before a quinidine dose so that the digoxin plasma levels will be reasonably reproducible. Any change in digoxin concentration sampled in this way should represent actual changes in digoxin disposition rather than transient changes within a quinidine dosing interval[83] (Fig. 10.4). One report also cited that amiodarone like quinidine may cause variations of digoxin concentrations during the dosing interval.[49] This report would suggest that amiodarone may, in fact, change the volume of distribution as a rise and fall of the digoxin concentration during the interval not associated with the administration of the digoxin dose must be because of transient changes in plasma and tissue concentrations and hence altered volume. This is a single report and, until more data are available to confirm and quantify this observation, the authors will continue to assume that amiodarone does not affect digoxin volume to a significant degree.

In the case of both amiodarone[76] and verapamil, if a reduction in digoxin dose is contemplated, it is not necessary to skip a daily dose. Instead, the maintenance regimen should be reduced by the appropriate amount at about the time the amiodarone or verapamil therapy is instituted.

Question #16 *What other drugs commonly used in patients receiving digoxin are likely to cause a significant change in its disposition?*

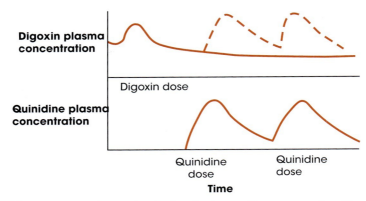

FIGURE 10.4   Displacement of digoxin by quinidine. The digoxin plasma concentration with no quinidine (*solid line*) and following the administration of two quinidine doses (*dashed line*). Note that as the quinidine plasma concentrations rise and then fall, the digoxin levels also rise and then fall. The elevation of digoxin levels appears to be minimal at quinidine concentrations less than 1 mg/L.[83]

Amiodarone is probably the most significant and common drug that interacts with digoxin. However, other compounds, such as propafenone and verapamil, also reduce digoxin clearance.[86,90–93] The decrease in digoxin clearance with the addition of propafenone ranges from less than 25% to more than 50%. Most of the change appears to be associated with the metabolic route of digoxin elimination. In addition, the decrease in metabolism appears to increase as the concentration of propafenone increases. Monitoring digoxin plasma levels may be helpful in evaluating the extent of the propafenone–digoxin interaction. Careful consideration should be given to those patients with renal dysfunction or who are to be given large doses of propafenone.

Although the change in clearance for verapamil is not remarkable, approximately a 25% reduction, there may be individual patients in whom a modest reduction in the digoxin maintenance dose is warranted. Broken line D in Figure 10.3 depicts the anticipated rise in digoxin concentration following the institution of verapamil therapy. Note that the slow rise in digoxin concentration suggests that the volume of distribution for digoxin is not altered. The clearance, although reduced, is not reduced to the same extent as that associated with concomitant amiodarone or quinidine therapy; this is consistent with the smaller increase in steady-state digoxin concentrations associated with verapamil. Nifedipine and diltiazem appear to have relatively little influence on digoxin disposition; verapamil has modest effects.

St. John wort can reduce digoxin concentrations by approximately 25%.[24–27] The most common explanation is a reduced bioavailability, but hepatic enzyme induction and an increase in clearance have also been proposed as a possible mechanism.[26,27,94] Note in Figure 10.3, line E, that the digoxin concentration decreases with the addition of an agent that either reduces bioavailability or increases clearance.

Macrolide antibiotics (e.g., clarithromycin, erythromycin) and ritonavir have been reported to increase digoxin serum levels.[95–99] In addition, depending on the assay procedure, other drugs, including herbal and nontraditional agents, may result in assay interference with digoxin, resulting in either false elevation or decrease in the reported digoxin concentration.[61,62,100]

Question #17 *A.P., a 75-year-old, 60-kg man, was admitted with complaints of increased shortness of breath and yellow sputum production. He has a medical history of chronic obstructive pulmonary disease and CHF. During his hospital stay, he developed atrial fibrillation and was given digoxin to slow his ventricular rate. He received 250 mcg IV every 3 hours × 3 doses (starting at 9:00 p.m., day 1) and was given a maintenance dose of 250-mcg tablets each morning (starting at 9:00 a.m., day 2). His serum creatinine is stable at 1.5 mg/dL. A digoxin level obtained at 9:00 a.m. on the morning of day 4 (2.5 days after the loading dose) was reported to be 1.5 mcg/L. A.P. had, therefore, received his initial IV loading dose and two oral maintenance doses when a plasma sample was drawn on the morning of day 4. What would you expect his digoxin concentration to be?*

To calculate the expected concentration, just before the third maintenance dose, one would first need to calculate A.P.'s expected digoxin pharmacokinetic parameters. Using Equation 10.5 for Cl_{Cr}, an estimate of 36.1 mL/min is calculated.

$$Cl_{Cr} \text{ for Males} = \frac{(140 - \text{Age})(\text{Weight in kg})}{(72)(SCr_{ss})}$$
$$= \frac{(140 - 75 \text{ yr})(60 \text{ kg})}{(72)(1.5 \text{ mg/dL})}$$
$$= 36.1 \text{ mL/min}$$

Then, using Equation 10.1 for digoxin V and Equation 10.4 for the digoxin clearance in patients with CHF, the corresponding values can be obtained.

$$V_{Digoxin} (L) = (3.8 \text{ L/kg})(\text{Weight in kg}) + (3.1)(Cl_{Cr} \text{ in mL/min})$$
$$= (3.8 \text{ L/kg})(60 \text{ kg}) + (3.1)(36.1 \text{ mL/min})$$
$$= 228 \text{ L} + 112 \text{ L}$$
$$= 340 \text{ L}$$

$$\begin{aligned}\text{Total } Cl_{Digoxin} \text{ (mL/min)} \\ \text{(Patients with CHF)}\end{aligned} = \begin{aligned}(0.33 \text{ mL/kg/min})(\text{Weight in kg}) \\ + (0.9)(Cl_{Cr} \text{ in mL/min})\end{aligned}$$
$$= (0.33 \text{ mL/kg/min})(60 \text{ kg}) + (0.9)(36.1 \text{ mL/min})$$
$$= 19.8 \text{ mL/min} + 32.5 \text{ mL/min}$$
$$= 52.3 \text{ mL/min}$$

The $Cl_{Digoxin}$ in mL/min can be converted to the more convenient units of L/day using Equation 10.11.

$$Cl \text{ (L/day)} = (Cl \text{ as mL/min})\left(\frac{1,440 \text{ min/day}}{1,000 \text{ mL/L}}\right)$$
$$= (52.3 \text{ mL/min})\left(\frac{1,440 \text{ min/day}}{1,000 \text{ mL/L}}\right)$$
$$= 75.3 \text{ L/day}$$

Using the calculated volume of distribution of 340 L and clearance of 75.3 L/day, Equation 10.16 estimates an elimination rate constant of 0.22 day^{-1}.

$$K = \frac{Cl}{V}$$
$$= \frac{75.3 \text{ L/day}}{340 \text{ L}}$$
$$= 0.22 \text{ day}^{-1}$$

Equation 10.17 estimates a half-life of approximately 3 days.

$$t\tfrac{1}{2} = \frac{(0.693)(V)}{Cl}$$
$$= \frac{(0.693)(340 \text{ L})}{75.3 \text{ L/day}}$$
$$= 3.1 \text{ days}$$

To calculate A.P.'s digoxin plasma concentration, one needs to consider the loading dose plus the two maintenance doses. To model this series of doses, refer to Chapter 2: Selecting the Appropriate Equation: Series of Individual Doses, and Fig. 2.7, in which the loading dose plus the two maintenance doses are depicted as D_1, D_2, and D_3. Because his loading dose of 750 mcg (250 mcg $\times$ 3 doses) was given over a total of 6 hours and A.P.'s expected digoxin half-life is 3.1 days, one can group the entire loading dose together as though it was administered as a single dose, all administered when the first 250 mcg dose was given (i.e., time from start to end of loading [tin] is $\leq 1/6 \, t\tfrac{1}{2}$).

$$C_{(Sum)} = \frac{(S)(F)(D_1)}{V}(e^{-Kt_1}) + \frac{(S)(F)(D_2)}{V}(e^{-Kt_2}) + \frac{(S)(F)(D_3)}{V}(e^{-Kt_3})\dots \quad \textbf{(Eq. 10.22)}$$

$$= \frac{(1)(1)(750 \text{ mcg})}{340 \text{ L}}(e^{-(0.22 \text{ day}^{-1})(2.5 \text{ days})}) + \frac{(1)(0.7)(250 \text{ mcg})}{340 \text{ L}}(e^{-(0.22 \text{ day}^{-1})(2 \text{ days})})$$
$$+ \frac{(1)(0.7)(250 \text{ mcg})}{340 \text{ L}}(e^{-(0.22 \text{ day}^{-1})(1 \text{ day})})$$
$$= (2.2 \text{ mcg/L})(0.58) + (0.51 \text{ mcg/L})(0.64) + (0.51 \text{ mcg/L})(0.8)$$
$$= 1.3 \text{ mcg/L} + 0.33 \text{ mcg/L} + 0.41 \text{ mcg/L}$$
$$= 2 \text{ mcg/L}$$

Note that the predicted digoxin concentration of 2 mcg/L is greater than the observed value of 1.5 mcg/L. Unfortunately, revision of pharmacokinetic parameters at this point would be difficult. After only 2.5 days and with a half-life of 3 days, it is relatively easy to see that we have gone beyond one-third of the half-life because the loading dose was administered. Generally, to accurately estimate volume of distribution following a loading dose, we would want a plasma sample within one-third of a half-life. Furthermore, A.P.'s maintenance dose has not been administered longer than two half-lives, which limits our ability to extract information about clearance. The observed plasma concentration may reflect a larger-than-expected V, a higher-than-expected Cl, or some combination of both of these factors. To more accurately determine A.P.'s digoxin clearance, it will be necessary to wait several more days to obtain a plasma concentration that might reasonably be expected to yield information about clearance. Given his expected half-life of approximately 3 days and the probability that his half-life is less than expected, an additional 2 or 3 days would probably be sufficient to begin to obtain some additional information that will help to predict A.P.'s final steady-state concentration.

In the example above, the time intervals were based on the number of days. In the clinical setting, many times, levels and doses are not administered in a way that days would be the most appropriate unit. Instead, hours may be more appropriate. If this is the case, it is important to have the units for clearance in L/hr and the units for elimination rate constant in hr^{-1} so that the units are consistent with the time in hours. The equations for calculating the concentrations would be the same and the end result would be the same, just the units would reflect hours and not days.

Question #18   *C.A. is a 60-year-old, 65-kg man with a serum creatinine of 1.3 mg/dL. He had been taking 0.25 mg of digoxin at 9:00 a.m. orally for his CHF. On the day of admission, a digoxin level of 0.8 mcg/L was measured just before his morning dose. His outpatient maintenance dose was continued. On the fifth day, just before his morning dose (four doses of digoxin having been administered each day at 9:00 a.m.), a second digoxin sample was obtained. Using the expected pharmacokinetic parameters, calculate C.A.'s digoxin concentration on the morning of the fifth day.*

Again, to calculate the expected plasma concentration, one would first have to estimate C.A.'s creatinine clearance and then use the appropriate equations to calculate his volume of distribution, clearance, elimination rate constant, and half-life.

Using Equation 10.5, we calculate a creatinine clearance of 55.6 mL/min.

$$\text{Cl}_{\text{Cr}} \text{ for Males} = \frac{(140 - \text{Age})(\text{Weight in kg})}{(72)(\text{SCr}_{\text{ss}})}$$

$$= \frac{(140 - 60 \text{ yr})(65 \text{ kg})}{(72)(1.3 \text{ mg/dL})}$$

$$= 55.6 \text{ mL/min}$$

Then, using Equation 10.1 for digoxin V and Equation 10.4 for the digoxin clearance in patients with CHF, the corresponding values can be obtained.

$$V_{\text{Digoxin}} (L) = (3.8 \text{ L/kg})(\text{Weight in kg}) + (3.1)(\text{Cl}_{\text{Cr}} \text{ in mL/min})$$

$$= (3.8 \text{ L/kg})(65 \text{ kg}) + (3.1)(55.6 \text{ mL/min})$$

$$= 247 \text{ L} + 172 \text{ L}$$

$$= 419 \text{ L}$$

$$\frac{\text{Total Cl}_{\text{Digoxin}} \, (\text{mL}/\min)}{(\text{Patients with CHF})} = \frac{(0.33 \, \text{mL}/\text{kg}/\min)(\text{Weight in kg})}{+ (0.9)(\text{Cl}_{\text{Cr}} \, \text{in mL}/\min)}$$

$$= (0.33 \, \text{mL}/\text{kg}/\min)(65 \, \text{kg}) + (0.9)(55.6 \, \text{mL}/\min)$$

$$= 21.5 \, \text{mL}/\min \; + \; 50 \, \text{mL}/\min$$

$$= 71.5 \, \text{mL}/\min$$

The $\text{Cl}_{\text{Digoxin}}$ in mL/min can be converted to the units of L/day using Equation 10.11.

$$\text{Cl} \, (\text{L}/\text{day}) = (\text{Cl as mL}/\min)\left(\frac{1,440 \, \text{min}/\text{day}}{1,000 \, \text{mL}/\text{L}}\right)$$

$$= (71.5 \, \text{mL}/\min)\left(\frac{1,440 \, \text{min}/\text{day}}{1,000 \, \text{mL}/\text{L}}\right)$$

$$= 103 \, \text{L}/\text{day}$$

Using the calculated volume of distribution and clearance, Equation 10.16 estimates an elimination rate constant of 0.25 day^{-1}.

$$K = \frac{\text{Cl}}{\text{V}}$$

$$K = \frac{103 \, \text{L}/\text{day}}{419 \, \text{L}}$$

$$= 0.25 \, \text{day}^{-1}$$

Equation 10.17 estimates a half-life of approximately 3 days.

$$t\tfrac{1}{2} = \frac{(0.693)(\text{V})}{\text{Cl}}$$

$$= \frac{(0.693)(419 \, \text{L})}{103 \, \text{L}/\text{day}}$$

$$= 2.8 \, \text{days}$$

To model the initial digoxin concentration decay and the four subsequent doses, several approaches could be used. One approach is to use Equation 10.23 to model the initial digoxin concentration and subsequent decay.

$$C_{(Sum)} = C_1(e^{-Kt_1}) + \frac{(S)(F)(D_1)}{V}(e^{-Kt_1}) + \frac{(S)(F)(D_2)}{V}(e^{-Kt_2}) + \frac{(S)(F)(D_3)}{V}(e^{-Kt_3})... \quad \textbf{(Eq. 10.23)}$$

In the above equation, the digoxin concentration of 0.8 would be C_1 the first t_1 the time from that concentration to the time of sampling (4 days), D_1 the initial dose of 250 mcg, and the second t_1 the time from that dose to the time of the sample (again 4 days). D_2 is the second dose, t_2 the second time interval (3 days), and so on. The calculations would then be as follows:

$$C_{(Sum)} = (0.8\ mcg/L)(e^{-0.25\ day^{-1}\ (4\ days)}) + \frac{(1)(0.7)(250\ mcg)}{419\ L}(e^{-(0.25\ day^{-1})(4\ days)})$$

$$+ \frac{(1)(0.7)(250\ mcg)}{419\ L}(e^{-(0.25\ day^{-1})(3\ days)})$$

$$+ \frac{(1)(0.7)(250\ mcg)}{419\ L}(e^{-(0.25\ day^{-1})(2\ days)})$$

$$+ \frac{(1)(0.7)(250\ mcg)}{419\ L}(e^{-(0.25\ day^{-1})(1\ day)})$$

Note that because S and F as well as each of the digoxin doses were the same, the above equation can be factored to the following:

$$C_{(Sum)} = (0.8\ mcg/L)(e^{-(0.25\ day^{-1})(4\ days)})$$

$$+ \frac{(1)(0.7)(250\ mcg)}{419\ L}\left[\begin{array}{l} (e^{-(0.25\ day^{-1})(4\ days)}) + e^{-(0.25\ day^{-1})(3\ days)} \\ + e^{-(0.25\ day^{-1})(2\ days)} + e^{-(0.25\ day^{-1})(1\ day)} \end{array} \right]$$

$$C_{(Sum)} = (0.8\ mcg/L)(0.37) + 0.42\ mcg/L[(0.37) + (0.47) + (0.61) + (0.78)]$$

$$= 0.3\ mcg/L + 0.42\ mcg/L[2.23]$$

$$= 0.3\ mcg/L + 0.94\ mcg/L$$

$$= 1.24\ mcg/L$$

An alternative approach is to use a model that takes advantage of digoxin's long half-life relative to the dosing interval (see Chapter 2: Selecting the Appropriate Equation, Fig. 2.5). In this model, one could choose to decay the initial digoxin plasma concentration and then add the four subsequent doses by treating them as a continuous infusion, as depicted in Equation 10.24:

$$C_t = (C_1)(e^{-Kt_1}) + \frac{(S)(F)(Dose/\tau)}{Cl}(1 - e^{-Kt_1}) \qquad \textbf{(Eq. 10.24)}$$

Note that, in the infusion part of the non–steady-state equation, Dose/τ is the rate of drug administration and t_1 is the duration of drug administration. Therefore, Dose/$\tau \times t_1$ should equal the total amount of drug administered. In this case, there were four doses administered for 1,000 mcg. Given that the rate of administration is 250 mcg/day, t_1 would be 4 days.

Using the appropriate doses, times, and pharmacokinetic parameters, a digoxin concentration of 1.37 mcg/L is calculated.

$$C_t = (0.8 \text{ mcg/L})(e^{-(0.25 \text{ day}^{-1})(4 \text{ days})})$$
$$+ \frac{(1)(0.7)(250 \text{ mcg/day})}{103 \text{ L/day}}(1 - e^{-(0.25 \text{ day}^{-1})(4 \text{ days})})$$
$$= (0.8 \text{ mcg/L})(0.37) + (1.7 \text{ mcg/L})(1 - 0.37)$$
$$= 0.3 \text{ mcg/L} + 1.07 \text{ mcg/L}$$
$$= 1.37 \text{ mcg/L}$$

The concentrations predicted by the first method (individual bolus doses) and the second method (digoxin given as an infusion) are similar, indicating that either method is a reasonable way to predict C.A.'s digoxin concentration on the morning of the fifth day. Also, note that the predicted steady-state concentration produced by a maintenance dose of 0.25 mg/day (250 mcg/day) would be ≈1.7 mcg/L (see above part of Equation 10.24 that represents Css ave or Equation 10.20).

$$\text{Css ave} = \frac{(S)(F)(\text{Dose}/\tau)}{Cl}$$
$$= \frac{(1)(0.7)(250 \text{ mcg/day})}{103 \text{ L/day}}$$
$$= 1.7 \text{ mcg/L}$$

Question #19   *C.A.'s digoxin level reported from the laboratory was 1.6 mcg/L. Because the observed digoxin concentration is greater than the predicted level (1.24 to 1.37 mcg/L), what would one expect C.A.'s digoxin clearance and subsequent steady-state digoxin concentration to be on his current regimen of 0.25 mg/day?*

Either of the two approaches in the previous question can be used to resolve this problem. Clearance could be calculated by first assuming C.A.'s digoxin volume of distribution to be 419 L. Then, using a trial and error method or iterative search, one could substitute various clearance values and the corresponding elimination rate constant values until the equation predicted the observed digoxin concentration of 1.6 mcg/L. Because this process could be laborious, an alternative approach is to use the mass balance technique and solve directly for C.A.'s clearance (see Interpretation of Plasma Drug Concentrations: Non-steady-state Revision of Clearance [Mass Balance] in Chapter 2). The expected steady-state digoxin concentration for C.A. could then be more easily calculated.

$$Cl = \frac{(S)(F)(\text{Dose}/\tau) - \dfrac{(C_2 - C_1)V}{t}}{C \text{ ave}}$$ **(Eq. 10.25)**

In this equation, t is the time interval between C_1 and C_2 and, therefore, is 4 days, because this is the interval between C_1 (0.8 mcg/L) and C_2 (1.6 mcg/L). C ave is calculated as the arithmetic mean of the two plasma concentrations.

$$C\text{ ave} = \frac{C_1 + C_2}{2} \qquad \textbf{(Eq. 10.26)}$$

$$= \frac{0.8\text{ mcg/L} + 1.6\text{ mcg/L}}{2}$$

$$= 1.2\text{ mcg/L}$$

Substituting the appropriate values in Equation 10.25, a digoxin clearance of 76 L/day can be calculated.

$$Cl = \frac{(S)(F)(Dose/\tau) - \dfrac{(C_2 - C_1)V}{t}}{C\text{ ave}}$$

$$= \frac{(1)(0.7)(250\text{ mcg/day}) - \dfrac{(1.6\text{ mcg/L} - 0.8\text{ mcg/L})(419\text{ L})}{4\text{ days}}}{1.2\text{ mcg/L}}$$

$$= \frac{91.2\text{ mcg/day}}{1.2\text{ mcg/L}}$$

$$= 76\text{ L/day}$$

Note that this calculated digoxin clearance and our assumed volume of distribution of 419 L is consistent with an expected half-life of approximately 3.8 days (Equation 10.17).

$$t\tfrac{1}{2} = \frac{(0.693)(V)}{Cl}$$

$$= \frac{(0.693)(419\text{ L})}{76\text{ L/day}}$$

$$= 3.8\text{ days}$$

Evaluating the revised half-life is an important step in our assessment of the clearance prediction of 76 L/day. As mentioned in Part I (see Chapter 2), there are three key issues or rules to be considered when using the mass balance approach when solving for clearance, using non–steady-state data:

1. t or time interval between C_1 and C_2 should be at least one half-life but not more than two half-lives. If t is very short, relative to the drug half-life, small differences in C_1 and C_2 can result in widely varying estimates of drug accumulation or drug loss. If t is much more than two half-lives, the second concentration would be approaching steady-state, and our C ave would be an underestimate of the average concentration within the time interval t. Hence, the rule is that t should be at least one but not more than two half-lives.

2. The plasma concentration values should be reasonably close to one another; therefore, $C_2/C_1 \leq 2$ if the concentration is increasing, and $C_2/C_1 \geq 0.5$ if the concentration is decreasing. If there is a large difference between C_1 and C_2, it means that relatively little of the dose administered between C_1 and C_2 has been eliminated. In this situation, volume of distribution and the total dose administered are the critical factors, and the drug concentrations contain very little information about clearance. If the concentration has declined more than one $t\frac{1}{2}$, that is, $C_2/C_1 < 0.5$, there will be a significant curve in the decay line, and the arithmetic mean of C_1 and C_2 [i.e., $(C_1 + C_2)/2$] will not be a good estimate of the average drug concentration over the time interval t. Ideally, C_1 and C_2 would be very close together and the net drug accumulation or loss would be approaching 0, suggesting near steady-state conditions and, therefore, ideal conditions for estimating clearance.
3. The rate of drug administration $[(S)(F)(Dose/\tau)]$ should be regular and result in a reasonably smooth progression from C_1 to C_2. If the doses are very irregular because either the interval is not consistent or the dose is changing, the accumulation pattern will not be a smooth transition from C_1 to C_2. Therefore, the C ave as calculated from the arithmetic mean of C_1 and C_2 [i.e., $(C_1 + C_2)/2$] will not accurately represent the true C ave between C_1 and C_2. Another potential problem with the mass balance approach is when the dosing interval is longer than the drug half-life. Under these conditions, there will be significant increases and decreases in the drug concentration within each dosing interval. The progression from C_1 to C_2 will not be smooth, and, as a result, the arithmetic mean $[(C_1 + C_2)/2]$ may be a poor estimate of the true average concentration.

Assuming we have met all the three rules described above and are using the revised clearance value and Equation 10.20, the expected steady-state digoxin concentration of approximately 2.3 mcg/L can be calculated.

$$\begin{aligned} \text{Css ave} &= \frac{(S)(F)(Dose/\tau)}{Cl} \\ &= \frac{(1)(0.7)(250 \text{ mcg/day})}{76 \text{ L/day}} \\ &= 2.3 \text{ mcg/L} \end{aligned}$$

Because this value is above the upper limit of the usually accepted therapeutic range for heart failure, one would most likely choose to reduce the digoxin maintenance dose at this time. This is especially true given that most patients with CHF do well clinically with digoxin concentrations in the range of 0.5 to 0.9 mcg/L and evidence that digoxin has a potentially harmful effect if digoxin concentration is ≥ 1.2 mcg/L.[5] An alternative approach would be to hold digoxin for approximately one half-life (3 to 4 days) and resample. Assuming the resampled digoxin level is about half (≈ 0.8 mcg/L), it would be further evidence that the final steady-state level would be in the range of 2.3 mcg/L. If the desire steady-state level is 0.6 mcg/L (one-fourth of the predicted steady-state level of 2.3), a reasonable new maintenance dose would be 0.0625 mg daily or 0.125 mg every other day. As a general rule for a patient being treated only for CHF, the initial maintenance dose should be 0.125 mg/day or lower depending on patient size, renal function, and other drugs.

Question #20   *When is DigiFab indicated and how is the dose determined?*

DigiFab, Digoxin Immune Fab (Ovine), is indicated for life-threatening digoxin intoxication, that is, severe ventricular arrhythmias or progressive bradyarrhythmias not responsive to treatment, or progressive elevation in serum potassium. Each vial of DigiFab binds 0.5 mg or 500 mcg of digoxin. If the total amount of digoxin is known, Equation 10.27 can be used to calculate the dose of DigiFab.

$$\frac{\text{DigiFab}}{\text{(No. of Vials)}} = \frac{\text{mcg of Digoxin in Body}}{500} \qquad \textbf{(Eq. 10.27)}$$

If the total body stores is uncertain but a digoxin concentration is known, Equation 10.28 can be used to calculate the number of vials of DigiFab that would be needed.

$$\frac{\text{DigiFab}}{\text{(No. of Vials)}} = (C_{\text{Digoxin}} \text{ in mcg/L}) \left(\frac{\text{Weight in kg}}{100} \right) \qquad \textbf{(Eq. 10.28)}$$

Equation 10.28 assumes a digoxin volume of 5 L/kg. In obese patients, it is not clear what weight to use, but the authors would recommend using the weight that best correlates with the digoxin volume of distribution, that is, IBW if obese. However, care should be taken not to "underdose" the patient. Also, care should be taken in young healthy individuals because their digoxin volume of distribution may be larger than the assumed value of 5 L/kg in Equation 10.28. Lastly, when the calculated DigiFab dose contains a fraction of a vial (e.g., 4.4 vials), most clinicians would round up to the next whole number of vials.

Another important issue is whether or not serum digoxin levels would be appropriate following the administration of DigiFab. The answer depends on the assay being used.[67,101] DigiFab is a digoxin antibody fragment (Fab) that binds the plasma digoxin, thereby creating disequilibrium between the plasma and tissue concentrations. The tissue digoxin then re-equilibrates with the plasma and that re-equilibrated plasma digoxin is then bound to the Fab. This process continues until all or almost all of the digoxin is pulled from the tissue and bound in the plasma to the Fab. While the total plasma digoxin is very high, almost all is bound to the Fab and essentially "inactive."

Some digoxin assays measure the unbound digoxin and some or all of the Fab-bound digoxin. These assays are of no clinical value following the administration of DigiFab and can be clinically confusing because the reported digoxin concentration represents both the unbound "active" and the Fab-bound "inactive" digoxin. With this type of assay, depending on how much of the Fab-bound digoxin is being analyzed, it is possible for the digoxin concentration to increase following the administration of DigiFab. Some digoxin assays measure only the unbound "active" digoxin concentration. These assays may be of some clinical value, but, in most cases, the unbound digoxin concentration will be very low.

REFERENCES

1. Smith TW. Digitalis toxicity: epidemiology and clinical use of serum concentration measurements. *Am J Med.* 1975;58:470.

2. Smith TW, Haber E. Digoxin intoxication: the relationship of clinical presentation to serum digoxin concentration. *J Clin Invest.* 1970;49:2377.

3. Hunt SA; American College of Cardiology; American Heart Association Task Force on Practice Guidelines (Writing Committee to Update the 2001 Guidelines for the Evaluation and Management of Heart Failure). ACC/AHA 2005 Guideline update for the diagnosis and management of chronic heart failure in the adult. *J Am Coll Cardiol.* 2005;46:e1–e82. http://content.onlinejacc.org. Accessed August 3, 2008.

4. Adams KF Jr, Gheorghiade M, Uretsky BF, et al. Clinical benefits of low serum digoxin concentrations in heart failure. *J Am Coll Cardiol.* 2002;39:946–953.

5. Adams KF Jr, Patterson JH, Gattis WA, et al. Relationship of serum digoxin concentration to mortality and morbidity in women in the digitalis investigation group trial: a retrospective analysis. *J Am Coll Cardiol.* 2005;46:497–504.

6. Ahmed A, Rich MW, Love TE, et al. Digoxin and reduction in mortality and hospitalization in heart failure: a comprehensive post hoc analysis of the DIG trial. *Eur Heart J.* 2006;27:178–186.

7. HFSA Guidelines for management of patients with heart failure caused by left ventricular systolic dysfunction-pharmacologic approaches. *J Card Fail.* 1999;5:357–382.

8. Sameri RM, Soberman JE, Finch CK, et al. Lower serum digoxin concentrations in heart failure and reassessment of laboratory report forms. *Am J Med Sci.* 2002;324:10–13.

9. Snow V, Weiss KB, LeFevre M, et al. Management of newly detected atrial fibrillation: a clinical practice guideline from the American academy of family physicians and the American college of physicians. *Ann Intern Med.* 2003;139:1009–1017.

10. Kock-Weser J, Duhme DW, Greenblatt DJ. Influence of serum digoxin concentration measurements on frequency of digitoxicity. *Clin Pharmacol Ther.* 1974;16:284.

11. Sheiner LB, Melmon KL, Rosenberg B. Instructional goals for physicians in the use of blood level data and the contribution of computers. *Clin Pharmacol Ther.* 1974;16:260.

12. Ogilvie RI, Ruedy J. An educational program in digitalis therapy. *JAMA.* 1972;222:50.

13. DiDomenico RJ, Bress AP, Na-Thalang K, et al. Use of a simplified nomogram to individualize digoxin dosing versus standard dosing practices in patients with heart failure. *Pharmacotherapy.* 2014;34(11):1121–1131.

14. Patel N, Ju C, Macon C, et al. Temporal trends of digoxin use in patients hospitalized with heart failure: analysis from the American Heart Association get with the guidelines-heart failure registry. *JACC Heart Fail.* 2016;4(5):348–356.

15. Virgadamo S, Charnigo R, Darrat Y, et al. Digoxin: a systematic review in atrial fibrillation, congestive heart failure and post myocardial infarction. *World J Cardiol.* 2015;7(11):808–816.

16. Allen LA, Fonarow GC, Simon DN, et al. Digoxin use and subsequent outcomes among patients in a contemporary atrial fibrillation cohort. *J Am Coll Cardiol.* 2015;65(25):2691–2698.

17. Scalese MJ, Salvatore DJ. Role of digoxin in atrial fibrillation. *J Pharm Pract.* 2016; pii: 0897190016642361. doi:10.1177/0897190016642361.

18. Huffman DH, Manion CV, Azarnoff DL. Absorption of digoxin from different oral preparations in normal subjects during steady state. *Clin Pharmacol Ther.* 1974;16:310.

19. Lisalo E. Clinical pharmacokinetics of digoxin. *Clin Pharmacokinet.* 1977;2:1.

20. Mallis GI, Schmidt DH, Lindenbaum J. Superior bioavailability of digoxin solution in capsules. *Clin Pharmacol Ther.* 1975;18:761.

21. Marcus FI, Dickerson J, Pippin S, et al. Digoxin bioavailability: formulations and rates of infusions. *Clin Pharmacol Ther.* 1976;20:253.

22. Rathore SS, Curtis JP, Wang Y, et al. Association of serum digoxin concentration and outcomes in patients with heart failure. *JAMA.* 2003;289:871–878.

23. Heart Failure Society of America. Executive summary: HFSA 2006 comprehensive heart failure practice guideline. *J Card Fail.* 2006;12:10–38.

24. Johne A, Brockmöller J, Bauer S, et al. Pharmacokinetic interaction of digoxin with an herbal extract from St John's wort *(Hypericum perforatum)*. *Clin Pharmacol Ther*. 1999;66:338–345.

25. Izzo AA, Ernst E. Interactions between herbal medicines and prescribed drugs: a systematic review. *Drugs*. 2001;61:2163–2175.

26. Dürr D, Stieger B, Kullak-Ublick GA, et al. St John's wort induces intestinal P-glycoprotein/MDR1 and intestinal and hepatic CYP3A4. *Clin Pharmacol Ther*. 2000;68:598–604.

27. Henderson L, Yue QY, Bergquist C, et al. St John's wort *(Hypericum perforatum):* drug interactions and clinical outcomes. *Br J Clin Pharmacol*. 2002;54:349–356.

28. Bizjak ED, Mauro VF. Digoxin–macrolide drug interaction. *Ann Pharmacother*. 1997;31:1077–1079.

29. Gooderham MJ, Bolli P, Fernandez PG. Concomitant digoxin toxicity and warfarin interaction in a patient receiving clarithromycin. *Ann Pharmacother*. 1999;33:796–799.

30. Wakasugi H, Yano I, Ito T, et al. Effect of clarithromycin on renal excretion of digoxin: interaction with P-glycoprotein. *Clin Pharmacol Ther*. 1988;64:123–128.

31. Lindenbaum J, Rund DG, Butler VP Jr, et al. Inactivation of digoxin by the gut flora: reversal by antibiotic therapy. *N Engl J Med*. 1981;305:789–794.

32. Partanen J, Jalava KM, Neuvonen PJ. Itraconazole increases serum digoxin concentration. *Pharmacol Toxicol*. 1996;79:274–276.

33. Henderson RP, Solomon CP. Use of cholestyramine in the treatment of digoxin intoxication. *Arch Intern Med*. 1988;148:745–746.

34. Neuvonen PJ, Kivisto K, Hirvisalo EL. Effects of resin and activated charcoal on the absorption of digoxin, carbamazepine and frusemide. *Br J Pharmacol*. 1988;25:229–233.

35. Reuning RH, Sams RA, Notari RE. Role of pharmacokinetics in drug dosage adjustment: I. Pharmacologic effect kinetics and apparent volume of distribution of digoxin. *J Clin Pharmacol*. 1973;13:127.

36. Abernethy DR, Greenblatt DJ, Smith TW. Digoxin disposition in obesity: clinical pharmacokinetic investigation. *Am Heart J*. 1981;102:740–744.

37. Jelliffe RW, Milman M, Schumitzky A, et al. A two-compartment population pharmacokinetic-pharmacodynamics model of digoxin in adults, with implications for dosage. *Ther Drug Monit*. 2014;36(3):387–393.

38. Shapiro W, Narahara K, Taubert K. Relationship of plasma digitoxin and digoxin to cardiac response following intravenous digitalization in man. *Circulation*. 1970;42:1065.

39. Walsh FM, Sode J. Significance of non-steady state serum digoxin concentrations. *Am J Clin Pathol*. 1975;63:446.

40. Lanoxin (digoxin) injection [package insert]. Cary, NC: Covis Pharmaceuticals Inc.; July 2015. https://dailymed.nlm.nih.gov/dailymed/fda/fdaDrugXsl.cfm?setid=3e66b3d0-d36e-4795-b707-e27ecae5723d&type=display. Accessed May 24, 2016.

41. Kramer WG, Lewis RP, Cobb TC, et al. Pharmacokinetics of digoxin: comparison of a two and a three compartment model in man. *J Pharmacokinet Biopharm*. 1974;2:299.

42. Sheiner LB, Rosenberg B, Marathe VV. Estimation of population characteristics of pharmacokinetic parameters from routine clinical data. *J Pharmacokinet Biopharm*. 1977;5:445.

43. Sheiner LB, Rosenberg B, Melmon KL. Modeling of individual pharmacokinetics for computer-aided drug dosage. *Comput Biomed Res*. 1972;5:441.

44. Smith TW, Haber E. Clinical value of the radioimmunoassay of the digitalis glycosides. *Pharmacol Rev*. 1973;25:219.

45. Fenster PE, White NW Jr, Hanson CD. Pharmacokinetic evaluation of the digoxin–amiodarone interaction. *J Am Coll Cardiol*. 1985;5:108–112.

46. Nademanee K, Kannan R, Hendrickson J, et al. Amiodarone–digoxin interaction: clinical significance, time course of development, potential pharmacokinetic mechanisms and therapeutic implications. *J Am Coll Cardiol*. 1984;4:111–116.

47. Trujillo TC, Nolan PE. Antiarrhythmic agents: drug interactions of clinical significance. *Drug Saf*. 2000;23:509–532.

48. Vallakati A, Chandra PA, Pednekar M, et al. Dronedarone-induced digoxin toxicity: new drug, new interactions. *Am J Ther*. 2013;20(6):e717–e719.

49. Devore KJ, Hobbs RA. Plasma digoxin concentration fluctuations associated with timing of plasma sampling and amiodarone administration. *Pharmacotherapy*. 2007;27:472–475.

50. See I, Shehab N, Kegler SR, et al. Emergency department visits and hospitalizations for digoxin toxicity: United States 2005 to 2010. *Circ Heart Fail*. 2014;7(1):28–34.

51. Jusko WH, Szefler SJ, Goldfarb AL. Pharmacokinetic design of digoxin dosage regimens in relation to renal function. *J Clin Pharmacol*. 1974;14:525.

52. Jusko WJ, Wintraub M. Myocardial distribution of digoxin and renal function. *Clin Pharmacol Ther*. 1974;16:449.

53. Wagner JG. Loading and maintenance doses of digoxin in patients with normal renal function and those with severely impaired renal function. *J Clin Pharmacol*. 1974;14:329.

54. Ohnhaus EE. Protein binding of digoxin in human serum. *Eur J Clin Pharmacol*. 1972;5:34.

55. Koup JR, Greenblatt DJ, Jusko WJ, et al. Pharmacokinetics of digoxin in normal subjects after intravenous bolus and infusion doses. *J Pharmacokinet Biopharm*. 1975;3:181.

56. Wintraub M, Au WY, Lasagna L. Compliance as a determinant of serum digoxin concentration. *JAMA*. 1973;224:481.

57. FDA Recall: Actavis Totowa (formerly known as Amide Pharmaceutical, Inc.) recalls all lots of Bertek and UDL laboratories Digitex® (digoxin tablets, usp) as precaution. April 25, 2008. https://wayback. archive-it.org/7993/20170406122157/https://www.fda.gov/Safety/Recalls/ArchiveRecalls/2008/ ucm112435.htm. Accessed July 27, 2017.

58. Lader S, Bye, A, Mardsen P. The measurement of plasma digoxin concentrations: a comparison of two methods. *Eur J Clin Pharmacol*. 1972;5:22.

59. Silber B, Sheiner LB, Powers JL, et al. Associated digoxin radioimmunoassay interference. *Clin Chem*. 1979;25:48.

60. Dasgupta A. Endogenous and exogenous digoxin-like immunoreactive substances: impact on the therapeutic drug monitoring of digoxin. *Am J Clin Pathol*. 2002;118:132–140.

61. Steimer W, Muller C, Eber B. Digoxin assays: frequent, substantial and potentially dangerous interference by spironolactone, canrenone, and other steroids. *Clin Chem*. 2002;48:507–516.

62. Dasgupta A. Therapeutic drug monitoring of digoxin: impact of endogenous and exogenous digoxin-like immunoreactive substances. *Toxicol Rev*. 2006;25:273–281.

63. Graves SW, Brown B, Valdes R Jr. An endogenous digoxin-like substance in patients with renal impairment. *Ann Intern Med*. 1983;99:604.

64. Pudek MR, Seccombe DW, Jacobson BE, et al. Seven different digoxin immunoassay kits compared with respect to interference by a digoxin-like immunoreactive substance in serum from premature and full-term infants. *Clin Chem*. 1983;29:1972.

65. Yatscoff RW, Desjardins PR, Dalton JG. Digoxin-like immunoreactivity in the serum of neonates and uremic patients, as measured in the Abbott TDX [Letter]. *Clin Chem*. 1984;30:588.

66. Avendaño C, Alvarez JS, Sacristan JA, et al. Interference of digoxin-like immunoreactive substances with TDx Digoxin II assay in different patients. *Ther Drug Monit*. 1991;13:523–527.

67. Valdes R Jr, Jortani SA, Gheorghiade M. Standards of laboratory practice: cardiac drug monitoring. *Clin Chem*. 1998;44:1096–1109.

68. Severijnen R, Bayat N, Bakker H, et al. Enteral drug absorption in patients with short small bowel: a review. *Clin Pharmacokinet*. 2004;43:951–962.

69. Luchi RJ, Gruber JW. Unusually large digitalis requirements. *Am J Med*. 1968;45:322.

70. Doherty JE, Perkins WH. Digoxin metabolism in hypo- and hyperthyroidism. *Ann Intern Med*. 1966;64:489.

71. Lawrence JR, Sumner DJ, Kalk WJ. Digoxin kinetics in patients with thyroid dysfunction. *Clin Pharmacol Ther*. 1977;22:7.

72. Croxson MS, Ibbertson HK. Serum digoxin in patients with thyroid disease. *Br Med J*. 1985;3:566.

73. Ackerman GL, Doherty JE, Flanigan WJ. Peritoneal and hemodialysis of tritiated digoxin. *Ann Intern Med*. 1967;67:4:718.

74. Benken ST, Lizza BD, Yamout H, et al. Management of digoxin therapy using pharmacokinetics in a patient undergoing continuous venovenous hemofiltration. *Am J Health Syst Pharm*. 2013;70(23):2105–2109.

75. Reetze-Bonorden P, Bohler J, Keller E. Drug dosage in patients during continuous renal replacement therapy. *Clin Pharmacokinet*. 1993;24:362–379.

76. Lesko LJ. Pharmacokinetic drug interactions with amiodarone. *Clin Pharmacokinet*. 1989;17:130–140.

77. Hardman JG, Limbird LE, Gilman AG, eds. *The Pharmacological Basis of Therapeutics*. 10th ed. New York, NY: McGraw-Hill; 2001.

78. Ejvinsson G. Effect of quinidine of plasma concentrations of digoxin. *Br Med J*. 1978;279.

79. Leahey EB Jr, Reiffel JA, Drusin RE, et al. Interactions between quinidine and digoxin. *JAMA*. 1978;240:533.

80. Bauer LA, Horn JR, Pettit H. Mixed-effect modeling for detection and evaluation of drug interactions: digoxin-quinidine and digoxin-verapamil combinations. *Ther Drug Monit*. 1996;18:46–52.

81. Leahey EB Jr, Bigger JT Jr, Butler VP Jr, et al. Quinidine-digoxin interaction: time course and pharmacokinetics. *Am J Cardiol*. 1981;48:1141.

82. Hager DW, Fenster P, Mayersohn M, et al. Digoxin-quinidine interaction. *N Engl J Med*. 1979;300:1238.

83. Powell JR, Fenster PE, Hager WD, et al. Quinidine-digoxin interaction. *N Engl J Med*. 1980;302:176.

84. Doering W. Quinidine-digoxin interaction. *N Engl J Med*. 1979;301:400.

85. Fichtl B, Doering W. The quinidine-digoxin interaction in perspective. *Clin Pharmacokinet*. 1983;8:137.

86. Bussey HI. The influence of quinidine and other agents on digitalis glycosides. *Am Heart J*. 1982;104:289.

87. Steiness E, Waldorff S, Hansen PB, et al. Reduction of digoxin-induced inotropism during quinidine administration. *Clin Pharmacol Ther*. 1980;27:791.

88. Schenck-Gustafsson K, Jogestrand T, Brodin LA, et al. Cardiac effects of treatment with quinidine and digoxin, alone and in combination. *Am J Cardiol*. 1983;51:777.

89. Belz GB, Doering W, Aust PE, et al. Quinidine-digoxin interaction: cardiac efficacy of elevated serum digoxin concentration. *Clin Pharmacol Ther*. 1982;31:548.

90. Nolan PE Jr, Marcus FI, Erstad BL, et al. Effects of coadministration of propafenone on the pharmacokinetics of digoxin in healthy volunteer subjects. *J Clin Pharmacol*. 1989;29:46–52.

91. Bigot MC, Debruyne D, Bonnefoy L, et al. Serum digoxin levels related to plasma propafenone levels during concomitant treatment. *J Clin Pharmacol*. 1991;31:521–526.

92. Belz GG, Doering W, Munkes R, et al. Interactions between digoxin and calcium antagonists and antiarrhythmic drugs. *Clin Pharmacol Ther*. 1983;33:410–417.

93. Pedersen KE, Christiansen BD, Kjaer K, et al. Verapamil-induced changes in digoxin kinetics and intraerythrocytic sodium concentration. *Clin Pharmacol Ther*. 1983;34:8.

94. Zhou S, Chan E, Pan SQ, et al. Pharmacokinetic interactions of drugs with St John's wort. *J Psychopharmacol*. 2004;18:262–276.

95. Hirata S, Izumi S, Furukubo T, et al. Interactions between clarithromycin and digoxin in patients with end-stage renal disease. *Int J Clin Pharmacol Ther*. 2005;43:30–36.

96. Rengeshausen J, Goggelmann C, Burhenne J, et al. Contribution of increased oral bioavailability and reduced nonglomerular renal clearance of digoxin to the digoxin-clarithromycin interaction. *Br J Clin Pharmacol*. 2003;56:32–38.

97. Eberl S, Renner B, Neubert A, et al. Role of p-glycoprotein inhibition for drug interactions: evidence from in vitro and pharmacoepidemiological studies. *Clin Pharmacokinet*. 2007;46:1039–1049.

98. Tanaka H, Matsumoto K, Ueno K, et al. Effect of clarithromycin on steady-state digoxin concentrations. *Ann Pharmacother*. 2003;37:178–181.

99. Ding R, Tayrouz Y, Riedel KD, et al. Substantial pharmacokinetic interaction between digoxin and ritonavir in healthy volunteers. *Clin Pharmacol Ther*. 2004;76:73–84.

100. Dasgupta A, Tso G, Wells A. Effect of Asian ginseng, Siberian ginseng and Indian ayurvedic medicine ashwagandha on serum digoxin measurement by digoxin III, a new digoxin immunoassay. *J Clin Lab Anal*. 2008;22:295–301.

101. McMillin GA, Owen WE, Lambert TL, et al. Comparable effects of Digibind and DigiFab in thirteen digoxin immunoassays. *Clin Chem*. 2002;48:1580–1584.

11

IMMUNOSUPPRESSANTS: CYCLOSPORINE, TACROLIMUS, SIROLIMUS, AND MYCOPHENOLIC ACID

Tony K. L. Kiang and Mary H. H. Ensom

Learning Objectives

By the end of the immunosuppressants: cyclosporine, tacrolimus, sirolimus, and mycophenolic acid chapter, the learner shall be able to:

1. Know the therapeutic range of the immunosuppressive drugs (cyclosporine, tacrolimus, sirolimus, and mycophenolate). The learner shall also be able to explain the consequences of subtherapeutic concentrations and list the toxicities associated with supratherapeutic concentrations.
2. List drugs that can alter the disposition of cyclosporine, tacrolimus, sirolimus, and mycophenolate. The learner shall also be able to increase cyclosporine, tacrolimus, sirolimus, or mycophenolate concentration and decrease cyclosporine, tacrolimus, sirolimus, or mycophenolate concentration.
3. Know the differences in the pharmacokinetic disposition between cyclosporine and the cyclosporine-modified formulations.
4. Adjust the dose to achieve a concentration within the therapeutic range, given the dosing history of a patient, for cyclosporine, tacrolimus, sirolimus, and mycophenolate.
5. Convert to an intravenous dosing regimen for a patient taking oral cyclosporine-modified formulations or tacrolimus. For a patient on intravenous cyclosporine or tacrolimus, the learner shall be able to convert to an oral dosing regimen.

6. Explain, using the criteria outlined in Chapter 3, Drug Dosing in Kidney Disease and Dialysis, why dialysis is not likely to remove significant amounts of cyclosporine, tacrolimus, sirolimus, and mycophenolate.
7. Describe the clinical pharmacogenomics of cyclosporine, tacrolimus, sirolimus, and mycophenolate and the available evidence that supports or does not support pharmacogenomics-guided dosing of each agent.

Immunosuppression plays a vital role in preventing and treating allograft rejection in the transplant recipient and in the treatment of various autoimmune disorders.

Many of the immunosuppressive drugs have a narrow therapeutic window and exhibit pharmacokinetic variability. There can be large fluctuations in the observed blood concentrations between patients receiving the same dose normalized for weight (interpatient variability) and within the same patient receiving the same dose (intrapatient variability). Subtherapeutic concentrations and wide fluctuations in drug concentrations are risk factors for allograft rejection and decreased graft survival, whereas supratherapeutic concentrations increase the likelihood of developing adverse effects. Therapeutic drug monitoring is essential in optimizing the patient's immunosuppressive drug regimen to minimize the risk of allograft rejection and dose-related adverse effects.

Immunosuppressive drug therapy is usually individualized to the patient and tailored to the specific organ(s) transplanted, time after transplant, indication for transplantation, and transplant center–specific immunosuppression protocols. Although there are many immunosuppressive drugs available, this chapter focuses on the four drugs that undergo therapeutic drug monitoring in the setting of organ transplantation: cyclosporine, tacrolimus, sirolimus, and mycophenolic acid (hereafter designated as mycophenolate). The clinical pharmacokinetic, pharmacodynamic, and pharmacogenomic data for each immunosuppressant are presented.

Cyclosporine

Cyclosporine, a calcineurin inhibitor, is a cyclical peptide used in clinical practice for the prevention of allograft rejection in solid organ transplant recipients, for the prevention of graft versus host disease in bone marrow transplant recipients, and for the management of various autoimmune disorders. The primary immunosuppressive effects of cyclosporine are to inhibit the production and secretion of interleukin-2 (IL-2) and other cellular growth factors by inhibiting the enzyme, calcineurin. IL-2 plays a vital role in the rejection process by signaling for cytotoxic T-lymphocyte activation and proliferation. Cyclosporine is used to prevent acute allograft rejection, not to treat rejection. Cyclosporine is usually given in combination with a corticosteroid and an antiproliferative agent such as azathioprine or mycophenolate mofetil as part of an immunosuppression regimen.[1,2]

KEY PARAMETERS: Cyclosporine[a]

Therapeutic concentration	See Table 11.2
F[b]	30% (range: 8%–60%)
V[c]	4–6 L/kg (reduced in cardiac transplant)
Cl[d]	5–10 mL/kg/min
$t\frac{1}{2}$	6–12 hr
fu[e] (fraction unbound in plasma)	2%–10%

[a]As with the therapeutic range, pharmacokinetic parameters will vary, depending on the biologic fluid and assay procedure used.
[b]Bioavailability exhibits both inter- and intraindividual variability.
[c]Cyclosporine is distributed into multiple compartments; however, toxicity is not known to be associated with drug concentrations in the distribution phase.
[d]Clearance is primarily by hepatic metabolism.
[e]Cyclosporine is extensively bound to many blood elements and, in plasma, is extensively bound to lipoproteins.

    Cyclosporine is available in several different formulations; the reader should refer to Table 11.1 for the various immunosuppressive drug formulations. The original formulation of cyclosporine, Sandimmune, is formulated in olive oil. Absorption of the oil-based formulation depends on the presence of food and bile for emulsification.

TABLE 11.1   Immunosuppressive Drug Formulations

DRUG	FORMULATIONS
Cyclosporine Sandimmune	25 and 100 mg capsules 100 mg/mL oral solution 50 mg/mL ampules for intravenous infusion
Cyclosporine modified Neoral, Gengraf, and others	25 and 100 mg capsules (50 mg available in generics) 100 mg/mL oral solution
Tacrolimus Prograf (or generic) Astagraf XL or Advagraf Envarsus XR	0.5, 1, and 5 mg capsules 5 mg/mL ampules for intravenous infusion 0.5, 1, and 5 mg extended release capsules 0.75, 1, and 4 mg extended release tablets
Sirolimus Rapamune	1 and 2 mg tablets 1 mg/mL oral solution
Mycophenolate mofetil Sodium Mofetil hydrochloride	250 mg capsule, 500 mg tablet, 200 mg/mL oral solution 180 and 360 mg delayed release tablets 500 mg vial for injection

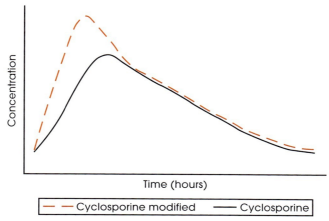

FIGURE 11.1   The typical concentration–time curves of cyclosporine and cyclosporine modified after an oral dose.

External bile drainage, cholestasis, or diarrhea may reduce the amount of bile for emulsification and impair cyclosporine absorption. In addition to poor and erratic absorption of cyclosporine, there is substantial intrapatient and interpatient pharmacokinetic variability. The newer formulation, Neoral, a microemulsion of cyclosporine, and other bioequivalent preparations (cyclosporine modified) have improved absorption and are less dependent on the presence of bile or food. The newer formulations will be collectively referred to as cyclosporine modified, and the Sandimmune formulation as cyclosporine. As compared to the cyclosporine formulation, the cyclosporine-modified formulations are absorbed faster (shorter time-to-maximal concentration, t_{max}), to a greater extent (greater area under the concentration–time curve and higher maximum concentration), and more consistently (decreased intrapatient and interpatient variability).[3] Figure 11.1 compares the typical concentration–time curves of cyclosporine and cyclosporine modified after an oral dose. Because cyclosporine and cyclosporine modified are absorbed differently, they are not considered bioequivalent formulations and therefore should not be used interchangeably. Because of the limitations in pharmacokinetic characteristics, the original cyclosporine formulation is no longer commonly used. Patients may be receiving Sandimmune brand if they are on a stable regimen and wish to continue with this particular formulation. Most patients who are initiated on a cyclosporine-based immunosuppression regimen are started with a cyclosporine-modified formulation.

The typical starting oral dose of cyclosporine or cyclosporine modified (used in combination with steroids and anti-metabolites) to prevent allograft rejection is approximately 4 to 14 mg/kg/day given as a divided dose twice a day (BID) (e.g., 2 to 7 mg/kg q12h). Renal transplant recipients are usually given higher doses of cyclosporine compared to liver and heart patients. If patients are unable to tolerate oral formulations, an intravenous (IV) formulation is available and usually dosed at one-third of the oral dose. Target cyclosporine blood trough concentrations will vary according to the organ(s) transplanted, time after transplant, and transplant center–specific immunosuppression protocols. For the treatment of rheumatoid arthritis or psoriasis, the starting dose is usually 2.5 mg/kg/day given as a divided dose BID.[1,2]

Cyclosporine and cyclosporine modified are available in oral liquid formulations for those unable to swallow the capsules. The oral syringe enclosed with the cyclosporine solution should be used to measure the dose. The cyclosporine-modified solution should be diluted with orange juice or apple juice in a glass container, stirred, and ingested immediately. The container should be rinsed with more diluent and should be consumed to ensure delivery of the entire dose.[1,2] Grapefruit juice should be avoided because it can reduce the metabolism or transport of cyclosporine by inhibiting cytochrome P450 3A4 (CYP3A4) and P-glycoprotein enzymes, respectively.[4] As indicated earlier, cyclosporine is also available as an IV solution (50 mg/mL) which may be used in patient unable to tolerate oral formulations.[1,2]

Cyclosporine preparations exhibit a narrow therapeutic window. The concentration range between subtherapeutic concentrations, at which patients are at risk of developing acute rejection, and toxic concentrations, where the patient is at risk of developing adverse effects, is narrow. Regular therapeutic drug monitoring, usually built into the posttransplant protocols in each individual transplant center, is essential for maintaining cyclosporine concentrations within a target blood concentration range to maximize immunosuppression and minimize dose-related adverse effects. The therapeutic target usually varies depending on time posttransplant (i.e., typically decreases rapidly over the initial year posttransplant) and is specific to each transplant center.

THERAPEUTIC AND TOXIC CONCENTRATIONS (BLOOD)

Cyclosporine is a lipid soluble compound that is approximately 20% bound to leukocytes and 40% bound to erythrocytes; 40% remains in the plasma fraction of blood, where it is highly bound to lipoproteins, which comprise a relatively small fraction of the plasma proteins.[5,6] Cyclosporine binding to these different blood elements is temperature dependent. Thus, assays performed on a sample other than whole blood must be done at 37°C. Otherwise, the therapeutic range needs to be temperature corrected for changes in protein binding. For this reason, whole blood is the preferred matrix for measurement.[7] Although cyclosporine is available in several different formulations, with different absorption characteristics, it is the parent compound, cyclosporine, that is measured in the blood.

As can be seen from Table 11.2, nonspecific assays measure not only cyclosporine but also its metabolites. Polyclonal and monoclonal fluorescence polarization immunoassays are most commonly used in clinical practice. Because the polyclonal assay also detects cyclosporine metabolites, the therapeutic range is substantially higher than that for the more specific monoclonal methods. As a general rule, high-performance liquid chromatography (HPLC) assay results have the same range as monoclonal methods. Although requiring more technical support, many institutions prefer the HPLC methods because they are less expensive than the monoclonal assays, and it is easier to discern assay interference and to detect metabolites. Clearly, clinicians must be aware of the assay method and biologic fluids used at their institution to ensure appropriate interpretation of cyclosporine concentrations. The lack of a single standard assay method has made it difficult to establish therapeutic ranges. When concentrations

TABLE 11.2   Cyclosporine Assay Methods and Therapeutic Range

ASSAY	SERUM/PLASMA[a] (mcg/L or ng/mL)	WHOLE BLOOD[a] (mcg/L or ng/mL)
Monoclonal radioimmunoassay (RIA)	50–125	150–400
Fluorescence polarization immunoassay (FPIA)		
Polyclonal	150–400	200–800
Monoclonal	50–125	150–400
High-performance liquid chromatography (HPLC)	50–125	150–400

[a]Therapeutic range is variable that depends on the dosing interval (τ), time of sampling, assay technique, and temperature.

in whole blood are measured, most clinicians accept trough concentrations of 150 to 400 mcg/L (ng/mL) as the target range, where allograft rejection and adverse effects are minimal. This range, however, may be different depending on the type of transplant, time after transplant, and the use of other concomitant immunosuppressive drugs. The goal of monitoring cyclosporine concentrations is to maximize the benefit-to-risk ratio so that the patient has an optimal chance of achieving a positive therapeutic outcome with minimal toxicity.

ADVERSE EFFECTS

The most common adverse effects (i.e., > 10% incidence) associated with cyclosporine are hypertension, headache, hypertrichosis, hirsutism, elevated triglycerides, nausea, gum hyperplasia, various types of infections, and renal dysfunction (elevated serum creatinine or renal insufficiency), which usually improve when the dose is decreased or the drug discontinued. Hypertension is likely the most common adverse reaction to cyclosporine, and some patients may benefit from antihypertensive co-therapies. Although the mechanism for nephrotoxicity is unclear, it may be related to cyclosporine-induced renal vasoconstriction. Because irreversible renal failure develops in some patients, the cyclosporine doses and target concentrations are often lowered in patients who show early signs of nephrotoxicity.[1,2,8]

BIOAVAILABILITY (F)

Cyclosporine is a highly lipophilic compound with limited and highly variable bioavailability. Cyclosporine undergoes presystemic metabolism via gut CYP450 or more specifically CYP3A4. In addition, cyclosporine is a substrate for P-glycoprotein, the drug efflux pump. These factors contribute in part to the incomplete and variable absorption. A low or variable bioavailability is a risk factor for allograft rejection.[9,10] The bioavailability of the oil-based formulation, Sandimmune, is highly variable (10% to 90%) and depends on graft type. Peak concentrations occur in about 2 to 6 hours for the cyclosporine formulation and 1 to 2 hours after an oral dose for the cyclosporine-modified formulations. Rapid gastrointestinal transit may also reduce the bioavailability and should be considered in a patient with diarrhea who is receiving oral cyclosporine.[11] One issue that is unique to liver transplant recipients during the immediate postoperative period is the lack of a sufficient amount of bile salts that are necessary for the adequate absorption of cyclosporine as a result of cholestasis or external biliary drainage. This problem can be overcome by administering the drug IV or by refeeding bile with the dose of cyclosporine to enhance solubility and absorption.[12] Bioavailability of cyclosporine modified is approximately 20% to 50% (also depends on graft type), but cyclosporine modified is probably more consistently absorbed than the original product. In addition, cyclosporine-modified formulations do not require bile for emulsification and are absorbed in a similar fashion, even in the setting of external biliary drainage.[13]

VOLUME OF DISTRIBUTION (V)

The volume of distribution of cyclosporine is approximately 4 to 6 L/kg. The V is reduced in heart transplant recipients and patients with end-stage renal disease. This relatively large V is consistent with the observation that cyclosporine is significantly bound to plasma and blood elements, that the unbound portion in the plasma is less than 10%, and that it is probably extensively bound to organ tissues outside the vascular space.[14–16] Part of the variability in reported V can be attributed to the fact that cyclosporine exhibits two-compartment modeling with a substantial α or distribution phase.[14] The assay method and the type of biologic fluid assayed will influence the measured concentration and, therefore, the derived pharmacokinetic parameters. The uncertainty surrounding cyclosporine's volume of distribution does not influence its clinical use to a large degree because loading doses are seldom administered (see Clinical Application of Cyclosporine Pharmacokinetics).

CLEARANCE (Cl)

Cyclosporine undergoes extensive metabolism via CYP3A4/5 in the liver and gut to multiple metabolites. These metabolites are generally thought to be less active than the parent compound. The whole blood clearance by cyclosporine is approximately 5 to 10 mL/kg/min in adult patients, indicating that it is probably a drug with a low extraction ratio. In other words, its total clearance is influenced primarily by the unbound cyclosporine concentration and hepatic intrinsic clearance, but independent of hepatic blood flow.[16,17] As such, drug interactions that result in protein binding displacement (i.e., altered free fraction), modulation of hepatic metabolism (i.e., induction or inhibition of CYP3A4), or functional genetic polymorphisms associated with binding and metabolism may result in differential effects on the total and the free cyclosporine concentration. These clearance values are based on whole blood determinations and are lower than those would be estimated using room temperature serum or plasma concentration data or those derived from nonspecific assay methods. With respect to altered intrinsic clearance, there are a number of drugs that have been reported to influence the metabolism of cyclosporine via CYP3A4 or P-glycoprotein induction or inhibition (Table 11.3).

TABLE 11.3   Immunosuppressive Drug–Drug Interactions

Drugs that inhibit cytochrome P450 (CP3A4) and P-glycoprotein[a] (and increase cyclosporine/sirolimus/tacrolimus concentrations)

Calcium channel blockers	*Antifungal agents*
Diltiazem	Fluconazole
Nicardipine	Itraconazole
Verapamil	Ketoconazole
Antibiotics	Posaconazole
Clarithromycin	Voriconazole
Erythromycin	*Antidepressants*
HIV protease inhibitors	Fluoxetine
Indinavir	Fluvoxamine
Ritonavir	Sertraline
Gastrointestinal prokinetic agents	Paroxetine
Cisapride	*Others*
Metoclopramide	Amiodarone
	Bromocriptine
	Cimetidine
	Danazol
	Ethinyl estradiol
	Grapefruit juice
	Methylprednisolone
	Nefazodone

Drugs that induce cytochrome P450 (CYP3A4) and P-glycoprotein[a] (and decrease cyclosporine/sirolimus/tacrolimus concentrations)

Antibiotics	*Anticonvulsants*
Caspofungin	Carbamazepine
Nafcillin	Phenobarbital
Rifabutin	Phenytoin
Rifampin	Primidone
Others	
St. John wort (*Hypericum perforatum*)	

[a]This is a partial list of drugs that can interact with cyclosporine, sirolimus, or tacrolimus.

HALF-LIFE (t½)

The average half-life calculated from the values indicated in the preceding sections and Equation 11.1 would suggest a value of approximately 7 hours.

$$t\,\tfrac{1}{2} = \frac{(0.693)(V)}{Cl}$$ **(Eq. 11.1)**

$$= \frac{(0.693)(4.5\ \text{L/kg})}{(7.5\ \text{mL/kg/min})\left(\dfrac{60\ \text{min/hr}}{1{,}000\ \text{mL/L}}\right)}$$

$$= 6.93\ \text{hr}$$

This half-life exhibits a wide range because of variability associated with the volume of distribution and clearance estimates for cyclosporine. The multicompartmental nature of cyclosporine may also result in an underestimation of the terminal half-life and associated pharmacokinetic parameters. The most commonly reported values for cyclosporine half-life are in the range of 10 to 27 hours for cyclosporine and 5 to 18 hours for the modified formulations.[1,2]

TIME TO SAMPLE

Although there are a number of ways to monitor cyclosporine therapy, the most widely used methods are to sample the trough (just before the dose) and 2-hour post-dose (C_2) concentrations. Cyclosporine concentrations as represented by the area under the concentration–time curve (AUC_{0-12}) is a more accurate method for predicting clinical outcomes because it directly reflects drug exposure, but this approach is usually not used in the clinic because, to determine the AUC_{0-12}, multiple blood samples over the 12-hour dosing interval are necessary. The added cost and inconvenience of multiple blood samples essentially means that the AUC_{0-12} method is never used routinely. Although there is generally a poor correlation between trough concentrations and AUC with the cyclosporine, cyclosporine-modified formulations show a stronger correlation between them.[18] The improved predictability of cyclosporine exposure makes the trough concentration a more reliable aid for therapeutic drug monitoring in a clinical setting for patients taking the modified formulations. Because most of the variability in cyclosporine absorption occurs within the first 4 hours after administration of cyclosporine modified, the AUC_{0-4} serves as a sensitive predictor for acute rejection.[19] The cyclosporine concentration at 2 hours after administration of modified formulations (e.g., C_2) is the most accurate single-sample time marker for AUC_{0-4},[20] but there is a 15-minute period before and after the 2-hour time point, during which the C_2 sample can be taken to remain within an acceptable margin of error. The precise timing of the sample dictates that this method of monitoring should be performed in a controlled environment, such as a hospital or clinic. Furthermore, abbreviated AUC (or limited sampling strategy [LSS]) algorithms utilize a limited number of sampling points and regression—or population pharmacokinetic—generated equations to estimate the AUC.[21] However, these LSSs should be validated and used only in patients who have similar characteristics compared to the subjects/conditions in which the equations were originally developed and validated. Despite improved accuracy of prediction, the requirement for multiple sampling for the AUC or LSS approaches means that the trough and C_2 concentrations are still the most commonly used method to monitor cyclosporine therapy today.

CLINICAL PHARMACOGENOMICS OF CYCLOSPORINE

Currently (May 2016), there are insufficient data to support a pharmacogenomics-guided dosing for cyclosporine[22–31] (see Pharmacogenomic Applications).

Clinical Application of Cyclosporine Pharmacokinetics

Complex computer programs or relatively straightforward approaches can be used to evaluate a patient's pharmacokinetic parameters; however, in most cases, the clinical result is essentially the same. When the cyclosporine concentration is low, the dose is increased; when the concentration is high, the dose is decreased. If the cyclosporine concentration is low, it is appropriate to evaluate patient adherence to the prescribed regimen and determine whether any drugs have been added that might decrease cyclosporine absorption or increase metabolism. If there are no easily correctable problems, most clinicians would increase the dose modestly (the extent of dose change typically is limited to within 25% of the original dose, although individual transplant centers might have their own protocols), recognizing that the change in concentration should be approximately proportional to the change in the maintenance dose. If the cyclosporine concentration is high, it is important to first determine whether the sample has been obtained at the appropriate time (i.e., trough or C_2). In addition, patient adherence should be assessed and the potential for any drug–drug interactions (i.e., CYP3A4 inhibition) that might account for the increased cyclosporine concentration. If the sample is valid, many clinicians will hold a dose and then restart on a proportionally lower maintenance dose, or simply lower the dose to bring the cyclosporine concentration into the desired range. The steady-state (i.e., after five half-lives) cyclosporine concentration should be verified to ensure that the patient has achieved therapeutic concentrations. Occasionally, patients have an isolated elevated or decreased cyclosporine concentration for which no logical explanation can be found. The patient should be assessed to determine whether he or she is clinically stable, and the clinician should then recheck the cyclosporine concentration as soon as reasonably possible.

Question #1   *R.I., a 39-year-old, 51-kg woman, received an unrelated renal transplant over a decade ago. Her serum creatinine had been stable in the range of 1.4 to 1.7 mg/dL. She has been receiving cyclosporine modified orally (PO), 125 mg BID. Cyclosporine concentrations have been 85 to 110 mcg/L (whole blood HPLC assay). Her last clinic appointment was 3 weeks ago. Other immunosuppressive medications included prednisone 10 mg/day and mycophenolate mofetil 1,000 mg BID. She returned to the clinic yesterday complaining of increasing fatigue since her last clinic appointment. Blood and urine cultures were taken, and she was admitted to the hospital with a serum creatinine of 2.8 mg/dL. How would you adjust R.I.'s cyclosporine-modified dose to increase the cyclosporine concentration to approximately 200 mcg/L?*

First, it is important to determine whether the rise in serum creatinine is caused by graft rejection or cyclosporine toxicity. If the increase in serum creatinine is presumed to be a sign of allograft rejection (i.e., after confirmatory investigations from renal ultrasound or biopsy), the patient would probably also receive additional acute immunosuppressant therapy, including methylprednisolone and/or antithymocyte globulin. Using approach number three as outlined in Interpretation of Plasma Drug Concentrations; Choosing a Model to Revise or Estimate a Patient's Clearance at Steady State in Chapter 2, a revised set of pharmacokinetic parameters can be calculated.

First, we would start by estimating a revised elimination rate constant.

$$K_{revised} = \frac{\ln\left(\dfrac{Css\ min + \dfrac{(S)(F)(Dose)}{V}}{Css\ min}\right)}{\tau} \qquad \textbf{(Eq. 11.2)}$$

The average cyclosporine concentration of approximately 100 mcg/L would be used as the Css min, F would be 0.3 (average value), and the dose would be expressed as 125,000 mcg. The V would have to be estimated (4.5 L/kg), and τ would be 12 hours. Using these values, the revised elimination rate constant is approximately 0.0807 inverse hours.

$$= \frac{\ln\left(\dfrac{100\ mcg/L + \dfrac{(1)(0.3)(125,000\ mcg)}{(4.5\ L/kg)(51\ kg)}}{100\ mcg/L}\right)}{12\ hr}$$

$$= \frac{\ln\left(\dfrac{263.4\ mcg/L}{100\ mcg/L}\right)}{12}$$

$$= 0.0807\ hr^{-1}$$

This $K_{revised}$ would correspond to a clearance of 18.5 L/hr:

$$Cl = (K_{revised})(V) \qquad \textbf{(Eq. 11.3)}$$

$$= (0.0807\ hr^{-1})(4.5\ L/kg)(51\ kg)$$
$$= (0.0807\ hr^{-1})(229.5\ L)$$
$$= 18.5\ L/hr$$

and a half-life of approximately 8 or 9 hours.

$$t\tfrac{1}{2} = \frac{0.693}{K} \qquad \text{(Eq. 11.4)}$$

$$= \frac{0.693}{0.0807 \text{ hr}^{-1}}$$

$$= 8.6 \text{ hr}$$

Using the revised pharmacokinetic parameters, a new dose can be calculated by rearranging Equation 11.5.

$$\text{Css min} = \frac{\dfrac{(S)(F)(\text{Dose})}{V}}{\left(1 - e^{-K\tau}\right)}\left(e^{-K\tau}\right) \qquad \text{(Eq. 11.5)}$$

$$\text{Dose} = \frac{(\text{Css min})(V)\left(1 - e^{-K\tau}\right)}{(S)(F)\left(e^{-K\tau}\right)} \qquad \text{(Eq. 11.6)}$$

Making the appropriate substitutions for Css min, V, S, F, K, and τ, a dose of approximately 250 mg can be calculated.

$$= \frac{(200 \text{ mcg/L})(4.5 \text{ L/kg})(51 \text{ kg})\left(1 - e^{-(0.0807)(12)}\right)}{(1)(0.3)\left(e^{-(0.0807)(12)}\right)}$$

$$= \frac{(200 \text{ mcg/L})(229.5 \text{ L})(1 - 0.38)}{(1)(0.3)(0.38)}$$

$$= 249,631 \text{ mcg or} \approx 250 \text{ mg q12h}$$

Note that this dose adjustment to 250 mg every 12 hours is double the original dose of 125 mg every 12 hours and should result in a proportional change in the steady-state trough concentration. This method of using the desired change in the plasma concentration as the same ratio change for maintenance dose is useful as long as the dosing interval is not altered. Because the dosing interval remains the same, this is the most common method of adjusting the cyclosporine dose. Most clinicians do not calculate the elimination rate constant or clearance values associated with steady-state cyclosporine trough concentrations. They simply make a proportional or clinically reasonable change and determine the steady-state concentration of cyclosporine after making the dose change. In this case, the steady-state cyclosporine (trough or C_2) concentration should be ordered 2 days after dose change, which correspond to greater than five half-lives as determined for this patient.

Question #2   *E.R., a 48-year-old, 59-kg male patient, received a living-related renal transplant many years ago. He is currently receiving Sandimmune 300 mg PO as the solution BID and, in addition, prednisone 5 mg/day and mycophenolate 1,000 mg BID. E.R.'s current serum creatinine is 2.1 mg/dL, and his steady-state cyclosporine trough concentration is 590 mcg/L. The physician has ruled out the possibility of rejection and believes that the recent rise in serum creatinine is because of cyclosporine toxicity. What questions would one ask E.R., and how would one adjust his cyclosporine regimen to achieve a new steady-state cyclosporine concentration of approximately 200 mcg/L?*

First, confirm that E.R. has been taking his Sandimmune 300 mg BID as prescribed and determine whether any new medications have been added to his regimen or if he has consumed grapefruits or grapefruit juice. In addition, verify the time of sampling relative to when he took his last dose to ensure that the concentration is in fact a trough and not a peak concentration. If there are no easily correctable reasons for the elevated cyclosporine concentration, at least one cyclosporine dose should be held and then E.R. should be restarted on a new regimen. The dose decrease should approximate the proportionate decrease in cyclosporine concentration that is desired:

$$\text{Desired Dose} = \frac{\text{Css Desired}}{\text{Css Current}} \times \text{Current Dose} \qquad \textbf{(Eq. 11.7)}$$

Using the current steady-state cyclosporine concentration of 590 mcg/L and the new target concentration of 200 mcg/L, the new cyclosporine dose is approximately 100 mg.

$$\begin{aligned}\text{Desired Dose} &= \frac{200\ \text{mcg/L}}{300\ \text{mcg/L}} \times 300\ \text{mcg} \\ &= 0.339 \times 300\ \text{mg} \\ &= 101.7\ \text{mg or} \approx 100\ \text{mg}\end{aligned}$$

This new dose assumes that the bioavailability remains the same and that the drug will be administered at the same interval of 12 hours. It is unclear why E.R. requires a lower than average cyclosporine dose (200 mg/day or ≈3.4 mg/kg/day). He may be absorbing more than the usual 30%, his hepatic metabolism may be unusually low, or he may be affected by a combination of both factors. The steady-state (i.e., >5 half-lives) trough cyclosporine concentration should be determined after the dose change to ensure that E.R.'s concentration is within the therapeutic target.

Question #3   *M.J., a new 78-kg liver transplant patient, is receiving 200 mg/day of cyclosporine as a continuous IV infusion (patient was intolerant to tacrolimus). Currently, his hepatic function tests appear to be stable, and for the past 3 days, he* *has been improving clinically with steady-state cyclosporine concentrations of approx-imately 220 mcg/L. What would be an appropriate oral cyclosporine dose for M.J.? The hepatologist is also asking whether genotyping would help guide dosing for this patient. Which genes would you target and why?*

Because the usual bioavailability for cyclosporine is approximately 30%, most clinicians give an oral dose that is three times the parenteral dose. In this case, it would be approximately 600 mg/day, or 300 mg every 12 hours. Some clinicians prefer dividing the dose to reduce the volume of cyclosporine liquid or the number of capsules per dose. Dividing the daily dose would maintain the same steady-state average concentration but increase the trough and decrease the peak concentrations. This is because when the same rate of drug administration is given as smaller doses more often, a constant infusion model is more closely approximated, and the peak and trough concentrations are moving toward the steady-state average (see Interpretation of Plasma Drug Concentrations; Revising Pharmacokinetic Parameters; Clearance in Fig. 2.11 of Chapter 2). Again, pharmacokinetic calculations could have been performed; however, the outcome would have been essentially the same as adjusting the dose in proportion to the desired change in steady-state plasma concentration.

In this case, we have the additional factor of a change in route and, therefore, bioavailability to consider:

$$\text{New Dose} = \frac{\text{Css Desired}}{\text{Css Current}} \times \frac{\text{F Current}}{\text{F New Dosage Form}} \times \text{Current Dose} \qquad \textbf{(Eq. 11.8)}$$

Assuming the reported cyclosporine concentration of 220 mcg/L is acceptable, the new dose will be approximately 600 mg/day.

$$= \frac{220 \text{ mcg/L}}{220 \text{ mcg/L}} \times \frac{1.0}{0.3} \times 200 \text{ mg}$$
$$= 1 \times 3.33 \times 200 \text{ mg}$$
$$= 666 \text{ mg} \approx 600 \text{ mg}$$

Again, if the dose is divided and given as 300 mg every 12 hours, trough concentrations will be somewhat higher than those produced by single daily doses. However, the bioavailability will probably be a more important influence on the trough cyclosporine concentration.

Currently, there is insufficient evidence to support genotype-guided dosing of cyclosporine. Select polymorphisms (e.g., CYP3A4*1B, CYP3A4*18) may be of interest, but further systematic studies are needed to establish the utility of genotyping (see Pharmacogenomics Applications).

Question #4   *A.H. is a 63-year-old woman who received a liver transplant 10 years ago. She was taking a stable regimen of Sandimmune 150 mg PO BID and prednisone 5 mg PO daily, with a cyclosporine concentration 150 mcg/L 1 month ago. Since then, she had a surgical procedure to relieve a bile duct obstruction. As a result of the procedure, A.H. received a T-tube drain (a tube that drains the bile into an external bag). Her cyclosporine concentration in the clinic yesterday was 25 mcg/L. A.H. states that she is compliant with her medication regimen and has not taken any new medications or changed the way that she takes her medications. What would account for A.H.'s low cyclosporine concentration?*

Cyclosporine (Sandimmune) is an oil-based formulation that requires bile for absorption. Because A.H. received a T-tube that drains the bile externally, there is insufficient bile in her gastrointestinal tract for emulsification of cyclosporine for absorption. A.H. could be re-fed her bile along with her cyclosporine dose or be changed to a cyclosporine-modified product. For patients who are being switched from the Sandimmune formulation to one of the cyclosporine-modified formulations, the same daily dose that was previously used for Sandimmune can be used (1:1 dose conversion). In patients who have poor or erratic absorption, the conversion from Sandimmune to cyclosporine modified may result in increased cyclosporine blood trough concentrations as a result of increased absorption with the cyclosporine-modified formulation. The dose of cyclosporine modified should be adjusted to obtain the desired cyclosporine blood trough concentration. The cyclosporine blood trough concentration should be monitored closely until a stable target concentration is achieved. For many patients, the dose required for cyclosporine modified will be somewhat less than the dose that was being given as Sandimmune.

Tacrolimus

Tacrolimus is a macrolide antibiotic with immunosuppressive effects. Whereas tacrolimus has a chemical structure similar to sirolimus, its mechanism of action is similar to that of cyclosporine. Tacrolimus, like cyclosporine, inhibits the activity of calcineurin, leading to a decrease in the production and release of IL-2. Tacrolimus is used as part of an immunosuppressive drug regimen to prevent allograft rejection.[32,33]

Tacrolimus is available as 0.5-, 1-, and 5-mg immediate release capsules (Prograf and various generic brands), 0.5, 1, and 5 mg extended release capsules (Astagraf XL or Advagraf), 0.75 mg, 1 mg, and 4 mg extended release tablets (Envarsusis), and a 5 mg/mL solution for IV administration. The recommended initial oral dose of tacrolimus is approximately 0.2 mg/kg/day (in combination with other immunosuppressants) in kidney transplant recipients, 0.075 mg/kg/day in heart transplant recipients, 0.1 to 0.15 mg/kg/day in liver transplant recipients, and 0.15 to 0.2 mg/kg/day in pediatric liver transplant recipients. The oral doses are usually given as divided doses every 12 hours.[32,33] The IV formulation is usually given as a continuous infusion. IV tacrolimus is not commonly

KEY PARAMETERS: Tacrolimus

Therapeutic concentration[a]	5–20 mcg/L
F	Mean 25% (range: 7%–32%)
V[b]	Mean 1 L/kg (range: 0.85–1.94 L/kg)
Cl[b]	0.04–0.083 L/kg/hr
t½	Immediate release: 2–36 hr Extended release: 35–41 hr
fu (fraction unbound in plasma[c])	0.01

[a]Whole blood trough concentration. Target concentrations may vary with the organ(s) transplanted and transplant center–specific immunosuppression protocols.
[b]Based on blood concentrations.
[c]The blood-to-plasma ratio is approximately 35 (range: 12–67), indicating extensive partitioning into blood cells. Tacrolimus is bound mainly to albumin and α_1-acid glycoprotein.

used because most patients can take it orally immediately after transplant. Tacrolimus, like cyclosporine and sirolimus, has a narrow therapeutic window and exhibits variability in its pharmacokinetic parameters. In addition, tacrolimus is a substrate for CYP3A4 and P-glycoprotein. There are many drugs known to be inhibitors or inducers of CYP3A4 and P-glycoprotein.[32,33] Table 11.3 lists commonly used drugs that can interact with tacrolimus. Similar to cyclosporine, therapeutic drug monitoring of tacrolimus is essential in optimizing immunosuppression and minimizing dose-related toxicity.

THERAPEUTIC AND TOXIC CONCENTRATIONS (BLOOD)

The therapeutic range of tacrolimus is 5 to 20 mcg/L (ng/mL). Subtherapeutic tacrolimus concentrations are associated with an increased risk for allograft rejection, and concentrations above the therapeutic range are associated with increased risk for toxic effects (such as renal dysfunction, neurotoxicity, and hypertension).[34] Owing to the narrow therapeutic range and the wide interindividual variability in tacrolimus pharmacokinetics, patients may experience rejection and/or exhibit signs of toxicity even within the therapeutic range. The target blood concentrations of tacrolimus will vary according to the organ(s) transplanted, time after transplant, and transplant center–specific immunosuppression protocols.

ADVERSE EFFECTS

Tacrolimus is associated with a wide range of adverse effects. The most common dose-related adverse effects include nephrotoxicity, posttransplant diabetes mellitus, neurotoxicity (headache, tremor, paresthesia, and seizure), hypertriglyceridemia, diarrhea, and hypertension. Other adverse effects include hyperkalemia, nausea, diarrhea, myocardial hypertrophy, alopecia, opportunistic infections, and malignancies. The IV formulation contains castor oil, which can cause anaphylactic reactions.[32,33]

BIOAVAILABILITY (F)

The oral bioavailability of tacrolimus is poor. The bioavailability ranges from 7% to 32%, suggesting large variability in patients.[35] The low bioavailability in part may be the result of presystemic metabolism in the gut wall by intestinal CYP3A4 and the activity of the drug efflux pump, P-glycoprotein.[36,37] Tacrolimus is a lipophilic compound whose absorption is dissolution rate limited. Unlike the unmodified cyclosporine formation, absorption of tacrolimus does not depend on the presence of bile salts, but may be impaired by gut motility and significantly increased by diarrhea. Food, especially that high in fat content, also decreases the rate and extent of tacrolimus absorption.[38] When tacrolimus is given with meals or after meals, the t_{max} increases five- to sevenfold, the C max decreases by 39% to 77%, and the AUC decreases by 27% to 37%. To minimize variability of absorption, tacrolimus should be given consistently with or without food, preferably on an empty stomach to maximize absorption. Tacrolimus is rapidly absorbed, with peak concentrations being reached in approximately 0.5 to 6 hours after oral administration.[32,33]

VOLUME OF DISTRIBUTION (V)

The volume of distribution of tacrolimus is greater than 20 L/kg when based on plasma concentration.[35] This indicates extensive distribution outside the plasma compartment. The blood-to-plasma ratio of 35 (range: 12 to 67) is consistent with extensive distribution into red blood cells. The volume of distribution is approximately 1 L/kg when based on blood concentration. The plasma protein binding of tacrolimus is approximately 99%. Tacrolimus is bound mainly to albumin and α_1-acid glycoprotein.

CLEARANCE (Cl)

Tacrolimus is extensively metabolized in the liver and gut via CYP3A4/5 to several hydroxylated and demethylated metabolites. Several of the metabolites have immuno-suppressive activity.[39] The presence of active metabolites should be taken into consideration when using a tacrolimus assay that measures both the parent compound and its metabolites, such as the microparticle enzyme immunoassay and enzyme-linked immunosorbent assay methods.

The systemic clearance of tacrolimus in plasma is very high, ranging from 0.6 to 5.4 L/kg/hr. However, the extensive distribution of tacrolimus into red blood cells limits its clearance from the blood. Systemic clearance of tacrolimus in blood ranges from 0.04 to 0.083 L/kg/hr. Clearance decreases as hepatic function progressively declines. In addition, recipients of a partial liver transplant (e.g., right lobe) have decreased tacrolimus dosing requirements compared with recipients of a whole liver transplant. The exact reason for this is not clear, but may be because of reduced metabolic capacity from the smaller graft size. The clearance of tacrolimus is higher in children compared with that in adults.[40] Children require higher doses of tacrolimus to achieve similar target concentrations.[41] With respect to altered intrinsic clearance, there are a number of drugs that have been reported to influence the metabolism of tacrolimus via CYP3A4 induction or inhibition (Table 11.3).

HALF-LIFE (t½)

The elimination half-life of tacrolimus is approximately 2 to 36 hours and is prolonged in patients with impaired hepatic function.[32,33]

TIME TO SAMPLE

Tacrolimus blood concentrations are usually drawn just before the dose (trough). Given the elimination half-life of about 2 to 36 hours, it is reasonable to wait 2 to 3 days after initiating or altering therapy before checking tacrolimus blood concentrations to ensure steady-state conditions.[32,33]

CLINICAL PHARMACOGENOMICS OF TACROLIMUS

There is sufficient evidence to support pharmacogenomics-guided dosing for tacrolimus, with respect to CYP3A5 genetic polymorphism[42] (see Pharmacogenomics Applications).

> **Question #5**   *C.F. is a 55-year-old man who just received a liver transplant. His current immunosuppression regimen is IV methylprednisolone 160 mg/day and mycophenolate mofetil 1,000 mg PO BID. His weight is 80 kg, and his serum creatinine is 1.1 mg/dL. The liver donor had previously been determined to have the CYP3A5*1/*1 (wild-type) genotype. What dose (immediate release vs. extended release) of tacrolimus would you recommend?*

The recommended starting dose for the immediate release formulations is approximately 0.1 mg/kg/day given as 0.05 mg/kg every 12 hours. Clinicians typically initiate tacrolimus therapy using the immediate release formulation. Only in settings of noncompliance or greater than normal variabilities (as determined in tacrolimus therapeutic drug monitoring) would patients be switched to the extended release formulations.

$$\text{Daily Dose} = 80 \text{ kg} \times 0.1 \text{ mg/kg/day} = 8 \text{ mg/day}$$
$$\text{Administered Dose} = 4 \text{ mg PO q12h}$$

In the absence of genetic (i.e., CYP3A5) information, many clinicians can elect to initiate therapy at lower doses and increase the dose over the next few days to determine whether the patient will tolerate tacrolimus. Typical starting doses range from 1 to 2 mg PO every 12 hours and would be increased over the next few days to a target dose of 4 mg PO every 12 hours if tolerated. Alternatively, some clinicians would just empirically start the patient at the target dose (i.e., 4 mg PO every 12 hours) and monitor concentrations after attaining steady state.

However, because prior genetic information is available for this patient's liver, genomic-guided dosing should be considered following the Clinical Pharmacogenetics Implementation Consortium (CPIC) published clinical guideline (see Pharmacogenomics Applications). Because this patient now carries the liver with the CYP3A5*1/*1 genotype, he would be classified an "extensive metabolizer," and should be started on a higher tacrolimus dose (i.e., 1.5 to 2 times the labeled dose, which would be 6 to 8 mg PO every 12 hours). Although pharmacogenomic-guided dosing has been proven to attain therapeutic tacrolimus concentrations more efficiently, these strategies have yet been associated with improved tacrolimus pharmacodynamics (i.e., reduced toxicity and graft loss). As such, standard therapeutic drug monitoring is still recommended in this setting.

Given the elimination half-life of approximately 2 to 36 hours, it is necessary to wait approximately five half-lives to reach steady state after initiating or altering therapy. It would be reasonable to wait 2 days before checking tacrolimus blood concentrations. Tacrolimus concentrations are usually drawn as trough concentrations (just before the dose).

Clinically, tacrolimus blood concentrations are monitored on a daily basis during the immediate posttransplant period. The frequency of tacrolimus concentration monitoring decreases because the patient's condition becomes more stable.

Question #6   *C.F. continues to improve clinically 4 days after the liver transplant. Owing to his CYP3A5 genotype (CYP3A5*1/*1), the team had started him on a higher tacrolimus dose of 6 mg PO BID (on day 1 posttransplant). Trough tacrolimus concentrations have been obtained serially daily in the morning (day 2: 8 mcg/L; day 3: 10 mcg/L; and day 4: 12 mcg/L). The transplant physician would like the patient to have a higher therapeutic target of tacrolimus because he has increased risk of organ rejection in this immediate posttransplant period. The team would like you to adjust the tacrolimus dose to achieve a trough concentration of 18 mcg/L. Please show your approach.*

The pharmacokinetics of tacrolimus is highly variable within an individual patient and between patients. A linear proportionality between dose and exposure may be assumed for the purpose of dose adjustments. Assuming nothing else has changed (i.e., renal function, hepatic function, and coadministered drugs) in this case, it is reasonable to increase the tacrolimus dose to 9 mg PO BID using Equation 11.7. After attaining steady state (~5 half-lives, usually 2 to 3 days), one should verify the trough concentration to ensure that the desired target has been obtained.

$$\text{Desired Dose} = \frac{\text{Css Desired}}{\text{Css Current}} \times \text{Current Dose}$$

$$= \frac{18 \text{ mcg/mL}}{12 \text{ mcg/mL}} \times 12 \text{ mg/day}$$

$$= 18 \text{ mg/day or } 9 \text{ mg q12h}$$

Question #7   *L.J. is a 45-year-old woman who had a liver transplant. She is receiving a stable regimen of tacrolimus 4 mg PO every 12 hours and prednisone 5 mg PO daily. Two weeks ago, her tacrolimus concentration on this regimen was 12 mcg/L. She was prescribed diltiazem XR 300 mg PO daily for hypertension 1 week ago, and now* *presents with headaches and tremors. Her serum creatinine is 1.4 mg/dL (baseline 1.1 mg/dL), and her tacrolimus concentration is 26 mcg/L. How can you account for the elevated tacrolimus concentration? How would you manage her tacrolimus dose to achieve a tacrolimus concentration of 10 to 15 mcg/L? What alternative antihypertensive agents would you recommend to minimize the interaction?*

L.J. is likely experiencing adverse effects as a result of elevated tacrolimus blood concentrations. Nephrotoxicity and neurotoxicity are related to elevated tacrolimus concentrations. In assessing the elevated tacrolimus concentration, one should determine whether the tacrolimus blood concentration was drawn at the appropriate time relative to when the last dose was taken. Concentrations drawn too early or too late (i.e., after dose given) may not represent trough concentrations. In addition, patient adherence should be assessed, and it should be determined whether the patient is taking any medications or foods that may interact with tacrolimus.

Tacrolimus is primarily metabolized by CYP3A4/5 in the liver and the gut, which account for a significant first-pass metabolism. In addition to being a substrate for CYP3A4/5, tacrolimus is also a substrate for P-glycoprotein, the drug efflux pump in the gut. P-glycoprotein is a membrane-localized drug transporter found on the luminal face of enterocytes that pumps drug from the cells back into the lumen of the gut. Diltiazem is an inhibitor of both CYP 3A4 and P-glycoprotein. The net effect is increased absorption (from decreased gut wall metabolism) with decreased drug efflux and decreased first-pass hepatic metabolism. L.J. can be managed by either discontinuing diltiazem and choosing another antihypertensive agent that does not inhibit CYP3A4 (e.g., the use of dihydropyridine calcium channel blockers such as amlodipine that does not interact with CYP3A4 or P-glycoprotein enzymes) or by decreasing the dose of tacrolimus. The pharmacokinetics of tacrolimus is highly variable within an individual patient and between patients. After attaining steady state, it is reasonable to decrease the tacrolimus dose by one-half and to target a tacrolimus concentration range of 10 to 15 mcg/L using Equation 11.7.

$$\text{Desired Dose} = \frac{\text{Css Desired}}{\text{Css Current}} \times \text{Current Dose}$$

$$= \left(\frac{12\ \text{mcg/mL}}{26\ \text{mcg/mL}}\right) 8\ \text{mg/day}$$

$$= (0.461)\, 8\ \text{mg/day}$$

$$= 3.7\ \text{mg/day} \approx 4\ \text{mg/day}$$

or

$$2\ \text{mg q12h}$$

Question #8 *D.J. is a 55-year-old male who received a kidney transplant 3 months ago. He presents with a 2-day history of fever and cough. A chest radiograph reveals a cavitary lesion consistent with pulmonary aspergillosis. D.J. is started on antifungal* *therapy with IV anidulafungin. After 2 weeks of therapy, D.J. has responded well to IV anidulafungin, and is to be transitioned to oral voriconazole. His immunosuppression regimen consists of tacrolimus 6 mg PO BID, prednisone 5 mg PO daily, and mycophenolic acid 720 mg PO BID. The most recent tacrolimus concentration was 8.5 mcg/L. Are there any dosage modifications to D.J.'s immunosuppressive regimen that should be considered prior to starting voriconazole? How should tacrolimus concentrations be monitored?*

Voriconazole is a potent inhibitor of cytochrome CYP3A4 and P-glycoprotein. Concomitant administration of voriconazole increases the exposure (AUC_τ) of tacrolimus by approximately threefold. It would be prudent to empirically decrease the dose of tacrolimus to approximately one-third the original dose to prevent the development of potentially toxic blood concentrations. For D.J., the dose of tacrolimus can be empirically decreased to 1 mg PO BID when voriconazole is started. Tacrolimus concentrations should be monitored closely and appropriate dosage adjustments made to maintain tacrolimus within the desired therapeutic range. The inhibitory effects of voriconazole will be fully apparent when it has reached steady state; thus, the timing of the tacrolimus concentration should correspond to this variable (i.e., voriconazole's half-life) as well. More importantly, the patient's renal function should be monitored closely. The dose of mycophenolate and prednisone may not need to be adjusted in the setting of stable graft function.

Question #9 *L.A., a 62-kg liver transplant recipient is receiving tacrolimus 4 mg PO BID, mycophenolate mofetil 1,000 mg PO BID, and prednisone 10 mg PO daily. Currently, his hepatic function tests appear to be stable, with a recent tacrolimus concentration of 11 mcg/L. He underwent surgery for a small bowel obstruction, and will not be able to take medications PO for a few days. What would be an appropriate IV tacrolimus dose for L.A.?*

Because the usual bioavailability of tacrolimus is approximately 25%, most clinicians give an IV dose approximately one-fourth to one-third of the oral dose. In this case, it would be approximately 2 mg/day. Although pharmacokinetic calculations could have been performed, the outcome would most likely be the same as adjusting the dose in proportion to the desired change in steady-state concentration. In this situation, we also have the additional factor of a change in route, and therefore, bioavailability to consider:

$$\text{New Dose} = \frac{\text{Css Desired}}{\text{Css Current}} \times \frac{\text{F Current}}{\text{F New Dosage Form}} \times \text{Current Dose}$$

Assuming the reported tacrolimus concentration of 11 mcg/L is reasonable, the IV dose will be 2 mg/day (0.032 mg/kg/day). This is consistent with an IV dosing of approximately 0.03 to 0.05 mg/kg/day for liver or kidney transplant recipients. The recommended IV dose for heart transplant recipients is 0.01 mg/kg/day.

$$= \frac{11 \,\text{mcg/L}}{11 \,\text{mcg/L}} \times \frac{0.25}{1.0} \times 8 \,\text{mg}$$
$$= 1 \times 0.25 \times 8 \,\text{mg}$$
$$= 2 \,\text{mg}$$

IV tacrolimus is usually given as a continuous infusion, but intermittent (i.e., 4 hours) infusion protocols are also available. The method of administration is usually dictated by institutional guidelines. Tacrolimus must be diluted in 0.9% normal saline or 5% dextrose water to a concentration of 0.004 to 0.02 mg/mL. The solution should be stored in glass or polyethylene containers, and infused using polyvinyl chloride-free tubing to minimize the potential for extraction of phthalates and adsorption of the drug onto the tubing. In general, IV tacrolimus is not frequently given. Most patients are able to tolerate medications by the oral route following transplantation.

Question #10   *P.S. is a 57-year-old male who received a kidney transplant 3 years ago. He reports decreased urine output and gaining approximately 5 pounds over the past week. His creatinine is now 3.7 mg/dL (was 1.3 mg/dL 6 weeks ago). His immunosuppression regimen consists of tacrolimus 6 mg PO BID and prednisone 5 mg PO daily. Other medications include metoprolol 25 mg PO BID, dapsone 100 mg PO daily, glipizide 5 mg PO BID, and naproxen 500 mg PO BID as needed for knee pain (started about 2 weeks ago). How would you assess P.S.'s renal function?*

Allograft rejection of the kidney and calcineurin inhibitor (tacrolimus or cyclosporine) toxicity can have a similar presentation (decreased urine output and rising serum creatinine). A tacrolimus concentration should be obtained to determine whether it is within the therapeutic range. A kidney ultrasound and biopsy will aid in determining whether allograft rejection is a cause of P.S.'s renal failure. Compliance with P.S.'s medication regimen should be assessed. The current immunosuppression regimens should be reassessed (e.g., the reason for not using an additional agent such as mycophenolate, azathioprine, or sirolimus should be clarified). In addition, P.S.'s medication list should be reviewed to determine whether any nephrotoxic drugs were recently started. Naproxen, like other nonsteroidal anti-inflammatory drugs (NSAIDs) can potentiate the nephrotoxic effects of calcineurin inhibitors such as tacrolimus and should be substituted with a non-nephrotoxic analgesic such as acetaminophen.

Question #11   *P.S. states that he has been taking his immunosuppressive medications as ordered. A tacrolimus concentration of 10.3 mcg/L and a clinical course consistent with NSAID-induced nephrotoxicity makes acute rejection less likely. Despite stopping the naproxen, P.S.'s renal function continues to deteriorate. It is decided that hemodialysis will be performed. Does the dose of tacrolimus need to be adjusted for hemodialysis?*

Tacrolimus is a large lipophilic molecule with a molecular weight of 822. Unit for molecular weight (g/mol) is highly protein bound (99%) and extensively partitions into whole blood (whole blood-to-plasma ratio of ~35). The large volume of distribution for tacrolimus suggests extravascular uptake. Tacrolimus is metabolized in the liver and gastrointestinal tract primarily by cytochrome P4503A4/5, with less than 1% of the administered dose excreted unchanged in the urine. Because tacrolimus is highly lipid soluble, almost completely metabolized, has a large volume of distribution, is extensively protein bound, and partitions into blood, it is not removed by hemodialysis or continuous hemofiltration.[43,44] A top-up dose of tacrolimus is also not recommended. Cyclosporine and sirolimus have similar physiochemical properties, and as such, are not removed by hemodialysis either. Even though tacrolimus does not accumulate in the setting of renal dysfunction nor is it removed by hemodialysis, many clinicians in this setting will target blood concentrations in the lower range in an effort to minimize any adverse effects on renal function.

Sirolimus

Sirolimus is a macrolide compound that has a chemical structure similar to tacrolimus. Although sirolimus and tacrolimus are structurally related, they have different mechanisms of action. Tacrolimus blocks the production of IL-2 by inhibiting calcineurin, whereas sirolimus prevents the IL-2-driven cell cycle progression. Sirolimus is usually given in combination with a calcineurin inhibitor, such as cyclosporine, and a corticosteroid, such as prednisone, to prevent allograft rejection.[45,46]

Sirolimus, like cyclosporine and tacrolimus, has a narrow therapeutic window and exhibits variability in its pharmacokinetic parameters. Sirolimus is also a substrate for CYP3A4 and P-glycoprotein. There are many drugs known to affect the intrinsic clearance of sirolimus. Table 11.3 lists commonly used drugs that can interact with sirolimus.

Sirolimus, rarely used in liver, lung, and cardiac transplants, is primarily used only in kidney (or kidney-pancreas) transplant recipients who have developed severe toxicities to calcineurin inhibitors, acquired BK virus-associated nephropathy during calcineurin inhibitor therapy, or exhibited signs of skin cancer. Dosing depends on the immunologic risk of the patient: for subjects with low immunologic risk, a weight-based regimen is typically used where patients less than 40 kg would receive a loading dose of 3 mg/m^2, then 1 mg/m^2 as maintenance; patients greater than 40 kg should receive a loading dose of 6 mg, followed by 2 mg/day of maintenance. In subjects classified as high immunologic risk, the suggested loading and maintenance doses are 15 mg and 5 mg/daily, respectively.[45,46]

Sirolimus is available as 0.5-, 1- and 2-mg tablets (Rapamune and various generics) and an oil-based oral solution (1 mg/mL). The solution should be mixed with at least 60 to 120 mL (2 to 4 ounces) of water or orange juice in a glass or plastic container. Owing to limited information on the stability of the diluted solution, other diluent liquids should be avoided, and the solution should be consumed immediately after mixing. After drinking the mixture, the container should be rinsed with a similar volume of water or orange juice and consumed to maximize delivery of the dose.[45,46]

THERAPEUTIC AND TOXIC CONCENTRATIONS (BLOOD)

The therapeutic range of sirolimus is 5 to 15 mcg/L. Concentrations less than 5 mcg/L are associated with an increased risk of rejection, and concentrations greater than 15 mcg/L are associated with an increased risk of adverse effects. The target concentration will vary according to the organ(s) transplanted, concurrent immunosuppression (i.e., lower target if given concurrently with calcineurin inhibitors and mycophenolate vs. higher target if sirolimus is used alone), and transplant center–specific immunosuppression protocols. Results from assays may differ depending on methodology. Chromatographic methods such as HPLC with ultraviolet detection or HPLC with tandem mass spectrometric detection will be approximately 20% lower than immunoassay techniques for whole blood concentrations.[47] Adjustments for the target concentrations should be made based on the assay used.

ADVERSE EFFECTS

The most common adverse effects (>10% incidence) associated with sirolimus are dose-dependent hypertension, headache, acne, hypertriglyceridemia, hypercholesterolemia, constipation, anemia, thrombocytopenia, and leukopenia. Other adverse effects include anemia, hypokalemia, impaired wound healing, formation of lymphoceles, rash, and increased risk of hepatic artery thrombosis in liver transplant recipients (therefore sirolimus is not first-line agent for this setting). Although sirolimus has a chemical structure similar to tacrolimus, it is not associated with the nephrotoxic effects commonly seen with tacrolimus; however, proteinuria and delayed recovery of renal function have been reported.[48-50]

KEY PARAMETERS: Sirolimus

Therapeutic concentration[a]	5–15 mcg/L
F[b]	
Liquid formulation	14%
Tablet formulation	18%
V[c]	Mean 12 L/kg (4–20 L/kg)
Cl[c,d]	139–221 mL/kg/hr
t½[e]	Mean 62 hr (46–78 hr)
fu (fraction unbound in plasma[f])	0.02–0.08

[a]Trough blood concentration. Target concentrations may vary with the organ(s) transplanted, concurrent immunosuppression regimens, and transplant center–specific immunosuppression protocols.
[b]High-fat meals will increase the bioavailability of sirolimus by 23% to 35% (tablets and liquid, respectively). Liquid and tablet formulations are not considered bioequivalent.
[c]Volume of distribution and clearance are calculated as V/F and Cl/F, respectively. Therefore, true values are lower than those reported (see Sirolimus; Volume of Distribution and Clearance).
[d]Sirolimus is extensively metabolized in the liver and is a substrate of CYP3A4/5 and P-glycoprotein.
[e]Half-life can be increased in extensive liver impairment.
[f]Primarily binds to albumin.

BIOAVAILABILITY (F)

Sirolimus is a lipophilic compound with limited oral absorption. The systemic bioavailability of the liquid formulation is approximately 14%. When sirolimus is given with a high-fat meal, the AUC is increased by approximately 35% (with a reduced Cmax] and increased time-to-reach Cmax). To minimize variability, sirolimus should be taken consistently with or without food. The bioavailability of the tablets is about 27% higher relative to the solution; that is, the tablets are approximately 18% absorbed (F ≈ 0.18). Whereas the tablets are not bioequivalent to the liquid formulation, the 2-mg dose is clinically equivalent, and no dose adjustment is clinically necessary.[45,46]

VOLUME OF DISTRIBUTION (V)

The volume of distribution of sirolimus is approximately 12 L/kg.[45,46] This large volume of distribution was calculated from oral dosing. The reported value is V/F, indicating that the actual volume of distribution is in the range of one-tenth (assuming an oral bioavailability of 10%) to one-fifth (assuming an oral bioavailability of 20%) the reported value. Sirolimus extensively distributes in tissues. The blood-to-plasma ratio of sirolimus is about 36, indicating that sirolimus partitions extensively into blood cells. Sirolimus in the plasma is also extensively protein bound (~92%) to albumin, α_1-acid glycoprotein, and lipoproteins.[51] Although sirolimus bioavailability is low, peak concentrations occur approximately 1 to 6 hours after an oral dose.

CLEARANCE (Cl)

Sirolimus undergoes extensive liver and gut metabolism.[45,46,51] The clearance of sirolimus is approximately 139 to 221 mL/kg/hr. Like volume of distribution, the reported clearance values were determined following oral doses without taking into account the limited bioavailability (i.e., the clearance value is Cl/F). Therefore, the actual clearance of sirolimus is probably in the range of one-tenth to one-fifth the reported value, assuming an oral bioavailability of 10% to 20%. Sirolimus, like cyclosporine and tacrolimus, is a substrate for CYP3A4/5 and P-glycoprotein. Drugs that inhibit CYP3A4/5, such as fluconazole, erythromycin, and diltiazem, can decrease the intrinsic clearance of sirolimus and result in increased blood concentrations. Similar to cyclosporine and tacrolimus, grapefruit and grapefruit juice can also inhibit CYP3A4 and P-glycoprotein but should be avoided. On the other hand, drugs that increase the intrinsic clearance (e.g., rifampin) of sirolimus can result in decreased sirolimus concentrations (Table 11.3).

HALF-LIFE (t½)

The elimination half-life of sirolimus is approximately 62 hours and may be increased in subjects with severe hepatic dysfunction.[51]

TIME TO SAMPLE

Because sirolimus has a relatively long half-life (~62 hours), it is reasonable to wait at least 1 to 2 weeks (or five half-lives to achieve steady state) when obtaining a whole blood concentration after initiating or changing therapy. Because the trough concentrations correlate well with the AUC (in kidney transplant patients) and sirolimus' pharmaco-dynamic effects, trough concentrations are most commonly used when monitoring sirolimus drug concentrations.[45,46]

CLINICAL PHARMACOGENOMICS OF SIROLIMUS

Currently (May 2016), there are insufficient data to support a pharmacogenomics-guided dosing for sirolimus[52–56] (see Pharmacogenomics Applications).

Question #12   *A.B. just received a cadaveric renal transplant. It is determined that A.B. will receive an immunosuppression regimen that utilizes sirolimus, cyclosporine modified, and prednisone. What dose of sirolimus should A.B. receive? Is genetic-guided dosing of sirolimus warranted in this case?*

Because sirolimus has a relatively long half-life, a loading dose is commonly used to achieve therapeutic concentrations in a timely fashion. The usual daily maintenance dose of sirolimus is 2 mg (although this depends on the nature of the transplant, e.g., immunologic risk, and patient's weight). The loading dose is typically three times the maintenance dose; in this case, 6 mg. A.B. should receive 6 mg of sirolimus as a loading dose immediately and then begin a maintenance dose of 2 mg/day starting the next day. Only a few studies have characterized the effects of CYP3A5, CYP3A4, and ATP binding cassette subfamily B member 1 (ABCB1) genetic polymorphisms on the pharmacokinetics of sirolimus. The current literature does not support pharmacogenomics-guided dosing of sirolimus. Conventional therapeutic drug monitoring (i.e., trough sirolimus concentrations) is recommended.

Question #13   *A.B. is to begin an immunosuppression regimen consisting of cyclosporine modified 300 mg PO BID, sirolimus 2 mg PO daily, and prednisone taper. Does it matter when A.B. takes his sirolimus?*

Sirolimus is typically given in combination with other immunosuppressive drugs (e.g., cyclosporine and prednisone). When sirolimus is administered simultaneously with cyclosporine-modified capsules, the C max and AUC of sirolimus are increased by 116% and 230%, respectively. When sirolimus is administered 4 hours after cyclosporine-modified capsules, the C max and AUC are increased by 37% and 80%, respectively. It is recommended by the manufacturer to administer sirolimus 4 hours after cyclosporine modified. The C max and AUC of cyclosporine did not change when sirolimus was administered simultaneously or 4 hours after cyclosporine modified. Clinically, the most important factor is for the patient to consistently take their medications at the same time of the day to minimize variations. Some patients may find it easier to take their dose of sirolimus with their dose of cyclosporine modified. Although this results in an increased exposure (AUC) to sirolimus, the most important factor is for the patient to do this consistently, so that the blood concentrations can be interpreted appropriately and the dosage regimen adjusted if necessary.[51,57]

Question #14   *A.B. is being given sirolimus in a liquid formulation during his hospital stay. He mixes his daily dose with orange juice but does not like the taste. Can A.B. be switched to the tablet formulation?*

Sirolimus is available in a liquid and tablet formulation. The liquid formulation must be mixed with water or orange juice and consumed immediately. Other liquids for dilution should not be used because of lack of stability data. Many patients complain of an unpleasant taste. The tablet formulation may be more convenient in an outpatient setting, because it does not need to be refrigerated or diluted with water or orange juice. A.B. can be switched from the liquid to the tablet formulation at the same dose of 2 mg/day. However, doses other than 2 mg may not be considered interchangeable between the two formulations and would need titration based on trough concentrations.

Question #15   *C.G. was taking a stable regimen of cyclosporine modified 200 mg PO BID, sirolimus 2 mg PO daily, and prednisone 10 mg PO daily. Her steady-state cyclosporine concentration was 200 mcg/L (via HPLC assay) and steady-state sirolimus concentration was 9 mcg/L on this regimen. C.G. was started on fluconazole 200 mg PO daily to treat a fungal infection. Two weeks later, her platelet count decreased from 200K to 75K, and her white blood cells decreased from 7K to 2.5K. Her latest cyclosporine blood concentration was 470 mcg/L, and sirolimus concentration was 22 mcg/L. What could account for her thrombocytopenia and leukopenia and elevated cyclosporine and sirolimus concentrations? How would you manage this interaction?*

Patient adherence should always be assessed. The timing of the drug concentrations should be verified. In addition, it should be determined whether there have been any changes to C.G.'s medication regimen and how C.G. takes her sirolimus. It appears that C.G. was on a stable immunosuppression regimen, with therapeutic, steady-state cyclosporine and sirolimus blood concentrations. She was recently started on fluconazole. Fluconazole is an inhibitor of CYP3A4 and P-glycoprotein. Like cyclosporine, sirolimus is a substrate for both CYP3A4 and P-glycoprotein. Fluconazole will decrease the metabolism of sirolimus and cyclosporine and result in increased blood concentrations. The elevated blood concentrations of sirolimus could account for her thrombocytopenia and leukopenia. Because C.G. is manifesting toxicity (leukopenia, thrombocytopenia) from a supratherapeutic concentration of sirolimus, a lower dose of sirolimus would be warranted. The blood concentration of sirolimus is dose proportional over a wide range. If her dose of sirolimus was lowered to 1 mg/day, her sirolimus concentration would be estimated to be approximately 11 mcg/L. Given the long half-life of sirolimus, a repeat trough concentration is warranted in 1 to 2 weeks after dose adjustment, in addition to repeat complete blood count. Alternatively, she could be given another appropriate antifungal regimen that did not inhibit CYP3A4 (e.g., micafungin) and be maintained on her current immunosuppression regimen. In this scenario, a steady-state concentration is still warranted to ensure that the trough sirolimus concentration is within therapeutic targets (after 1 to 2 weeks of stopping fluconazole).

Mycophenolate

Mycophenolate suppresses the functions of B and T lymphocytes, thereby mediating its immunosuppression effects via the inhibition of inosine monophosphate dehydrogenase.[58,59] It is primarily used in the kidney, liver, heart, lung transplantations, although off-label usage in other conditions such as autoimmune hepatitis, lupus, and psoriasis is also practiced. Similar to the other immunosuppressants discussed in this chapter, mycophenolate is almost always used as part of a combined immunosuppressive regimen (e.g., in conjunction with calcineurin inhibitors with or without corticosteroids). Mycophenolate can be administered as a prodrug (mycophenolate mofetil, CellCept, and generics) or as the sodium salt of mycophenolic acid (Myfortic or various generics). The prodrug formulation is inert, but once in the vasculature undergoes rapid activation (via hydrolysis) to form the acid. On the other hand, the sodium formulation does not require bioactivation, but is formulated only as an oral enteric-coated product for the purpose of minimizing gastrointestinal irritation.

Because of the different pharmacokinetic characteristics, the oral dosage forms (CellCept and Myfortic, or various generics) are not considered interchangeable.[58,59] Mycophenolate mofetil is available as 250 or 500 mg capsules/tablets and a 200 mg/mL suspension. The enteric-coated mycophenolate sodium is available as 180 and 360 mg tablets. Mycophenolate mofetil for injection (as hydrochloride) is supplied as a 500 mg vial for reconstitution. Whereas the injection is supplied as a 500 mg vial for reconstitution. However, the IV formulation is reserved only for patients who cannot tolerate oral intake. A loading dose of mycophenolate is usually not indicated, and the recommended initial doses in adults (oral or IV) are 1 g BID (kidney graft) or 1.5 g BID (liver and heart transplants), whereas pediatric patients are dosed based on body-surface

KEY PARAMETERS: Mycophenolate

Therapeutic concentration	30–60 mg · hr/L based on exposure values. Various limited sampling strategies for estimating area under the curve have been proposed.[60]
F	70%–90% (depending on the formulation and time posttransplant)
V	3.6–4 L (mofetil), 54–112 L (enteric-coated sodium)
Cl	173–193 mL/min
t½[b]	8–18 hr
fu (fraction unbound in plasma)	0.01–0.03

[a]Target exposure ranges may vary with the organ(s) transplanted and transplant center–specific immunosuppression protocols.
[b]Large variability is potentially secondary to the propensity for mycophenolate to undergo enterohepatic recirculation.

area (600 mg/m^2). The enteric-coated sodium formulation is typically not the first-line formulation for newly transplanted patients, and the typical dosing is 720 mg BID (comparable, but not bioequivalent, to 1 g BID mycophenolate mofetil).[58,59] Dose adjustments of mycophenolate based on renal or hepatic function are usually not necessary unless renal function is significantly deteriorated (i.e., glomerular filtration <25 mL/min/1.73 m^2 in which case a maximum daily dose of 2 g is suggested), but temporarily withholding the drug may be considered in patients developing severe neutropenia.[58,59] Similar to tacrolimus, mycophenolate is not likely removed by hemodialysis based on its physiochemical properties. Mycophenolate is primarily metabolized by UDP-glucuronosyltransferase (UGT) enzymes and transported by multidrug-resistant transporter 2 proteins (MRP2); thus, molecular drug interactions with xenobiotics that affect these metabolic pathways may be possible. Although mycophenolate exhibits wide intra- and interindividual variability in its pharmacokinetic parameters, therapeutic drug monitoring is not commonly practiced and remains a controversial topic.[60]

THERAPEUTIC AND TOXIC CONCENTRATIONS

The therapeutic range (30 to 60 mg · hr/L) of mycophenolate AUC has only been established in kidney transplant patients, but this range has not been extensively validated. As such, routine therapeutic drug monitoring in solid organ transplant patients remains controversial.[60] Currently, most of the data favor the use of mycophenolate AUC (estimated by LSSs) over trough concentration data for mycophenolate therapeutic drug monitoring, because the latter does not correlate well with drug exposure in a variety of transplant types. Although various LSSs have been proposed to estimate mycophenolate exposure in solid organ transplant patients (the majority of the data have been reported in kidney transplants), these predictive equations should be used only in similar patient populations for which the equations were originally developed/validated.[60] Overall, in contrast to cyclosporine, tacrolimus, and sirolimus, routine mycophenolate therapeutic drug monitoring is usually not instituted in most transplant centers. However, LSS-estimated mycophenolate exposure may be used in select kidney transplant recipients with unexplained organ rejection or adverse drug effect to guide dose adjustments to tailor to the empirical therapeutic target (30 to 60 mg · hr/L).

ADVERSE EFFECTS

Mycophenolate is associated with a wide range of adverse effects.[58,59] The most common dose-related effects are gastrointestinal pain, nausea, vomiting, diarrhea, abnormal liver function tests, and elevated serum creatinine. Less frequently, neutropenia, which is more likely to occur within the first 18 months after engraftment, can be associated with mycophenolate use. The gastrointestinal side effects may be alleviated by administering with food, dividing the total daily dose into more frequent intervals, or administering a proton pump inhibitor. Alternatively, patients who do not tolerate mycophenolate mofetil may be switched to the enteric-coated formulation. With respect to neutropenia, frequent monitoring (complete blood count and absolute neutrophil count) during the first posttransplant year after initiation of mycophenolate should be instituted. In the event of suspected mycophenolate-induced neutropenia, the dose of mycophenolate may have to be reduced until other causes of neutropenia (e.g., cytomegalovirus infection, other drugs such as cotrimoxazole or valganciclovir) can be ruled out.

BIOAVAILABILITY (F)

The oral bioavailability of mycophenolate, which is dependent on formulation and time posttransplant, is relatively high compared to that of cyclosporine and tacrolimus.[58,59] Mycophenolate mofetil reaches t_{max} at 1 to 1.5 hours, relatively faster than the enteric-coated formulation (t_{max}, 2 to 3 hours). The bioavailability of mycophenolate mofetil is also higher (i.e., >90%) than the enteric-coated formulation (~70%), but the prodrug (mofetil salt) requires bioactivation in the vasculature in a reaction that is rapid and complete. Because the overall exposure of mycophenolate increases in relation to posttransplant time, dose reduction may be needed to attain the same exposure. The presence of food does not affect the overall exposure of mycophenolate but has been documented to decrease the maximum concentration by up to 40%. To minimize the variability in absorption, mycophenolate (both formulations) should be given consistently with or without food. In the presence of gastrointestinal upset, clinicians usually recommend ingesting mycophenolate with small amounts of food.

VOLUME OF DISTRIBUTION (V)

The volume of distribution of mycophenolate (3.6 to 4 L/kg for mycophenolate mofetil and 54 to 112 L for enteric-coated sodium) depends on the formulation.[61] Mycophenolate is primarily distributed in plasma and extensively bound to albumin. The free fraction of mycophenolate is approximately 1% to 3% under normal conditions.

CLEARANCE (Cl)

Mycophenolate mofetil is an inactive prodrug that requires bioactivation (by hydrolysis) to generate the active mycophenolic acid. Mycophenolate is extensively metabolized in the liver by UDP-glucuronosyltransferase (UGT) enzymes, primarily UGT2B9 and UGT1A9, in the formation of both inactive and active glucuronide metabolites, respectively.[58,59,61] The inactive glucuronide constitutes the major, whereas the acyl-glucuronide is the minor metabolite. Both glucuronide metabolites undergo enterohepatic recirculation in a reaction catalyzed by MRP2 enzymes. The enterohepatic recirculation results in the formation of secondary "peaks" observed in the blood concentration–time curves of mycophenolate.[61] Mycophenolate has a reported clearance value of 173 to 193 mL/min. Because mycophenolate is a substrate of various phase II conjugative enzymes and transporters, its clearance can be altered by drug interactions mediated by modulators of these enzyme and transporter systems. However, in contrast to cyclosporine, tacrolimus, and sirolimus (where the enzyme of interest is the extensively studied CYP3A4/5), fewer data are available documenting the effects of UGT or MRP2 interaction on the clinical pharmacokinetics of mycophenolate.

HALF-LIFE (t½)

The elimination half-life of mycophenolate is approximately 8 to 18 hours.[58,59] As indicated in Clearance section, the half-life of mycophenolate may be prolonged if it is administered with an inhibitor (of UGT enzymes or MRP2 transporters) and vice versa for a coadministered inducer.

TIME TO SAMPLE

The utility of therapeutic drug monitoring for mycophenolate is still undergoing debate.[60] With respect to the method of monitoring, the majority of the literature favors the use of mycophenolate AUC, estimated with LSSs (usually three to four sampling points in the initial 4 to 6 hours period after dose), over trough concentration data. This is because poor correlations between trough concentration and mycophenolate exposure have been documented in most transplant populations. Various LSSs have been proposed to estimate mycophenolate exposure in solid organ transplant patients, and the majority of the data have been reported in kidney transplant recipients. Population pharmacokinetic-based algorithms (i.e., Bayesian approaches) are also available, but these methods usually require more sophisticated software programs that may not be practical in the clinical setting. The LSS-associated equations should be used only in similar patient populations for which the equations were originally developed/validated[60]; therefore, equations developed for mycophenolate mofetil cannot be used for the enteric-coated formulation (and vice versa).

CLINICAL PHARMACOGENOMICS OF MYCOPHENOLATE

Currently (May 2016), there are insufficient data to support a pharmacogenomics-guided dosing for mycophenolate[62-67] (see Pharmacogenomic Applications).

Question #16   *C.J. (50 years old, 70 kg) just received a cadaveric kidney transplant (panel reactive antibody 5%), and the transplant team wants to start her on mycophenolate, tacrolimus, and valganciclovir (cytomegalovirus mismatch). She was not prescribed a regular maintenance steroids regimen because of the low immunologic risk. She has a history of hypertension and takes amlodipine 5 mg PO daily. All of her blood work is within normal limits. Her current GFR is 15 mL/min. The site protocol also starts the patient on cotrimoxazole three times weekly as antibacterial prophylaxis and pantoprazole 40 mg PO daily as gastrointestinal prophylaxis. On what dose of mycophenolate would you start C.J.? Is genetic testing warranted in this setting?*

A loading dose of mycophenolate is typically not administered. Because C.J. is able to tolerate oral intake of medications, the conventional starting dose (not based on weight) for C.J. would be mycophenolate mofetil 1 g PO BID. Currently, there is insufficient evidence to recommend routine therapeutic drug monitoring of mycophenolate, unless there are specific reasons that the team suspects which can alter the pharmacokinetics of mycophenolate (e.g., decreased absorption or altered elimination) or there are occurrences of unexplained organ rejection/adverse events. If therapeutic drug monitoring is warranted, an LSS-based predictive equation to estimate the exposure of mycophenolate can be used. Trough concentrations are usually not reliable surrogate makers for exposure. Likewise, currently, there is insufficient evidence to support pharmacogenomics-guided dosing of mycophenolate.

Question #17   *It has been 1-month posttransplant and C.J.'s renal function has deteriorated to ~10 mL/min. Her serum creatinine has been trending up slightly over 2 weeks. Her current immunosuppressants are mycophenolate mofetil 1 g PO BID and tacrolimus 2.5 mg PO BID (trough concentration within target). Her blood pressure is adequately controlled on amlodipine. She is seronegative with respect to cytomegalovirus and BK virus. Her clinical blood work is within normal limits. She has not experienced any adverse effects from drugs. The team suspects acute graft rejection and has ordered a renal ultrasound to be followed by renal biopsy. Is it appropriate to monitor mycophenolate exposure in this setting? How would you adjust the dose?*

It may be appropriate to monitor mycophenolate exposure in the setting where no other causes can explain the patient's acute rejection episode. The best approach to determine mycophenolate exposure is to estimate AUC using LSS equations.[60] However, the LSS-associated equations should be used only in similar patient populations for which the equations were originally developed/validated.[60] The only LSS equation available in the literature today (May 2016) describing the use of mycophenolate in a similar population (coadministered with tacrolimus in the absence of steroids) uses three sampling time points[68]:

$$\text{Mycophenolate Exposure} = 9.328 + 1.311(C_{1hr}) + 1.455(C_{2hr}) + 2.901(C_{4hr}) \quad \textbf{(Eq. 11.9)}$$

In order to use this equation to estimate C.J.'s mycophenolate exposure, serum mycophenolate concentrations would have to be obtained precisely at 1, 2, and 4 hours after the ingestion of dose.

Question #18   *The laboratory reports the following mycophenolate concentrations: timing of dose (9 a.m.), 4 mg/L (1 hour post-dose), 1.5 mg/L (2 hours post-dose), and 1 mg/L (4 hours post-dose). Calculate C.J.'s mycophenolate exposure based on this information.*

$$\text{Mycophenolate Exposure} = 9.328 + 1.311\,(4\text{ mg/L}) + 1.455\,(1.5\text{ mg/L}) + 2.901\,(1\text{ mg/L})$$
$$= \sim\!20\text{ mg} \cdot \text{hr/L}$$

Because the therapeutic target of mycophenolate AUC in kidney transplant is usually 30 to 60 mg · hr/L, one can adjust the mycophenolate dose using Equation 11.7, assuming there is a proportional dose–exposure relationship:

$$\text{Desired Dose} = \frac{\text{Exposure Desired}}{\text{Exposure Current}} \times \text{Current Dose}$$

$$= \frac{30 \text{ mg} \cdot \text{hr/L}}{20 \text{ mg} \cdot \text{hr/L}} \times 2 \text{ g/day}$$

$$= 3 \text{ g/day or } 1.5 \text{ g q12h}$$

Question #19 *C.J.'s kidney rejection episode was reversed with steroid pulse, and her renal function has gradually normalized (GFR of 50 mL/min) at 2 months posttransplant. Her current immunosuppressants are mycophenolate mofetil 1.5 g PO BID and tacrolimus 3 mg PO BID (trough concentrations within target). Her blood pressure is adequately controlled (130/80 mm Hg) on amlodipine 10 mg PO daily. She is still on valganciclovir 900 mg PO daily and cotrimoxazole DS tablet three times weekly. Her clinic blood work is within normal limits, but she complains of stomach cramps and occasional diarrhea for the past 1 month (timing associated with the dose increase of mycophenolate), which became more intensified/intolerable in the past week. The symptoms are more intense after the ingestion of her BID medication regimens. How would you manage this complaint?*

A thorough history of C.J.'s stomach ailments should be taken. If other differential causes (e.g., gastric ulceration, infection) are ruled out by the transplant team, then a drug-associated adverse effect should be considered. Although all of her current medications can potentially cause these symptoms, stomach cramp and diarrhea are often associated with mycophenolate mofetil. The timing of gastrointestinal upset also corresponds with the increase in mycophenolate dose. She can be tried off mycophenolate mofetil and started on enteric-coated mycophenolate sodium, which has been shown to have reduced gastrointestinal adverse effects. Because the two oral formulations are not bioequivalent, the closest comparable dose is 1,080 mg PO BID.

Question #20 *A year after C.J.'s transplant, her renal function has remained stable (GFR of 60 mL/min). Her current immunosuppression regimen includes enteric-coated mycophenolate sodium 1,080 mg PO BID, tacrolimus 3.5 mg PO BID (trough concentrations within target), and prednisone 5 mg PO BID. Her cotrimoxazole had been taken off 2 weeks ago because of a significant drop in white blood cell count. Her valganciclovir was stopped 3 months ago because of several, consecutive sero-negative cytomegalovirus readings in the blood. Her blood pressure is well controlled with amlodipine. Her current clinic blood work still reveals a depressed white blood cell and neutrophil count. She is afebrile and otherwise asymptomatic. Virology indicates no detectable amounts of BK or cytomegalovirus in the blood. How would you advise the team?*

Neutropenia commonly occurs within the first 1.5 years posttransplant and may be because of a host of reasons. In the setting where the differential causes have been ruled out (e.g., virus-associated neutropenia), drug causes should be considered. Because the team had already stopped cotrimoxazole (the first agent likely to be discontinued in the setting of neutropenia), the possibility of over immunosuppression from her other drugs should be considered. In this scenario, the next mostly likely target for drug-induced neutropenia would be mycophenolate, because mycophenolate exposure values are known to increase over posttransplant time. The patient's mycophenolate dose can be dropped by 25% to 50%. Because no LSSs are yet available to estimate mycophenolate exposure in patients taking enteric-coated mycophenolate sodium (in the absence of steroids) in kidney transplant patients, one cannot resort to LSS-guided therapeutic drug monitoring in this scenario. The patient's clinical status (e.g., complete white blood cell count and renal function) should be monitored closely.

Pharmacogenomic Applications

Cyclosporine, tacrolimus, and sirolimus are primarily metabolized by hepatic/gut CYP3A4/5 and also act as substrates of the P-glycoprotein efflux pumps. Mycophenolate is a substrate of UGT enzymes and MRP2 transporters. Genetic polymorphisms of these enzymes and transporters that result in functional phenotypic alterations can theoretically affect the clearance of these agents. However, currently (as of May 2016), clinical guidelines from the CPIC, which provides peer-reviewed practice recommendations (https://www.pharmgkb.org/page/cpic), are not available for cyclosporine, sirolimus, and mycophenolate. In the case of cyclosporine and sirolimus, potential but no definitive associations have been drawn between CYP3A4, CYP3A5, and ABCB1 polymorphisms and altered pharmacokinetics/pharmacodynamics in humans.[22–31,52–56] Likewise, studies on the effects of UGT or MRP2 polymorphisms have not reported conclusive effects for mycophenolate.[62] Despite reports of potential associations between UGT1A9*3, UGT2B7*2, and MRP2 (24C > T) polymorphisms with elevated mycophenolate exposure,[63–67] little is known if these translate to altered pharmacodynamics (e.g., increased organ rejection or mycophenolate-associated toxicities). Overall, the absence of clear links between known genetic polymorphisms and altered pharmacokinetics/pharmacodynamics means that genomic-guided dosing for these agents cannot yet be recommended.

On the other hand, a CPIC guideline is available for tacrolimus in the context of CYP3A5 polymorphism.[42] Specifically, patients carrying the CYP3A5*3/*6/*7 alleles (the most common mutations for this gene) exhibit reduced catalytic activity toward tacrolimus compared to the wild-type (CYP3A5*1). It has been recommended that three different phenotypic categories can be assigned to subjects based on their genotype: wild-type homozygous individuals would be classified as "extensive metabolizer," those carrying a wild-type and a mutant allele classified as "intermediate metabolizer," and patients with two mutant alleles classified as "poor metabolizer".[42] A higher tacrolimus dose is recommended (i.e., 1.5 to 2 times the labeled dose) for both extensive and intermediate metabolizers, whereas the original labeled doses are suggested for the poor metabolizers. Although this approach has been proven to attain therapeutic tacrolimus concentrations more efficiently, these pharmacogenomic dosing strategies have yet been associated with improved tacrolimus pharmacodynamics (i.e., reduced toxicity and graft loss). As such, the CPIC guideline does not recommend the routine testing of CYP3A5 for individuals being prescribed tacrolimus, and standard therapeutic drug monitoring is still recommended irrespective of the availability of the CYP3A5 genomic data. However, if CYP3A5 genetic information were already available, then clinicians can provide tacrolimus dose adjustments according to the guideline, in conjunction with therapeutic drug monitoring.[42]

ACKNOWLEDGMENT

The important work of David J. Quan to a previous version of this chapter is acknowledged.

REFERENCES

1. *Sandimmune (cyclosporine)* [package insert]. East Hanover, NJ: Novartis Pharmaceuticals Corp. http://www.pharma.us.novartis.com/product/pi/pdf/sandimmune.pdf. March 2015. Accessed May 10, 2016.

2. *Lexicomp Clinical Drug Information* [intranet database]. Neoral (cyclosporine). Indianapolis, IN: Wolters Kluwer Inc. http://online.lexi.com/action/home. Accessed May 10, 2016.

3. Wahlberg J, Wilczek HE, Fauchald P, et al. Consistent absorption of cyclosporine from a microemulsion formulation assessed in stable renal transplant recipients over a one-year study period. *Transplantation*. 1995;60:648–652.

4. Yee GC, Stanley DL, Pessa LJ, et al. Effect of grapefruit juice on blood cyclosporine concentration. *Lancet*. 1995;345:955–956.

5. LeMarie M, Tillement JP. Role of lipoproteins and erythrocytes in the in vivo binding and distribution of cyclosporin A in the blood. *J Pharm Pharmacol*. 1982;34:715–718.

6. Niederberger W, Lemaire M, Maurer G, et al. Distribution and binding of cyclosporine in blood and tissue. *Transplant Proc*. 1983;15:2419–2421.

7. Oellerich M, Armstrong VW, Kahan B, et al. Lake Louise Consensus Conference on Cyclosporin Monitoring in Organ Transplantation: report of the consensus panel. *Ther Drug Monit*. 1995;17: 642–654.

8. De Groen PC, Aksamit AJ, Rakela J, et al. Central nervous system toxicity after liver transplantation: the role of cyclosporine and cholesterol. *N Engl J Med*. 1987;317:861–866.

9. Kahan BD, Welsh M, Schoenberg L, et al. Variable absorption of cyclosporine: a biopharmaceutical risk factor for chronic renal allograft rejection. *Transplantation*. 1996;62:599–606.

10. Lindholm A, Kahan BD. Influence of cyclosporine pharmacokinetics trough concentrations, and AUC monitoring on outcomes after kidney transplantation. *Clin Pharmacol Ther*. 1993;54:205–218.

11. Atkinson K, Biggs JC, Britton K, et al. Oral administration of cyclosporine A for recipients of allogeneic marrow transplants: implications of clinical gut dysfunction. *Br J Haematol*. 1984;56:223–231.

12. Merion RM, Gorski DH, Burtch GD, et al. Bile refeeding after liver transplantation and avoidance of intravenous cyclosporine. *Surgery*. 1989;106:604.

13. Levy G, Altraif I, Rezieg M, et al. Cyclosporine in liver transplant patients. *Transplant Proc*. 1994;26:3184–3187.

14. Gupta SK, Bakran A, Johnson RW, et al. Pharmacokinetics of cyclosporine: influence of the rate–duration profile of an intravenous infusion in renal transplant patients. *Br J Clin Pharmacol*. 1989;27:353.

15. Lindholm A, Henricsson S, Lind M, et al. Intraindividual variability in the relative systemic availability of cyclosporine after oral dosing. *Eur J Clin Pharmacol*. 1988;34:461.

16. Ptachcinski RJ, Venkataramanan R, Rosenthal JT, et al. Cyclosporine kinetics in renal transplantation. *Clin Pharmacol Ther*. 1985;38:296.

17. Yee GC, McGuire TR, Gmur DJ, et al. Blood cyclosporine pharmacokinetics in patients undergoing marrow transplantation: influence of age, obesity, and hematocrit. *Transplantation*. 1988;46:399.

18. Kahan BD, Dunn J, Fitts C, et al. The Neoral formulation: improved correlation between cyclosporine trough levels and exposure in stable renal transplant recipients. *Transplant Proc.* 1994;26:2940.

19. Levy G, Thervet E, Lake J, et al. Patient management by Neoral C_2 monitoring: an international consensus statement. *Transplantation.* 2002;73(suppl):S12–S18.

20. Nashan B, Cole E, Levy G, et al. Clinical validation studies of Neoral C_2 monitoring: a review. *Transplantation.* 2002;73(suppl):S3–S11.

21. Koristkova B, Grundmann M, Brozmanova H, et al. Validation of sparse sampling strategies to estimate cyclosporine A area under the concentration–time curve using either a specific radioimmunoassay or high-performance chromatography method. *Ther Drug Monit.* 2010;32:586–593.

22. Hesselink D, van Schaik RH, van der Heiden I, et al. Genetic polymorphisms of the CYP3A4, CYP3A4, and MDR-1 genes and pharmacokinetic of the calcineurin inhibitors cyclosporine and tacrolimus. *Clin Pharmcol Ther.* 2003;74:245–254.

23. Bouamar R, Hesselink DA, van Schaik RH, et al. Polymorphisms in CYP3A4, CYP3A4, and ABCB1 are not associated with cyclosporine pharmacokinetics nor with cyclosporine clinical end points after renal transplantation. *Ther Drug Monit.* 2011;33:178–184.

24. Von Ahsen N, Richter M, Grupp C, et al. No influence of the MDR-1 C3435T polymorphism or a CYP3A4 promoter polymorphism (CYP3A4-V allele) on dose-adjusted cyclosporine A trough concentrations or rejection incidence in stable renal transplant recipients. *Clin Chem.* 2001;47:1048–1052.

25. Hesselink D, van Gelder T, van Schaik RH, et al. Population pharmacokinetics of cyclosporine in kidney and heart transplant recipients and the influence of ethnicity and genetic polymorphisms in the MDR-1, CYP3A4, and CYP3A4 genes. *Clin Pharmacol Ther.* 2004;76:545–556.

26. Qiu XY, Jiao Z, Zhang M, et al. Association of MDR1, CYP3A4*18B, and CYP3A5*3 polymorphisms with cyclosporine pharmacokinetics in Chinese renal transplant recipients. *Eur J Clin Pharmacol.* 2008;64:1069–1084.

27. Qiu F, He XJ, Sun YX, et al. Influence of ABCB1, CYP3A4*18B and CYP3A5*3 polymorphisms on cyclosporine A pharmacokinetics in bone marrow transplant recipients. *Pharmacol Rep.* 2011;63:815–825.

28. Zhao Y, Song M, Guan D, et al. Genetic polymorphisms of CYP3A4 genes and concentration of the cyclosporine and tacrolimus. *Transplant Proc.* 2005;37:178–181.

29. Chu XM, Hao HP, Wang GJ, et al. Influence of CYP3A5 genetic polymorphism on cyclosporine A metabolism and elimination in Chinese renal transplant recipients. *Acta Pharmacol Sin.* 2006;27:1504–1508.

30. Staatz CE, Goodman LK, Tett SE. Effect of CYP3A and ABCB1 single nucleotide polymorphisms on the pharmacokinetics and pharmacodynamics of calcineurin inhibitors: Part I. *Clin Pharmacokinet.* 2010;49:141–175.

31. Crettol S, Venetz J, Fontana M, et al. Influence of ABCB1 genetic polymorphisms on cyclosporine intracellular concentration in transplant recipients. *Pharmacogenet Genomics.* 2008;18:307–315.

32. *Lexicomp Clinical Drug Information* [intranet database]. Prograf (tacrolimus). Indianapolis, IN: Wolters Kluwer Inc. http://www.online.lexi.com. Accessed May 10, 2016.

33. Tacrolimus. In: McEvoy GK, ed. AHFS Drug Information 2015. Bethesda, MD: American Society of Health-System Pharmacists, Inc. http://www.online.lexi.com. Accessed May 10, 2016.

34. Kershner RP, Fitzsimmons WE. Relationship of FK506 whole blood concentrations and efficacy and toxicity after liver and kidney transplantation. *Transplantation.* 1996;62:920–926.

35. Venkataramanan R, Swaminathan A, Prasad T, et al. Clinical pharmacokinetics of tacrolimus. *Clin Pharmacokinet.* 1995;29:404–430.

36. Tuteja S, Alloway RR, Johnson JA. The effect of gut metabolism on tacrolimus bioavailability in renal transplant recipients. *Transplantation.* 2001;71:1303–1307.

37. Mancinelli LM, Frassetto L, Floren LC, et al. The pharmacokinetics and metabolic disposition of tacrolimus: a comparison across ethnic groups. *Clin Pharmacol Ther.* 2001;69:24–31.

38. Kimikawa M, Kamoya K, Toma H, et al. Effective oral administration of tacrolimus in renal transplant recipients. *Clin Transplant.* 2001;15:324–329.

39. Plosker GL, Foster RH. Tacrolimus: a further update of its pharmacology and therapeutic use in the management of organ transplantation. *Drugs.* 2000;59:323–389.

40. Wallemacq PE, Verbeeck RK. Comparative clinical pharmacokinetics of tacrolimus in paediatric and adult patients. *Clin Pharmacokinet.* 2001;40:283–295.

41. McDiarmid SV, Colonna JO, Shaked A, et al. Differences in oral FK506 dose requirements between adult and pediatric liver transplant patients. *Transplantation.* 1993;55:1328–1332.

42. Birdwell KA, Decker B, Barbarino JM, et al. Clinical Pharmacogenetics Implementation Consortium (CPIC) guidelines for CYP3A5 genotype and tacrolimus dosing. *Clin Pharmacol Ther.* 2015;98:19–24.

43. Venkataramanan R, Jain A, Cadoff E, et al. Pharmacokinetics of FK 506: preclinical and clinical studies. *Transplant Proc.* 1990;22(suppl 1):52–56.

44. Kishino S, Takekuma Y, Sugawara M, et al. Influence of continuous haemodiafiltration on the pharmacokinetics of tacrolimus in liver transplant recipients with small-for-size grafts. *Clin Transplant.* 2003;17:412–416.

45. *Lexicomp Clinical Drug Information* [intranet database]. Rapamune (sirolimus). Indianapolis, IN: Wolters Kluwer Inc. http://www.online.lexi.com. Accessed May 10, 2016.

46. Sirolimus. In: McEvoy GK, ed. *AHFS Drug Information 2015.* Bethesda, MD: American Society of Health-System Pharmacists, Inc. http://www.online.lexi.com. Accessed May 10, 2016.

47. Shaw LM, Kaplan B, Brayman KL. Advances in therapeutic drug monitoring for immunosuppressants: a review of sirolimus. *Clin Ther.* 2000;22(suppl B):B1–B13.

48. Kahan BD, Napoli KL, Kelly PA, et al. Therapeutic drug monitoring of sirolimus: correlations with efficacy and toxicity. *Clin Transplant.* 2000;14:97–109.

49. McTaggart RA, Gottlieb D, Brooks J, et al. Sirolimus prolongs recovery from delayed graft function after cadaveric renal transplantation. *Am J Transplant.* 2004;4:953–961.

50. van den Akkher JM, Wetzels JM, Hoitsma AJ. Proteinuria following conversion from azathioprine to sirolimus in renal transplant recipients. *Kidney Int.* 2006;70:1355–1357.

51. Zimmerman J, Kahan BD. Pharmacokinetics of sirolimus in stable renal transplant patients after multiple oral dose administration. *J Clin Pharmacol.* 1997;37:405–415.

52. Le Meur Y, Djebli N, Szelag JC, et al. CYP3A5*3 influences sirolimus oral clearance in de novo and stable renal transplant recipients. *Clin Pharmacol Ther.* 2006;80:51–60.

53. Anglicheau D, Le Corre D, Lechaton S, et al. Consequences of genetic polymorphisms for sirolimus requirements after renal transplant in patients on primary sirolimus therapy. *Am J Transplant.* 2005;5:595–603.

54. Woillard JB, Kamar N, Coste S, et al. Effect of CYP3A4*22, POR*28, and PPARA rs4253728 on sirolimus in vitro metabolism and trough concentrations in kidney transplant recipients. *Clin Chem.* 2013;59:1761–1969.

55. Sam WJ, Chamberlain CE, Lee SJ, et al. Associations of ABCB1 3435C>T and IL-10-1082G>A polymorphisms with long-term sirolimus dose requirements in renal transplant patients. *Transplantation.* 2011;92:1342–1347.

56. Woillard JB, Kamar N, Rousseau A, et al. Association of sirolimus adverse effects with mTOR, p70S6K or Raptor polymorphisms in kidney transplant recipients. *Pharmacogenet Genomics.* 2012;22:725–732.

57. Kaplan B, Meier-Kriesche HU, Napoli KL, et al. The effects of relative timing of sirolimus and cyclosporine microemulsion formation coadministration on the pharmacokinetics of each agent. *Clin Pharmacol Ther.* 1998;63:48–53.

58. *Lexicomp Clinical Drug Information* [intranet database]. Mycophenolate. Indianapolis, IN: Wolters Kluwer Inc. http://www.online.lexi.com. Accessed May 16, 2016.

59. Mycophenolate. In: McEvoy GK, ed. *AHFS Drug Information 2015.* Bethesda, MD: American Society of Health-System Pharmacists, Inc. http://www.online.lexi.com. Accessed: May 16, 2016.

60. Kiang T, Ensom MH. Therapeutic drug monitoring of mycophenolate in adult solid organ transplant patients: an update. *Expert Opin Drug Metab Toxicol.* 2016;12:545–553.

61. Staatz C, Tett S. Clinical pharmacokinetics and pharmacodynamics of mycophenolate in solid organ transplant recipients. *Clin Pharmacokinet.* 2007;46:13–58.

62. Barraclough KA, Lee KJ, Staatz CE. Pharmacogenetic influences on mycophenolate therapy. *Pharmacogenomics.* 2010;11:369–390.

63. Levesque E, Delage R, Benoit-Biancamano MO, et al. The impact of UGT1A8, UGT1A9, and UGT2B7 genetic polymorphisms on the pharmacokinetic profile of mycophenolic acid after a single oral dose in healthy volunteers. *Clin Pharmacol Ther.* 2007;81:392–400.

64. van Schaik RH, van Agteren M, de Fijter JW, et al. UGT1A9-275T>A/-2152C>T polymorphisms correlate with low MPA exposure and acute rejection in MMF/tacrolimus-treated kidney transplant patients. *Clin Pharmacol Ther.* 2009;86:319–327.

65. Johnson LA, Oetting WS, Basu S, et al. Pharmacogenetic effect of the UGT polymorphisms on myco-phenolate is modified by calcineurin inhibitors. *Eur J Clin Pharmacol.* 2008;64:1056.

66. Baldelli S, Merlini S, Perico N, et al. C-440T/T-331C polymorphisms in the UGT1A9 gene affect the pharmacokinetics of mycophenolic acid in kidney transplantation. *Pharmacogenomics.* 2007;8:1127–1141.

67. Naesens M, Kuypers DR, Verbeke K, et al. Multidrug resistance protein 2 genetic polymorphisms in-fluence mycophenolic acid exposure in renal allograft recipients. *Transplantation.* 2006;82:1074–1084.

68. Poulin E, Greanya ED, Partovi N, et al. Development and validation of limited sampling strategies for tacrolimus and mycophenolate in steroid-free renal transplant regimens. *Ther Drug Monit.* 2011;33:50–55.

12

LITHIUM

Erin D. Knox and Julie A. Dopheide

Learning Objectives

By the end of lithium chapter, the learner shall be able to:

1. Discuss how the physiochemical properties of lithium impact its absorption, distribution, and clearance.
2. Describe the clinical significance of small fluctuations in plasma lithium concentrations.
3. Explain the rationale for waiting a minimum of 8 hours before obtaining plasma lithium concentrations.
4. List at least three different drug classes that can influence the total body clearance of lithium and predict the relative change in lithium plasma concentration when each drug class is coadministered with lithium.
5. Recommend a daily dose of lithium carbonate that will achieve a therapeutic plasma concentration given the specific age, total body weight, and serum creatinine of an individual patient.
6. Given a lithium level above or below the desired range, recommend a dosing adjustment to achieve a therapeutic level.
7. List five reasons why a measured plasma lithium concentration may be higher or lower than predicted based upon patient-specific parameters.
8. Describe how age, obesity, and pregnancy may affect the pharmacokinetic disposition of lithium.
9. Explain the impact of hemodialysis on the pharmacokinetic parameters of lithium, and describe the timing of posthemodialysis samples.
10. Describe strategies to enhance lithium elimination in a patient experiencing lithium toxicity.
11. Describe pharmacokinetic changes and necessary dosing adjustments when lithium is administered in a pregnant or postpartum woman.

Lithium, a monovalent cation, was first approved by the Food and Drug Administration (FDA) in 1970 for bipolar disorder, with current approval in patients aged 12 years and older. Lithium is effective for mania, relapse prevention, and to a lesser extent depression, as well as mixed phases of illness. It has antisuicide and neuroprotective properties[1] and is used for the treatment of a variety of psychiatric and neurologic conditions.[1,2]

Lithium carbonate, formulated in tablets and capsules, and lithium citrate, available as an oral solution, are widely prescribed. (Table 12.1) Lithium orotate and lithium aspartate are regulated as dietary supplements by the FDA and are uncommonly used.[3] Usual daily doses of lithium needed to achieve a therapeutic level may range from 600 to 2,100 mg and are dependent on body mass, hydration status, renal function, concurrent medications, and age.

Because lithium possesses a relatively narrow therapeutic range and displays rather predictable pharmacokinetics, it serves as an excellent candidate for routine therapeutic drug monitoring.

THERAPEUTIC AND TOXIC PLASMA CONCENTRATIONS

The therapeutic plasma level range of lithium is 0.5 to 1.2 mEq/L according to several decades of research.[1,2] In the treatment of acute mania, lithium levels between 1.0 and 1.5 mEq/L may be needed for stabilization; however, plasma levels above 1.0 mEq/L are associated with a higher incidence of intolerable side effects, such as cognitive dulling or impaired coordination.[1,4] For relapse prevention or maintenance treatment of bipolar disorder, a plasma concentration of 0.8 to 1.0 mEq/L is more effective than 0.4 to 0.6 mEq/L[5]; most patients and providers find that maintaining a level between 0.6 and 0.8 mEq/L provides relapse prevention with good tolerability.[1,6]

Early common side effects of lithium pharmacotherapy include nausea, polyuria, polydipsia, and diarrhea. Many of the effects subside over time, or may be minimized by altering administration schedules or changing formulations. Gastrointestinal effects may occur with lithium initiation or administration of large single doses; nausea and vomiting may decrease with continued treatment or may be managed by administering smaller divided doses with meals. Polyuria and polydipsia can be lessened by changing administration from divided doses to a single dose at bedtime. When plasma concentrations of 1.0 mEq/L or greater are targeted, more severe adverse effects are possible.

TABLE 12.1 Commercially Available Preparation: Lithium

FORMULATION	STRENGTH (mg)	mEq EQUIVALENCE
Lithium carbonate Immediate-release capsules or tablets	300	8.12 mEq
Lithium carbonate Controlled- or slow-release tablets	300 450	8.12 mEq 12.18 mEq
Lithium citrate Oral solution	~300	8 mEq/5 mL

KEY PARAMETERS: Lithium

Therapeutic range	0.5–1.2 mEq/L (predose level)
F	1 (100%)
V	0.7 L/kg
Cl	$0.25 \times Cl_{Cr}$
t½	
α	6 hr
β	18–24 hr
fu (fraction unbound in plasma)	1

Amdisen[9]; Finley et al.[10]; Thornhill[11]; Yukawa et al.[12]

Sensitivity to side effects may be more common in the elderly, even in the setting of lower plasma levels.[7] Long-term adverse effects may develop with lithium therapy, including hypothyroidism, fine intentional tremor, weight gain, acne, worsening psoriasis, and nephrotoxicity.

Acute toxicity is seen with levels >1.5 mEq/L, but can also be evident at lower levels.[2,8] Severe nausea, vomiting, and diarrhea may be early signs of toxicity, which can progress to confusion, coarse tremor, seizures, coma, arrhythmia, or death as levels exceed 2.5 mEq/L (CANMAT, 2013).[2,7]

BIOAVAILABILITY (F)

Lithium is rapidly absorbed, with peak plasma concentrations observed within 1 hour for the solution, 1 to 3 hours for the immediate-release, and 3 to 6 hours for the extended- or controlled-release preparations. Gastrointestinal absorption of lithium solution or regular-release tablets and capsules appears to be nearly complete (95% to 100%). The absorption of slow-release lithium products may be more variable and can be as low as 85%.[11]

VOLUME OF DISTRIBUTION (V)

Lithium is not protein bound and distributes throughout the body as a free ion. After being absorbed in the upper gastrointestinal tract, lithium undergoes a complex and extended distribution phase. The volume of distribution for lithium is approximately 0.7 L/kg.[13] Lithium will, however, concentrate in various intracompartmental spaces and subsequently equilibrates very slowly with the extracellular fluid volume.[13] Overall, lithium disposition appears to follow a two-compartment model, displaying an initial volume of distribution of 0.25 to 0.3 L/kg and a final volume of distribution at equilibrium of ≈0.7 L/kg. The elevated plasma lithium concentrations observed during the initial distribution phase do not appear to correlate with efficacy or toxicity.[13]

CLEARANCE (Cl)

Lithium is not metabolized but eliminated from the body almost exclusively via the kidneys, with minimal amounts lost through feces and sweat. Nearly 100% of the absorbed drug is filtered through the glomerulus, and 70% to 80% is reabsorbed in the proximal tubule.[9] The renal tubular reabsorption of lithium is very closely linked with sodium reabsorption and is influenced by the same factors regulating sodium balance (e.g., dehydration, hypotension, sodium depletion, etc.). In patients with a normal sodium balance, lithium clearance is approximately 25% of creatinine clearance.[12] A wide variety of medications and disease states can influence lithium clearance, most commonly through an alteration in renal function or sodium balance. The most clinically relevant pharmacokinetic drug–drug interactions are listed in Table 12.2.

TABLE 12.2   Drug–Drug Interactions: Lithium

MEDICATION CLASS	IMPACT ON LITHIUM LEVELS	DEGREE OF IMPACT ON LITHIUM LEVEL[a]	COMMENTS
Angiotensin-converting enzyme inhibitors (ACE inhibitors) Angiotensin receptor blockers (ARBs)	Increase	Moderate to severe	Avoid coadministration
NSAIDs or cyclooxegenase-2 inhibitors	Increase	Low, moderate, or severe	Low if taking one-time dose; severe if taking routine doses
Thiazide diuretics	Increase	Moderate	Avoid coadministration or lower lithium dose by 50% and monitor
Methylxanthines (theophylline, aminophylline, caffeine)	Decrease	Low to moderate	Counsel patient to look for signs of relapse
Salt restriction	Increase	Moderate	Counsel patient to maintain consistent salt intake and TDM.

[a]Low impact: may not be significant as change in level may only be 20%.
Moderate impact: coadministration could result in toxicity; case reports demonstrate possible level increases from 25% to 50%.
Severe impact: coadministration may result in severe toxicity; case reports describe variable level increases from 50% to 350%; some cases requiring dialysis.
ACEInh—Finley et al.[10]; Bisogni et al.[38]; ARB—Nagamine[39]; Bisogni et al.[38]; NSAIDs—DeWinter et al.[14]; Reimann et al.[15]; Ragheb and Powell[40]; thiazides—Finley et al.[10]; Bisogni et al.[38]; COX-2—Phelan et al.[41]; methylxanthines—Perry et al.[42]; Finley et al.[10]
NSAIDs, nonsteroidal anti-inflammatory drugs; TDM, therapeutic drug monitoring.

TISSUE PENETRATION

Lithium has been measured in most body tissues and is excreted most significantly in urine but is also present in bile, saliva, sweat, and feces. Cerebrospinal fluid concentrations of lithium are approximately 44% of plasma levels when at steady state, with no difference observed in the concentrations of gray and white brain matter.[16] Lithium may also concentrate in thyroid or bone tissue, with little deposited in adipose tissue.[9]

HALF-LIFE (t½)

The initial distribution or α half-life of lithium is approximately 6 hours, and the final elimination or β half-life is 18 to 24 hours.[10] Plasma half-lives of 48 hours or longer may be seen in patients with significant renal impairment. The half-life of lithium may be influenced by duration of therapy; one study of patients on maintenance lithium therapy (n = 30) demonstrated a half-life of nearly twice that of those on lithium for less than 1 year.[17]

TIME OF SAMPLING

Because lithium distribution follows a two-compartment pharmacokinetic model, it is imperative that lithium plasma levels be obtained at consistent and reproducible times. The current standard of practice is to obtain samples before any morning dose of lithium and ideally 12 hours after the last dose was taken.[7] The terminal or β half-life of approximately 24 hours dictates that steady-state lithium levels will be achieved within 5 days for most healthy adults. Although lithium levels appear to plateau within 4 to 5 days, full therapeutic effects are not generally observed for 14 to 21 days after therapy has been initiated, likely owing to the time it takes for active transport across the blood–brain barrier.[16]

SPECIAL POPULATIONS

Children

Lithium has demonstrated efficacy for bipolar disorder in children and adolescents,[18,19] and two studies examine lithium's pharmacokinetics in youth. A single-dose study in 39 patients aged 7 to 17 years (mean age 11.8 years) gave lithium 600 mg to youth weighing 20 to 30 kg and 900 mg to youth >30 kg, then performed pharmacokinetic modeling. Clearance was higher in children (140 mL/min) compared to adolescents (125 mL/min), and youth had shorter calculated multiple-dose elimination half-lifes (13 to 15 hours) compared to pharmacokinetic studies in adults (17 to 27 hours).[20]

Seniors or older adults

Lithium is an effective therapy for bipolar disorder in older adults (>65 years) although they are at increased risk for neurologic side effects and levels should be kept below

1.0 mEq/L. Most seniors are maintained at levels below 0.8 mEq/L to minimize risk of toxicity.[6,21] When compared to younger patients, individuals aged 65 years and older eliminate lithium more slowly and have a smaller V_d. Studies have suggested that older adult women (ages 67 to 80) on lithium may require a 33% to 50% lower dose when compared to a similarly sized adult[22] although levels can be consistent over time. A study monitoring repeat levels in 40- to 49-year olds, 50- to 59-year olds, 60 to 69-year olds, and 70+ found no variability in levels that could be correlated to age over a 2-year period.[6]

Pregnancy

For lithium responders, the benefits of continuing therapy in the second and third trimesters can outweigh the risk of teratogenicity, which is greatest in the first trimester. However, close monitoring of the lithium level is needed because of an increase in volume of distribution and enhanced renal clearance of lithium during pregnancy. During pregnancy, lithium clearance has been estimated to be up to 50% higher than preconception, necessitating significant dose increases to maintain target plasma concentrations. As a result of increased clearance and larger V_d during pregnancy, lower steady-state plasma concentrations have been documented for lithium in the second and third trimesters. More frequent plasma concentration monitoring may be needed until individualized target doses are established. Of note, in the immediate postpartum period, renal clearance and V_d quickly return to baseline and therefore, to avoid toxicity, it is prudent to cut the lithium dose in half or hold the dose for 24 hours and retitrate lithium to pre-pregnancy dosing.[23]

INITIAL DOSE SELECTION

Given lithium's predictable pharmacokinetics, several authors have suggested various dosing methods to achieve the desired steady-state serum levels.[24,25] These methods include loading dose calculations of 30 mg/kg/day and nomograms developed from 12- or 24-hour lithium trough levels.[24-27] An extensive review of some 273 papers describing lithium prediction methods found limited reproducibility of methods and higher side effect burden of loading doses.[28] National guidelines recommend initiating lithium in low divided doses of 300 mg two to four times daily depending on weight (15 to 18.5 mg/kg/day) and titrating to desired plasma levels.[2,7,9,29]

Question #1   *J.L., a 37-year-old, 74-kg man, is being treated with lithium and quetiapine for acute mania. His current lithium carbonate dose is 300 mg given orally three times a day. His most recent serum creatinine is measured to be 0.95 mg/dL. Calculate the expected lithium plasma concentration once he has achieved steady state.*

The first step in calculating J.L.'s lithium concentration would be to estimate his renal function using Equation 12.1:

$$Cl_{Cr} \text{ for Males (mL/min)} = \frac{(140 - Age)(\text{Weight in kg})}{(72)(SCr_{ss})} \qquad \text{(Eq. 12.1)}$$

$$Cl_{Cr} \text{ for Males (mL/min)} = \frac{(140 - 37)(74)}{(72)(0.95)}$$

$$= 111 \text{ mL/min}$$

$$Cl_{Cr} (\text{L/hr}) = 111 \text{ mL/min} \left[\frac{60 \text{ min/hr}}{1,000 \text{ mL/L}} \right]$$

$$= 6.66 \text{ L/hr}$$

Next, the corresponding lithium clearance should be calculated using Equation 12.2 as follows:

$$\text{Lithium Clearance} = [0.25][\text{Creatinine Clearance}] \qquad \text{(Eq. 12.2)}$$

$$= [0.25][6.66 \text{ L/hr}]$$

$$= 1.67 \text{ L/hr}$$

J.L.'s total lithium dose of 900 mg corresponds to $\approx$24.4 mEq of lithium, based on the following calculation:

$$\begin{array}{c}\text{Lithium Dose} \\ \text{(mEq)}\end{array} = \left[\begin{array}{c}\text{Lithium Carbonate Dose} \\ \text{(mg)}\end{array} \right] \left[\frac{8.12 \text{ mEq}}{300 \text{ mg}} \right] \qquad \text{(Eq. 12.3)}$$

$$= [900 \text{ mg}] \left[\frac{8.12 \text{ mEq}}{300 \text{ mg}} \right]$$

$$= 24.36 \approx 24.4 \text{ mEq}$$

The average steady-state lithium concentration can then be calculated using Equation 12.4. Note that F is 1 and S is 1 because the salt factor for the dose of lithium carbonate has already been corrected or accounted for in Equation 12.3.

$$Css \text{ ave} = \frac{(S)(F)(\text{Dose}/\tau)}{Cl} \qquad \text{(Eq. 12.4)}$$

$$= \frac{(1)(1)(24.4 \text{ mEq}/24 \text{ hr})}{1.67 \text{ L/hr}}$$

$$= 0.61 \text{ mEq/L}$$

Question #2   *J.L.'s trough concentration on the morning of day 6 (after 5 full days of 900 mg/day) was 0.5 mEq/L. Calculate a new dosing regimen designed to achieve a trough concentration of 0.8 mEq/L.*

Equation 12.5 can be used to estimate J.L.'s lithium clearance.

$$Cl = \frac{(S)(F)(Dose/\tau)}{Css\ ave}$$

(Eq. 12.5)

$$= \frac{(1)(1)\left(24.4\ mEq/24\ hr\right)}{0.5\ L/hr}$$

$$= 2.03\ L/hr$$

J.L.'s specific lithium clearance then can be used with Equation 12.6 to calculate the daily maintenance dose (in mEq).

$$Maintenance\ Dose = \frac{(Cl)\left(Css\ ave\right)(\tau)}{(S)(F)}$$

(Eq. 12.6)

$$= \frac{\left(2.03\ L/hr\right)(0.8\ mEq/L)(24\ hr)}{(1)(1)}$$

$$= 38.98\ mEq$$

Equation 12.7 can then be used to convert the lithium dose expressed as mEq/24 hours to the equivalent dose expressed in milligrams of lithium carbonate.

$$\frac{Lithium\ Carbonate\ Dose}{(mg)} = \left[\frac{Lithium\ Dose}{(mEq)}\right]\left[\frac{300\ mg}{8.12\ mEq}\right]$$

(Eq. 12.7)

$$= [38.98\ mEq]\left[\frac{300\ mg}{8.12\ mEq}\right]$$

$$= 1440\ mg \quad or \quad \approx 1500\ mg$$

This daily dose of 1,500 mg of lithium carbonate may be scheduled as a total daily dose of five 300 mg lithium carbonate tablets or capsules: two 300 mg formulations in the morning and three 300 mg formulations in the evening. Despite the long half-life, lithium is usually initiated in multiple daily doses to reduce acute nausea, vomiting, and diarrhea. Once patients have achieved a desirable plasma concentration and their bipolar illness is considered to be stabilized, common practice is to consolidate the total daily dose into single, once-daily administration. This is done as an attempt to minimize polyuria and long-term structural damage to the kidney, as well as to improve adherence.[1]

A repeat lithium plasma concentration should be obtained once steady state is reached with this new dosing regimen. Because J.L. has good renal function and his apparent lithium clearance is close to the projected value, based on lithium's half-life of 24 hours or less, steady state will occur within 4 to 5 days.

An additional variable that should be considered is a possible alteration in lithium clearance during acute mania. Some authors have suggested up to a 50% increase in lithium clearance during acute manic episodes largely because of increased cardiac output and renal perfusion.[30] This variation in clearance can significantly impact patients who are stabilized during acute mania because lithium levels may increase once euthymia is achieved, which is often after hospital discharge. Therefore, it may be judicious to repeat lithium trough levels 2 to 4 weeks after stabilization of manic symptoms.

Question #3   *J.A., a 51-year-old woman, is receiving 300 mg of lithium carbonate twice daily. At 10:30 a.m., her blood was drawn, and the plasma lithium concentration was reported to be 2.4 mEq/L. List six common reasons why lithium levels may be elevated, and discuss how J.A. should be managed.*

Potential reasons for lithium elevation are as follows:

1. Plasma level obtained during distribution phase (i.e., not a true trough, or less than 8 to 12 hours from last dose)
2. Over compliance (e.g., administration of "prn" (as needed) doses or taking more than prescribed)
3. Drug interactions (e.g., diuretics, nonsteroidal anti-inflammatory drugs, angiotensin-converting enzyme inhibitors)
4. Renal compromise
5. Dehydration
6. Sodium depletion

The successful management of JA must first address an appropriate interpretation of her lithium level. The initial steps should be to confirm that the sample was drawn at the right time (i.e., 8 to 12 hours postdose) and to verify that steady-state has been achieved. The significant two-compartment modeling and the prolonged lithium α half-life of 6 hours dictate that lithium levels should be obtained at least 8, and ideally 12 hours, after the previous dose. If the level was drawn at an appropriate time, the next step would be to assess the patient's clinical presentation. Typically, patients with levels in excess of 2.0 mEq/L will present with significant signs and symptoms of lithium toxicity (e.g., diarrhea, coarse tremor, ataxia, etc.). If JA's presentation is not consistent with toxicity, it is likely that this elevated lithium concentration of 2.4 mEq/L was obtained during the α distribution phase. Plasma concentrations measured in this phase generally do not correlate with the efficacy or toxicity of lithium.

Question #4   *Immediately after the elevated lithium level is reported, J.A.'s psychiatrist examines her and finds that she is quite lethargic and confused, unable to recall when she last took her lithium. She complains of intermittent vomiting and diarrhea and has difficulty walking without assistance. A neurologic examination reveals coarse intentional hand tremors bilaterally and increased deep tendon reflexes. How should J.A. be managed at this time?*

Lithium intoxication is quite serious and is usually considered a medical emergency. If the lithium exposure is acute, whole bowel irrigation is the first step to remove unabsorbed lithium from the gastrointestinal tract, because lithium is not effectively adsorbed by charcoal.[31,32] Laboratory draws should be performed immediately, which should include renal and electrolyte panels, as well as lithium levels; additionally, an electrocardiogram should be obtained. During acute overdose, the lithium levels may be drawn during the distribution phase, and interpretation of these elevated levels is impossible. Initiating intravenous normal saline is also necessary to improve hydration and renal function, as well as restoring sodium balance, thereby accelerating lithium clearance.

Although hemodialysis (HD) was previously recommended empirically whenever plasma levels exceeded 2.0 or 2.5 mEq/L, the indication for starting HD is now controversial. Although HD increases lithium removal from the central compartment (lithium clearance values for HD are ~150 to 200 mL/min), it is debatable if this actually accelerates clinical recovery. Moreover, the initial HD session is usually more effective at removing lithium than subsequent HD session, most likely because of lithium's removal from the central compartment. However, lithium remains in the body, sequestered in other tissue. Thus, the decision to initiate an invasive procedure like HD in patients with elevated lithium levels should be based more on severity of patient presentation and less on plasma concentrations. In general, HD should be reserved for patients with significantly impaired renal function and lithium levels >4.0 mEq/L, or in the presence of a decreased level of consciousness, seizures, or life-threatening arrhythmias.[33] If the decision is made to initiate HD, it is vital to remember that lithium will undergo an additional distribution phase at the end of the procedure owing to the removal of lithium from the central compartment. Consequently, it is judicious to wait a minimum of 6 to 8 hours before rechecking post-HD plasma levels.

In the case of JA, her symptoms of lithium intoxication are moderate in severity, and HD would not be indicated.[33] Lithium should be discontinued, with a repeat level and renal panel obtained in the next few hours to ensure that the plasma concentration is not increasing further (owing to previously unabsorbed lithium remaining in her gastrointestinal tract). Plasma lithium levels should also be obtained 24 to 48 hours later to estimate the lithium half-life and clearance. In the interim, JA should be rehydrated either via intravenous normal saline or oral replacement, and the cause of her toxicity should be thoroughly investigated.

Question #5   *How would you estimate an appropriate dosing regimen for a patient who is obese?*

Given the overall prevalence of obesity, and that people suffering from bipolar illness are more likely to be obese than the general population,[34] it is common to encounter patients whose total body weight exceeds ideal body weight. Pharmacokinetic studies of lithium in obese patients suggest that their clearance correlates more closely with their actual body weight than ideal body weight.[35] This observation is not well explained; lithium clearance primarily depend on renal function, which is strongly correlated with ideal body weight. The volume of distribution for lithium among obese patients is only marginally increased, as expected, because lithium is an ion that does not concentrate in adipose tissue.[9] Consequently, actual body weight should be used to estimate clearance when selecting an obese patient's lithium dose.

Question #6   *Are there any alternative methods for determining lithium concentrations?*

Lithium's primary therapeutic actions are generally believed to be in the central nervous system; however, plasma levels are more convenient to obtain and, therefore, are routinely used to monitor efficacy and toxicity. Various alternatives to plasma levels have been investigated. Several studies have evaluated the correlation between efficacy and the erythrocyte lithium concentrations, as well as the erythrocyte–plasma lithium concentration ratio; these results remain inconclusive. Saliva lithium concentrations have been evaluated for clinical monitoring as an alternative to blood samples; however, the saliva to plasma ratio has significantly more interpatient variability, limiting the clinical utility of this method.[26,36] Future monitoring of lithium's therapeutic efficacy may be evaluated through brain imaging techniques. Early research has found a strong correlation of clinical improvement with brain concentrations (quantified using magnetic resonance spectroscopy of lithium isotopes).[37] The clinical application and cost-effectiveness of this approach has yet to be fully evaluated.

REFERENCES

1. Curran G, Ravindran A. Lithium for bipolar disorder: a review of the recent literature. *Expert Rev Neurother.* 2014;14(9):1079–1098.
2. Hirschfeld RM, Bowden CL, Gitlin MJ, et al. Treatment of patients with bipolar disorder. *APA Practice Guideline 2002* (2010).
3. Lithium. In: Natural Medicines [database on the Internet]. Somerville, MA: Therapeutic Research Center; 2016 [cited 22 June 2016]. https://naturalmedicines.therapeuticresearch.com. Subscription required to view.
4. Severus WE, Kleindienst N, Seemuller F, et al. What is the optimal serum lithium level in the long-term treatment of bipolar disorder—a review? *Bipolar Disord.* 2008;10:231–237.
5. Gelenberg AJ, Carroll JA, Baudhuin MG, et al. The meaning of serum lithium levels in maintenance therapy of mood disorders: a review of the literature. *J Clin Psychiatry.* 1989;50:17–22.
6. van Melick EJ, Souverein PC, den Breeijen JH, et al. Age as a determinant of instability of serum lithium concentrations. *Ther Drug Monit.* 2013;35(5):643–648.
7. Yatham LN, Kennedy SH, Parikh SV, et al. Canadian Network for Mood and Anxiety Treatments (CANMAT) and International Society for Bipolar Disorders (ISBD) collaborative update of CANMAT guidelines for the treatment of patients with bipolar disorder: update 2013. *Bipolar disord.* 2013;15(1):1–44.
8. Malhi GS, Tanious M, Gershon S. The *lithiumeter*: a measured approach. *Bipolar Disord.* 2011;13:219–226.

9. Amdisen A. Serum level monitoring and clinical pharmacokinetics of lithium. *Clin Pharmacokinet.* 1977;2(2):73–92.

10. Finley PR, Warner MD, Peabody CA. Clinical relevance of drug interactions with lithium. *Clin Pharmacokinet.* 1995;29(3):172–191.

11. Thornhill DP. Serum levels and pharmacokinetics of ordinary and sustained-release lithium carbonate in manic patients during chronic dosage. *Int J of Clin Pharmacol Ther Toxicol.* 1986;24(5):257–261.

12. Yukawa E, Nomiyama N, Higuchi S, et al. Lithium population pharmacokinetics from routine clinical data: role of patient characteristics for estimating dosing regimens. *Ther Drug Monit.* 1993;15:75–82.

13. Jermain DM, Crimson ML. Population pharmacokinetics of lithium. *Clin Pharm.*1991;10(5):376–381.

14. Dewinter S, Meersseman W, Verelst S, et al. Drug-related admissions due to interaction with an old drug, lithium. *Acta Clin Belg.* 2013;68(5):356–358.

15. Reimann IW, Diener UD, Frolich JC. Indomethacin but not aspirin increases plasma lithium ion levels. *Arch Gen Psychiatry.* 1983;40(3):283–286.

16. Terhaag B, Scherber A, Schaps P, et al. The distribution of lithium into cerebrospinal fluid, brain tissue and bile in man. *Int J Clin Pharmacol Biopharm.* 1978;16(7):333–335.

17. Goodnick PJ, Fieve RR, Meltzer HL, et al. Lithium elimination half-life and duration of therapy. *Clin Pharmacol Ther.* 1981;29(1):47–50.

18. Findling RL, Robb A, McNamara NK, et al. Lithium in the acute treatment of bipolar I disorder: a double-blind, placebo-controlled study. *Pediatrics.* 2015;136(5):885–894.

19. McClellan J, Kowatch R, Findling R. Practice parameter for the assessment and treatment of children and adolescents with bipolar disorder. *J Am Acad Child Adolesc Psychiatry.* 2007;46(1):107–125.

20. Findling RL, Landersdorfer CB, Kafantaris V, et al. First-dose pharmacokinetics of lithium carbonate in children and adolescents. *J Clin Psychopharmacol.* 2010;30(4):404–410.

21. Sajatovic M, Strejilevich SA, Gildengers AG, et al. A report on older-age bipolar disorder from the International Society for Bipolar Disorders Task Force. *Bipolar Disord.* 2015;17(7):689–704.

22. Hardy BG, Shulman KI, Mackenzie SE, et al. Pharmacokinetics of lithium in the elderly. *J Clin Psychopharmacol.* 1987;7(3):153–158.

23. Deligiannidis KM. Pharmacotherapy for mood disorders in pregnancy: a review of pharmacokinetic changes and clinical recommendations for therapeutic drug monitoring. *J Clin Psychopharmacol.* 2014;34(2):244–255.

24. Cooper TB, Bergner PE, Simpson GM. The 24-hour serum lithium level as a prognosticator of dosage requirements. *Am J Psychiatry.* 1973;130(5):601–603.

25. Perry PJ, Alexander B, Dunner FJ, et al. Pharmacokinetic protocol for predicting serum lithium levels. *J Clin Psychopharmacol.* 1982;2(2):114–117.

26. Neu C, Dimascio A, Williams D. Saliva lithium levels: clinical applications. *Am J Psychiatry.* 1975;132(1):66–68.

27. Kook KA, Stimmel GL, Wilkins JN, et al. Accuracy and safety of a priori lithium loading. *J Clin Psychiatry.* 1985;46(2):49–51.

28. Sienaert P, Geeraerts I, Wyckaert S. How to initiate lithium therapy: a systematic review of dose estimation and level prediction methods. *J Affect disord.* 2013;146(1):15–33.

29. Groves GE, Clothier JL, Hollister LE. Predicting lithium dose by the body-weight method. *Int Clinc Psychopharmacol.* 1991;6(1):19–23.

30. Kukopulos A, Minnai G, Muller-Oerlinghausen B. The influence of mania and depression on the pharmacokinetics of lithium: a longitudinal single-case study. *J Affect disord.* 1985;8(2):159–166.

31. Favin FD, Klein-Schwartz W, Oderda GM, et al. In vitro study of lithium carbonate adsorption by activated charcoal. *J Toxicol: Clin Toxicol.* 1988;26(7):443–450.

32. Smith SW, Ling LJ, Halstenson CE. Whole-bowel irrigation as a treatment for acute lithium overdose. *Ann Emerg Med.* 1991;20(5):536–539.

33. Decker BS, Goldfarb DS, Dargan PI, et al. Extracorpeal treatment for lithium poisoning: systematic review and recommendations from the EXTRIP Workgroup. *Clin J Am Soc Nephrol.* 2015;10(5): 875–887.

34. Vancampfort D, Vansteelandt K, Correll CU, et al. Metabolic syndrome and metabolic abnormalities in bipolar disorder: a meta-analysis of prevalence rates and moderators. *Am J Psychiatry*. 2013;170(3):265–274.

35. Reiss RA, Haas CE, Karki SD, et al. Lithium pharmacokinetics in the obese. *Clin Pharmacol Ther*. 1994;55:392–398.

36. Obach R, Borja J, Prunonosa J, et al. Lack of correlation between lithium pharmacokinetic parameters obtained from plasma and saliva. *Ther Drug Monit*. 1988;10:265–268.

37. Kato T, Inubushi T, Takahashi S. Relationship of lithium concentrations in the brain measured by lithium-7 magnetic resonance spectroscopy to treatment response in mania. *J Clin Psychopharmacol*. 1994;14:330–335.

38. Bisogni V, Rossitto G, Reghin F, et al. Antihypertensive therapy in patients on chronic lithium treatment for bipolar disorders. *J Hypertens*. 2016;34(1):20–28.

39. Nagamine T. Lithium intoxication associated with angiotensin II type 1 receptor blockers in women. *Clin Neuropsychopharmacol Ther*. 2013;4:23–25.

40. Ragheb M, Powell A. Lithium interaction with sulindac and naproxen. *J Clin Psychopharmacol*. 1986:6(3):150–154.

41. Phelan KM, Mosholder AD, Lu S. Lithium interaction with cyclooxygenase 2 inhibitors rofecoxib and celecoxib and other nonsteroidal anti-inflammatory drugs. *J Clin Psychiatry*. 2003;64(11):1328–1334.

42. Perry PJ, Calloway RA, Cook BL, et al. Theophylline precipitated alterations of lithium clearance. *Acta Psychiatr Scand*. 1984;69(6):528–537.

13

PHENOBARBITAL

John E. Murphy

Learning Objectives

By the end of the phenobarbital chapter, the learner shall be able to:

1. Describe the concentration–effect relationship for phenobarbital in the treatment of seizures.
2. Describe the impact of the long half-life of phenobarbital on the time to steady state.
3. Determine the impact of the following on average population values for phenobarbital and use the alterations to predict doses and intervals to produce desired concentrations or to predict concentrations from dosing already being used for a patient.
   a. Drug interactions (those discussed in the chapter)
   b. Patient age
4. Adjust the dose of phenobarbital after a measured steady-state phenobarbital concentration by (a) calculating the patient's actual clearance and then determining the new dose and (b) by simple ratio.
5. Estimate a patient's half-life from a measured phenobarbital concentration or estimated clearance. Use the estimated half-life to determine time to steady state.
6. Estimate a patient's clearance and eventual steady-state concentration from a phenobarbital concentration measured prior to steady state after the patient has received a loading dose followed by maintenance doses or just maintenance doses.

7. Determine whether a patient who develops hypoalbuminemia will require a dosage adjustment until the condition is corrected.
8. Determine the impact of hemodialysis and peritoneal dialysis on the need for additional doses of phenobarbital postdialysis.
9. Estimate a patient's steady-state phenobarbital concentration (Css ave) using two concentrations measured prior to steady state on a consistent dosing regimen using the mass balance technique.

Phenobarbital is a long-acting barbiturate used in the treatment of seizure disorders, insomnia, and anxiety. It is most commonly administered orally but may also be administered intramuscularly and intravenously (IV).

The usual adult maintenance dose of 2 mg/kg/day produces a steady-state concentration of approximately 20 mg/L. Limited evidence suggests that dosing should be based on total body weight.[1] Phenobarbital has a half-life of approximately 5 days; therefore, therapeutic concentrations are not achieved for 2 to 3 weeks following the initiation of an appropriate maintenance regimen. When therapeutic concentrations of 20 mg/L are required immediately for children and adults, a loading dose of 15 to

---

KEY PARAMETERS: Phenobarbital

Therapeutic concentrations	15–40 mg/L
Bioavailability (F)	1.0 (>0.9)
S (for Na salt)	0.9
V	
Neonates	0.9 L/kg (0.7–1.0)
Children and adults	0.7 L/kg (0.6–0.7)
Cl	
Children	0.008 L/kg/hr (0.2 L/kg/day)
Adults and neonates	0.004 L/kg/hr (0.1 L/kg/day)
Elderly (>65 yr)	0.003 L/kg/hr (0.07 L/kg/day)
$t\frac{1}{2}$	
Children	2.5 days
Adults	5 days
fu (fraction unbound in plasma)	0.5

20 mg/kg can be administered, usually in three divided doses of 5 mg/kg given every 2 to 3 hours, although the entire loading dose may be given at once.[2]

THERAPEUTIC AND TOXIC CONCENTRATIONS

In adults, phenobarbital concentrations of 10 to 30 mg/L are generally required for seizure control.[3] The overall therapeutic range is now considered to be 15 to 40 mg/L.[4] The upper end of the therapeutic range is limited by the appearance of side effects such as central nervous system depression and ataxia,[5] although some patients may exhibit no symptoms of chronic toxicity even when phenobarbital concentrations exceed 40 mg/L.[6] Phenobarbital concentrations in excess of 100 mg/L are considered potentially lethal, although patients with higher concentrations have survived.[6-8] Many patients develop excessive sedation when phenobarbital concentrations are rapidly pushed into the therapeutic range. For this reason, when it is clinically feasible, prescribers may prefer to start patients on about 25% of the target maintenance dose for the first week of therapy and then increase the maintenance dose by another 25% for each of the subsequent 3 weeks, finally achieving the full maintenance dose regimen on the fourth week of therapy. The technique of slowly increasing the maintenance dose allows many patients to adjust to their phenobarbital concentrations; however, it does prolong the time required to achieve concentrations in the usually accepted therapeutic range.[9] With adequate monitoring and concern for the sedative effects of phenobarbital, full loading doses have been used to quickly bring a patient to the therapeutic range.[2]

BIOAVAILABILITY (F)

Although it has not been well studied, available data indicate that at least 80% and probably greater than 90% of phenobarbital administered orally is absorbed. Complete bioavailability (F = 1.0) is supported by the observation that similar concentrations are observed when the same dose of phenobarbital is given orally and parenterally. Intramuscular dosing has been shown to be 100% bioavailable,[10] and administration of the injectable product as a rectal solution results in 90% bioavailability.[11] A solution and suspension have been shown to be equivalent to tablet dosage forms.[12]

Phenobarbital is frequently administered as the sodium salt (injection), which is approximately 91% phenobarbital acid (S ≅ 0.91); however, a correction for the salt form is seldom made because the degree of error is small and the therapeutic range is relatively broad. When phenobarbital sodium is administered parenterally, it is usually administered at a rate of no more than 50 mg/min to avoid toxicities associated with the propylene glycol diluent.[13] Proportionally slower infusion rates based on the size of the patient should be used in children.

VOLUME OF DISTRIBUTION (V)

The volume of distribution for phenobarbital in children and adults is approximately 0.7 L/kg.[14,15] In newborns, it is slightly higher at approximately 0.9 L/kg (0.7 to 1 L/kg).[16,17]

CLEARANCE (Cl)

Phenobarbital is primarily metabolized by the liver; less than 20% is eliminated by the renal route.[18] N-glucoside and cytochrome P450 2C9 and 2C19 oxidation make up the bulk of metabolism, and genetic polymorphisms may alter clearance.[19] However, polymorphisms of CYP2C19 did not affect clearance in one study of neonates and infants.[20] The average total clearance for phenobarbital in adults and newborns is ≈ 4 mL/kg/hr (0.004 L/kg/hr) or 0.1 L/kg/day. The clearance value of approximately 0.1 L/kg/day in adults and neonates results in the following clinical observation: for every 1 mg/kg/day of administered, a steady-state phenobarbital concentration of about 10 mg/L is achieved.

$$Css\ ave = \frac{(S)(F)(Dose/\tau)}{Cl}$$

(Eq. 13.1)

$$= \frac{(1)(1)(1\,mg/kg/day)}{0.1\,L/kg/day}$$

$$= 10\,mg/L$$

This clinical guideline suggests that in adult and newborn patients, maintenance doses of 2 mg/kg/day should result in steady-state concentrations of ≈ 20 mg/L. The clearance in children aged 1 to 18 years is approximately twice the average adult clearance.[21–23] Therefore, these patients generally require maintenance doses of phenobarbital that are about twice those of the average adult relative to body weight, or a maintenance dose of 4 to 5 mg/kg/day will be needed to achieve steady-state concentrations of 20 mg/L. The elderly exhibit diminished clearance of ≈ 3 mL/kg/hr (0.003 L/kg/hr) or 0.07 L/kg/day.[24] A maintenance dose of approximately 1.5 mg/kg/day would be needed in the elderly for steady-state concentrations of ≈ 20 mg/L.

HALF-LIFE (t½)

The half-life of phenobarbital is ≈ 5 days in most adult patients, but may be as short as 2 to 3 days in some individuals, especially children, or in patients exposed to drug interactions with agents that induce the metabolism of phenobarbital.

TIME TO SAMPLE

With a half-life of approximately 5 days, samples obtained within the first 1 to 2 weeks of therapy yield limited information about the eventual steady-state concentrations. For this reason, routine phenobarbital concentrations should be monitored 2 to 3 weeks after the initiation or a change in the phenobarbital regimen. Samples obtained before this time should be used either to determine whether an additional loading dose is needed (e.g., when concentrations are much lower than desired) or whether the maintenance dose should be withheld or reduced (e.g., phenobarbital concentrations are greater than desired or the steady-state concentration estimated from the measured concentration is higher than desired).

Once steady state has been achieved, the time of sampling within a dosing interval of phenobarbital is not critical; concentrations can be obtained at almost any time relative to the phenobarbital dose. As a matter of consistency, however, trough concentrations are generally recommended. If phenobarbital is being administered by the IV route, care should be taken to sample at least 1 hour after the end of the infusion to avoid the distribution phase.

Question #1   *P.M., a 2-week-old, 3.2-kg male neonate, has developed idiopathic tonic–clonic seizure activity. An IV loading dose of phenobarbital sodium of 20 mg/kg was given followed by maintenance doses of 1.5 mg/kg every 12 hours. Estimate the postload phenobarbital concentration and the average steady-state concentration from the maintenance dose.*

Because this is a loading dose problem, and there is no existing initial drug concentration, Equation 13.2 should be used to estimate C_0:

$$C_0 = \frac{(S)(F)(\text{Loading Dose})}{V} \qquad \textbf{(Eq. 13.2)}$$

F can be assumed to be 1 because this is an IV dose and $S = 0.9$ for phenobarbital sodium. V is estimated to be 0.9 L/kg (see Key Parameters, this chapter) or 2.9 L. After the loading dose of 64 mg (20 mg/kg $\times$ 3.2 kg), the predicted postload concentration (ideally taken about 1 hour after the loading dose to avoid any distribution phase) is as follows:

$$C_0 = \frac{(0.9)(1)(64 \text{ mg})}{2.88 \text{ L}}$$
$$C_0 = 20 \text{ mg/L}$$

The loading dose and volume of distribution could each be used without multiplying by the patient's weight to get the dose in milligram (64 mg) and the volume in liter (2.9 L), because weight will cancel out of the numerator and denominator.

$$C_0 = \frac{(0.9)(1)(20 \text{ mg/kg})}{0.9 \text{ L/kg}}$$
$$C_0 = 20 \text{ mg/L}$$

Although Equation 13.3 is representative of the actual dosing and monitoring situation, it is not necessary to use it to account for the difference between the concentration drawn at 1 hour and that assumed to have occurred at C_0, because very little elimination will occur in such a short time when the drug has a very long half-life.

$$C_1 = \frac{(S)(F)(\text{Loading Dose})}{V}\left(e^{-Kt_1}\right) \qquad \textbf{(Eq. 13.3)}$$

To illustrate this, the half-life can be estimated using Equation 13.4:

$$t\frac{1}{2} = \frac{(0.693)(V)}{Cl} \qquad \textbf{(Eq. 13.4)}$$

$$t\frac{1}{2} = \frac{(0.693)(0.9\,L/kg)}{0.004\,L/kg/hr} = 156\,\text{hours}\ \ \text{or}\ \ 6.5\,\text{days}$$

The fraction of drug or concentration remaining (e^{-Kt}) after t time (in this case, 1 hour) would be 0.996, indicating negligible elimination. The difference in prediction would be 20 mg/L versus 20 mg/L $\times$ 0.996 = 19.92 mg/L. As with many aspects of equation use in pharmacokinetics, when one event occurs quickly relative to another, the equations may be simplified with little error.[25]

Because clearance is the major determinant of the eventual steady-state concentrations achieved by the maintenance dose, this parameter must be estimated for P.M. There is, of course, intersubject variability in all pharmacokinetic parameters. However, the average clearance of phenobarbital should be used until concentrations are measured. In newborns, the population clearance is 0.004 L/kg/hr. Thus, the expected clearance for P.M., who weighs 3.2 kg, is 0.013 L/hr:

$$\text{Clearance Newborn Phenobarbital} = \left(0.004\,L/kg/hr\right)(\text{Weight in kg}) \qquad \textbf{(Eq. 13.5)}$$

$$= (0.004\,L/kg/hr)(3.2\,kg)$$
$$= 0.013\,L/hr$$

The predicted average steady-state concentration of the maintenance dose of 1.5 mg/kg (4.8 mg) every 12 hours is determined from Equation 13.1:

$$Css\ ave = \frac{(S)(F)(Dose/\tau)}{Cl}$$
$$= \frac{(0.9)(1)(4.8\,mg/12\,hr)}{\left(0.013\,L/hr\right)}$$
$$= 28\,mg/L$$

As before, the maintenance dose and clearance could be left as mg/kg and L/kg/hr because weight would cancel out in the numerator and denominator.

With the long half-life estimated in this patient, the dose could easily be given once daily. However, once switched to oral dosing, the elixir is not readily taken by infants because of the taste and volume (5 mL delivers either 15 or 20 mg depending on the manufacturer). Mixing the smaller volume that can be used with twice daily dosing in formula or breast milk seems to increase palatability and increase the potential to deliver a complete dose.

Question #2 *P.M. has a postload concentration of 22 mg/L, 1 hour after the dose. Because the baby is still having seizures, the team monitoring P.M.'s progress decides to increase his concentration to 30 mg/L. Calculate an additional loading dose to take his concentration to 30 mg/L (assume that little elimination has occurred in the time from sample collection to the decision to increase P.M.'s phenobarbital concentration) and adjust his maintenance dose to provide a predicted Css ave of 30 mg/L.*

It is important to remember that the patient's volume of distribution can now be determined, and this should be used rather than the population average volume to determine the new dose. A second critical point to remember is that the baby should not be given a dose to take him from 0 to 30 mg/L, but rather from the concentration of 22 to 30 mg/L, or an incremental change in concentration of 8 mg/L.

Calculating the baby's volume of distribution using Equation 13.6 gives:

$$V = \frac{(S)(F)(\text{Loading Dose})}{C_0} \qquad \textbf{(Eq. 13.6)}$$

$$= \frac{(0.9)(1)(64\text{ mg})}{22\text{ mg/L}}$$

$$= 2.62\text{ L}$$

$$= 2.62\text{ L} \div 3.2\text{ kg} = 0.8\text{ L/kg}$$

The additional incremental loading dose is then determined using Equation 13.7 as:

$$\text{Incremental Loading Dose} = \frac{(V)(C_{\text{desired}} - C_{\text{initial}})}{(S)(F)} \qquad \textbf{(Eq. 13.7)}$$

$$= \frac{(2.62\text{ L})(30\text{ mg/L} - 22\text{ mg/L})}{(0.9)(1)}$$

$$= 23\text{ mg}$$

Because doses and concentrations are proportional for first-order drugs like phenobarbital, the incremental dose could simply have been solved by ratio. The loading dose of 64 mg produced a postload concentration of 22 mg/L. To increase the concentration by 8 mg/L, the ratio is:

$$(64\text{ mg})\left(\frac{8\text{ mg/L}}{22\text{ mg/L}}\right) = 23\text{ mg}$$

The new maintenance dose can also be solved this way because the dose of 4.8 mg every 12 hours was estimated to produce a Css ave of 28 mg/L.

$$(4.8\,\text{mg})\left(\frac{30\,\text{mg/L}}{28\,\text{mg/L}}\right) = 5.1\,\text{mg every 12h}$$

Or, the revised desired Css ave of 30 mg/L can be put into Equation 13.8 to solve for the new maintenance dose.

$$\text{Maintenance Dose} = \frac{(\text{Cl})(\text{Css ave})(\tau)}{(\text{S})(\text{F})} \qquad \textbf{(Eq. 13.8)}$$

$$= \frac{(0.0134/\text{h})(3.2\,\text{kg})(30\,\text{mg/L})(12\,\text{hr})}{(0.9)(1)}$$

$$= 5.1\,\text{every 12h}$$

Question #3   *P.M. has his concentration measured halfway through the dosage interval (Css ave) after 6 weeks of dosing at 5.1 mg of phenobarbital elixir every 12 hours; it is reported as 23 mg/L. The baby now weighs 4 kg. Determine the baby's phenobarbital clearance assuming that the concentration is at steady state. S = 1, assume F = 1.*

By rearranging Equations 13.1, we can solve for clearance:

$$\text{Cl} = \frac{(\text{S})(\text{F})(\text{Dose}/\tau)}{(\text{Css ave})} \qquad \textbf{(Eq. 13.9)}$$

$$= \frac{(1)(1)(5.1\,\text{mg/12 hr})}{(23\,\text{mg/L})}$$

$$= 0.0185\,\text{L/hr} \div 4\,\text{kg}$$

$$= 0.0046\,\text{L/kg/hr}$$

Owing primarily to the baby's weight gain and continuation of the 5.1 mg dose, the concentration dropped despite limited difference in clearance per body weight from predicted. If necessary, because of continuing seizure activity, a small loading dose could be given followed by an increase in maintenance dose to bring the concentration back to near 30 mg/L (or to any other desired concentration). If the baby remains seizure free, the current dose may be continued with the understanding that the Css ave will likely continue to decrease with increasing weight and/or increasing clearance.

Question #4 *W.R., a 39-year-old, 70-kg man, developed generalized seizures several months after an automobile accident in which he sustained head injuries. Phenobarbital is to be initiated. Calculate an oral loading dose of phenobarbital to produce a concentration of 20 mg/L.*

Because this is a loading dose problem, and there is no existing initial drug concentration, Equation 13.10 may be used.

$$\text{Loading Dose} = \frac{(V)(C_0)}{(S)(F)} \qquad \textbf{(Eq. 13.10)}$$

If S = 1, F is assumed to be 1, and the volume of distribution is assumed to be 0.7 L/kg (see Key Parameters, this chapter) or 49 L (0.7 L/kg × 70 kg = 49 L), then the calculated loading dose will be 980 mg or approximately 1 g as given in the following equation.

$$\text{Loading Dose} = \frac{(49\,\text{L})(20\,\text{mg/L})}{(1)(1)}$$
$$= 980\,\text{mg or} \approx 1\,\text{g}$$

This 1-g dose is very close to the usual loading dose of 15 mg/kg. It may be administered orally, intramuscularly, or IV.

Generally, the loading dose is divided into three or more portions and administered over several hours. The necessity for dividing the loading dose when administered orally or intramuscularly is not clear. It is probably done to act as a precaution against toxicity should a two-compartmental distribution exist or to avoid cardiovascular toxicity from the propylene glycol diluent in the injectable dosage form. Patients receiving loading doses will generally be sedated at first. Caution should be exercised in patients with respiratory depression.

Question #5 *Estimate an oral maintenance dose for W.R. to maintain a phenobarbital concentration of 20 mg/L. How should the dose be administered?*

Because clearance is the major determinant of the maintenance dose, this parameter must be estimated for W.R. Although there is some intersubject variability, the average clearance of phenobarbital in adults is 0.004 L/kg/hr or 0.1 L/kg/day. Thus, the expected clearance for W.R., who weighs 70 kg, is 7 L/day.

If S = 1 and F is assumed to be 1, the daily maintenance dose of phenobarbital can be calculated using Equation 13.8 as:

$$\text{Maintenance Dose} = \frac{(Cl)(Css\,ave)(\tau)}{(S)(F)}$$
$$= \frac{(7\,\text{L/day})(20\,\text{mg/L})(1\,\text{day})}{(1)(1)}$$
$$= 140\,\text{mg}$$

In practice, the daily dose is often divided into two or more portions; however, with a half-life of 5 days (Equation 13.4), once daily dosing should suffice.[14] If the entire dose is given at bedtime, some of the side effects associated with sedation may be reduced.

$$t\tfrac{1}{2} = \frac{(0.693)(V)}{Cl}$$

$$= \frac{(0.693)(49\ L)}{7\ L/day}$$

$$= 4.85\ days\ or\ \approx 5\ days$$

Interestingly, the calculated dose corresponds to the empiric clinical guideline described earlier that has been used for many years: the phenobarbital steady-state concentration produced by a maintenance dose in adults and neonates will be approximately equal to 10 times the daily dose in mg/kg:

$$W.R.'s\ Maintenance\ Dose\ (mg/kg) = \frac{140\ mg}{70\ kg}$$

$$= 2\ mg/kg$$

According to the clinical guideline, the concentration in mg/L produced by this dose will be 20 mg/L (2 × 10).

Question #6   *If W.R. does not receive a loading dose, how long will it take to achieve a minimum therapeutic concentration of 15 mg/L following the initiation of the maintenance dose? How long will it take to achieve a steady-state concentration of 20 mg/L?*

To answer a question involving time, knowledge of the half-life is required. The half-life for phenobarbital in W.R. is approximately 5 days, as calculated in Question 5. If it is assumed that three to five half-lives are a sufficient approximation of steady state (87.5% to 96.9% of steady-state), approximately 15 to 25 days will be required to approach the final plateau concentration of 20 mg/L. Because the minimum therapeutic concentration of 15 mg/L is three-quarters (75%) of the predicted steady-state concentration of 20 mg/L, two half-lives or 10 days will be required for the phenobarbital concentration to accumulate to 15 mg/L. This can be illustrated using the following equations:

$$K = \frac{0.693}{t\tfrac{1}{2}}$$

(Eq. 13.11)

$$= \frac{0.693}{5\ days}$$

$$= 0.139\ days^{-1}$$

$$C_1 = \frac{(S)(F)(Dose/\tau)}{Cl}(1 - e^{-Kt_1})$$

(Eq. 13.12)

where Css ave is the average steady-state concentration (in this case, 20 mg/L), and t_1 is the duration of the maintenance dose therapy (in this case, 10 days).

$$= (20 \text{ mg/L})(1 - e^{-(0.139d^{-1})(10 \text{ days})})$$
$$= (20 \text{ mg/L})(0.75)$$
$$= 15 \text{ mg/L}$$

The time can also be calculated by manipulating Equation 13.12.

After the passage of sufficient time to reach steady state (i.e., 3 to 5 $t\frac{1}{2}$s, where e^{-Kt} approaches 0, leaving $1 - e^{-Kt}$ to ~ $1 - 0$ or 1), Equation 13.12:

$$C_1 = \frac{(S)(F)(Dose/\tau)}{Cl}(1 - e^{-Kt_1})$$

becomes Equation 13.1:

$$Css \text{ ave} = \frac{(S)(F)(Dose/\tau)}{Cl}$$

Therefore, Equation 13.12 can be rewritten as follows:

$$C_1 = Css \text{ ave} (1 - e^{-Kt_1}) \qquad \text{(Eq. 13.13)}$$

And then, it follows that

$$\frac{C_1}{Css \text{ ave}} = 1 - e^{-Kt_1} \qquad \text{(Eq. 13.14)}$$

By taking the natural log (ln) of both sides of Equation 13.14 and rearranging the terms, the time to achieve a certain C_1 can be estimated:

$$t = \frac{-\ln\left(1 - \dfrac{C_1}{Css \text{ ave}}\right)}{K} \qquad \text{(Eq. 13.15)}$$

$$= \frac{-\ln\left(1 - \dfrac{15}{20}\right)}{0.139 \text{ days}^{-1}}$$
$$= 10 \text{ days}$$

Question #7   *If W.R. had valproic acid (VPA) 1,000 mg/day added to his overall therapy, how would this affect the original maintenance dose prediction?*

The addition of VPA to phenobarbital therapy has been noted to lead to increased phenobarbital concentrations. VPA was reported to decrease phenobarbital clearance by 25% on average at VPA doses of 1,000 mg/day and by 50% at VPA doses of 2,000 mg/day.[26] This would indicate the potential to increase phenobarbital concentrations by 33% to 100% (1.33 to 2-fold). Because W.R. is receiving VPA doses of 1,000 mg/day, the dose suggested could be empirically decreased by 25% to account for the interaction. The patient could be told that if VPA is discontinued, a phenobarbital dose increase might be necessary and that an increase in the VPA dose may require further reduction in the phenobarbital dose. Because the interaction is of moderate impact at present and the predicted concentration at the lower end of the therapeutic range, it would also be reasonable to simply monitor the steady-state concentrations and patient side effects and make dosing adjustments if necessary.

Question #8   *K.P., a 62-year-old, 57-kg woman, was admitted for poor seizure control. Before admission, she had been receiving an unknown dose of phenobarbital. On admission, the phenobarbital concentration was 5 mg/L. She was subsequently started on 60 mg of phenobarbital every 8 hours (180 mg/day). Five days later, the phenobarbital trough concentration was 17 mg/L. Estimate her final steady-state concentration on the present regimen.*

There are several ways to approach this problem. Because Css ave is defined by clearance, one could use the average clearance for phenobarbital (0.1 L/kg/day × 57 kg = 5.7 L/day) and insert this value into Equation 13.1:

$$\text{Css ave} = \frac{(S)(F)(\text{Dose}/\tau)}{\text{Cl}}$$
$$= \frac{(1)(1)\,(180\ \text{mg/day})}{5.7\ \text{L/day}}$$
$$= 31.6\ \text{mg/L}$$

Another method could be used to estimate the steady-state value. The concentration of 17 mg/L reported on the fifth day is assumed to represent the sum of the fraction of the initial concentration (5 mg/L) remaining at this time plus the accumulated concentration resulting from five daily doses of 180 mg. If K.P.'s half-life for phenobarbital is 5 days, the fraction of the initial concentration remaining after one half-life will be 0.5 and contribution to the reported concentration at 5 days will be 2.5 mg/L (5 mg/L × 0.5). The remaining portion of the reported concentration (14.5 mg/L) represents 50% of the steady-state concentration that will be produced by the 180 mg/day dose (after one half-life, 50% of steady-state has been achieved). Therefore, the predicted Css ave would be 29 mg/L (2 × 14.5 mg/L). The following calculations illustrate how this can be determined by equations when the measured concentration does not conveniently fall exactly on a multiple of the half-life.

Equation 13.16 is used to calculate the concentration (C_1) remaining from the initial 5 mg/L:

$$C_1 = C_0(e^{-Kt_1})$$ **(Eq. 13.16)**

$$C_{1 \text{ at 5 days}} = 5 \text{ mg/L}(e^{-(K)(5 \text{ days})})$$

$$= 5 \text{ mg/L}\left(e^{-\left(\frac{0.693}{5 \text{ days}}\right)(5 \text{ days})} \right)$$

$$= 2.5 \text{ mg/L}$$

Although there are a number of models, Equation 13.17, which describes the concentration C_2 following the Nth dose, can be used to determine the contribution of the five doses of 180 mg given each day (see Chapter 1).

$$C_2 = \left[\frac{\dfrac{(S)(F)(\text{Dose})}{V}}{(1-e^{-K\tau})} \right](1-e^{-K(N)\tau})(e^{-Kt_2})$$ **(Eq. 13.17)**

$$C_2 = \left[\frac{\dfrac{(1)(1)(180 \text{ mg})}{(0.7 \text{ L/kg})(57 \text{ kg})}}{(1-e^{-(0.139 \text{ days}^{-1})(1 \text{ day})})} \right]\left(1-e^{-(0.139 \text{ days}^{-1})(5)(1 \text{ day})}\right)\left(e^{-(0.139 \text{ days}^{-1})(1 \text{ day})}\right)$$

$$C_2 = 15.2 \text{ mg/L}$$
$$C_1 + C_2 = 2.5 \text{ mg/L} + 15.2 \text{ mg/L}$$
$$= 17.7 \text{ mg/L (vs. measured concentration of 17 mg/L)}$$

One could also use the empiric clinical guideline discussed in Question 5 regarding the prediction of Css ave from the mg/kg dose of phenobarbital. In this case, the mg/kg dose would be 180 mg/57 kg or 3.16 mg/kg. The predicted Css ave would be 31.6 mg/L (3.16×10).

All these estimates are based on the assumption that K.P.'s pharmacokinetic parameters for phenobarbital are similar to those reported in the literature. Because the estimates for Css ave are at the upper end of the therapeutic range, it would be reasonable to obtain another concentration 15 to 20 days after the initiation of the maintenance dose. In addition, because the repeat concentration will be obtained after more than three to four half-lives have passed, K.P.'s clearance for phenobarbital can be estimated more reliably (see Interpretation of Plasma Drug Concentrations in Chapter 2).

When the concentration on the fifth day was predicted from the average pharma-cokinetic parameters, the value was quite close to what was measured. Thus, her actual parameters appear to be similar to the averages.

Question #9   *N.P., a 35-year-old, 80-kg man, is being treated for a seizure dis-order secondary to a motor vehicle accident. He has been receiving 200 mg/day of phenobarbital (100 mg twice daily) for the past 15 days. The phenobarbital serum concentration just before the morning dose on day 16 (i.e., at the trough of the 30th and just before to the 31st dose) was reported to be 29 mg/L. Calculate the pheno-barbital concentration you would have predicted on that day if N.P. has average pharmacokinetic parameters for phenobarbital.*

The average pharmacokinetic parameters for N.P. are as follows: Cl = 8 L/day (0.1 L/kg/day × 80 kg) and V = 56 L (0.7 L/kg × 80 kg).

Using the values above for Cl and V, Equation 13.18 can be used to calculate an elimination rate constant (K) of 0.143 days^{-1}:

$$K = \frac{Cl}{V} \qquad \text{(Eq. 13.18)}$$

$$= \frac{8\ L/day}{56\ L}$$
$$= 0.143\ day^{-1}$$

and using the K value from above in Equation 13.19, a half-life of 4.85 days is calculated:

$$t\tfrac{1}{2} = \frac{0.693}{K} \qquad \text{(Eq. 13.19)}$$

$$t\tfrac{1}{2} = \frac{0.693}{0.143\ day^{-1}}$$
$$= 4.85\ days$$

Because N.P. has been receiving his phenobarbital maintenance dose for 15 days or approximately three half-lives, the phenobarbital concentration is assumed to be almost a steady-state concentration. Equation 13.20 can be used to predict the trough concentration at steady state. Using the previously calculated parameters, the steady-state trough concentration should be approximately 24 mg/L based on the following calculation.

$$\text{Css min} = \left[\frac{\dfrac{(S)(F)(Dose)}{V}}{(1 - e^{-K\tau})} \right] (e^{-K\tau}) \qquad \textbf{(Eq. 13.20)}$$

$$= \left[\frac{\dfrac{(1)(1)(100 \text{ mg})}{56 \text{ L}}}{(1 - e^{-(0.143 \text{ days}^{-1})(0.5 \text{ days})})} \right] \left(e^{-(0.143 \text{ days}^{-1})(0.5 \text{ days})} \right)$$

$$= \left[\frac{1.78 \text{ mg/L}}{0.069} \right] (0.93)$$

$$= \left[25.9 \text{ mg/L} \right] (0.93)$$

$$= 24 \text{ mg/L}$$

Question #10 *Considering the measured phenobarbital concentration of 29 mg/L in N.P., what method is most appropriately used to adjust his pharmacokinetic parameters? Do these patient-specific parameters suggest that a maintenance dose adjustment is necessary if the goal is to maintain the phenobarbital concentration at 25 mg/L?*

The measured trough concentration of phenobarbital is greater than the predicted concentration; therefore, N.P.'s phenobarbital clearance is likely to be lower than expected. If this is true, then his phenobarbital half-life is likely to be longer than 5 days (see Equation 13.3), and a non–steady-state approach will have to be used to revise his clearance value.

$$\uparrow t_{1/2} = \frac{(0.693)(V)}{\downarrow Cl}$$

Although there are a number of models, Equation 13.17, which describes the concentration (C_2, t_2 hours following the Nth dose), fits this situation nicely (see Chapter 2).

$$C_2 = + \left[\frac{\dfrac{(S)(F)(Dose)}{V}}{(1 - e^{-K\tau})} (1 - e^{-K(N)\tau})(e^{-Kt_2}) \right]$$

Tau (τ) is the dosing interval of 0.5 days, N the number of doses administered (30), and t_2 the time elapsed since the last dose (0.5 days). To calculate the concentration at the time of sampling (C_2), the elimination rate constant should be adjusted first by reducing the expected clearance value in Equation 13.18.

$$K = \frac{Cl}{V}$$

Unfortunately, there is not a direct solution to this problem, and a trial and error method must be used to find the clearance value that will produce the observed phenobarbital concentration of 29 mg/L. For example, if a phenobarbital clearance of 6 L/day is used in Equation 13.18 and volume is assumed to be equal to the average value, an elimination rate constant of 0.107 days^{-1} is calculated.

$$K = \frac{Cl}{V}$$
$$= \frac{6 \text{ L/day}}{56 \text{ L}}$$
$$= 0.107 \text{ days}^{-1}$$

and

$$t\tfrac{1}{2} = \frac{0.693}{K}$$
$$= \frac{0.693}{0.107 \text{ days}^{-1}}$$
$$= 6.5 \text{ days}$$

The elimination rate constant (0.107 days^{-1}), when placed in Equation 13.17, results in an expected phenobarbital concentration of approximately 26 mg/L.

$$C_2 = \left(\frac{\frac{(S)(F)(Dose)}{V}}{\left(1 - e^{-K\tau}\right)} \right)\left(1 - e^{-K(N)\tau}\right)\left(e^{-Kt_2}\right)$$

$$= \left(\frac{\frac{(1)(1)(100 \text{ mg})}{56 \text{ L}}}{\left(1 - e^{-(0.107 \text{ days}^{-1})(0.5 \text{ days})}\right)} \right)\left(1 - e^{-(0.107 \text{ days}^{-1})(30)(0.5 \text{ days})}\right)\left(e^{-(0.107 \text{ days}^{-1})(0.5 \text{ days})}\right)$$

$$= \frac{1.78 \text{ mg/L}}{0.052}(1 - 0.2)(0.948)$$
$$= 25.9 \text{ mg/L or} \approx 26 \text{mg/L}$$

Further decreasing the phenobarbital clearance to 5 L/day in Equation 13.18 results in an elimination rate constant of 0.0893 days^{-1}, and when this elimination rate constant is used in Equation 13.17, a phenobarbital concentration of 28.7 mg/L is calculated.

$$K = \frac{Cl}{V}$$
$$= \frac{5 \text{ L/day}}{56 \text{ L}}$$
$$= 0.0893 \text{ days}^{-1}$$

and

$$t\tfrac{1}{2} = \frac{0.693}{K} = \frac{0.693}{0.0893 \text{ days}^{-1}}$$

$$= 7.8 \text{ days}$$

$$C_2 = \left(\frac{\dfrac{(S)(F)(Dose)}{V}}{\left(1 - e^{-K\tau}\right)} \right) \left(1 - e^{-K(N)\tau}\right)\left(e^{-Kt_2}\right)$$

$$= \left(\frac{\dfrac{(1)(1)(100 \text{ mg})}{0.0893 \text{ L}}}{\left(1 - e^{-(0.0893 \text{ days}^{-1})(0.5 \text{ days})}\right)} \right) \left(1 - e^{-(0.0893 \text{ days}^{-1})(30)(0.5 \text{ days})}\right)\left(e^{-(0.0893 \text{ days}^{-1})(0.5 \text{ days})}\right)$$

$$= \frac{1.78 \text{ mg/L}}{0.0437}(0.738)(0.956)$$

$$= 28.7 \text{ mg/L or} \approx 29 \text{ mg/L}$$

The convergence of the predicted and observed concentrations suggests that N.P.'s phenobarbital clearance is approximately 5 L/day, assuming that volume did not change. It is possible to create other scenarios where both volume and clearance are different from the population values that would create a concentration outcome similar to that measured. Assuming that the clearance of 5 L/day is reasonably accurate, the predicted steady-state phenobarbital concentration (Equation 13.1) would then be approximately 40 mg/L on the current dosing regimen of 200 mg/day as calculated in the following equation.

$$Css \text{ ave} = \frac{(S)(F)(Dose/\tau)}{Cl}$$

$$= \frac{(1)(1)(200 \text{ mg/day})}{5 \text{ L/day}}$$

$$= 40 \text{ mg/L}$$

If a steady-state concentration of approximately 25 mg/L is desired, a reduction in the maintenance dose to approximately 125 mg/day would be necessary as shown in Equation 13.8.

$$Maintenance \text{ Dose} = \frac{(Cl)(Css \text{ ave})(\tau)}{(S)(F)}$$

$$= \frac{(5 \text{ L/day})(25 \text{ mg/L})(1 \text{ day})}{(1)(1)}$$

$$= 125 \text{ mg}$$

This could also be solved quickly by concentration change to dose ratio (because 40 mg/L is predicted to occur with a 200 mg/day dose, a 25 mg/L concentration requires a proportionally smaller dose):

$$\left(\frac{25 \text{ mg/L}}{40 \text{ mg/L}}\right)(200 \text{ mg}) = 125 \text{ mg}$$

Even though the calculations used accounted for non–steady-state conditions, because N.P.'s revised phenobarbital clearance is based on a measured drug concentration obtained very close to two estimated half-lives (i.e., 2×7.8 days $\approx$ 15 days) after therapy was initiated, the revised and expected steady-state concentrations must be considered somewhat uncertain.

Although it may be appropriate to reduce the phenobarbital dose, additional concentration monitoring would be prudent in 24 to 40 days to ensure that the steady-state concentration is actually about 25 mg/L on a daily dose of 125 mg.

Question #11   *Calculate a revised concentration for N.P. using a non–steady-state continuous infusion model.*

Because of the relatively long half-life and short dosing interval, the continuous infusion model is usually satisfactory as compared to use of Equation 13.17 when predicting phenobarbital concentrations. In this case, Equation 13.12 is used to predict phenobarbital concentrations obtained before steady state had been achieved (see Fig. 13.1 and Fig. 2.11).

$$C_1 = \frac{(S)(F)(Dose/\tau)}{Cl}(1 - e^{-Kt_1})$$

A helpful check in using Equation 13.12 is to multiply the duration of the infusion (t_1) by the infusion rate (dose divided by τ). This product should equal the total amount of drug that has been administered to the patient. For example, in N.P., the "infusion" rate of 100 mg divided by 0.5 days times the duration of the infusion of 15 days results in a total administered dose of 3,000 mg.

$$\text{Total Amount of Drug Administered} = (Dose/\tau)(t_1) \qquad \textbf{(Eq. 13.21)}$$

$$= (100 \text{ mg}/0.5 \text{ days})(15 \text{ days})$$
$$= 3,000 \text{ mg}$$

This amount (3,000 mg) is equal to the total amount of phenobarbital actually administered (i.e., 100 mg $\times$ 30 doses). Early in a regimen, the total amount of drug

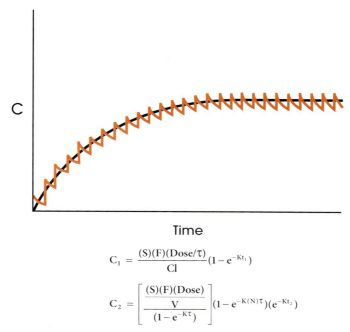

$$C_1 = \frac{(S)(F)(Dose/\tau)}{Cl}(1 - e^{-Kt_1})$$

$$C_2 = \left[\frac{\dfrac{(S)(F)(Dose)}{V}}{(1 - e^{-K\tau})} \right] (1 - e^{-K(N)\tau})(e^{-Kt_2})$$

FIGURE 13.1   Concentration–time curve for the accumulation and eventual attainment of steady state for a drug administered with a dosing interval that is much shorter than the elimination half-life. The solid smooth line represents the accumulation pattern during a continuous input model as expressed in Equation 13.12, and the saw-toothed pattern indicates the accumulation pattern for a drug administered intermittently, as in Equation 13.17. Note that the concentrations predicted by the intermittent input model are very similar to the accumulation pattern of the continuous input model.

administered and the duration of the theoretical infusion are somewhat disparate. For example, immediately after the administration of the second phenobarbital dose, a total of 200 mg has been administered, whereas the total time elapsed is only 1.5 days. However, use of Equation 13.21 suggests that only 100 mg has been administered. Whereas this problem is most apparent early in therapy, it is seldom an issue after multiple doses have been administered. This is because a variation in one dosing interval represents a relatively small percentage error with respect to the total amount of drug administered.

Using Equation 13.12, the previously calculated clearance of 5 L/day, and the corresponding elimination rate constant of 0.0893 day^{-1}, a phenobarbital concentration of 29.6 mg/L is calculated.

$$C_1 = \frac{(1)(1)(100 \text{ mg}/0.5 \text{ days})}{5 \text{ L/day}}(1 - e^{-(0.0893 \text{ days}^{-1})(15 \text{ days})})$$

$$= (40 \text{ mg/L})(0.74)$$

$$= 29.6 \text{ mg/L}$$

The similarities between the predicted phenobarbital concentration using the continuous infusion and the intermittent bolus model suggest that either model could be used, particularly after a good number of doses have been given, with the continuous infusion model requiring fewer computations.

Question #12   *J.R., an epileptic male who has been managed chronically with phenobarbital 120 mg/day, has recently developed hypoalbuminemia secondary to nephrotic syndrome. Will his phenobarbital concentration be affected by decreases in his albumin concentration or renal function?*

Only 40% to 50% of phenobarbital is bound to plasma proteins; therefore, fu (the fraction of phenobarbital that is unbound) is 0.5 to 0.6.[27,28] The concentration of a drug that is bound to protein to the extent of 50% or less is not likely to be significantly affected by changes in plasma protein concentrations or protein binding affinity.

The renal clearance for phenobarbital is probably less than 20% of the total clearance in patients with normal renal function and uncontrolled urine pH (i.e., the urine pH is not intentionally adjusted).[15] Therefore, it is unlikely that patients with renal failure will require significant adjustments in their phenobarbital dosage regimens.

Thus, J.R.'s phenobarbital concentrations are not likely to be significantly affected by his hypoalbuminemia or poor renal function.

Question #13   *R.T. is a 28-year-old, 70-kg man with chronic renal failure and a seizure disorder. He has been maintained with 60 mg of phenobarbital twice daily and has had steady-state concentrations of ≈20 mg/L. Over the past 3 months, his renal function has progressively worsened and he is to be started on 3 hours of high-flux hemodialysis three times weekly. Will he require an adjustment of his maintenance regimen? (see Dialysis of Drugs in Chapter 3.) If he was eventually switched to continuous peritoneal dialysis (CAPD), would that create a need for adjustment of his maintenance regimen?*

To determine whether a significant amount of drug is lost during each dialysis period, the three steps outlined in "Dialysis of Drugs" in Chapter 3 should be examined. First, the apparent volume of distribution for unbound drug should be estimated using Equation 13.22. Using a volume of distribution of 0.7 L/kg or 49 L for this 70 kg patient and a fu of 0.5 for phenobarbital, the apparent unbound volume of distribution for phenobarbital in R.T. is approximately 98 L. Because this is less than the upper limit of 250 L for a dialyzable drug, dialysis possibly could remove a significant amount of phenobarbital.

$$\text{Unbound Volume of Distribution} = \frac{V}{fu} \qquad \text{(Eq. 13.22)}$$

$$= \frac{49\,\text{L}}{0.5}$$

$$= 98\,\text{L}$$

Second, R.T.'s clearance of phenobarbital must be estimated. The usual clearance of 0.1 L/kg/day, or 7 L/day for the 70-kg patient, represents a total body clearance of approximately 5 mL/min. This value is low enough (i.e., <500 to 700 mL/min) that dialysis could significantly increase the total clearance.

$$\text{Clearance (mL/ min)} = (7 \, \text{L/day}) \left(\frac{1,000 \, \text{mL/L}}{1,440 \, \text{min /day}} \right)$$

$$= 4.9 \, \text{mL/ min or} \approx 5 \, \text{mL/ min}$$

Third, estimate the drug's half-life using Equation 13.4. The apparent half-life of approximately 5 days is long, suggesting that drug may be removed by dialysis (see Dialysis of Drugs, Estimating Drug Dialyzability, Criterion 3 in Chapter 3) (i.e., hemodialysis is more likely to significantly alter the dosing regimen if the drug half-life is very long).

$$t\tfrac{1}{2} = \frac{(0.693)(V)}{Cl}$$

$$= \frac{(0.693)(49 \, L)}{7 \, \text{L/days}}$$

$$= 4.9 \, \text{days}$$

Because the unbound volume of distribution and phenobarbital clearance of R.T. are relatively small, and the half-life is much greater than the lower limit of 1 to 2 hours, a significant amount of phenobarbital could be cleared during a dialysis period. For this reason, the actual clearance of phenobarbital during standard hemodialysis will have to be determined from the literature. The clearance of phenobarbital by hemodialysis has not been studied extensively; however, two older cases on the use of "standard" hemodialysis in the treatment of phenobarbital overdoses indicated that the clearance of phenobarbital by standard hemodialysis was approximately 3 L/hr.[8,29] Two case reports indicated that in renal replacement therapy, newer hemodialysis membranes are much more efficient.[30,31] For this patient, the first step would be to calculate his phenobarbital clearance (Cl) using Equation 13.9:

$$Cl = \frac{(S)(F)(Dose/\tau)}{Css \, ave}$$

$$= \frac{(1)(1)(60 \, \text{mg/0.5 day})}{20 \, \text{mg/L}}$$

$$= 6 \, \text{L/day or } 0.25 \, \text{L/hr}$$

Using Equation 13.23, an estimate of 10 L/hr[32] as the clearance by high-flux dialysis (Cl_{dial}) and the patient's calculated clearance (Cl_{pat}) of 0.25 L/hr, a dialysis replacement dose can be calculated. Equation 13.23 was selected to calculate the replacement dose because of the long half-life and relatively short dosing interval for phenobarbital (see Dialysis of Drugs in Chapter 3 and Fig. 3.1).

$$\text{Postdialysis Replacement Dose} = (V)(\text{Css ave})\left(1 - e^{-\left(\frac{Cl_{pat} + Cl_{dial}}{V}\right)(T_{dial})}\right) \quad \textbf{(Eq. 13.23)}$$

$$= (49 \text{ L})(20 \text{ mg/L})\left(1 - e^{-\left(\frac{0.25 \text{ L/hr} + 10 \text{ L/hr}}{49 \text{ L}}\right)(3 \text{ hr})}\right)$$

$$= (980 \text{ mg})(1 - e^{-(0.209 \text{ hr}^{-1})(3 \text{ hr})})$$

$$= (980 \text{ mg})(1 - 0.53)$$

$$= 460 \text{ mg}$$

This replacement dose of approximately 450 mg represents the amount of drug eliminated from the body during the dialysis period by both metabolic and dialysis clearance. In this case, the vast majority of the drug eliminated during the 3-hour dialysis period represents drug eliminated by the dialysis route. For this reason, the total daily phenobarbital dose on days of dialysis would be 120 mg (maintenance dose) plus the postdialysis dose of ≈450 mg. If less efficient dialyzers are used, the postdialysis dose would be less. For example, if the clearance of 3 L/hr from the older case reports is used in the above calculations with a 3-hour dialysis period, the replacement dose would be approximately 175 mg. This illustrates one of the problems of using literature on dialysis clearance to predict doses. That is, dialyzers and dialysis procedures have become more efficient over time. It is, therefore, important to seek data on the actual dialysis membrane and procedures being used or to measure before and after concentrations to determine actual loss in a given patient. In addition, it is possible that the actual drug loss during high-flux dialysis will be less for R.T. than was estimated. One possible flaw in the estimation is that the amount eliminated in Equation 13.23 assumes that the Cl_{dial} is eliminating phenobarbital from the entire volume of distribution, when, in fact, it is the plasma that is being cleared. If plasma is cleared faster than it can re-equilibrate from the deeper tissues, the amount of drug loss will be less than predicted, and there will be a significant rebound in the plasma concentration following dialysis. The more efficient the dialysis membrane, the more likely it is that Equation 13.23 will overestimate the amount of drug loss.

Standard replacement doses of phenobarbital after dialysis are frequently in the range of 200 to 300 mg. Although this replacement dose appears to be large when compared with the maintenance dose, it is not unusual. If there is concern about the size of the postdialysis replacement dose, one could administer a smaller dose of 100 to 200 mg after dialysis and continue to monitor the patient during subsequent dialysis periods to ensure that the phenobarbital concentration does not continue to decline because of additional elimination by the dialysis route.

If R.T. receives CAPD, then further dose adjustments will be needed. In hemodialysis, where dialysis is intermittent, the majority of the phenobarbital clearance during dialysis is primarily Cl_{dial} and hence the need for a replacement dose postdialysis. With CAPD, the dialysis clearance values are lower but continuous. As a result, both the clearance by CAPD and the patient's metabolism are important contributors to the elimination of phenobarbital. With CAPD, it appears that 35% to 50% of the daily dose is removed in the dialysate. Thus, the predicted daily dose would usually be increased by about 40% to compensate for the additional loss caused by peritoneal dialysis.[27] The clearance owing to dialysis in CAPD is greatly affected by dextrose concentration, dwell time, and the number of cycles. For example, in the case cited, loss of phenobarbital was only ≈7 mg during a 12-hour daytime period with one cycle versus ≈45 mg during six cycles at night.[33] Thus, steady-state concentrations should be used to guide therapy, and if the peritoneal exchange process is altered significantly (i.e., volume or exchange dwell time), additional dose adjustments may be necessary.

Question #14   *H.P., a 7-year-old, 30-kg boy, is to be given oral phenobarbital for his seizure disorder. Calculate the maintenance dose of phenobarbital that will produce a steady-state concentration of ≈25 mg/L.*

To calculate H.P.'s phenobarbital maintenance dose, one would first assume his clearance to be ≈6 L/day (0.2 L/kg/day × 30 kg). This clearance value, although larger-than-usual adult value, is consistent for children. Using Equation 13.8 with a target concentration of 25 mg/L, and a salt form (S) fraction of 1, a daily maintenance dose of 150 mg can be calculated.

$$\text{Maintenance Dose} = \frac{(\text{Cl})(\text{Css ave})(\tau)}{(S)(F)}$$

$$= \frac{(6 \text{ L/day})(25 \text{ mg/L})(1 \text{ day})}{(1)(1)}$$

$$= 150 \text{ mg}$$

Depending on the clinical situation, one could administer a loading dose to rapidly achieve therapeutic concentrations or start the patient on his maintenance dose without a loading dose. In the latter situation, the urgency of the clinical situation will determine whether the initial maintenance dose should be 150 mg/day or one-quarter of the target maintenance dose (≈38 mg/day) for the first week, increased by ≈38 mg/day weekly until the final maintenance dose of 150 mg/day is being administered. As noted previously, excessive sedation can be a consequence of starting the patient with either a loading dose or even the full maintenance dose. H.P. should be monitored for both therapeutic and potential side effects during this period of dose titration.

Question #15   *H.P. is able to take phenobarbital tablets and is given the commercially available dose of 65 mg twice daily for a total daily dose of 130 mg. What impact would the use of this dose have on the predicted Css ave?*

Using Equation 13.1, the Css ave can be predicted from the actual dose used:

$$Css\ ave = \frac{(S)(F)(Dose/\tau)}{Cl}$$

$$= \frac{(1)(1)(130\ mg/day)}{6\ L/day}$$

$$= 21.7\ mg/L$$

Or, because in Equation 13.1, Css ave and dose are proportional so long as S, F, and τ are held constant, the new Css ave could have been calculated as a ratio of the doses times the predicted concentration:

$$Css\ ave = (25\ mg/L)\left(\frac{130\ mg}{150\ mg}\right) = 21.7\ mg/L$$

Question #16   *S.M., a 45-year-old, 60-kg woman, was recently prescribed 120 mg/day of phenobarbital. Ten days ago, her concentration was 15 mg/L; today her phenobarbital concentration is 24 mg/L. Based on the data provided, what would you calculate her steady-state phenobarbital concentration to be?*

To calculate S.M.'s phenobarbital concentration, one will first have to determine her clearance. Unfortunately, because phenobarbital has a long half-life, it is unlikely that the present concentration of 24 mg/L represents steady state. Therefore, some type of iterative search or indirect procedure must be used to estimate clearance. One method is to combine Equations 13.16 and 13.12 where C_0 is the initial phenobarbital concentration of 15 mg/L and, in Equation 13.12, the infusion rate is essentially represented by the daily dose of 120 mg/day. In both Equations 13.16 and 13.12, the time interval "t" between C_0 and the current concentration of 24 mg/L would be 10 days.

$$C_1 = C_0\left(e^{-Kt_1}\right) + \frac{(S)(F)(Dose/\tau)}{Cl}\left(1 - e^{-Kt_1}\right)$$

$$24\ mg/L = (15\ mg/L)(e^{-(K)(10\,days)}) + \left[\frac{(1)(1)(120\ mg/day)}{Cl}\right](1 - e^{-(K)(10\,days)})$$

Unfortunately, the resolution to this problem first requires assuming S.M.'s volume of distribution (0.7 L/kg × 60 kg or = 42 L) and then iteratively solving for the clearance (Cl) and K (Cl/V = Cl/42 L) until the result is a calculated concentration equal to the observed C_1 of 24 mg/L. As discussed previously, this is a sometimes laborious procedure, and an alternative approach that could be of use is the mass balance equation, Equation 13.24:

$$Cl = \frac{(S)(F)(Dose/\tau) - \dfrac{(C_2 - C_1)V}{t}}{C\ ave} \qquad \textbf{(Eq. 13.24)}$$

In the above equation, if one substitutes S.M.'s maintenance dose of phenobarbital, the corresponding C_1 of 15 mg/L and C_2 of 24 mg/L, and assuming that the C ave is $\approx$19.5 mg/L, or halfway between the initial and present phenobarbital concentrations [(15 mg/L + 24 mg/L)/2], a clearance of $\approx$4.2 L/day is calculated.

$$Cl = \frac{\left(\dfrac{(1)(1)(120 \text{ mg})}{1 \text{ day}}\right) - \left(\dfrac{(24 \text{ mg/L} - 15 \text{ mg/L})(42 \text{ L})}{10 \text{ day}}\right)}{19.5 \text{ mg/L}}$$

$$= \frac{120 \text{ mg/day} - \dfrac{378 \text{ mg}}{10 \text{ days}}}{19.5 \text{ mg/L}}$$

$$= \frac{82.2 \text{ mg/day}}{19.5 \text{ mg/L}}$$

$$= 4.2 \text{ L/day}$$

This clearance value of 4.2 L/day corresponds to a half-life of approximately 7 days (Equation 13.3, assuming V = 42 L).

$$t\tfrac{1}{2} = \frac{(0.693)(V)}{Cl}$$

$$= \frac{(0.693)(42 \text{ L})}{4.2 \text{ L/days}}$$

$$= 6.9 \text{ days}$$

Using Equation 13.11 and the t½ from above, the elimination rate constant (K) can be calculated.

$$K = \frac{0.693}{t\tfrac{1}{2}}$$

$$= \frac{0.693}{6.9 \text{ days}}$$

$$= 0.1 \text{ days}^{-1}$$

As discussed in Part I (see Chapter 2), there are several conditions that should be met if the prediction calculated by use of the mass balance equation is to be reasonably accurate. First, the time between the first and second concentrations should be at least one but no longer than two drug half-lives. Second, if concentrations are rising, C_2 should be less than twice C_1. Third, the rate of drug administration should be reasonably regular and smooth. By examining the drug half-life, the change in concentrations, and the dosing regimen, it is clear that all three of these conditions have been met; therefore, one would anticipate that the clearance value predicted should be reasonably accurate.

If there was concern about the validity of the revised clearance derived from the mass balance equation, the clearance value of 4.2 L/day along with the corresponding elimination rate constant of 0.1 days^{-1} could be used in Equations 13.16 and 13.12 to confirm that both the iterative search and mass balance equations generate essentially the same answer.

$$C_1 = C_0(e^{-Kt}) + \frac{(S)(F)(Dose/\tau)}{Cl}(1-e^{-Kt_1})$$

$$= (15\ mg/L)(e^{-(0.1\,days)(10\,days)}) + \left[\frac{(1)(1)(120\ mg/day)}{4.2\ L/day}\right](1-e^{-(0.1\,days^{-1})(10\,days)})$$

$$= \left[15\ mg/L(0.368)\right] + \left[(28.57\ mg/L)(1-0.368)\right]$$

$$= 5.52\ mg/L + 18\ mg/L$$

$$= 23.52\ mg/L$$

As can be seen from this calculation, the predicted concentration using the exponential equations results in a value very close to the observed concentration of 24 mg/L. This comparison is useful when there is concern that the assumptions implicit in the mass balance equation have oversimplified a more complex problem. Our comparison indicates that both approaches are equivalent.

To calculate the expected steady-state concentration of approximately 29 mg/L, Equation 13.1 would be used in conjunction with our revised phenobarbital clearance of 4.2 L/day.

$$Css\ ave = \frac{(S)(F)(Dose/\tau)}{Cl}$$

$$= \frac{(1)(1)\,(120\ mg/day)}{4.2\ L/day}$$

$$= 28.57\ or \approx 29\ mg/L$$

REFERENCES

1. Wilkes L, Danziger LH, Rodvold KA, et al. Phenobarbital pharmacokinetics in obesity: a case report. *Clin Pharmacokinet*. 1992;22:481–484.

2. Wilmshurst JM, van der Walt J, Ackermann S, et al. Rescue therapy with high-dose oral phenobarbitone loading for refractory status epilepticus. *J Paediatr Child Health*. 2010;46:17–22.

3. Buchthal F, Svensmark O, Simonsen H. Relation of EEG and seizures to phenobarbital in serum. *Arch Neurol*. 1968;19:567.

4. Jannuzzi G, Cian P, Fattore C, et al. A multicenter randomized controlled trial on the clinical impact of therapeutic drug monitoring in patients with newly diagnosed epilepsy. *Epilepsia*. 2000;41:222–230.

5. Plass GL, Hine CH. Hydantoin and barbiturate blood levels observed in epileptics. *Arch Int Pharmacodyn Ther*. 1960;128:375.

6. Sushine I. Chemical evidence of tolerance to phenobarbital. *J Lab Clin Med*. 1957;50:127.

7. Baselt RC, Wright JA, Cravey RH. Therapeutic and toxic concentrations of more than 100 toxicologically significant drugs in blood, plasma, or serum: a tabulation. *Clin Chem*. 1975;21:44.

8. Kennedy AC, Briggs JD, Young N, et al. Successful treatment of three cases of very severe barbiturate poisoning. *Lancet*. 1969;1:995.

9. Levy RH, Wilensky AJ, Anderson GD. Carbamazepine, valproic acid, phenobarbital and ethosuximide. In: Evans WE, Schentag JJ, Jusko WJ, eds. *Applied Pharmacokinetics: Principles of Therapeutic Drug Monitoring*. 3rd ed. Vancouver, WA: Applied Therapeutics Inc.; 1992.

10. Wilensky AJ, Friel PN, Levy RH, et al. Kinetics of phenobarbital in normal subjects and epileptic patients. *Eur J Clin Pharmacol*. 1982;23:87–92.

11. Graves NM, Holmes GB, Kriel RL, et al. Relative bioavailability of rectally administered phenobarbital sodium parenteral solution. *DICP*. 1989;23:565–568.

12. Yska JP, Essink GW, Bosch FH, et al. Oral bioavailability of phenobarbital: a comparison of a solution in myvacet 9–08, a suspension, and a tablet. *Pharm World Sci*. 2000;22:67–71.

13. Gal P. Phenobarbital and primidone. In: Taylor WJ, Diers-Caviness MH, eds. *A Textbook for the Clinical Application of Therapeutic Drug Monitoring*. Irving, TX: Abbott Laboratories Diagnostics Division; 1986:237–252.

14. Havidberg E, Dam M. Clinical pharmacokinetics of anticonvulsants. *Clin Pharmacokinet*. 1976;1:151.

15. Alvin J, McHorse T, Hoyumpa A, et al. The effect of liver disease in man on the disposition of phenobarbital. *J Pharmacol Exp Ther*. 1975;192:224.

16. Battino D, Estienne M, Avanzini G. Clinical pharmacokinetics of antiepileptic drugs in paediatric patients. Part I: Phenobarbital, primidone, valproic acid, ethosuximide and mesuximide. *Clin Pharmacokinet*. 1995;29:257–286.

17. Touw DJ, Graafland O, Cranendonk A, et al. Clinical pharmacokinetics of phenobarbital in neonates. *Eur J Pharmaceut Sci*. 2000;12:111–116.

18. Linton AL, Luke RG, Briggs JD, et al. Methods of forced diuresis and its application in barbiturate poisoning. *Lancet*. 1967;2:377.

19. Goto S, Seo T, Murata T, et al. Population estimation of the effects of cytochrome P450 2C9 and 2C19 polymorphisms on phenobarbital clearance in Japanese. *Ther Drug Monit*. 2007;29:118–121.

20. Lee SM, Chung JY, Lee YM, et al. Effects of cytochrome P450 (CYP)2C19 polymorphisms on pharmacokinetics of phenobarbital in neonates and infants with seizures. *Arch Dis Childhood*. 2012;97:569–572.

21. Gladtke E. Pharmacokinetics of phenobarbital in childhood. *Eur J Clin Pharmacol*. 1977;12:305.

22. Painter MJ, Pippenger C, MacDonald H, et al. Phenobarbital and diphenylhydantoin levels in neonates with seizures. *J Pediatr*. 1978;92:315.

23. Botha JH, Gray AL, Miller R. Determination of phenobarbitone population clearance values for South African children. *Eur J Clin Pharmacol*. 1995;48:381–383.

24. Messina S, Battino D, Croci D, et al. Phenobarbital pharmacokinetics in old age: a case-matched evaluation based on therapeutic drug monitoring data. *Epilepsia*. 2005;46:372–377.

25. Murphy JE, Winter ME. Clinical pharmacokinetic pearls: using bolus versus infusion equations. *Pharmacotherapy*. 1996;16:698–700.

26. Vucicevic K, Jovanovic M, Golubovic B, et al. Nonlinear mixed effects modelling approach in investigating phenobarbital pharmacokinetic interactions in epileptic patients. *Eur J Clin Pharmacol*. 2015;71:183–190.

27. Waddell WJ, Butler TC. The distribution of phenobarbital. *J Clin Invest*. 1957;36:1217.

28. Houghton GW, Richens A, Toseland PA, et al. Brain concentrations of phenytoin, phenobarbitone, and primidone in epileptic patients. *Eur J Clin Pharmacol*. 1975;9:73.

29. Henderson LW, Merrill JP. Treatment of barbiturate intoxication. *Ann Intern Med*. 1966;64:876.

30. Quan DJ, Winter ME. Extracorporeal removal of phenobarbital by high-flux hemodialysis. *J Appl Ther Res*. 1998;2:75–79.

31. Rosenborg S, Saraste L, Wide K. High phenobarbital clearance during continuous renal replacement therapy. *Medicine*. 2014;93:1–2.

32. Palmer BF. Effectiveness of hemodialysis in the extracorporeal therapy of phenobarbital overdose. *Am J Kidney Dis*. 2000;36:640–643.

33. Porto I, John EG, Heilliczer J. Removal of phenobarbital during continuous cycling peritoneal dialysis in a child. *Pharmacotherapy*. 1997;17:832–835.

PHENYTOIN

Michael E. Winter

Learning Objectives

By the end of the phenytoin chapter, the learner shall be able to:

1. Describe the effect of uremia and hypoalbuminemia on the:
   a. Unbound plasma phenytoin concentration.
   b. Bound plasma phenytoin concentration.
   c. Total plasma phenytoin concentration.
   d. Fraction unbound (fu).
   e. Total body stores of phenytoin.
2. Calculate the phenytoin concentration that would have been observed had the patient had normal plasma binding, given a phenytoin concentration in a patient with hypoalbuminemia and normal renal function or receiving dialysis.
3. Calculate the patient's therapeutic range adjusted for altered binding that would correspond to the usual therapeutic range of 10 to 20 mg/L in patients with normal binding, given a patient with hypoalbuminemia and normal renal function or receiving dialysis.
4. Estimate the plasma phenytoin concentration that would have been observed if the patient had normal binding (i.e., no valproic acid present), given a patient receiving valproic acid and phenytoin with simultaneous valproic acid and phenytoin concentrations.
5. Know the salt form (S) for phenytoin capsules, injectable (phenytoin and fosphenytoin), chewable tablets, and suspension.
6. List the conditions that are known or likely to be associated with decreased phenytoin oral bioavailability.
7. Determine whether the patient meets the criteria for obesity and calculate the expected volume of distribution for the obese and nonobese patients, given a patient history.

8. Describe the elements of capacity-limited metabolism (Km and Vm) and how Km and Vm relate to clearance.
9. Describe or demonstrate the relationship between a change in the phenytoin maintenance dose and the new Css ave when:
   a. Css ave is below Km.
   b. Css ave is the same as Km.
   c. Css ave is much greater than Km.
   d. The maintenance dose is greater than Vm.
10. Explain or use examples to demonstrate why the concept of t½ for phenytoin has little to no usefulness in the clinical setting.
11. Do the following if a dosing history is given:
    a. Predict the time expected to achieve 90% of steady state (t90%).
    b. Determine whether or not a measured plasma concentration is likely to represent steady state (90% t).
    c. List the conditions necessary for the t90% and 90% t equations to be employed and the potential errors that can be encountered when using the two equations.
    d. Calculate the time required for a phenytoin concentration to decline from an initial concentration to a defined second concentration, assuming no drug input.
12. Identify, given a patient's phenytoin dosing regimen, based on the product being administered, route of administration, and time of the phenytoin plasma sample, whether or not it would be appropriate to consider the steady-state phenytoin concentration as a Css ave and, if not, how to approximate the Css ave.
13. Do the following if a patient history with one Css ave phenytoin level is given:
    a. Use a reasonable assumed Km to calculate a revised Vm.
    b. Use the revised Vm and assumed Km to calculate either a new Css ave from a selected dosing regimen or a new dosing regimen from the selected Css ave.
14. Determine whether phenytoin is a possible candidate for a patient, given a patient's HLA-B15:02 status, and explain how initial maintenance doses might be adjusted, given the CYP2C9 genetic status.
15. Explain why, in some patients, the phenytoin concentration remains stable and does not significantly for several days following the discontinuation of oral phenytoin.
16. Use the "orbit graph" (see Fig. 14.2) to determine the most probable Vm and Km and then determine a new dosing regimen to achieve a desired Css ave, given a patient history with one Css ave.
17. Calculate and estimate graphically (see Fig. 14.3) the unique Km and Vm values that are consistent with the data provided, given a patient history with two different phenytoin maintenance doses and corresponding Css aves.
18. Do the following if an initial phenytoin concentration and a second "non–steady-state" phenytoin concentration are given:
    a. Use the mass balance technique to estimate a revised estimate of Vm.

    b. Use the revised Vm to design a new dosing regimen to achieve a desired Css ave.

    c. Describe the rules or condition necessary to improve accuracy of the mass balance technique when applied to phenytoin.

19. Recognize the altered binding condition and calculate the corresponding normal binding concentrations, given a patient with hypoalbuminemia and either normal renal function or receiving dialysis, and then:

    a. Determine whether dosing adjustments would be appropriate.

    b. Revise the Vm (one Css ave) or Km and Vm (two dosing regimens with Css aves).

    c. Revise the dosing regimen (incremental loading and maintenance doses) to achieve a desired normal binding concentration.

    d. Calculate the Css ave that would be assayed given the altered binding condition.

    e. Calculate the "therapeutic range" of the altered binding condition that would correspond to the normal binding concentrations of 10 to 20 mg/L.

20. Explain, using the criteria outlined in Dialysis of Drugs: Estimating Drug Dialyzability in Chapter 3, why dialysis is not likely to remove significant amounts of phenytoin.

21. Calculate the amount of phenytoin removed by chronic renal replacement therapy (CRRT), given the target unbound phenytoin concentration and the effluent flow rate for a patient receiving CRRT.

Phenytoin is primarily used as an anticonvulsant and has been used in the past for the treatment of certain types of cardiac arrhythmias.[1] It is usually administered orally in single or divided doses of 200 to 400 mg/day. When a rapid therapeutic effect is required, a loading dose of 15 mg/kg can be administered by oral or intravenous (IV) routes. Although phenytoin for injection can be administered intramuscularly (IM), this route should be avoided because of slow and erratic absorption. Fosphenytoin is a more soluble ester of phenytoin and is usually administered by the IV or IM route. Absorption of fosphenytoin by the IM route is more rapid than the oral sodium phenytoin but slower than the IV route of administration.[2]

Individualizing the dose of phenytoin is complicated by two major problems. First, binding of phenytoin to plasma proteins is decreased in patients with renal failure or hypoalbuminemia, and, in certain cases, phenytoin can be displaced by other drugs. Second, the metabolic capacity of phenytoin is limited; therefore, changes in the maintenance dose result in disproportionate changes in steady-state plasma concentrations. The capacity-limited metabolism of phenytoin also eliminates the clinical usefulness of half-life (t½) as a pharmacokinetic parameter and makes estimates of the time required to achieve steady state difficult. Although phenytoin is still commonly used, the difficulty with the capacity-limited metabolism, multiple drug–drug interactions, as well as the long-term side effect profile has limited its use in epilepsy to a second- or third-line agent.[3]

KEY PARAMETERS: Phenytoin

Therapeutic plasma concentration	10–20 mg/L
F[a]	1
S[b]	0.92, 1
V	0.65 L/kg
Cl	
Vm[c]	7 mg/kg/day
Km[d]	4 mg/L
t½[e]	Concentration dependent
fu (fraction unbound in plasma)	0.1

[a]Oral bioavailability is generally assumed to be 1 (100% absorbed). However, bioavailability is difficult to estimate, and different drug products are not considered to be interchangeable or therapeutically equivalent.
[b]For capsules and the injectable preparations (phenytoin and fosphenytoin), salt factor (S) = 0.92; for the suspension and chewable tablet, S = 1.
[c]Adult value, Vm values are >7 mg/kg/day and age dependent for children.
[d]Adult value, Km values are variable for children.
[e]For time required to achieve steady state (see "Half-Life t½" section).

THERAPEUTIC AND TOXIC PLASMA CONCENTRATIONS

Phenytoin plasma concentrations of 10 to 20 mg/L are generally accepted as therapeutic.[4–9] Plasma concentrations in the range of 5 to 10 mg/L can be therapeutic for some patients, but concentrations <5 mg/L are not likely to be effective.[10]

A number of long-term phenytoin side effects, such as gingival hyperplasia, folate deficiency, peripheral neuropathy, and cutaneous reactions, do not appear to be easily related to plasma phenytoin concentrations. Patients with the HLA-B15:02 gene have a higher risk of developing Stevens–Johnson syndrome or toxic epidermal necrolysis to the extent that phenytoin is not recommended for these patients.[11] In contrast, central nervous system (CNS) side effects do correlate to some degree with plasma concentration. Far-lateral nystagmus (ocular tremor on far-lateral gaze) usually occurs in patients with plasma phenytoin concentrations >20 mg/L. The concentration range associated with this effect, however, is broad, with some patients showing symptoms at concentrations of 15 mg/L and others having no nystagmus at concentrations >30 mg/L. Although far-lateral nystagmus is often used to monitor phenytoin therapy, it is seldom considered a true drug side effect or toxicity and is not a reason to reduce the phenytoin dose. As an example, if a patient has always presented with far-lateral nystagmus but is no longer exhibiting nystagmus, it is an indication that the phenytoin concentration is probably lower than on previous visits. Other CNS symptoms such as ataxia and diminished mental capacity are frequently observed in patients with concentrations exceeding 30 and 40 mg/L, respectively.[5] In addition, precautions should be taken when phenytoin for injection is administered by the IV route because the propylene glycol diluent has cardiac depressant properties.[4] Fosphenytoin is more soluble than phenytoin for injection and does not contain propylene glycol as a diluent. However, fosphenytoin does have similar effects on the myocardium and cardiovascular system (bradycardia and hypotension) but to a lesser extent. Clinicians should be aware that the maximum recommended rate of IV administration is 50 mg/min for phenytoin for injection and 150 mg/min for fosphenytoin, and slower rates of infusion (½ to ⅓ the maximum rate) are often used, especially when larger loading doses are administered.

Alterations in plasma protein binding

The usual phenytoin therapeutic range of 10 to 20 mg/L represents the total drug concentration that consists of unbound (or free) drug concentration plus the phenytoin, which is bound to plasma albumin. The usual fu or free fraction of phenytoin is 0.1. Therefore, approximately 90% of phenytoin in the plasma is bound to serum albumin; about 10% is unbound and free to equilibrate with the tissues where the pharmacologic effects and metabolism occur. It is important to keep in mind that although most of the phenytoin in plasma is bound to plasma albumin, most of the phenytoin is not in plasma. Therefore, any phenytoin displaced off the plasma albumin, whereas a large percentage of the drug in plasma, is a small percentage of phenytoin in the tissue. The displaced phenytoin will re-equilibrate with the tissue, resulting in large decrease in the total plasma concentration but very little change in the unbound or free plasma phenytoin concentration and very little change in the pharmacologic effect. Following re-equilibration of the displaced phenytoin, the unbound plasma phenytoin concentration will remain relatively unchanged. The total plasma phenytoin concentration will be decreased because the bound concentration has decreased. As a result, the total level will appear to be low relative to its potential for pharmacologic effect (therapeutic and/or toxic).

There are two approaches one can use to interpret phenytoin levels when protein binding is significantly altered. The first is to adjust all the parameters (i.e., therapeutic range, volume of distribution, and Km) to those that would be observed in the presence of altered plasma binding. The second is to convert the measured or observed plasma concentration with low binding into that which would be observed under normal binding conditions (C Normal Binding). In this instance, the parameters (i.e., therapeutic range, volume of distribution, and Km) associated with normal plasma protein binding would also be used in any calculations. Although either of these approaches is acceptable, it is the author's belief that the second method is least likely to result in calculation errors. Therefore, this latter approach is used throughout this chapter when alterations in plasma binding are encountered.

The three factors that are known to significantly alter the plasma protein binding of phenytoin are hypoalbuminemia, renal failure, and displacement by other drugs.

Hypoalbuminemia. In patients with low serum albumin, Equation 14.1 can be used to determine the plasma concentration that would have been observed with a normal plasma protein concentration.

$$\text{C Normal Binding} = \frac{C'}{(1-\text{fu})\left[\dfrac{P'}{P_{NL}}\right] + \text{fu}} \qquad \textbf{(Eq. 14.1)}$$

C′ is the observed plasma concentration reported by the laboratory; fu is the normal free fraction of drug (phenytoin fu = 0.1) [12–15]; P′ is the patient's serum albumin in units of g/dL; P_{NL} is the normal serum albumin (4.4 g/dL); and C Normal Binding is the plasma drug concentration that would have been observed if the patient's serum albumin concentration had been normal. Placing the corresponding values for fu and a normal serum albumin results in Equation 14.2.

$$\frac{\text{Phenytoin Concentration}}{\text{Normal Plasma Binding}} = \frac{\text{Patient's Phenytoin Concentration with Altered Plasma Binding}}{\left[0.9 \times \dfrac{\text{Patient's Serum Albumin}}{4.4 \text{ g/dL}} + 0.1 \right]} \qquad \textbf{(Eq. 14.2)}$$

This equation is most useful when a patient has a low serum albumin concentration but does not have significantly diminished renal function and is not taking other drugs known to displace phenytoin. In clinical practice, if one is willing to assumes that 0.9 is approximately 1 and 0.1 is approximately 0, the adjustment factor is simply the patients albumin divided by the normal albumin. This simplification should not be used if the patient's albumin is <2 g/dL because it suggests that, at the unbound phenytoin, concentration would be zero if there were no albumin, and this of course is not true.

Renal Failure. In patients with end-stage renal disease, the free fraction of phenytoin increases from 0.1 to 0.2 to 0.35.[12,16–19] Some of this change in plasma binding is because of the decrease in serum albumin concentration associated with end-stage renal disease, and some of the binding changes are because of a change in the binding affinity of phenytoin to serum albumin. When the creatinine clearance is >25 mL/min, the change in the binding affinity appears to be minimal, no adjustment for renal function need to be made, and Equation 14.2 should be used. However, if the creatinine clearance is <10 mL/min and the patient is undergoing hemodialysis treatments, binding changes can be significant.[20]

In the latter circumstance, Equation 14.2 can be altered to accommodate changes in both the serum albumin concentration and the affinity of phenytoin for serum albumin. Hence, Equation 14.3 is given as follows:

$$\frac{\text{Phenytoin Concentration}}{\text{Normal Plasma Binding}} = \frac{\text{Dialysis Patient's Phenytoin Concentration with Altered Plasma Binding}}{\left[(0.9)(0.48) \times \dfrac{\text{Patient's Serum Albumin}}{4.4 \text{ g/dL}} + 0.1 \right]}$$

$$\textbf{(Eq. 14.3)}$$

The above equations should only be used in patients with end-stage renal disease receiving hemodialysis treatments because the factor that represents the decreased affinity for phenytoin binding to serum albumin (0.48) was derived from this type of patient. Note that, in Equation 14.3, fu is again assumed to be 0.1 [i.e., 0.9 = (1 − fu)] because the Phenytoin Concentration Normal Plasma Binding (C Normal Binding) calculated by Equation 14.3 is correct for both serum albumin and renal dysfunction. In addition, it should be recognized that Equations 14.2 and 14.3 are only approximate estimates of normal plasma binding phenytoin concentrations, and there can be considerable variance among individual patients. The accuracy of Equations 14.2 and 14.3 has been studied, and variances have been identified. This is especially true in critically ill patients.[21,22] Regardless of what equation is used to adjust for altered binding, the general concept that phenytoin binding needs to be considered when evaluating phenytoin concentration, is important to remember when using phenytoin concentrations to adjust a patient's dosing regimen. In patients with diminished renal function who are not undergoing intermittent hemodialysis, binding affinity is unpredictably altered when the creatinine clearance is between 10 and 25 mL/min. The plasma concentration of drugs cannot be interpreted accurately for this group of patients using Equation 14.3.[20]

When discussing alterations in plasma binding with a nonpharmacist clinician, it is often useful to consider what would be the target phenytoin concentration in a patient with decreased plasma binding. That is, what is the lower and upper concentration in your patient with altered binding that would be equivalent to the usual range of 10 to 20 mg/L when binding is normal. These values can be calculated by rearranging Equations 14.2 and 14.3.

For patients with hypoalbuminemia and a creatinine clearance >25 mL/min, the equivalent lower and upper end of the concentration range would be as follows:

$$\text{Patient's Therapeutic Range with Low Albumin That Would Be Equal to 10 mg/L} = \text{(Eq. 14.4)}$$

$$10 \text{ mg/L} \times \left[\left(0.9 \times \frac{\text{Patient's Serum Albumin}}{4.4 \text{ g/dL}}\right) + 0.1\right]$$

$$\text{Patient's Therapeutic Range with Low Albumin That Would Be Equal to 20 mg/L} = \text{(Eq. 14.5)}$$

$$20 \text{ mg/L} \times \left[\left(0.9 \times \frac{\text{Patient's Serum Albumin}}{4.4 \text{ g/dL}}\right) + 0.1\right]$$

For patients with hypoalbuminemia who are receiving dialysis, the equivalent lower and upper end of the concentration range would be as follows:

$$\text{Patient's Therapeutic Range with Low Albumin and on Dialysis That Would Be Equal to 10 mg/L} = \text{(Eq. 14.6)}$$

$$10 \text{ mg/L} \times \left[\left(0.9 \times 0.48 \times \frac{\text{Patient's Serum Albumin}}{4.4 \text{ g/dL}}\right) + 0.1\right]$$

$$\text{Patient's Therapeutic Range with Low Albumin and on Dialysis That Would Be Equal to 20 mg/L} = \text{(Eq. 14.7)}$$

$$20 \text{ mg/L} \times \left[\left(0.9 \times 0.48 \times \frac{\text{Patient's Serum Albumin}}{4.4 \text{ g/dL}}\right) + 0.1\right]$$

Drug Displacement. Drugs can also displace phenytoin from plasma protein binding sites. As explained in Desired Plasma Concentration (C) in Chapter 1, it is usually difficult to estimate the extent of drug displacement from protein binding sites because the concentration of the displacing agent is seldom known. One exception to this rule is the situation in which serum concentrations of both valproic acid and phenytoin are being monitored. When the serum valproic acid concentration is <20 mg/L, the displacement of phenytoin appears to be minimal, and adjustment of the phenytoin concentration is probably not warranted. When the valproic acid concentration increases, phenytoin displacement from plasma protein binding sites increases. At valproic acid concentrations of approximately 70 mg/L, phenytoin serum concentrations decrease by 40% (see Equation 14.8 and Chapter 15).[15,23,24]

In a study by Kerrick et al.,[25] an equation was developed to help correct or adjust for the displacement of phenytoin by valproic acid. Equation 14.8 is a modification of their original equation:

$$\frac{\text{Phenytoin Concentration}}{\text{Normal Plasma Binding}} = \frac{\left[0.095 + (0.001)(\text{Valproic Acid Concentration})\right]\left(\text{Phenytoin Concentration}\right)}{0.1} \qquad \textbf{(Eq. 14.8)}$$

where the Phenytoin Concentration Normal Plasma Binding is the concentration that would have been reported if there had been no displacement by valproic acid (i.e., fu = 0.1). The valproic acid and phenytoin concentrations are the concentrations that are reported by the laboratory. Note, however, that Equation 14.8 has the requirement that the two drug concentrations be measured (obtained) at the same time. In addition, there should not be any other factors present that would alter plasma binding (e.g., hypoalbuminemia, renal failure, other displacing drugs).

BIOAVAILABILITY (F)

Phenytoin is completely absorbed (F = 1.0) from most currently available products[26]; however, the various dosage forms and different manufacturers' products are not considered to be interchangeable.[8,27–30] Although most data suggests that generic phenytoin products are safe and effective, it is usually recommended that changing manufacturer or dosage form should be avoided to rule out the possibility that small differences in absorption might result in a therapeutic failure or toxicity.[31] It is the author's recommendation that if a change in manufacturer is necessary, it would be best to make the change at a time when the patient's daily routine is normal (e.g., not at the start of school, vacations, new job, etc.) because changes in the daily routine are more likely to result in nonadherence, making it more uncertain as to whether a change is clinical status is the result of differences in absorption or adherence. In addition, there are different salt forms of phenytoin. The capsule and injectable preparations consist of the sodium salt (S = 0.92) of phenytoin, whereas the chewable tablet and suspension contain the acid form (S = 1.0) of phenytoin. Although the fosphenytoin injectable product has a salt factor other than 0.92, the content of the fosphenytoin vial is labeled as mg of P.E. or "phenytoin equivalent"; therefore, a salt factor (S) of 0.92 should be used in calculations with this product. The rate of phenytoin absorption following oral administration is slow because of the limited aqueous solubility of phenytoin. This is true regardless of whether the prompt or extended absorption oral products are used.[27] Serum concentrations of phenytoin extended absorption products usually peak 3 to 12 hours after oral administration when given as the usual daily maintenance doses.[27]

Phenytoin is absorbed slowly, and the bioavailability could be less than 100% in patients with short gastrointestinal (GI) transit times.[32] Phenytoin concentrations are significantly decreased in patients receiving liquid dietary supplements (nasogastric feedings) and neonates.[33–35] Presumably, rapid GI motility decreases the apparent bioavailability of phenytoin, although the specific mechanism has not been identified. In some patients receiving nasogastric feedings, phenytoin doses of up to 1,200 mg/day were required to achieve therapeutic concentrations. Discontinuation of the enteral feedings resulted in a significant increase in the phenytoin plasma concentrations. It is recommended that patients receiving nasogastric feedings be closely monitored, because concentrations within the usual therapeutic range are difficult to achieve and maintain. Similar potential problems may occur when phenytoin is administered concomitantly with antacids.[33,36]

The bioavailability of phenytoin is difficult to evaluate because of the drug's capacity-limited metabolism.[37] The slow absorption of phenytoin also tends to diminish the change in concentration following an oral dose. In most patients receiving oral phenytoin, the change in concentration (ΔC) will be about half that observed when giving the drug by the IV route. The slow rate of absorption also results in delayed peak concentrations that occur between 3 and 12 hours after administration of normal maintenance doses. When loading doses of 1 g are administered orally as the extended absorption product, serum concentrations usually peak in about 24 hours, and if the dose is increased to 1,600 mg, the peak may be delayed by as much as 30 hours.[38,39] The time required to achieve the peak concentration can be decreased if a phenytoin "prompt absorption" product is administered.[27] Fosphenytoin can be administered orally, and absorption appears to be relatively rapid and complete with peak concentrations at about 1 hour if conditions are optimal, for example, empty stomach, no delay in gastric emptying.[40] However, the time to peak is still delayed, and the IV route is preferred when rapid achievement of therapeutic concentrations is required.

While the absorption of phenytoin is almost certainly a complex process, one approach the author has used is to assume an absorption rate of approximately 50 mg/hr for the extended absorption product Dilantin capsules. This absorption rate is consistent with the observations stated above and is sometimes useful when estimating a time when the peak concentration will occur following oral administration. In addition, although it is common practice to divide 15 mg/kg loading doses into 5 mg/kg increments administered every 2 hours, there are no studies documenting that this procedure is optimal in terms of the dose size or interval between doses.

VOLUME OF DISTRIBUTION (V)

The volume of distribution for phenytoin in patients with normal renal function and with normal serum albumin concentrations is approximately 0.65 L/kg.[12,41,42] Although the apparent volume of distribution for phenytoin is increased in patients with diminished plasma binding, the loading dose should not be changed because the increase in the volume of distribution resulting from changes in plasma binding is accompanied by equal and opposite decrease in the desired phenytoin concentration. Also, as previously stated, the amount of phenytoin in the plasma represents only a small fraction of the total amount of phenytoin in the body. The approach taken in this chapter is to correct any measured concentrations altered by binding to the concentration that would be observed under normal plasma binding conditions. Under these conditions, a "normal binding" volume of distribution of 0.65 L/kg, which represents normal plasma binding (fu = 0.1), should be used in all computations.

In obese patients, the volume of distribution for phenytoin is a complex relationship between plasma protein binding, lipid solubility, and tissue perfusion. Equation 14.9 is based on a study by Abernathy and Greenblatt.[43]

For obese patients:

$$V_{\text{Phenytoin in L}} = 0.65 \text{ L/kg} \left[\text{IBW} + 1.3(\text{TBW} - \text{IBW}) \right] \qquad \textbf{(Eq. 14.9)}$$

where TBW is the patient's total body weight in kilogram and IBW is the patient's ideal body weight in kilogram.

$$\frac{\text{Ideal Body Weight}}{\text{for Males in kg}} = 50 + (2.3)(\text{Height in inches} > 60) \qquad \textbf{(Eq. 14.10)}$$

$$\frac{\text{Ideal Body Weight}}{\text{for Females in kg}} = 45 + (2.3)(\text{Height in inches} > 60) \qquad \textbf{(Eq. 14.11)}$$

CAPACITY-LIMITED METABOLISM

For most drugs, the rate of metabolism (and/or excretion) is proportional to the plasma concentration. Clearance is defined as the volume of plasma that is completely cleared of drug per unit of time (see Clearance [Cl] in Chapter 1). For first-order drugs, clearance can be viewed as a fixed proportionality constant that makes the steady-state plasma concentration equal to the rate of drug administration (R_A), as illustrated by Equation 14.12:

$$R_A = (\text{Cl})(\text{Css ave}) \qquad \textbf{(Eq. 14.12)}$$

R_A is (S)(F)(Dose/τ). This view of first-order pharmacokinetics, however, does not apply to phenytoin because the clearance of phenytoin decreases as Css ave increases.

The clearance of phenytoin from plasma occurs primarily by metabolism, and the rate of phenytoin metabolism approaches its maximum at therapeutic concentrations. Thus, the metabolism of phenytoin is described as being capacity limited.[5,42,44–47]

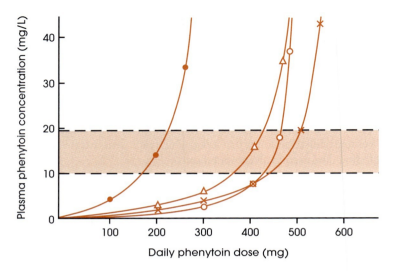

FIGURE 14.1 Changes in steady-state phenytoin plasma concentrations with maintenance dose. Note that for each patient, the plasma phenytoin concentration at steady state increases disproportionately with an increase in the rate of administration, especially as the dose approaches Vm. The patients in the figure represent the following Vm and Km values: *Filled circle*, 300 mg/day, 7 mg/L; *open triangle*, 500 mg/day, 4 mg/L; *open circle*, 500 mg/day, 2 mg/L; and *cross*, 600 mg/day, 4 mg/L. Also note that for patients with a low Km value, the range of doses that result in a Css ave between 10 and 20 mg/L is very narrow.

Capacity-limited metabolism results in clearance values that decrease with increasing plasma concentrations. Therefore, when the maintenance dose is increased, the plasma concentration rises disproportionately[44,48–53] (Fig. 14.1). This disproportionate rise in the steady-state plasma level makes dosage adjustment difficult.

The model that appears to fit the metabolic pattern for phenytoin elimination is the one originally proposed by Michaelis and Menten. The velocity (V) or rate at which an enzyme system can metabolize a substrate (S) can be described by the following equation:

$$V = \frac{(Vm)(S)}{Km + S} \qquad \textbf{(Eq. 14.13)}$$

where Vm is the maximum metabolic capacity or maximum rate of metabolism, and Km is the substrate concentration at which V will be one-half of Vm. When the average steady-state phenytoin concentration (Css ave) is substituted for the substrate concentration (S) and the daily dose or administration rate of phenytoin [R_A or (S)(F) (Dose/τ)] for V,[49,51–53] Equation 14.13 can be rewritten as:

$$(S)(F)(Dose/\tau) = \frac{(Vm)(Css\ ave)}{Km + Css\ ave} \qquad \textbf{(Eq. 14.14)}$$

In Equation 14.14, the "clearance" that makes (S)(F)(Dose/τ) equal to Css ave is a value that will change as the Css ave changes. As a result, there will be a disproportionate change in the Css ave resulting from a change in the administration rate.

$$(S)(F)(Dose/\tau) = \frac{(Vm)}{Km + Css\ ave}\ (Css\ ave)$$

Equation 14.14 can also be rearranged as follows:

$$Css\ ave = \frac{(Km)[(S)(F)(Dose/\tau)]}{Vm - [(S)(F)(Dose/\tau)]} \qquad \textbf{(Eq. 14.15)}$$

In accordance with the original definition of Vm and Km for Equations 14.13 through 14.15, Vm is the maximum rate of metabolism (metabolic capacity), and Km is the plasma concentration at which the rate of metabolism is one-half the maximum. The units for Vm and Km are usually mg/day and mg/L, respectively.

Equation 14.15 illustrates the sensitive and disproportionate relationship between the rate of phenytoin administration and Css ave when the rate of administration approaches Vm, the maximum metabolic capacity. If the maintenance dose was equal to Vm, then Vm − (S)(F)(Dose/τ) would be 0, and Css ave would be infinity:

$$\begin{aligned} Css\ ave &= \frac{(Km)[(S)(F)(Dose/\tau)]}{Vm - [(S)(F)(Dose/\tau)]} \\ &= \frac{(Km)[(S)(F)(Dose/\tau)]}{0} \\ &= [\infty] \end{aligned}$$

If (S)(F)(Dose/τ) is greater than Vm, Css ave will be a negative number, indicating that steady state can never be achieved. Equation 14.15 is, therefore, invalid as a predictor of Css ave when (S)(F)(Dose/τ) is equal to or exceeds Vm.

As can be seen from Equation 14.15, the relationship between steady-state phenytoin concentrations and the maintenance dose can be extremely sensitive. Understanding and being able to use pharmacokinetic parameters for phenytoin helps clinicians make initial dose adjustments and use clinical guidelines more effectively. For example, the following dose increments have been suggested using phenytoin concentrations as a guide: increasing the daily dose by 100 mg/day when Css ave concentrations are <7 mg/L; by 50 mg/day when Css ave concentrations are 7 to <12 mg/L; and a maximum increase of 30 mg/day when Css ave concentrations are >12 mg/L.[54] Although these guidelines are consistent with the usual pharmacokinetic parameters, any increase in dose should be considered carefully in the context of patient adherence and any potential alterations in plasma binding. One should also keep in mind that adding 100 mg/day to patients with a Css ave of 6 mg/L taking 200 mg/day will probably result in a more dramatic rise in the new steady-state phenytoin concentration than for patients with a Css ave of 6 mg/L taking 400 mg/day.

Another factor that can influence phenytoin metabolism and, therefore, the maintenance dose is genetic disposition. The majority of patients (~90%) are genetically classified as normal/extensive metabolizers of phenytoin. Approximately 10% of patients have a CYP2C9 heterozygous variant and are classified as intermediate metabolizers, and about 1% have a homozygous CYP2C9 variant and are classified as poor metabolizers. It is generally recommended that normal/extensive metabolizers start on phenytoin maintenance doses of approximately 5 mg/kg/day and that intermediate and poor metabolizers have their daily dose reduced by 25% and 50%, respectively.[11,55] Knowing that genetic disposition is helpful as a starting point, but careful monitoring of phenytoin concentrations over the first few weeks is important because with this nonlinear drug, small differences in maintenance doses/metabolism can result in significant differences in steady-state phenytoin concentrations.

Because phenytoin can be very sensitive to any change in either the bioavailability or metabolism, relatively minor drug–drug interactions can have significant effects on the steady-state phenytoin concentrations. There are a large number of drugs known to alter the pharmacokinetics of phenytoin (see Table 14.1), but the ability to predict from patient to patient the extent of the interaction is limited. It would be expected, however, that the higher the phenytoin concentration, the more likely that the drug–drug interaction will be significant (see Equation 14.15). Also, although not discussed here, phenytoin can alter the pharmacokinetics of other drugs, most commonly by enzyme induction and as a result of a decrease in efficacy, for example, statins and oral contraceptives.[56,57]

Km values are usually between 1 and 20 mg/L.[48,50–52,91] Vm appears to be between 5 and 15 mg/kg/day in most patients.[48,51,52] The relationship between Km and Vm is not clear, but if one of these parameters is low, the other is frequently low as well.[48,49,52] The average values for Km and Vm are difficult to establish. It is the author's opinion that approximately 4 mg/L for Km and 7 mg/kg/day for Vm are reasonable initial estimates for the average adult patient. While it is true that the elderly are more likely to have decreased serum albumin, may be more sensitive to the side effects, in general, the elderly do not appear to have significantly altered phenytoin pharmacokinetic parameters.[92]

For pediatric patients, the Vm value is usually larger than 7 mg/kg/day. Vm values are approximately 10 to 13 mg/kg/day for children aged 6 months to 6 years, and 8 to 10 mg/kg/day for children aged 7 to 16 years.[93–95] Km values for children vary considerably in the literature; some authors have suggested values of 2 to 3 mg/L,[94,96] whereas others have suggested that a Km value of 6 to 8 mg/L is more appropriate.[93,97] An average Km value of 7 mg/L, although uncertain, is not an unreasonable estimate for children between 6 months and 16 years of ages. While most standard pediatric references suggest starting with maintenance doses of approximately 5 mg/kg/day, most will require maintenance doses of 7 to 10 mg/kg/day. In addition, doses are almost always divided, either every 12 or, in some cases, every 8 hours. The divided dose schedule is in part because of the higher Vm and more rapid metabolism, and, in addition, many pediatric patients can only take either the suspension or the chewable tablets, and both of these products are prompt release and not intended for once-daily dosing.

TABLE 14.1   Drugs That Alter Phenytoin Pharmacokinetics[a]

DRUG	EFFECT ON PHENYTOIN CONCENTRATION	MECHANISM
Amiodarone[58,59]	Increase	Inhibition of metabolism
Antacids[b,60–62]	Decrease	Decreased absorption
Carbamazepine[63,64]	Increase or decrease	Induction of metabolism
Chloramphenicol[65,113]	Increase	Inhibition of metabolism
Cimetidine[66,114]	Increase	Inhibition of metabolism
Ciprofloxacin[67,68]	Decrease	Induction of metabolism
Cisplatinum[69]	Decrease	Decreased absorption[c]
Disulfiram[70,71]	Increase	Inhibition of metabolism
Efavirenz[72]	Increase	Inhibition of metabolism
Fluconazole[73]	Increase	Inhibition of metabolism
Fluoxetine[74]	Increase	Inhibition of metabolism
Folic acid[75–77]	Decrease	Induction of metabolism
Isoniazid[78,79,112]	Increase	Inhibition of metabolism (most significant in phenotypically slow acetylators)
Phenobarbital[d,80,81]	Increase or decrease	Inhibition or induction of metabolism
Rifampin[82]	Decrease	Induction of metabolism
Salicylates[e,83]	Decrease	Plasma protein displacement
Sertraline[84]	Increase	Inhibition of metabolism
Sulfonamides[85,86]	Increase	Inhibition of metabolism and plasma protein displacement
Ticlopidine[87,88]	Increase	Inhibition of metabolism
Trimethoprim[89]	Increase	Inhibition of metabolism
Valproic acid[f,23–25]	Decrease	Plasma protein displacement
Voriconazole[90]	Increase	Inhibition of metabolism

[a]The drugs listed are examples of those that influence phenytoin.
[b]A decrease in absorption is not consistently observed. Both drugs should not be administered at the same time; antacid and phenytoin doses should be taken at least 2-hour apart whenever possible.
[c]There are a number of chemotherapy drugs that appear to alter either phenytoin absorption or metabolism.
[d]The direction of change (if any) for the phenytoin concentration depends on which phenobarbital effect is predominant (i.e., induction or inhibition of metabolism).
[e]Plasma protein displacement results in a decrease in the reported total phenytoin concentration but has little effect on the unbound phenytoin concentration or therapeutic effect. Note that high salicylate concentrations, that is, >50 mg/L, are required for displacement and single daily doses of 80 to 325 mg should not result in altered binding of phenytoin.
[f]Valproic acid displaces phenytoin from its plasma protein binding. It is not clear, however, as to whether valproic acid also inhibits phenytoin metabolism.

CONCENTRATION-DEPENDENT CLEARANCE

The relationship between phenytoin clearance and phenytoin plasma concentration (Css ave) can be seen by studying Equation 14.14 and comparing it to the equivalent first-order equation. In the following first-order equation, clearance (Cl) is a constant value with the units of volume/time and can be thought of as the proportionality constant that makes the Css ave equal to $(S)(F)(Dose/\tau)$.

$$(S)(F)(Dose/\tau) = (Cl)(Css\ ave) \qquad \textbf{(Eq. 14.16)}$$

If we replace Cl in the equation for a first-order drug with the term $(Vm)/(Km + Css\ ave)$, we again have Equation 14.14 as:

$$(S)(F)(Dose/\tau) = \frac{(Vm)(Css\ ave)}{Km + Css\ ave}$$

where the clearance of phenytoin is as follows:

$$Cl_{Phenytoin} = \frac{Vm}{Km + C} \qquad \textbf{(Eq. 14.17)}$$

Note, in Equation 14.17, that the Css ave has been replaced by C to represent any phenytoin concentration. If C is very small compared to Km, clearance will be a relatively constant value (Vm/Km), and the metabolism will appear to follow first-order pharmacokinetics. Most drugs that are metabolized appear to fall into this category (i.e., the concentrations used therapeutically are well below the value of Km). However, if the drug concentration approaches or exceeds Km, clearance will decrease, and the metabolism will no longer appear to follow a first-order process. As clearance decreases with increasing phenytoin concentration, the velocity or metabolic rate will increase, but not in proportion to the increase in plasma concentration (see Fig. 14.1). Because Km values for phenytoin are generally below the usual therapeutic range, nearly all patients will display capacity-limited metabolism for phenytoin.

Alterations in plasma binding will also alter the apparent Km value. This is because Km values are reported as total phenytoin concentration, and it is only the unbound concentration that can cross cell membranes and be available for metabolism. Again, as previously discussed, changes in plasma binding have a profound effect on the total phenytoin concentration but not on the unbound phenytoin concentration. The general approach taken in this chapter is to adjust the measured concentration to that which would be observed under normal plasma binding conditions and to use pharmacokinetic parameters (V, Km, and C or Css ave), which are based on normal plasma binding.

CONCENTRATION-DEPENDENT HALF-LIFE

The usual reported half-life (t½) for phenytoin is ≈ 22 hours[45]; however, the t½ is not a constant value because the clearance of phenytoin changes with the plasma concentration. If Equation 14.17 (the clearance equation for phenytoin):

$$Cl_{Phenytoin} = \frac{Vm}{Km + C}$$

is substituted into the usual equation for half-life:

$$t\tfrac{1}{2} = \frac{(0.693)(V)}{Cl} \qquad \textbf{(Eq. 14.18)}$$

the half-life of phenytoin can be derived:

$$t\tfrac{1}{2}_{phenytoin} = \frac{(0.693)(V)}{Vm}(Km + C) \qquad \textbf{(Eq. 14.19)}$$

Based on Equation 14.19, it can be predicted that the half-life of phenytoin will increase as the plasma concentration increases, an observation that has been confirmed.[46] The value and applicability of this observation are very limited, however.

Limited utility of half-life

The clinical usefulness of the phenytoin half-life is limited because the time required to achieve steady state can be much longer than the usual three to four times the apparent half-life. Likewise, the time required for a plasma concentration to decay following discontinuation of the maintenance dose will be less than predicted by the apparent half-life. The problems associated with capacity-limited metabolism can best be explained by first examining the relationship between the rate of drug administration and elimination for a first-order drug. For a first-order drug, when the rate of administration (R_A) exceeds the rate of drug elimination from the body (R_E), the amount of drug in the body increases and the drug accumulates. If the rate of elimination exceeds the rate of drug administration, the amount of drug in the body will decrease.

$$R_A - R_E = \frac{\Delta \text{ Amount of Drug in Body}}{t} \qquad \textbf{(Eq. 14.20)}$$

The rate of drug elimination for a first-order drug is the product of clearance (Cl) and plasma concentration (C). When the pharmacokinetic parameter, clearance, and plasma concentration are substituted into Equation 14.20, the change in the amount of drug in the body per unit of time (Δ Amount of Drug in Body/t) is small when the product of Cl times C approaches the rate of drug administration. This proportional relationship between C and rate of elimination is the key to the usefulness of t½. Inspecting Equation 14.21:

$$R_A - (Cl)(C) = \frac{\Delta \text{ Amount of Drug in Body}}{t} \qquad \textbf{(Eq. 14.21)}$$

it can be seen that when C is 50% of Css ave, Δ Amount of Drug in Body/t is 50% of R_A; when C is 90% of Css ave, Δ Amount of Drug in Body/t is 10% of R_A. This relationship means that when Δ Amount of Drug in Body/t is small (i.e., very slow rate of accumulation) for a first-order drug, then C must be close to Css ave.

For capacity-limited drugs, however, clearance [Vm/(Km + C)] is not a constant factor. This expression for clearance is inserted into Equation 14.21 to form Equation 14.22.

$$R_A - \frac{(Vm)}{(Km + C)}(C) = \frac{\Delta \text{ Amount of Drug in Body}}{t} \qquad \textbf{(Eq. 14.22)}$$

As C exceeds Km, the rate of drug elimination approaches Vm, which is a fixed value (see Capacity-Limited Metabolism). In such cases, it may be possible to have a rate of elimination that is very close to the rate of drug administration, resulting in a slow yet very prolonged accumulation process.

When R_A is equal to or greater than Vm, accumulation would continue forever or at least until the patient develops toxicity symptoms and phenytoin is withheld. Capacity-limited accumulation problems are most dramatic when the plasma concentration greatly exceeds the Km value. In clinical practice, this means when either the Km value is low or there is a clinical need to achieve high phenytoin concentrations, accumulation will be slow, and time required to achieve steady state will be prolonged.

As an example, consider a patient with a Vm of 300 mg/day, a Km of 4 mg/L, and an R_A of 300 mg/day of phenytoin. Under these conditions, in which the rate of phenytoin administration is equal to Vm, the phenytoin concentrations will continue to increase indefinitely. At a phenytoin concentration of 36 mg/L, the rate of elimination should be 270 mg or 90% of the administration rate, and the accumulation is only 10% of the maintenance dose.

$$R_A - \frac{(Vm)}{(Km + C)}(C) = \frac{\Delta \text{ Amount of Drug in Body}}{t}$$

$$300 \text{ mg/day} - \frac{(300 \text{ mg/day})}{(4 \text{ mg/L} + 36 \text{ mg/L})}(36 \text{ mg/L}) = \frac{\Delta \text{ Amount of Drug in Body}}{t}$$

$$300 \text{ mg/day} - 270 \text{ mg/day} = 30 \text{ mg/day}$$

If this was a first-order drug, the concentration of 36 mg/L would be 90% of Css ave, and there would be very little additional accumulation to the final Css ave of 40 mg/L. However, this is not a first-order drug, and, in the example given, although R_E is 90% of R_A, at a C of 36 mg/L, the final theoretical Css ave would be infinity because R_A is equal to Vm.

Again, the key point with phenytoin accumulation is that in a patient with relatively stable concentrations over several days or even weeks, it can be assumed that the rate of elimination is close to the rate of administration, but unlike with first-order drugs, the phenytoin concentrations may or may not be at or near steady state.

Time to reach steady state

The time required to achieve 90% of steady state can be calculated as follows[98]:

$$t90\% = \frac{(Km)(V)}{\left[Vm - (S)(F)(Dose/day)\right]^2}\left[(2.3\,Vm) - (0.9)(S)(F)(Dose/day)\right] \quad \textbf{(Eq. 14.23)}$$

The t90% is the time required for a patient to achieve 90% of the steady-state plasma concentration on a dosing regimen, given Km, V, and Vm. The units are mg/L for Km, L for V, and mg/day for Vm and dose.

Equation 14.23 assumes that the initial plasma concentration is zero. If the initial plasma concentration is between zero and the steady-state concentration, 90% of steady state will be achieved sooner than predicted by Equation 14.23. Nevertheless, it is still reasonable to use Equation 14.23 to predict the time to achieve steady-state concentrations even when the initial plasma concentration is greater than zero but still relatively low. When therapy with phenytoin is initiated, at first, the drug accumulates rapidly over a short time period so that initial plasma concentrations do not, in most cases, significantly reduce the time required to achieve 90% of steady state. Equation 14.23 should not be used, however, when the initial plasma concentration is greater than the desired steady-state concentration. Because very small differences in Vm or Km or V can result in significant differences in time to t90%, perhaps the most valuable use of Equation 14.23 is to remind us that accumulation can be slow but prolonged, and time required to achieve steady state can be very long, especially when steady-state concentrations are high relative to Km.

When does a phenytoin concentration represent a steady-state value?

When a phenytoin plasma concentration is measured, there is frequently a question as to whether the concentration is likely to represent a steady-state level. This question can be answered using Equation 14.24:

$$90\%\,t = \frac{\left[115 + (35)(C)\right][C]}{(S)(F)(Dose/day)} \quad \textbf{(Eq. 14.24)}$$

where C is in mg/L, and the dose per day is in mg/day. This equation is for adults, and the dose per day should be normalized for a 70-kg patient. The 90% t value, which is calculated by this equation, represents the minimum amount of time the patient must have been receiving the maintenance regimen before it can be assumed that the measured

C is at steady state. Equation 14.24 is relatively conservative in that in its derivation, a Km value of 2 mg/L has been assumed; therefore, the 90% t value is longer than what would be required if the Km value was actually greater than 2 mg/L. Therefore, steady state may already have been achieved in a patient who has been receiving the mainte-nance regimen for a shorter period than calculated in Equation 14.24. Also, note that C in Equation 14.24 must reflect normal plasma protein binding.

Rate of decline: Phenytoin levels

The decline of phenytoin concentration after discontinuation of therapy can be described by Equation 14.25:

$$t = \frac{\left[Km\left(\ln \frac{C_1}{C_2} \right) + (C_1 - C_2) \right]}{\dfrac{Vm}{V}} \qquad \text{(Eq. 14.25)}$$

where C_1 is the initial plasma concentration, and C_2 is the plasma concentration at the end of the time interval t. When both C_1 and C_2 are much greater than Km, the rate of metabolism will approach Vm; therefore, the time required to decline from C_1 to C_2 is primarily controlled by the maximum rate of metabolism (Vm) and the apparent volume of distribution (V).

This equation can be used to estimate the Vm value in a patient who has either intentionally or accidentally received excessive phenytoin doses. In this instance, a decline in the phenytoin concentration can be observed over several days. Care should be taken, however, to ensure that no further drug is being administered to the patient. One must also consider that absorption of phenytoin may continue for several days after an acute overdose or following discontinuation of an oral maintenance regimen.[39,99] Given that the usual Vm is about 7 mg/kg/day for patients who have normal/extensive metabolism and V is approximately 0.65 L/kg, the maximum expected decrease in a phenytoin concentration in adults would be approximately 10 mg/L/day.

$$\frac{Vm}{V} = \frac{7 \text{ mg/kg/day}}{0.65 \text{ L/kg}} \approx 10 \text{ mg/L/day}$$

Again, this assumes the average value for Vm and V, no additional absorption of phenytoin, and that the beginning (C_1) and ending (C_2) phenytoin concentrations both are well above the patient's Km.

There is data to suggest that phenytoin toxic patients with either intermediate or poor metabolism that activated charcoal will increase the rate of phenytoin decline.[100] While the decline in phenytoin concentration was accelerated when activated charcoal was administered, some of the effect may have been because of the sorbitol, adminis-tered with the activated charcoal, acting as a laxative and eliminating phenytoin that remained in the GI tract. Regardless as to a patient's genetic status or whether activated charcoal is to be used, some type of bowel prep should be considered in patients with significant phenytoin toxicity to make sure that no phenytoin remains in the GI tract following withholding the daily oral maintenance dose.

TIME TO SAMPLE

Depending on the disease state being treated and the clinical condition of the patient, the time of sampling for phenytoin can vary greatly. In patients requiring rapid achievement and maintenance of therapeutic phenytoin concentrations, it is usually wise to monitor phenytoin concentrations within 2 to 3 days of initiating therapy. This is to ensure that the patient's metabolism is not remarkably different from that which would be predicted by average literature-derived pharmacokinetic parameters. A second phenytoin concentration would normally be obtained in another 3 to 5 days; subsequent doses of phenytoin can then be adjusted. If the plasma phenytoin concentrations have not changed over a 3- to 5-day period, the monitoring interval can usually be increased to once weekly in the acute clinical setting. In stable patients requiring long-term therapy, phenytoin plasma concentrations are generally monitored at 3- to 12-month intervals.[7,9,101]

The time required to achieve steady state with phenytoin can be prolonged. Therefore, plasma levels of phenytoin should be monitored before steady state to avoid sustained periods of low or high phenytoin concentrations. Nevertheless, these early phenytoin concentrations must be used cautiously in the design of new dosing regimens.

In patients receiving oral phenytoin extended absorption dosage form, especially in divided daily doses, the time of sampling within the dosing interval is not critical because the slow absorption of phenytoin minimizes the fluctuations between peak and trough concentrations. Trough concentrations are generally recommended for routine monitoring. In patients who are receiving phenytoin doses IV, trough concentrations can be adjusted by Equation 14.26 to calculate the average plasma concentration of phenytoin.

$$\text{Css ave} = [\text{Css min}] + \left[(0.5)\frac{(S)(F)(\text{Dose})}{V} \right] \qquad \textbf{(Eq. 14.26)}$$

Following IV administration, sampling within the first 1 to 2 hours after the end of the infusion should be avoided to ensure complete distribution (see Volume of Distribution: Two-Compartment Models in Chapter 1). In addition, if fosphenytoin is administered, there may be an assay cross-reactivity between fosphenytoin, which is an inactive prodrug, and the hydrolyzed phenytoin, which is the active drug.[8]

In patients receiving phenytoin orally as an extended absorption dosage form, the average concentration can be approximated by multiplying the change in concentration anticipated with the IV dose by 0.25. This 0.25 factor assumes that the fluctuation in plasma concentrations following oral administration is approximately half of that which would be expected if the drug were administered IV. It also assumes that the average concentration lies approximately halfway between the peak and trough concentrations.

$$\text{Css ave} = [\text{Css min}] + \left[(0.25)\frac{(S)(F)(\text{Dose})}{V} \right] \qquad \textbf{(Eq. 14.27)}$$

Use of Equation 14.27 is most appropriate when patients are receiving single daily doses of >5 mg/kg and when the phenytoin concentration is <5 mg/L. In patients with phenytoin concentrations >5 mg/L or in those receiving their phenytoin in divided daily doses, use of Equation 14.27 is less critical because the Css peak and Css trough are both relatively close to Css ave.

Question #1   *Calculate the phenytoin loading dose required to achieve a plasma concentration of 20 mg/L in B.F., a 70-kg man. Describe how this loading dose should be administered by the oral and IV routes.*

Equation 14.28 can be used to estimate the loading dose that will produce a plasma concentration of 20 mg/L. If the volume of distribution for phenytoin is assumed to be 0.65 L/kg (see Key Parameters, this chapter), the volume of distribution for B.F. would be 45.5 L (70 kg × 0.65 L/kg). In this case, we are assuming that B.F. has not been receiving phenytoin and, therefore, the $C_{observed}$ or the phenytoin concentration that is present is zero. The salt factor (S) is 0.92 for the oral capsules and injectable phenytoin dosage forms (phenytoin for injection and fosphenytoin), and the bioavailability is 100% (F = 1.0).

$$\text{Loading Dose} = \frac{(V)(C_{desired} - C_{observed})}{(S)(F)} \qquad \textbf{(Eq. 14.28)}$$

$$\text{Loading Dose} = \frac{(45.5\ \text{L})(20\ \text{mg/L} - 0\ \text{mg/L})}{(0.92)(1)}$$
$$= 989\ \text{mg}$$

This loading dose of 989 mg is reasonably close to the usual, recommended loading dose of 1,000 mg or 15 mg/kg.

If this loading dose is administered IV as phenytoin for injection, it should be administered slowly to avoid the cardiovascular toxicities associated with the propylene glycol diluent.[4] A maximum rate of 50 mg/min should be used until the entire loading dose is administered or toxicities are encountered.[1] An administration rate of 50 mg/min for the 1,000-mg dose would mean that the total dose could be administered over 20 minutes. However, because of the potential for cardiovascular side effects, most clinicians administer 1,000-mg loading doses with close monitoring over 45 minutes to 1 hour (i.e., about 15 to 25 mg/min). Also, note that this infusion rate is not size adjusted, and children require much slower infusion rates but are generally given the loading dose at a maximum infusion rate of approximately 1 mg/kg/min but preferably over about the same time as an adult (i.e., 45 minutes to 1 hour). If the dose were to be given as fosphenytoin, the total dose would be the same with a maximum infusion rate of 150 mg/min. If possible, fosphenytoin would be given at a slower rate (e.g., 75 mg/min) with similar cardiovascular monitoring.

If the 1,000-mg loading dose is to be given orally, a 400-mg dose followed by two 300-mg doses (≈5 mg/kg) at 2-hour intervals is recommended so that the entire loading dose is administered over 4 hours. The oral loading dose is divided into three separate doses to decrease the possibility of nausea and vomiting, which may be associated with a single large dose, and to decrease the time to peak concentration.[38,39] When the loading dose is administered orally, slow absorption causes the peak concentration to be delayed and lower than the expected 20 mg/L even if a prompt absorption product is used.[30,38,39] Following oral administration of the extended absorption capsules, the peak concentration is usually about one-half of the value calculated by the IV bolus dose model as predicted by the following equation:

$$\Delta C = (0.5)\frac{(S)(F)(Dose)}{V} \qquad \textbf{(Eq. 14.29)}$$

The above equation is based on the slow absorption associated with the phenytoin extended oral products, and the fluctuation in plasma concentration will probably be more than predicted by Equation 14.29 with the prompt absorption products.[30] Although the peak concentration is very likely to be less than 20 mg/L following oral administration, it is uncommon to give larger oral doses to compensate for the delay in absorption. Oral absorption is relatively unpredictable, and increasing the oral dose is not likely to reliably correct the problem. If it were imperative, from a clinical standpoint, to achieve a phenytoin level of 20 mg/L, it would be best to give the phenytoin by the IV route.

Question #2   *S.B. is a 37-year-old, 70-kg man with a seizure disorder that has only partially been controlled with 300 mg/day of phenytoin capsules. His plasma phenytoin concentration has been measured twice over the past year and was 8 mg/L both times. Calculate a maintenance dose to achieve a new steady-state concentration of 15 mg/L.*

To establish the new daily dose, it is necessary to assume a value of Vm or Km for S.B. The usual approach is to rearrange Equation 14.14:

$$(S)(F)(Dose/\tau) = \frac{(Vm)(Css\ ave)}{Km + Css\ ave}$$

and solve for Vm:

$$Vm = \frac{(S)(F)(Dose/\tau)(Km\ +\ Css\ ave)}{(Css\ ave)} \qquad \textbf{(Eq. 14.30)}$$

If Km is assumed to be 4 mg/L, S to be 0.92 (phenytoin capsules are the sodium salt), and F to be 1.0, then Vm would be 414 mg/day of acid phenytoin.

$$Vm = \frac{(0.92)(1)(300\ mg/day)(4\ mg/L + 8\ mg/L)}{(8\ mg/L)}$$

$$Vm = 414\ mg/day\ of\ acid\ phenytoin$$

To calculate the dose required to achieve a steady-state concentration of 15 mg/L, Equation 14.14:

$$(S)(F)(Dose/\tau) = \frac{(Vm)(Css\ ave)}{Km + Css\ ave}$$

can be rearranged as follows:

$$Dose = \frac{(Vm)(Css\ ave)(\tau)}{(Km + Css\ ave)(S)(F)} \qquad \textbf{(Eq. 14.31)}$$

Using the assumed Km of 4 mg/L and the calculated Vm of 414 mg/day of acid phenytoin, the daily dose required to achieve a steady-state concentration of 15 mg/L would be:

$$Dose = \frac{(414\ mg/day)(15\ mg/L)(1\ day)}{(4\ mg/L + 15\ mg/L)(0.92)(1)}$$
$$= 355\ mg\ of\ phenytoin\ sodium$$

This 18% dosage adjustment should result in a nearly 100% increase in the steady-state plasma level if the assumed Km of 4 mg/L is correct. A daily dose of 355 mg would be difficult to administer; therefore, this initial dosing estimate would probably be rounded off to 350 mg/day, and doses of 300 and 400 mg could be prescribed for alternate days. To aid with adherence, it is a common practice to prescribe the 300-mg dose (odd number of capsules) on the odd days of the month and 400 mg (even number of capsules) on the even days of the month. For those months with 31 days, most clinicians tell the patient to simply take the odd number of capsules 2 days in a row.

An alternative approach is illustrated in Figure 14.2. This method allows one to estimate the most probable combination of Km and Vm values for a patient, given the current dosing regimen and measured average steady-state phenytoin concentration.

If the steps outlined in Figure 14.2 are followed, a Km value of 5 mg/L and a Vm value of 6.4 mg/kg/day (448 mg/day for this 70-kg patient) can be determined. When these values are used in Equation 14.31 (or when Fig. 14.2 is used), a new dose of ≈350 mg/day is calculated. This method of using the "orbit graph" is perhaps slightly superior to the first in which a Km value of 4 mg/L was assumed. This is because the "orbit" method attempts to define the most likely set or combination of Km and Vm values for the patient, given the dosing history and measured phenytoin concentration.

Figure 14.2 can only be used for adult patients, and the phenytoin concentrations used in plotting lines A and B must represent normal plasma protein binding conditions. Figure 14.2 also requires that the phenytoin concentration be an average steady-state value.

Question #3 *Calculate a loading dose that would rapidly increase S.B.'s plasma phenytoin concentration from 8 to 15 mg/L.*

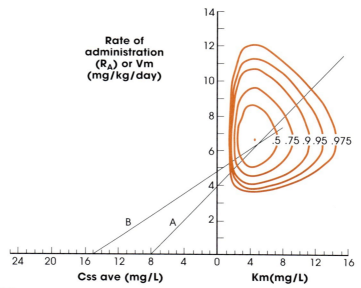

FIGURE 14.2 Orbit graph. The most probable values of Vm and Km for a patient may be estimated using a single steady-state phenytoin concentration and a known dosing regimen. The eccentric circles or "orbits" represent the fraction of the sample patient population whose Km and Vm values are within that orbit. (1) Plot the daily dose of acid phenytoin (mg/kg/day) on the vertical line (rate of administration [R_A]). (2) Plot the steady-state concentration (Css ave) on the horizontal line. (3) Draw a straight line connecting Css ave and daily dose through the orbits (line A). (4) The coordinates of the midpoint of the line crossing the innermost orbit through which line A passes are the most probable values for the patient's Vm and Km. (5) To calculate a new maintenance dose, draw a line from the point determined in Step 4 to the new desired Css ave (line B). The point at which line B crosses the vertical line (rate of administration [R_A]) is the new maintenance dose (mg/kg/day) of acid phenytoin. Line A represents a Css of 8 mg/L on 3.94 mg/kg/day or 276 mg/day of phenytoin acid (0.92 × 300 mg/day of sodium phenytoin) for a 70-kg person. The new steady-state concentration was 15 mg/L. From reference[58], the original figure is modified so that R_A, R_E, and Vm are in mg/kg/day of phenytoin acid. (Reprinted with permission from Burton ME. *Applied Pharmacokinetics: Principles of Therapeutic Drug Monitoring.* 4th ed. Baltimore, MD: Lippincott Williams & Wilkins; 2006.)

Equation 14.28 can be used to calculate an incremental loading dose. If V is 45.5 L (70 kg × 0.65 L/kg), S = 0.92, and F = 1.0, the loading dose required to increase S.B.'s plasma concentration from 8 to 15 mg/L would be:

$$\text{Loading Dose} = \frac{(V)(C_{desired} - C_{observed})}{(S)(F)}$$

$$= \frac{(45.5 \text{ L})(15 \text{ mg/L} - 8 \text{ mg/L})}{(0.92)(1)}$$

$$= 346 \text{ mg}$$

This loading dose should be given in addition to the new maintenance dose of 350 mg/day so that his total dose today will be approximately 700 mg (a new maintenance dose of 350 mg plus the small loading dose of 350 mg).

Question #4   *L.C., a 40-year-old, 80-kg man who has been receiving 300 mg/day of sodium phenytoin for the past 3 weeks (21 days), has a phenytoin level of 14 mg/L. Is this reported level likely to represent a steady-state concentration?*

Administration of the loading dose will result in a more rapid increase of the phenytoin concentration into the desired concentration range while S.B. is receiving the new maintenance dose. If 1 week after the loading dose and starting on the new maintenance dose the plasma concentration is <10 mg/L, it would suggest that the maintenance dose should again be adjusted. If a loading dose is not given and, at the end of 1 week, the plasma concentration is <10 mg/L, it would be difficult to determine why the level was low. One possibility would be that the phenytoin level has not yet reached steady state, and further accumulation on the new regimen would result in levels near our target of 15 mg/L. A second possibility is that our estimates are incorrect, and steady state has been achieved at a lower than expected concentration. In this case, an adjustment in the maintenance dose would be appropriate. Administration of the small or incremental loading dose limits the time when the patient has a low phenytoin level and decreases the risk of a seizure. In addition, it helps us to determine in a relatively short time (1 to 2 weeks) whether we have selected a reasonable maintenance dose for S.B. that, with time, may require at most only minor adjustments as true steady state is achieved.

If phenytoin was eliminated according to first-order pharmacokinetics, 21 days would have been more than enough time for steady state to have been achieved based on a half-life of 15 to 24 hours.

Phenytoin, however, exhibits capacity-limited metabolism; therefore, the time required to achieve steady state is frequently much longer than one would estimate using first-order pharmacokinetic principles. Equation 14.24 should be used to calculate the minimum number of days phenytoin must be administered before it can be reasonably assumed that the measured concentration represents a steady-state level. First, the daily dose of phenytoin should be normalized to 262.5 mg for a 70-kg individual using a ratio of 300 mg/80 kg in proportion to $\times$ mg/70 kg:

$$\left[\frac{300 \text{ mg}}{80 \text{ kg}}\right][70 \text{ kg}] = 262.5 \text{ mg}$$

When this value is placed into Equation 14.24 along with an assumed F of 1 and an S of 0.92, the 90% t value can be calculated.

$$
\begin{aligned}
90\% \text{ t} &= \frac{[115 + (35)(C)][C]}{(S)(F)(\text{Dose/day})} \\
&= \frac{[115 + (35)(14)][14]}{(0.92)(1)(262.5)} \\
&= 35 \text{ days}
\end{aligned}
$$

The calculated 90% t value of 35 days is longer than the actual duration of therapy (21 days), suggesting that steady state may not yet have been achieved. If an additional loading dose was administered within the first 21 days of therapy, or if the Km value is >2 mg/L, then the plasma level obtained at 21 days may actually represent a steady-state concentration. Owing to this uncertainty, additional phenytoin plasma concentrations should be monitored to detect possible accumulation of phenytoin into a potentially toxic concentration range. While the phenytoin concentration may not yet be at steady state, it is unlikely that the phenytoin concentrations will change rapidly even if it is not yet at steady state. Therefore, some time (e.g., 2 weeks or so) could be allowed before additional levels are obtained. In addition, the patient should be educated about the potential side effects so that if they do occur, their health care provider can be contacted.

Question #5   *A.P., a 52-year-old, 60-kg woman, received a 1,000-mg IV loading dose of phenytoin followed by a daily maintenance regimen of 300 mg. Eight days following the initial loading dose, A.P.'s plasma phenytoin level was 11 mg/L. Should her dose be adjusted at this time to achieve the desired phenytoin concentration of 10 to 20 mg/L?*

According to Equation 14.32, the 1-g loading dose administered to A.P. should have resulted in an initial concentration of 23.5 mg/L:

$$C_0 = \frac{(S)(F)(\text{Loading Dose})}{V}$$ (Eq. 14.32)

$$= \frac{(0.92)(1)(1,000 \text{ mg})}{(0.65 \text{ L/kg})(60 \text{ kg})}$$

$$= \frac{920 \text{ mg}}{39 \text{ L}}$$

$$= 23.5 \text{ mg/L}$$

Therefore, the plasma concentration of 11 mg/L 8 days later has declined significantly and, given the nonlinearity of phenytoin, it is unlikely to represent steady state. The concentration of 11 mg/L will probably continue to decline if the maintenance regimen remains at 300 mg/day.

The first step in calculating the new maintenance dose would be to estimate the rate at which the body had been eliminating phenytoin as it declined from the initial concentration of 23.5 mg/L to the observed concentration of 11 mg/L. The amount eliminated per unit of time can be calculated using Equation 14.33, which considers the rate of phenytoin administration $(S)(F)(Dose/\tau)$ and the net change in the amount of phenytoin in the body $[(C_2 - C_1)(V)/t]$.

$$\frac{\text{Amount Eliminated}}{t} = (S)(F)(Dose/\tau) - \left[\frac{(C_2 - C_1)(V)}{t}\right]$$ (Eq. 14.33)

In the above equation, C_1 is the initial phenytoin concentration, which is either predicted or measured, and C_2 is the second phenytoin concentration; t is the time interval between C_1 and C_2. It should be pointed out that both C_1 and C_2 phenytoin concentrations should represent the same plasma protein binding circumstances as V in Equation 14.32 (i.e., 0.65 L/kg). As suggested earlier, the author recommends calculating a plasma concentration that represents normal binding conditions rather than correcting the volume of distribution for the altered plasma binding. Assuming the phenytoin levels represent normal plasma binding, the elimination rate for phenytoin during this 8-day interval would be 337 mg/day of acid phenytoin, which corresponds to approximately 366 mg/day of sodium phenytoin.

$$\frac{\text{Amount Eliminated}}{t} = (S)(F)(\text{Dose}/\tau) - \left[\frac{(C_2 - C_1)(V)}{t} \right]$$

$$= \left[(0.92)(1)(300 \text{ mg/day}) \right] - \left[\frac{(11 \text{ mg/L} - 23.5 \text{ mg/L})(39 \text{ L})}{8 \text{ day}} \right]$$

$$= 276 \text{ mg/day} - [-61 \text{ mg/day}]$$

$$= 276 \text{ mg/day} + 61 \text{ mg/day}$$

$$= 337 \text{ mg/day of acid phenytoin,}$$

or

$$= 366 \text{ mg/day of sodium phenytoin} \left(\frac{337 \text{ mg/day}}{0.92} \right)$$

This elimination rate represents an average of A.P.'s actual elimination rate (>366 mg/day when her phenytoin concentration was 23 mg/L and <366 mg/day when her phenytoin concentration was 11 mg/L). Therefore, a dose of ≈ 360 mg/day should maintain an average phenytoin concentration somewhere between 23 and 11 mg/L.

Question #6   *T.L., a 70-kg patient, initially received a phenytoin loading dose to achieve a concentration of 20 mg/L and then received the usual maintenance dose of 300 mg/day. Ten days later, he had CNS symptoms that were consistent with phenytoin toxicity. A level was drawn and reported as 26 mg/L. What would be a new maintenance dose that would eventually achieve a Css ave of approximately 15 mg/L?*

This problem is similar to the previous example. First, using a volume of distribution of 45.5 L (0.65 L/kg × 70 kg) and Equation 14.33, we can calculate the average rate of phenytoin elimination as the level rose from 20 to 26 mg/L over the 10 days of treatment.

$$\frac{\text{Amount Eliminated}}{t} = (S)(F)(\text{Dose}/\tau) - \left[\frac{(C_2 - C_1)(V)}{t} \right]$$

$$= \left[(0.92)(1)(300 \text{ mg/day}) \right] - \left[\frac{(26 \text{ mg/L} - 20 \text{ mg/L})(45.5 \text{ L})}{10 \text{ day}} \right]$$

$$= 276 \text{ mg/day} - [27.3 \text{ mg/day}]$$

$$= 248.7 \text{ mg/day of acid phenytoin}$$

If, as in the previous example, we administered 248.7 mg/day of acid phenytoin, the final steady-state level would probably be about 23 mg/L or halfway between the initial concentration of 20 mg/L and the level at 10 days of 26 mg/L. In this case, the desired steady-state phenytoin concentration is not between C_1 and C_2, thus additional steps are required to estimate the new maintenance dose that will achieve a Css ave between 10 and 20 mg/L. Using the amount eliminated per unit of time and the average of C_1 and C_2 in the following equation, we can approximate the patient's Vm.

$$Vm = \frac{\left[\frac{Amount\ Eliminated}{t}\right]\left[Km + \left(\frac{C_1 + C_2}{2}\right)\right]}{\left(\frac{C_1 + C_2}{2}\right)}$$ **(Eq. 14.34)**

Assuming a Km value of 4 mg/L, a Vm of 292 mg/day of acid phenytoin is calculated.

$$Vm = \frac{[248.7\ mg/day]\left[4\ mg/L + \left(\frac{20\ mg/L\ +\ 26\ mg/L}{2}\right)\right]}{\left(\frac{20\ mg/L\ +\ 26\ mg/L}{2}\right)}$$

$$= \frac{[248.7\ mg/day][27\ mg/L]}{(23\ mg/L)}$$

$$= 292\ mg/day\ of\ acid\ phenytoin$$

This new Vm of 292 mg/day of acid phenytoin and the assumed Km value of 4 mg/L would then be used in Equation 14.31 to calculate the new phenytoin maintenance dose of 250 mg/day of phenytoin administered as the sodium salt.

$$Dose = \frac{(Vm)(Css\ ave)(\tau)}{(Km\ +\ Css\ ave)(S)(F)}$$

$$= \frac{(292\ mg/day)(15\ mg/day)(1\ day)}{(4\ mg/L\ +\ 15\ mg/L)(0.92)(1)}$$

$$= 250\ mg/day$$

This approach is more uncertain than the example in Question 5 for several reasons. In both cases, we had to assume a volume of distribution and, in both cases, there is likely to be some assay error in the reported drug concentrations. However, in this second case, we assumed a value for Km and, more importantly, we are extrapolating to a new concentration that is outside the concentration range we used to estimate the rate of phenytoin elimination. Given the nonlinear metabolism of phenytoin, any errors are compounded in the extrapolation to a new steady-state concentration range.

In addition, if the following three rules are not met, Equations 14.33 and 14.34 are less likely to accurately predict the patient's rate of metabolism, Vm, and any subsequent maintenance dose adjustments.

1. The time between C_1 and C_2 should be ≥ 3 days.

2. C_2 should be $\leq 2 \times C_1$ if the plasma concentrations are rising. C_2 should be $\geq \frac{1}{2}$ of C_1 if the plasma concentrations are declining.
3. The phenytoin dose, dosage form, and route of administration should be consistent.

If any of the three rules above is broken, Equations 14.33 and 14.34 do not necessarily become invalid, but their accuracy is less than the usual uncertainties associated with phenytoin dose adjustments.

Question #7   *If T.L.'s phenytoin dose was held, what would be the expected time required for T.L. to have his phenytoin level decline to approximately 15 mg/L?*

If T.L.'s dose is held, the decay time can be calculated using Equation 14.25.

$$t = \frac{\left[Km\left(\ln \frac{C_1}{C_2} \right) \right] + (C_1 - C_2)}{\frac{Vm}{V}}$$

If we substitute our literature estimates of 45.5 L for volume of distribution (0.65 L/kg $\times$ 70 kg), 4 mg/L for Km, and our patient-specific estimate of Vm, the time required to decline to 15 mg/L would be 2 days.

$$t = \frac{\left[Km\left(\ln \frac{C_1}{C_2} \right) \right] + (C_1 - C_2)}{\frac{Vm}{V}}$$

$$t = \frac{\left[4 \text{ mg/L}\left(\ln \frac{26 \text{ mg/L}}{15 \text{ mg/L}} \right) \right] + (26 \text{ mg/L} - 15 \text{ mg/L})}{\frac{292 \text{ mg/day}}{45.5 \text{ L}}}$$

$$t = \frac{[4 \text{ mg/L}(0.55)] + (11 \text{ mg/L})}{6.4 \text{ mg/L/day}}$$

$$= 2 \text{ days}$$

Note that because both C_1 and C_2 are well above our estimate of Km (4 mg/L), we could have estimated the daily drop in phenytoin concentration by Vm/V because at these concentrations, the rate of metabolism is relatively fixed at a value approaching Vm. Therefore, this simple method would suggest that the phenytoin concentration should decrease by approximately 6.4 mg/L in 1 day (292 mg/day/45.5 L). Therefore, in 2 days, the phenytoin concentration would fall by 12.8 mg/L, a value close to our desired decline of 11 mg/L (i.e., 26 to 15 mg/L). In either case, it is important that, for our estimates to be reasonably correct, the patient does not continue to receive (or absorb from previously administered oral doses) additional phenytoin. In any case, the patient should be monitored closely. If after only 1 day the symptoms of phenytoin toxicity have cleared, it might be appropriate to initiate the new maintenance dose at that time (to avoid the risk of seizures). If after holding the dose for 2 days the symptoms are still present, it would be appropriate to obtain another phenytoin level to confirm that the levels are declining as we expected. In addition, if the patient was at "high seizure risk" and the toxicity symptoms were not considered serious, many clinicians might elect to simply reduce the maintenance dose and allow the levels to decline slowly.

Question #8 *R.M., a 32-year-old, 80-kg nonobese man, had been taking 300 mg/day of acid phenytoin; however, his dose was increased to 350 mg/day of acid phenytoin, because his seizures were poorly controlled and because his plasma concentration was only 8 mg/L. Now he complains of minor CNS side effects, and his reported plasma phenytoin concentration is 20 mg/L. Renal and hepatic function are normal. Assume that both of the reported plasma concentrations represent steady-state levels and that R.M. has complied with the prescribed dosing regimens. Calculate R.M.'s apparent Vm and Km and a new daily dose of phenytoin that will result in a steady-state level of approximately 15 mg/L.*

The relationship between daily dose and Css can be made linear by plotting daily dose (R_A) versus daily dose divided by Css ave (clearance) for at least two steady-state plasma levels. The graph for R.M. is plotted in Figure 14.3, in which the rate-in intercept (390 mg/day) is Vm and the slope of the line (−2.5 mg/L) is the negative value of Km.

Using these values, the daily dose of phenytoin that will achieve a steady-state level of 15 mg/L can be calculated using Equation 14.31.

$$\text{Dose} = \frac{(\text{Vm})(\text{Css ave})(\tau)}{(\text{Km} + \text{Css ave})(\text{S})(\text{F})}$$

$$= \frac{(390 \text{ mg/day})(15 \text{ mg/L})(1 \text{ day})}{(2.5 \text{ mg/L} + 15 \text{ mg/L})(1)(1)}$$

$$= 334 \text{ mg}$$

The most convenient dose for calculated value of 334 mg/day, administered as acid phenytoin, would be 325 mg/day, which could be administered as the suspension. The suspension is available as 125 mg/5 mL (25 mg/mL) and, therefore, the volume to administer would be 13 mL. The suspension should be shaken vigorously and measured accurately to ensure that the proper dose is delivered. In addition, the suspension is not recommended to be given on a once-daily basis, and the dose should be divided to at least a twice-daily regimen (i.e., 162.5 mg or 6.5 mL twice daily).

If, for the convenience of once-daily dosing, the acid phenytoin dose was to be converted to a sodium phenytoin extended absorption product, the following equation could be used to calculate an equivalent dose)also see Bioavailability [F]: Chemical Form [S] in Chapter 1):

$$\frac{\text{Dose of New}}{\text{Dosage Form}} = \frac{\begin{array}{c}\text{Amount of Drug Absorbed} \\ \text{from Current Dosage Form}\end{array}}{(\text{S})(\text{F}) \text{ of New Dosage Form}} \qquad \textbf{(Eq. 14.35)}$$

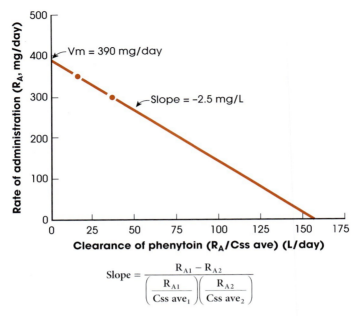

$$Slope = \frac{R_{A1} - R_{A2}}{\left(\dfrac{R_{A1}}{Css\ ave_1}\right)\left(\dfrac{R_{A2}}{Css\ ave_2}\right)}$$

FIGURE 14.3   The rate of administration (R_A) or the daily dose of phenytoin (mg/day) versus the clearance of phenytoin (R_A/Css ave, L/day) is plotted for two or more different daily doses of phenytoin. A straight line of the best fit is drawn through the points plotted. The intercept on the rate of administration axis is Vm (mg/day), and the slope of the line is the negative value of Km.

Assuming S to be 0.92 and F to be 1 for phenytoin sodium, the equivalent dose would be 363 mg.

$$\frac{Dose\ of\ New}{Dosage\ Form} = \frac{334\ mg}{(0.92)(1)\ of\ New\ Dosage\ Form}$$

$$= 363\ mg$$

This dose might be rounded off to 350 mg/day (300 mg alternating with 400 mg given as 100-mg capsules), or 360 mg/day given as three of the 100-mg capsules and two of the 30-mg capsules.

If it were decided to round off the dose to the average dose of 350 mg/day, the expected Css ave can be calculated using Equation 14.15:

$$Css\ ave = \frac{(Km)\big[(S)(F)(Dose/\tau)\big]}{Vm - \big[(S)(F)(Dose/\tau)\big]}$$

Using the patient-specific Km value of 2.5 mg/L and Vm of 390 mg/day of acid phenytoin for R.M., we calculate a Css ave on 350 mg/day of phenytoin sodium of 11.8 mg/L.

$$Css\ ave = \frac{(2.5\ mg/L)\big[(0.92)(1)(350\ mg/1\ day)\big]}{390\ mg/day - \big[(0.92)(1)(350\ mg/1\ day)\big]}$$

$$= 11.8\ mg/L$$

Assuming the concentration of 11.8 mg/L is satisfactory, the patient could be converted from the current acid phenytoin to phenytoin sodium extended absorption. In most cases, the Dilantin capsule product would be used, although there are other forms of phenytoin extended absorption available. However, regardless of which product is used, it is important to remember that phenytoin products are not considered to be interchangeable. If a change in dosage form is to be considered, a careful discussion with both the patient and the patient's provider should take place before any changes are made. It is also recommended that follow-up of phenytoin levels be obtained to ensure that the conversion from one dosage form to another results in the expected outcome.

An alternate approach to plotting the data for R.M. would be to calculate the negative value of Km using Equation 14.36:

$$-\text{Km} = \frac{R_1 - R_2}{\left(\dfrac{R_1}{\text{Css}_1}\right) - \left(\dfrac{R_2}{\text{Css}_2}\right)} \qquad \textbf{(Eq. 14.36)}$$

where R_1 and R_2 represent the first and second maintenance doses, respectively. Css_1 and Css_2 represent the steady-state concentrations produced by these doses. Again, assuming S and F to be 1.0, a value of -2.5 mg/L is calculated.

$$
\begin{aligned}
-\text{Km} &= \frac{R_1 - R_2}{\left(\dfrac{R_1}{\text{Css}_1}\right) - \left(\dfrac{R_2}{\text{Css}_2}\right)} \\[2mm]
&= \frac{300\ \text{mg/day} - 350\ \text{mg/day}}{\left(\dfrac{300\ \text{mg/day}}{8\ \text{mg/L}}\right) - \left(\dfrac{350\ \text{mg/day}}{20\ \text{mg/L}}\right)} \\[2mm]
&= \frac{-50\ \text{mg/day}}{(37.5\ \text{L/day}) - (17.5\ \text{L/day})} \\[2mm]
&= -2.5\ \text{mg/L}
\end{aligned}
$$

The value of 2.5 mg/L can then be used in Equation 14.30 with either of the maintenance doses and the corresponding steady-state levels to calculate Vm:

$$
\begin{aligned}
\text{Vm} &= \frac{(S)(F)(\text{Dose}/\tau)(\text{Km} + \text{Css ave})}{(\text{Css ave})} \\[2mm]
&= \frac{(1)(1)(300\ \text{mg/day})(2.5\ \text{mg/L} + 8\ \text{mg/L})}{(8\ \text{mg/L})} \\[2mm]
&= 393.75 \text{ or} \approx 390\ \text{mg/day}
\end{aligned}
$$

With only two data points, the calculated and graphically determined values for Km and Vm should be exactly the same. Small differences sometimes occur, however, because of differences in mechanical drawing skills or rounding off errors in the calculation.

Question #9 *How long will it take for R.M.'s phenytoin concentration of 20 mg/L to decline to 15 mg/L?*

As with Question 7, the important clinical decision is whether to hold the dose and allow the phenytoin levels to decline as rapidly as possible or to start a new lower dosing regimen and let the phenytoin concentrations decline slowly with time. The decision would be based on a balance between the severity of the phenytoin side effects and R.M.'s seizure risk. The phenytoin half-life will be of no value in predicting the time required for the plasma concentration to decay because the apparent half-life will change as the plasma concentration changes.

The time required for the phenytoin plasma concentration to fall from an initial concentration (C_1) to a lower concentration (C_2), if we hold the dose, can be calculated using Equation 14.25.

$$t = \frac{\left[Km\left(\ln \frac{C_1}{C_2} \right) \right] + (C_1 - C_2)}{\frac{Vm}{V}}$$

For R.M., who has a volume of distribution of 52 L (0.65 L/kg $\times$ 80 kg), a Vm of 390 mg/day, and a Km of 2.5 mg/L, the time required for the initial plasma concentration of 20 mg/L to decline to 15 mg/L will be about 0.76 days:

$$t = \frac{\left[Km\left(\ln \frac{C_1}{C_2} \right) \right] + (C_1 - C_2)}{\frac{Vm}{V}}$$

$$= \frac{\left[2.5 \text{ mg/L} \left(\ln \frac{20 \text{ mg/L}}{15 \text{ mg/L}} \right) \right] + (20 \text{ mg/L} - 15 \text{ mg/L})}{\frac{390 \text{ mg/day}}{52 \text{ L}}}$$

$$= 0.76 \text{ days}$$

This rate of decline assumes that phenytoin will not continue to be absorbed from the GI tract for a significant period following discontinuation of the drug. In the author's experience, however, the initial rate of decline for 1 to 3 days is often less than expected because of prolonged absorption.[39,99]

Question #10 *E.W., a 56-year-old, 60-kg woman, has chronic renal failure and a seizure disorder. She undergoes hemodialysis treatments three times a week, has a serum albumin of 3.3 g/dL, and takes 300 mg/day of phenytoin. Her reported steady-state plasma phenytoin concentration is 5 mg/L. What would be her phenytoin concentration if she had a normal serum albumin concentration and normal renal function? Should her daily phenytoin dose be increased?*

It is critical to carefully evaluate measured phenytoin plasma concentrations in uremic patients because plasma protein binding is altered in these individuals. In patients with normal renal function, about 90% of the measured plasma phenytoin concentration is bound to albumin and 10% is free (fu normal binding $= 0.1$).[12–14,20] Because binding affinity and albumin concentrations are decreased in uremic patients, the fraction of the total phenytoin concentration that is unbound or free in patients with very poor renal function increases from 0.1 to a range of 0.2 to 0.35[12,16–20] (see also Figs. 1.3 through 1.5, and Desired Plasma Concentration in Chapter 1).

Because the fraction free (fu) for phenytoin is increased in uremic individuals, lower plasma concentrations will produce pharmacologic effects that are equivalent to those produced by higher levels in nonuremic individuals. E.W.'s case can be used as an illustration.

Using E.W.'s serum albumin of 3.3 g/dL and her phenytoin concentration of 5 mg/L (Dialysis Patient's Phenytoin Concentration with Altered Plasma Binding) in Equation 14.3, a phenytoin concentration of 11.9 mg/L is calculated.

$$\frac{\text{Phenytoin Concentration}}{\text{Normal Plasma Binding}} = \frac{\text{Dialysis Patient's Phenytoin Concentration with Altered Plasma Binding}}{\left[(0.9)(0.48)\left(\dfrac{\text{Patient's Serum Albumin}}{4.4 \text{ g/dL}}\right)\right] + 0.1}$$

$$= \frac{5 \text{ mg/L}}{\left[(0.9)(0.48)\left(\dfrac{3.3 \text{ g/dL}}{4.4 \text{ g/dL}}\right)\right] + 0.1}$$

$$= \frac{5 \text{ mg/L}}{0.42}$$

$$= 11.9 \text{ mg/L} \approx 12 \text{ mg/L}$$

Therefore, E.W.'s measured plasma phenytoin concentration of 5 mg/L with altered binding is comparable to a concentration of 12 mg/L in a patient with normal plasma binding. That is, we would expect the reported concentration of 5 mg/L to have the same unbound or free phenytoin concentration as a concentration of 12 mg/L, which represents normal plasma binding. The usually accepted therapeutic range for phenytoin in patients with normal binding is 10 to 20 mg/L, and E.W.'s adjusted or normal binding concentration of 12 mg/L would be expected to correspond to the low end of this range. If E.W.'s seizure disorder is well controlled, no adjustment in the maintenance dose is necessary even though the reported concentration of 5 mg/L appears to be well below the usual "therapeutic range." However, if seizures are poorly controlled and phenytoin doses must be adjusted, the comparable plasma concentration for a patient with normal plasma binding (12 mg/L) should be used in all calculations because the values for phenytoin parameters reported in the literature were determined in patients with normal plasma protein binding.

Question #11   *Is it necessary to make dose adjustments or to administer a phenytoin replacement dose following dialysis?*

Using the principles outlined in Estimating Drug Dialyzability under Dialysis of Drugs in Chapter 3, it can be seen that the unbound volume of distribution is very large.

$$\text{Unbound Volume of Distribution} = \frac{V}{fu} \qquad \textbf{(Eq. 14.37)}$$

$$= \frac{0.65 \text{ L/kg}}{0.1}$$

$$= 6.5 \text{ L/kg}$$

Given that the unbound volume of distribution is 6.5 L/kg or 390 L (6.5 L/kg × 60 kg), a very small percentage of the total body phenytoin would be removed during hemodialysis. In addition, there are studies supporting this prediction.[16,17,102] It is also known that dialysis does not change the protein binding characteristics of the uremic patient.[16,17,102] Therefore, doses should not be adjusted for E.W. based on dialysis. Even though the binding has been decreased, it is important to remember that the unbound concentration for the uremic patient is not affected by the decreased albumin, nor the decreased affinity of phenytoin for albumin. Also, changes in plasma protein binding occur within a few days after the development of acute renal failure.[103] Conversely, there is some evidence that following a renal transplant, the plasma protein binding of phenytoin increases rapidly over the first 2 to 4 postoperative days and is almost normal 2 weeks after a successful transplant.[18]

Question #12   *Mr. T.B. is a 60-kg man in the intensive care unit receiving chronic renal replacement therapy (CRRT). His serum albumin is 4.2 and his serum creatinine is 3.8. His CRRT effluent flow is 2 L/hr (1 L/hr of ultrafiltration and 1 L/hr of dialysate). The patient is receiving phenytoin for a seizure disorder. At the start of CRRT, his phenytoin level was 9.8 mg/L. In addition to TB's phenytoin maintenance dose, should he receive an additional CRRT phenytoin replacement dose?*

The answer is possibly. Unlike hemodialysis and plasmapheresis, CRRT does remove some phenytoin. Data suggests that the concentration of phenytoin in the CRRT effluent is approximately equal to the unbound phenytoin concentration in plasma.[104] The amount removed by CRRT would depend on the target unbound phenytoin concentration and the CRRT effluent flow rate. CRRT effluent flow rate usually ranges from 0.5 to 4 L/hr and is continuous until the CRRT is discontinued. In most cases, CRRT is a temporary procedure and is seldom continued for more than a few days to a week.

In order to calculate T.B.'s phenytoin removal by CRRT, we first need to estimate his unbound phenytoin concentration. We could use the reported phenytoin level of 9.8 mg/L and then one of the equations to correct the reported value to a normal binding value (e.g., Equations 14.2 and 14.3). The difficulty is that if TB's renal dysfunction is recent Equation 14.3 for patients on dialysis may not be appropriate and in addition, as previously stated, estimating corrected phenytoin concentrations in critical care patients is difficult. A simpler approach might be to consider that an unbound concentration of 1 to 2 mg/L is associated with normal binding concentrations of 10 to 20 mg/L. Using the middle of the usual targeted unbound concentration of 1.5, we could use Equation 14.38 to calculate a daily phenytoin CRRT replacement dose.

$$\text{Amount of Phenytoin Removed by CRRT} = (C_{\text{UNBOUND}})(\text{Effluent Flow L/hr})(\text{Number of Hours})$$

(Eq. 14.38)

Substituting 1.5 mg/L for the C_{UNBOUND}, 2 L/hr for the effluent flow, and 24 hours for the number of hours in a day, the amount removed per day would be 72 mg.

$$\text{Amount of Phenytoin Removed by CRRT} = (1.5 \text{ mg/L})(2 \text{ L/hr})(24 \text{ hr})$$
$$= 72 \text{ mg/day}$$

Although 72 mg is not a large amount, it could be significant if CRRT is to be continued for several days. Because the duration of CRRT is uncertain, it would be logical to add approximately 70 mg to TB's daily maintenance dose and to adjust the CRRT replacement dose if the effluent flow rate is changed or to discontinue the replacement dose if CRRT is discontinued.

Question #13   *I.A. is a 52-year-old, 77-kg man with chronic renal failure who is receiving hemodialysis three times a week. Because of a seizure disorder, he has been receiving 300 mg of extended absorption phenytoin sodium each evening for the past year. He has had three seizures over the past year and one in the past month. His phenytoin concentration has been reported to be 3 mg/L on several occasions. His serum albumin is 2.7 g/dL, and his SCr fluctuates between 3 and 5 mg/dL. Should I.A. have his phenytoin dose increased? What would you recommend?*

Although a Cl_{Cr} of more than 10 mL/min can be calculated using the creatinine clearance equations, it would not be appropriate to use these equations. When a patient is receiving any type of dialysis, the creatinine clearance equations are invalid (see Creatinine Clearance [Cl_{Cr}] in Chapter 3). Therefore, to calculate I.A.'s phenytoin concentration that represents normal plasma, we should use Equation 14.3 as he is a dialysis patient.

$$\frac{\text{Phenytoin Concentration}}{\text{Normal Plasma Binding}} = \frac{\text{Dialysis Patient's Phenytoin Concentration with Altered Plasma Binding}}{\left[(0.9)(0.48)\left(\dfrac{\text{Patient's Serum Albumin}}{4.4 \text{ g/dL}}\right)\right] + 0.1}$$

$$= \frac{3 \text{ mg/L}}{\left[(0.9)(0.48)\left(\dfrac{2.7 \text{ g/dL}}{4.4 \text{ g/dL}}\right)\right] + 0.1}$$

$$= \frac{3 \text{ mg/L}}{[0.265] + 0.1}$$

$$= \frac{3 \text{ mg/L}}{0.365}$$

$$= 8.2 \text{ mg/L or} \approx 8 \text{ mg/L}$$

The normal plasma binding concentration of 8 mg/L is below the usual target concentration range of 10 to 20 mg/L. Assuming I.A. should have his concentration increased to prevent further seizures, we will need to calculate his Vm using an assumed average value of 4 mg/L for Km and the normal plasma binding concentration of 8 mg/L in Equation 14.30 to calculate Vm:

$$Vm = \frac{(S)(F)(Dose/\tau)(Km + Css\,ave)}{(Css\,ave)}$$

$$Vm = \frac{(0.92)(1)(300\,mg/day)(4\,mg/L + 8\,mg/L)}{(8\,mg/L)}$$

$$= 414\,mg/day\,of\,acid\,phenytoin$$

Note again in the above equation that the Phenytoin Concentration Normal Plasma Binding of 8 mg/L is used and not the observed value of 3 mg/L, which represents altered binding.

This revised Vm estimate of 414 mg/day of acid phenytoin, along with our assumed Km, can then be used in Equation 14.31 to calculate a new maintenance dose of 355 mg/day of phenytoin sodium to achieve a target level of 15 mg/L.

$$Dose = \frac{(Vm)(Css\,ave)(\tau)}{(Km + Css\,ave)(S)(F)}$$

$$Dose = \frac{(414\,mg/day)(15\,mg/L)(1\,day)}{(4\,mg/L + 15\,mg/L)(0.92)(1)}$$

$$= 355\,mg$$

If the patient is started on this new regimen of 350 mg/day (probably as 300 mg on odd days and 400 mg on even days), it will require some time to accumulate to the new steady-state concentration. To avoid the prolonged period of accumulation toward the new steady state, a small loading dose could be administered. This incremental loading dose can be calculated using Equation 14.28.

$$Loading\,Dose = \frac{(V)(C_{desired} - C_{observed})}{(S)(F)}$$

Again the normal binding concentration of 8 mg/L will be used for $C_{observed}$, and the V represents the usual value of 0.65 L/kg or 50 L for this 77-kg nonobese patient (0.65 L/kg × 77 kg).

$$Loading\,Dose = \frac{(50\,L)(15\,mg/L - 8\,mg/L)}{(0.92)(1)}$$

$$= 380\,mg\,or\,about\,400\,mg$$

This small loading dose of 400 mg, if given orally, may not increase I.A.'s phenytoin level to 15 mg/L, but should increase it to above 10 mg/L and shorten the time required for I.A. to achieve his new steady-state concentration on 350 mg/day. Remember that I.A. should receive both his loading dose and his new maintenance dose so that today he will receive a total of about 700 or 800 mg, probably as 300 or 400 mg increments separated by at least 2 hours.

Question #14 *What would you expect the measured or observed phenytoin concentration to be in I.A. when he achieves the new steady-state concentration?*

The value reported by the laboratory can be calculated by placing the targeted normal plasma binding concentration of 15 mg/L in Equation 14.3 and solving for the Patient's Phenytoin Concentration with Altered Plasma Binding.

$$\frac{\text{Phenytoin Concentration}}{\text{Normal Plasma Binding}} = \frac{\text{Dialysis Patient's Phenytoin Concentration with Altered Plasma Binding}}{\left[(0.9)(0.48)\left(\frac{\text{Patient's Serum Albumin}}{4.4 \text{ g/dL}}\right)\right] + 0.1}$$

$$15 \text{ mg/L} = \frac{\text{Dialysis Patient's Phenytoin Concentration with Altered Plasma Binding}}{\left[(0.9)(0.48)\left(\frac{2.7 \text{ g/dL}}{4.4 \text{ g/dL}}\right)\right] + 0.1}$$

$$15 \text{ mg/L} = \frac{\text{Dialysis Patient's Phenytoin Concentration with Altered Plasma Binding}}{0.365}$$

$$(15 \text{ mg/L})(0.365) = \text{Dialysis Patient's Phenytoin Concentration with Altered Plasma Binding}$$

$$5.5 \text{ mg/L} = \text{Dialysis Patient's Phenytoin Concentration with Altered Plasma Binding}$$

This phenytoin concentration of 5.5 mg/L for I.A. would be expected to have the same unbound or free phenytoin concentration as a level of 15 mg/L in a patient with normal binding.

It might also be reasonable to provide the clinicians caring for I.A. with a "therapeutic range" that they could use to compare to the assayed or reported phenytoin concentration. Equations 14.6 and 14.7 could be used to calculate a "therapeutic range" for I.A. that is approximately 3.5 to 7 mg/L.

Using Equation 14.6:

$$\text{Patient's Therapeutic Range with Low Albumin and on Dialysis That Would Be Equal to 10 mg/L} = 10 \text{ mg/L} \times \left[\left(0.9 \times 0.48 \times \frac{\text{Patient's Serum Albumin}}{4.4 \text{ g/dL}}\right) + 0.1\right]$$

$$\text{Patient's Therapeutic Range with Low Albumin and on Dialysis That Would Be Equal to 10 mg/L} = 10 \text{ mg/L} \times \left[\left(0.9 \times 0.48 \times \frac{2.7 \text{ g/dL}}{4.4 \text{ g/dL}}\right) + 0.1\right]$$

$$\frac{\text{Patient's Therapeutic Range with}}{\text{Low Albumin and on Dialysis That Would Be Equal to 10 mg/L}} =$$
$$10 \text{ mg/L} \times [0.365]$$

$$\frac{\text{Patient's Therapeutic Range with}}{\text{Low Albumin and on Dialysis That Would Be Equal to 10 mg/L}} = 3.65 \text{ mg/L}$$

and using Equation 14.7:

$$\frac{\text{Patient's Therapeutic Range with}}{\text{Low Albumin and on Dialysis That Would Be Equal to 20 mg/L}} =$$
$$20 \text{ mg/L} \times \left[\left(0.9 \times 0.48 \frac{\text{Patient's Serum Albumin}}{4.4 \text{ g/dL}} \right) + 0.1 \right]$$

$$\frac{\text{Patient's Therapeutic Range with}}{\text{Low Albumin and on Dialysis That Would Be Equal to 20 mg/L}} =$$
$$20 \text{ mg/L} \times \left[\left(0.9 \times 0.48 \times \frac{2.7 \text{ g/dL}}{4.4 \text{ g/dL}} \right) + 0.1 \right]$$

$$\frac{\text{Patient's Therapeutic Range with}}{\text{Low Albumin and on Dialysis That Would Be Equal to 20 mg/L}} =$$
$$20 \text{ mg/L} \times [0.365]$$

$$\frac{\text{Patient's Therapeutic Range with}}{\text{Low Albumin and on Dialysis That Would Be Equal to 20 mg/L}} = 7.3 \text{ mg/L}$$

Question #15   *Because phenytoin is bound to plasma protein to a significant extent, will a substantial amount of drug be lost during plasmapheresis or plasma exchange?*

Although 90% of the phenytoin in the serum is bound to albumin, the vascular space represents only a small fraction of the total volume of distribution for phenytoin. Of the total amount of drug in the body, only 5% is within the vascular space. Because most of the phenytoin is actually in the tissue compartments, plasmapheresis or plasma volume exchange should not result in a significant loss of phenytoin from the body. Most studies indicate that somewhere between 5% and 10% of phenytoin is lost from the body during plasmapheresis.[105] Of course, if the procedure was to be repeated many times, the cumulative effect could result in a significant amount of drug loss and the requirement of a replacement dose.

Question #16   *S.T. is a 47-year-old, 60-kg man with glomerular nephritis. His creatinine clearance is reasonably good, but he has a serum albumin concentration of 2.0 g/dL. S.T. is receiving 300 mg/day of phenytoin and has a steady-state phenytoin concentration of 6 mg/L. What would his phenytoin concentration be if his serum albumin was normal?*

The fraction of a drug concentration that is bound to plasma proteins is a function of the drug's affinity for the binding sites on the plasma protein and the number of binding sites available. The number of binding sites is proportional to the amount or concentration of plasma protein to which the drug is bound. Phenytoin is an acidic drug and appears to be bound primarily to albumin.[13] The relationship between a phenytoin concentration which is observed (Patient's Phenytoin Concentration with Altered Plasma Binding) when a patient has a low serum albumin relative to the phenytoin concentration that would be observed if the serum albumin were normal is described by Equation 14.2 (also see Desired Plasma Concentration in Chapter 1).

$$\frac{\text{Phenytoin Concentration}}{\text{Normal Plasma Binding}} = \frac{\text{Patient's Phenytoin Concentration with Altered Plasma Binding}}{\left[0.9 \times \dfrac{\text{Patient's Serum Albumin}}{4.4\ \text{g/dL}}\right] + 0.1}$$

The plasma phenytoin concentration that corresponds to a concentration that would be observed if S.T.'s albumin concentration was normal is calculated as follows:

$$\frac{\text{Phenytoin Concentration}}{\text{Normal Plasma Binding}} = \frac{6\ \text{mg/L}}{\left[0.9 \times \dfrac{2.0\ \text{g/dL}}{4.4\ \text{g/dL}}\right] + 0.1}$$

$$= \frac{6\ \text{mg/L}}{0.509}$$

$$= 11.8\ \text{mg/L}$$

The Phenytoin Concentration Normal Plasma Binding value of 11.8 mg/L should be used when comparing S.T.'s phenytoin concentration to the usual therapeutic range of 10 to 20 mg/L or in any of our calculations.

Question #17 *A.R., a 66-year-old, 60-kg man, was admitted to the hospital because of poor seizure control. He had been receiving 350 mg/day of phenytoin acid as an outpatient. On admission, he had a phenytoin plasma concentration of 3 mg/L. Nonadherence was suspected, and a dose of 350 mg/day as sodium phenytoin was ordered. Five days after administration, a second phenytoin level was reported as 18 mg/L. Has steady state been achieved? Is it reasonable to assume that A.R.'s Vm is close to the average values reported in the literature (i.e., 7 mg/kg/day)?*

The usual guideline of three to four half-lives as the time required to achieve steady state does not hold true for phenytoin because its metabolism is capacity limited. The rate of phenytoin accumulation is the difference between the rate of metabolism and the rate of administration. Unlike drugs following first-order elimination, the rate of elimination is not proportional to the plasma concentration. Therefore, the time required to reach steady state can be prolonged. This will be especially true when the plasma concentrations are much greater than Km. After the daily dose of 350 mg for this 60-kg patient is corrected to 408.3 mg/day for a 70-kg patient:

$$\left[\frac{350 \text{ mg}}{60 \text{ kg}}\right][70 \text{ kg}] = 408.3 \text{ mg}$$

Equation 14.24 can be used to calculate a 90% t value of 35.7 days.

$$\begin{aligned}
90\% \text{ t} &= \frac{[115 + (35)(C)][C]}{(S)(F)(\text{Dose/day})} \\
&= \frac{[115 + (35)(18)][18]}{(0.92)(1)(408.3)} \\
&= 35.7 \text{ days}
\end{aligned}$$

A.R. has been receiving this maintenance regimen for only 5 days; therefore, the plasma concentration of 18 mg/L is very unlikely to represent a steady-state condition. Equation 14.33 can be used to estimate the amount of drug eliminated per day.

$$\begin{aligned}
\frac{\text{Amount Eliminated}}{t} &= (S)(F)(\text{Dose}/\tau) - \left[\frac{(C_2 - C_1)(V)}{t}\right] \\
&= [(0.92)(1)(350 \text{ mg/day})] - \left[\frac{(18 \text{ mg/L} - 3 \text{ mg/L})(0.65 \text{ L/kg} \times 60 \text{ kg})}{5 \text{ day}}\right] \\
&= 322 \text{ mg/day} - \left[\frac{(15 \text{ mg/L})(39 \text{ L})}{5 \text{ day}}\right] \\
&= 322 \text{ mg/day} - [117 \text{ mg/day}] \\
&= 205 \text{ mg/day}
\end{aligned}$$

If a Km of 4 mg/L is assumed, a Vm of about 283 mg/day or 4.7 mg/kg/day is calculated for A.R. using Equation 14.34.

$$\begin{aligned}
\text{Vm} &= \frac{\left[\frac{\text{Amount Eliminated}}{t}\right]\left[\text{Km} + \left(\frac{C_1 + C_2}{2}\right)\right]}{\left(\frac{C_1 + C_2}{2}\right)} \\
&= \frac{\left[\frac{205 \text{ mg}}{1 \text{ day}}\right]\left[4 \text{ mg/L} + \left(\frac{3 \text{ mg/L} + 18 \text{ mg/L}}{2}\right)\right]}{\left(\frac{3 \text{ mg/L} + 18 \text{ mg/L}}{2}\right)} \\
&= \frac{\left[\frac{205 \text{ mg}}{1 \text{ day}}\right][4 \text{ mg/L} + 10.5 \text{ mg/L}]}{(10.5 \text{ mg/L})} \\
&= 283 \text{ mg/day}
\end{aligned}$$

or

$$= \frac{283 \text{ mg/day}}{60 \text{ kg}} = 4.7 \text{ mg/kg/day}$$

This Vm value of approximately 4.7 mg/kg/day is less than the average value of 7 mg/kg/day but is not unreasonable, and it can be used as a first approximation of a new maintenance dose. Note that even though C_2 was not $\leq 2 \times C_1$, the mass balance approach can be used as an initial adjustment, and the estimate of 4.7 mg/kg/day is probably a better guess than the literature average of 7 mg/kg/day for A.R.'s Vm.

Question #18 *Why does changing from oral to IM phenytoin for injection result in a sudden and dramatic decrease in phenytoin levels? Is there a difference between phenytoin for injection and fosphenytoin?*

Phenytoin is a relatively insoluble compound that crystallizes within the muscle following IM administration.[106] The phenytoin crystals are slowly absorbed, and the absorption rate is decreased initially. The subsequent decline in the plasma concentration of phenytoin will be more than proportional to the reduction in absorption from the IM injection because phenytoin metabolism is capacity limited. In one study,[97] a change from oral to IM administration resulted in an initial 40% to 60% decrease in the phenytoin plasma level, whereas the metabolite elimination decreased by only 16% to 20%. Therefore, the IM route of administration for phenytoin should be avoided.

Fosphenytoin for injection is a more soluble ester of phenytoin and has a much more reliable and rapid absorption pattern when administered by the IM route than phenytoin for injection. When administered by the IM route, the majority of patients achieve plasma concentrations in the therapeutic range within 30 minutes.[7,107] Whereas IM fosphenytoin is more rapidly absorbed than oral phenytoin, most clinicians prefer the IV route when rapid attainment of therapeutic concentrations is required, regardless of whether phenytoin for injection or fosphenytoin is used.

Question #19 *What effect does phenobarbital have on steady-state phenytoin concentrations? What other drugs might interact with phenytoin?*

Clinically, the addition of phenobarbital does not change steady-state phenytoin concentrations.[81] Phenobarbital, however, may induce the metabolism of phenytoin and, thereby, increase the metabolic capacity of phenytoin (i.e., increase Vm). Furthermore, competition between phenobarbital and phenytoin for the same metabolic enzymes could have the effect of increasing Km. If Vm is increased, phenytoin clearance will increase, and the phenytoin concentration will decrease. Increasing Km will have the opposite effect; therefore, there may be no consistent effect on the phenytoin concentration (see Equation 14.15).

$$Css\ ave\ =\ \frac{(Km)\big[(S)(F)(Dose/\tau)\big]}{Vm-\big[(S)(F)(Dose/\tau)\big]}$$

Similar problems exist in evaluating the mechanism for the increased phenytoin concentrations associated with drugs such as isoniazid, chloramphenicol, and cimetidine.[100–103] In the case of isoniazid, animal data suggest that there is noncompetitive inhibition of metabolic enzymes that reduces Vm.[108] The interaction appears to be more significant in patients who are phenotypically slow acetylators of isoniazid.[108]

Valproic acid, phenylbutazone, and salicylates reportedly displace phenytoin from albumin.[109] This protein displacement would decrease the total phenytoin concentration, but not the free or unbound concentration. Assuming no change in metabolism, the result of the altered binding would be a decreased bound concentration, no change in the free concentration, an increased free fraction, and a decrease in the total concentration, which would be associated with a corresponding and equally offsetting decreased therapeutic range. While monitoring of unbound phenytoin concentrations would seem to be the most logical approach, it is still an uncommon practice.[110]

The number of drugs reported to interact with phenytoin is large[111] (see Table 14.1). Many of the drugs are easily recognized because they are commonly reported to either increase (e.g., carbamazepine) or decrease (e.g., amiodarone) the metabolism of other drugs. Phenytoin is a more complex issue in that because of capacity-limited metabolism, even small changes in either absorption (F) or metabolism (Vm or Km) can result in significant changes in the final steady-state concentration of phenytoin. The potential for even small changes in metabolism to result in substantial changes in the steady-state concentration makes it difficult to predict which drugs will result in clinically significant drug–drug interaction with phenytoin (see Table 14.1).

> **Question #20**   *Ms. A.C. is a 48-year-old Asian woman who was admitted to the emergency department for an acute seizure. She weighs 55 kg. In reviewing AC's medical record, you note that her recent lab results indicated a normal serum albumin and creatinine. In addition, she has had genetic screening and, of note is, that she is HLA-B15:02 negative but is classified as an intermediate metabolizer for CYP2C9. What would you recommend for her phenytoin loading and maintenance dose?*

Because Ms. A.C. is HLA-B12:02 negative, phenytoin is not contraindicated, and if it is decided that it is appropriate, she can be given phenytoin. The phenytoin loading dose is a function of the target concentration and the volume of distribution, and V is not altered by genetics. Therefore, she should receive the standard 15 mg/kg or about 800 mg (15 mg/kg × 55 kg = 825 mg) loading dose. If the loading dose administered IV as either sodium phenytoin for injection or fosphenytoin, the initial phenytoin concentration should be approximately 17 mg/L as calculated by Equation 14.32 (S = 0.9, F = 1, loading dose = 800 mg, and V = 42 L (0.65 L/kg × 55 kg).

$$C_0 = \frac{(S)(F)(\text{loading dose})}{V}$$

$$= \frac{(0.9)(1)(800 \text{ mg})}{42 \text{ L}}$$

$$= 17 \text{ mg/L}$$

Most patients are started on a phenytoin daily maintenance dose of 300 mg (approximately 5 mg/kg/day). Because Ms. A.C. has been identified as an intermediate CYP2C9 metabolizer, her maintenance dose should be reduced by 25%, suggesting a maintenance dose of 225 mg/day. Because this specific dose would be difficult to prescribe, given the dosage forms available, and because we do not know with any certainty that her final maintenance dose will be 225 mg, AC should probably be started on 200 mg/day of extended-release sodium phenytoin. As with all patients starting phenytoin, she will require relatively frequent plasma monitoring over the next few days to a weeks. A.C. should probably have an initial level within 3 days to ensure that our initial dose is approximately correct. If our initial dose was much higher or lower that the dose that will maintain a therapeutic phenytoin concentration, it would be important to identify early that her phenytoin levels were declining or rising rapidly. Assuming her phenytoin level at 2 or 3 days is near our predicted 17 mg/L, the next sample should be in about a week. Then, depending on whether the phenytoin levels appear to be relatively stable, less frequent monitoring would be required. If the phenytoin concentrations are changing significantly, then more frequent monitoring with dose adjustments may be necessary (see Time to Sample and Questions #5 and #6).

REFERENCES

1. Bigger JT Jr, Schmidt DH, Kutt H. Relationship between the plasma level of diphenylhydantoin sodium and its cardiac antiarrhythmic effects. *Circulation*. 1968;38:363.
2. Pyror FM, Gidal B, Ramsay RE, et al. Fosphenytoin: pharmacokinetics and tolerance of intramuscular loading doses. *Epilepsia*. 2001;42(2):245–250.
3. National Institute for Clinical Excellence. Clinical Guideline. October 20, 2004, p. 65. http://www.nice.org.uk/nicemedia/pdf/CG020NICEguideline.pdf. Accessed July 15, 2008.
4. Louis S, Kutt H, McDowell F. The cardiocirculatory changes caused by intravenous Dilantin and its solvent. *Am Heart J*. 1967;74:523.
5. Kutt H, Winters W, Kokenge R, et al. Diphenylhydantoin metabolism, blood levels and toxicity. *Arch Neurol*. 1964;11:642.
6. Lund L. Effects of phenytoin in patients with epilepsy in relation to its concentration in plasma. In: David DS, Prichard NBC, eds. *Biological Effects of Drugs in Relation to Their Concentration in Plasma*. Baltimore, MD: University Park Press; 1972:227.
7. AHFS. Phenytoin. In: McEvoy GK, ed. *American Hospital Formulary Service Drug Information 2002*. Bethesda, MD: American Society of Health-System Pharmacists; 2002:2133–2139.
8. Kugler AR, Annesley TM, Nordblom GD, et al. Cross-reactivity of fosphenytoin in two human plasma phenytoin immunoassays. *Clin Chem*. 1998;44:1474–1480.
9. Yukawa E. Optimization of antiepileptic drug therapy. The importance of serum drug concentration monitoring. *Clin Pharmacokinet*. 1996;31:120–130.

10. Lascelles PT, Kocen RS, Reynolds EH. The distribution of plasma phenytoin levels in epileptic patients. *J Neurol Neurosurg Psychiatry*. 1970;33:501.

11. Caudle RE, Rettie AE, Whirl-Carrillo M, et al. Clinical pharmacogenetics implementation consortium guidelines for CYP2C9 and HLA-B genotypes and phenytoin dosing. *Clin Phamacol Ther*. 2014;96:542–548.

12. Odar-Cederlof I, Borgå O. Kinetics of diphenylhydantoin in uremic patients: consequence of decreased protein binding. *Eur J Clin Pharmacol*. 1974;7:31.

13. Koch-Weser J, Sellers EM. Binding of drugs to serum albumin. *N Engl J Med*. 1976;294:311.

14. Lund L, Berlin A, Lunde KM. Plasma protein binding of diphenylhydantoin in patients with epilepsy. *Clin Pharmacol Ther*. 1972;13:196.

15. Joerger M, Huitema AD, Boogerd W, et al. Interactions of serum albumin, valproic acid and carbamazepine with the pharmacokinetics of phenytoin in cancer patients. *Basic Clin Pharmacol Toxicol*. 2006;96:133–140.

16. Adler DS, Martin E, Gambertoglio JG, et al. Hemodialysis of phenytoin in a uremic patient. *Clin Pharmacol Ther*. 1975;18:65–69.

17. Reidenberg MM, Odar-Cedelöf L, von Bahr C, et al. Protein binding of diphenylhydantoin and desmethylimipramine in plasma from patients with poor renal function. *N Engl J Med*. 1971;285:264.

18. Odar-Cederlof I. Plasma protein binding of phenytoin and warfarin in patients undergoing renal transplantation. *Clin Pharmacokinet*. 1977;2:147.

19. Reidenberg MM. The binding of drugs to plasma proteins and the interpretation of measurements of plasma concentrations of drugs in patients with poor renal function. *Am J Med*. 1977;62:466.

20. Liponi DF, Winter ME, Tozer TN, et al. Renal function and therapeutic concentrations of phenytoin. *Neurology*. 1984;34:395.

21. Kiang, TK, Ensom MH. A comprehensive review on the predictive performance of the Sheiner-Tozer derivative equations for the correction of phenytoin concentrations. *Ann Pharmacotherap*. 2016;50(4):311–325.

22. Sadeghi K, Hadi F, Ahmadi A. Total phenytoin concentration is not well correlated with active free drug in critically-ill head trauma patients. *J Res Pharm Pract*. 2013;2(3):105–109.

23. Mattson RH, Cramer JA, Williamson PD, et al. Valproic acid in epilepsy: clinical and pharmacological effects. *Ann Neurol*. 1978;3:20–25.

24. Monks A, Richens A. Effect of single dose of sodium valproate on serum phenytoin levels and protein binding in epileptic patients. *Clin Pharmacol Ther*. 1980;27:89–95.

25. Kerrick JM, Wolff DL, Graves NM. Predicting unbound phenytoin concentrations in patients receiving valproic acid: a comparison of two prediction methods. *Ann Pharmacother*. 1995;29:470–474.

26. Jusko WJ, Koup JR, Alvan G. Nonlinear assessment of phenytoin bioavailability. *J Pharmacokinet Biopharm*. 1976;4:327.

27. Gugler R, Manion CV, Azarnoff DL. Phenytoin: pharmacokinetics and bioavailability. *Clin Pharmacol Ther*. 1976;19:135.

28. Wilder BJ, Leppik I, Hietpas TJ, et al. Effect of food on absorption of Dilantin Kapseals and Myland extended phenytoin sodium capsules. *Neurology*. 2001;57(4):571–573, 582–589.

29. Rosenbaum DH, Rowan AJ, Tuchman L, et al. Comparative bioavailability of generic phenytoin and Dilantin. *Epilepsia*. 1994;35:656–660.

30. Goff DA, Spunt AL, Jung D, et al. Absorption characteristics of three phenytoin sodium products after administration of oral loading doses. *Clin Pharm*. 1984;3:634–638.

31. Jankovic SM, Ignjatovic RD. Is bioavailability altered in generic vs brand anticonvulsants? *Expert Opin Drug Metab Toxicol*. 2015;11(3):329–332.

32. Cacek AT. Review of alterations in oral phenytoin bioavailability associated with formulation, antacids, and food. *Ther Drug Monit*. 1986;8:166.

33. Bauer LA. Interference of oral phenytoin absorption by continuous nasogastric feedings. *Neurology*. 1982;32:570.

34. Faraji B, Yu PP. Serum phenytoin levels of patients on gastrostomy tube feeding. *J Neurosci Nurs*. 1998;30:55–59.

35. Doak KK, Haas CE, Dunnigan KJ, et al. Bioavailability of phenytoin acid and phenytoin sodium with enteral feedings. *Pharmacotherapy.* 1998;18:637–645.

36. Carter BL, Garnett WR, Pellock JM, et al. Effect of antacids on phenytoin bioavailability. *Ther Drug Monit.* 1981;3(4):33–40.

37. Neuvonen PJ. Bioavailability of phenytoin: clinical pharmacokinetic and therapeutic implications. *Clin Pharmacokinet.* 1978;3:20.

38. Wilder BJ, Serrano EE, Ramsay RE. Plasma diphenylhydantoin levels after loading and maintenance doses. *Clin Pharmacol Ther.* 1973;14:797.

39. Jung D, Powell JR, Walson P, et al. Effect of dose on phenytoin absorption. *Clin Pharm Ther.* 1980;28:479.

40. Kaucher KA, Acquisto NM, Rao GG, et al. Relative bioavailability of orally administered fosphenytoin sodium injection compared with phenytoin sodium injection in healthy volunteers. *Pharmacotherapy.* 2015;35(5):482–488.

41. Havidberg E, Dam M. Clinical pharmacokinetics of anticonvulsants. *Clin Pharmacokinet.* 1976;1:151.

42. Glazko AJ, Chang T, Baukema J, et al. Metabolic disposition of diphenylhydantoin in normal human subjects following intravenous administration. *Clin Pharmacol Ther.* 1969;10:498.

43. Abernathy DR, Greenblatt DJ. Phenytoin disposition in obesity: determination of loading dose. *Arch Neurol.* 1985;42:568–571.

44. Bochner F, Hooper WD, Tyrer JH, et al. Effects of dosage increments on blood phenytoin concentrations. *J Neurol Neurosurg Psychiatry.* 1972;35:873.

45. Arnold K, Gerber N. The rate of decline of diphenylhydantoin in human plasma. *Clin Pharmacol Ther.* 1970;11:121.

46. Houghton GW, Richens A. Rate of elimination of tracer doses of phenytoin at different steady-state serum phenytoin concentrations in epileptic patients. *Br J Clin Pharmacol.* 1974;1:155.

47. Lund L, Alvan G, Berlin A, et al. Pharmacokinetics of single and multiple doses of phenytoin in man. *Eur J Clin Pharmacol.* 1974;7:81.

48. Mawer GE, Mullen PW, Rodgers M, et al. Phenytoin dose adjustments in epileptic patients. *Br J Clin Pharmacol.* 1974;1:163.

49. Lambie DG, Johnson RH, Nanda RN, et al. Therapeutic and pharmacokinetic effects of increasing phenytoin in chronic epileptics on multiple drug therapy. *Lancet.* 1976;2:386.

50. Richens A. A study of the pharmacokinetics of phenytoin (diphenylhydantoin) in epileptic patients, and the development of a nomogram for making dose increments. *Epilepsia.* 1975;16:627.

51. Ludden TM, Allen JP, Valutsky WA, et al. Individualization of phenytoin dosage regimens. *Clin Pharmacol Ther.* 1977;21:287.

52. Martin E, Tozer TN, Sheiner LB, et al. The clinical pharmacokinetics of phenytoin. *J Pharmacokinet Biopharm.* 1977;5:579.

53. Mullen PW. Optimal phenytoin therapy: a new technique for individualizing dosage. *Clin Pharmacol Ther.* 1978;23:228.

54. Privitera MD. Clinical rules for phenytoin dosing. *Ann Pharmacother.* 1993;27:1169–1173.

55. Franco V, Perucca E. CYP2C0 polymorphisms and phenytoin metabolism: implications for adverse effects. *Clin Toxicol.* 2015;53(2):131–133.

56. Khandwala HM. Lipid lowering inefficiency of high-dose statin therapy due to concurrent use of phenytoin. *South Med J.* 2006;99:1385–1387.

57. Thomas SV. Management of epilepsy and pregnancy. *J Post Grad Med.* 2006;52:57–64.

58. Nolan PE Jr, Marcus FI, Hoyer GL, et al. Pharmacokinetic interaction between intravenous phenytoin and amiodarone in healthy volunteers. *Clin Pharmacol Ther.* 1989;46:43–50.

59. Shackleford EJ, Watson FT. Amiodarone–phenytoin interaction. *Drug Intell Clin Pharm.* 1987;21:921.

60. Garrett WR, Carter BL, Pellock JM. Bioavailability of phenytoin administered with antacids. *Ther Drug Monit.* 1979;1:435–437.

61. O'Brien WM, Orme ML, Breckenridge AM. Failure of antacids to alter the pharmacokinetics of phenytoin. *Br J Clin Pharmacol.* 1978;6:276–277.

62. Smart HL, Somerville KW, Williams J, et al. The effects of sucralfate upon phenytoin absorption in man. *Br J Clin Pharmacol.* 1985;20:238–240.

63. Hansen JM, Siersbaek-Nielsen K, Skovsted L. Carbamazepine-induced acceleration of diphenylhydantoin and warfarin metabolism in man. *Clin Pharmacol Ther.* 1971;12:539–543.

64. Brown TR, Szabo GK, Evans JE, et al. Carbamazepine increases phenytoin serum concentrations and reduces phenytoin clearance. *Neurology.* 1988;38:1146–1150.

65. Harper JM, Yost RL, Stewart RB, et al. Phenytoin–chloramphenicol interaction: a retrospective study. *Drug Intell Clin Pharm.* 1979;13:425–429.

66. Phillips P, Hansky J. Phenytoin toxicity secondary to cimetidine administration. *Med J Aust.* 1984;141:602.

67. Pollak PT, Slayter KL. Hazards of doubling phenytoin dose in the face of an unrecognized interaction with ciprofloxacin. *Ann Pharmacother.* 1997;31:61–64.

68. Dillard ML. Ciprofloxacin-phenytoin interaction. *Ann Pharmacother.* 1992;26:263.

69. Sylvester RK, Lewis FB, Caldwell KC, et al. Impaired phenytoin bioavailability secondary to cisplatinum, vinblastine and bleomycin. *Ther Drug Monit.* 1984;6:302–305.

70. Olesen OV. Disulfiram (Antabuse) as inhibitor of phenytoin metabolism. *Acta Pharmacol Toxicol (Copenh).* 1966;24:317–322.

71. Brown CG, Kaminsky MJ, Feroli ER, et al. Delirium with phenytoin and disulfiram administration. *Ann Emerg Med.* 1983;12:310–313.

72. Robertson SM, Penzak SR, Lane J, et al. A potentially significant interaction between efavirenz and phenytoin: a case report and review of the literature. *Clin Infect Dis.* 2005;15:e15–e18.

73. Blum RA, Wilton JH, Hilloigoss DM, et al. Effect of fluconazole on the disposition of phenytoin. *Clin Pharmacol Ther.* 1991;49:420–425.

74. Jalil P. Toxic reaction following the combined administration of fluoxetine and phenytoin: two case reports. *J Neurol Neurosurg Psychiatry.* 1992;55:412.

75. Lewis DP, Van Dyke DC, Willhite LA, et al. Phenytoin-folic acid interaction. *Ann Pharmacother.* 1995;29:726–735.

76. Seligmann H, Potasman I, Weller B, et al. Phenytoin-folic acid interactions: a lesson to be learned. *Clin Neuropharmacol.* 1999;22:268–272.

77. Berg MJ, Stumbo PJ, Chenard CA, et al. Folic acid improves phenytoin pharmacokinetics. *J Am Diet Assoc.* 1995;95:352–356.

78. Miller RR, Porter J, Greenblatt DJ. Clinical importance of the interaction of phenytoin and isoniazid. *Chest.* 1979;75:356–358.

79. Brennan RW, Dehejia H, Kutt H, et al. Diphenylhydantoin intoxication attendant to slow inactivation of isoniazid. *Neurology.* 1970;20:687–693.

80. Kutt H, Haynes J, Verebely K, et al. The effect of phenobarbital on plasma diphenylhydantoin level and metabolism in man and in rat liver microsomes. *Neurology.* 1969;19:611–616.

81. Morselli PL, Rizzo M, Garaltini S, et al. Interaction between phenobarbital and diphenylhydantoin in animals and in epileptic patients. *Ann N Y Acad Sci.* 1971;179:88–107.

82. Kay L, Kampmann JP, Svendsen TL, et al. Influence of rifampicin and isoniazid on the kinetics of phenytoin. *Br J Clin Pharmacol.* 1985;20:323–326.

83. Odar-Cederlöf I, Borga O. Impaired plasma protein binding of phenytoin in uremia and displacement effect of salicylic acid. *Clin Pharmacol Ther.* 1976;20:36–47.

84. Haselberger MB, Freedman LS, Tolbert S. Elevated serum phenytoin concentrations associated with coadministration of sertraline. *J Clin Psychopharmacol.* 1997;17:107–109.

85. Lumholtz B, Siersbaek-Nielsen K, Skovsted L, et al. Sulfamethizole-induced inhibition of diphenylhydantoin, tolbutamide and warfarin metabolism. *Clin Pharmacol Ther.* 1975;17:731–734.

86. Lunde PK, Rane A, Yaffe SJ. Plasma protein binding of diphenylhydantoin in man. Interaction with other drugs and the effect of temperature and plasma dilution. *Clin Pharmacol Ther.* 1970;11:846–855.

87. Privitera M, Welty TE. Acute phenytoin toxicity followed by seizure breakthrough from a ticlopidine-phenytoin interaction. *Arch Neurol.* 1996;53:1191.

88. Donahue S, Flockhart, DA, Abernethy, DR. Ticlopidine inhibits phenytoin clearance. *Clin Pharmacol Therap*. 1999;66:563–568.

89. Hansen JM, Kampmann JP, Siersbaek-Nielsen K, et al. The effect of different sulfonamides on phenytoin metabolism in man. *Acta Med Scand Suppl*. 1979;624:106–110.

90. Purkins L, Wood N, Ghahramani P, et al. Coadministration of voriconazole and phenytoin: pharmacokinetic interaction, safety, and toleration. *Br J Clin Pharmacol*. 2003;56:37–44.

91. Atkinson AJ Jr, Shaw JM. Pharmacokinetic study of a patient with diphenylhydantoin toxicity. *Clin Pharmacol Ther*. 1973;14:521.

92. Ahn JE, Cloyd JC, Brundage RC, et al. Phenytoin half-life and clearance during maintenance therapy in adults and elderly patients with epilepsy. *Neurology*. 2008;71:38–43.

93. Bauer LA, Blouin RA. Phenytoin Michaelis-Menten pharmacokinetics in Caucasian pediatric patients. *Clin Pharmacokinet*. 1983;8:545.

94. Grasela TH, Sheiner LB, Rambeck B, et al. Steady-state pharmacokinetics of phenytoin from routinely collected patient data. *Clin Pharmacokinet*. 1983;8:355.

95. Dodson WE. Nonlinear kinetics of phenytoin in children. *Neurology*. 1982;32:42–48.

96. Chiba K, Ishizaki T, Miura H, et al. Michaelis-Menten pharmacokinetics of diphenylhydantoin and application in the pediatric age patient. *J Pediatr*. 1980;96:479.

97. Wilder BJ, Serrano EE, Ramsey E, et al. A method for shifting from oral to intramuscular diphenylhydantoin administration. *Clin Pharmacol Ther*. 1974;16:507.

98. Tozer TN, Winter ME. Phenytoin. In: Burton ME, Evans WE, Shaw LM, et al, eds. *Applied Pharmacokinetics: Principles of Therapeutic Drug Monitoring*. 4th ed. Baltimore, MD, Lippincott Williams and Wilkins; 2006.

99. Wilder BJ, Buchanan RA, Serrano EE. Correlation of acute diphenylhydantoin intoxication with plasma levels and metabolite excretion. *Neurology*. 1973;23:1329.

100. Chan BS, Sellors K, Chiew AL, et al. Use of multi-dose activated charcoal in phenytoin toxicity secondary to genetic polymorphism. *Clin Toxicol (Phila)*. 2015;53(2):131–133.

101. Warner A, Privitera M, Bates D. Standards of laboratory practice: antiepileptic drug monitoring. *Clin Chem*. 1998;44:1085–1095.

102. Martin E, Gambertoglio JG, Adler DS, et al. Removal of phenytoin by hemodialysis in uremic patients. *JAMA*. 1977;238:1750–1753.

103. Andreasen F, Jakobsen P. Determination of furosemide in blood plasma and its binding to proteins in normal plasma and in plasma from patients with acute renal failure. *Acta Pharmacol Toxicol (Copenh)*. 1974;35:49.

104. Oltrogge KM, Peppard WJ, Saleh M, et al. Phenytoin removal by continuous venovenous hemofiltraton. *Ann Pharmacother*. 2013;47(9):1218–1222.

105. Matzke GR. Does plasma exchange alter drug therapy? [editorial]. *Clin Pharm*. 1984;3:421.

106. Wilensky AJ, Lowden JA. Inadequate serum levels after intramuscular administration of diphenylhydantoin. *Neurology*. 1973;23:318.

107. Uthman BM, Wilder BJ, Ramsay RE. Intramuscular use of fosphenytoin: an overview. *Neurology*. 1996;46(6 suppl 1):S24–S28.

108. Kutt H, Verebely K, McDowell F. Inhibition of diphenylhydantoin metabolism in rats and in rat liver microsomes by antitubercular drugs. *Neurology*. 1968;18:706.

109. Richens A, Dunlop A. Serum phenytoin levels in the management of epilepsy. *Lancet*. 1975;2:247.

110. Dasgupta A. Usefulness of monitoring free (unbound) concentrations of therapeutic drugs in patient management. *Clin Chim Acta*. 2007;377:1–13.

111. e Facts and Comparison eAnswers [electronic resource] Check Interactions. http://online.factsand comparisons.com.ucsf.idm.oclc.org/index.aspx. Accessed May 17, 2016).

112. Kutt H, Winters W, McDowell FH. Depression of parahydroxylation of diphenylhydantoin by antituberculosis chemotherapy. *Neurology*. 1966;16:594.

113. Rose JQ, Choi HK, Schentag JJ, et al. Intoxication caused by interaction of chloramphenicol and phenytoin. *JAMA*. 1977;237:2630.

114. Bartle WR, Walker SE, Shapero T. Dose-dependent effect of cimetidine on phenytoin kinetics. *Clin Pharmacol Ther*. 1983;33:649.

15

VALPROIC ACID

Irving Steinberg

Irving Steinberg

Learning Objectives

By the end of the valproic acid chapter, the learner shall be able to:

1. Assess bioavailability factors and differences in absorption rates of various dosage forms of valproic acid, and the impact on therapeutic choices and dosing strategies.
2. Describe the therapeutic concentration range of valproic acid and the specific target concentrations for each indication.
3. Comprehend all clinical and pharmacokinetic aspects of the saturable protein binding of valproic acid, execute proper interpretation of serum concentrations in the context of changes in protein binding and drug clearance, and calculate a free valproic acid level, given a total drug level and albumin concentration or binding displacing drug.
4. Understand the volume of distribution range in various populations, the factors that impact these values, and calculate the serum concentration resulting from a loading dose.
5. Elucidate the varied metabolic pathways of valproic acid, the patient–drug interaction (and relevant mechanism), pharmacogenetic factors that influence its clearance, and active/toxic metabolite production. Describe typical clearance rates and elimination half-life values in various patient groups.
6. Calculate the clearance of valproic acid given a steady-state level, or using two levels within a dosage interval, and construct a dosage regimen to meet therapeutic levels and pharmacologic success.
7. Describe the impact of the presence of an interacting drug or changes in protein binding on clearance.
8. Detail the concentration- or dose-related adverse effects of valproic acid.
9. Utilize population pharmacokinetic models to calculate parameter estimates and initial and revised valproic acid dosage regimens.

Valproic acid (VPA), a simple branch-chain aliphatic acid, is among the most versatile central nervous system (CNS) active drugs in the pharmacopeia, and whose clinical uses and dosing strategies continue to be explored and refined.[1] It remains a drug of choice for various generalized and focal epilepsy disorders (classic and atypical absence, tonic–clonic, atonic and myoclonic seizures, Dravet syndrome, juvenile myoclonic epilepsy, and focal onset seizures),[2] as well as approved use in bipolar disorder treatment and migraine prophylaxis. The unusual nature of VPA is highlighted by:

a. concentration-dependent protein binding within the therapeutic range, and dose-dependent pharmacokinetic parameters[3,4];
b. large variability in concentration to dose ratio that depends on numerous demographic and clinical factors[5,6];
c. a great multitude of metabolic pathways with primary phase 1 and phase 2 reactions whose balance is age dependent and genetically determined[7];
d. significant adverse effects that are concentration- or dose dependent.

Drug interactions are numerous and mostly feature inhibiting the clearance of other hepatically eliminated drugs via cytochrome p450 and glucuronidation mechanisms. Likewise, other such medicines and genetic polymorphisms may interfere with the clearance of VPA, and increase its adverse event risk profile.

MECHANISM OF ACTION (MOA)

Enhanced inhibitory neurotransmission by γ-amino butyric acid by VPA is done via increased synthesis, and decreased degradation and turnover.[8] Additionally, anti-seizure effects derive from blockade of voltage-gated sodium channels and calcium channels. Likely, the effects on serotonergic and dopaminergic receptor transmission modulate the benefits seen in migraine prophylaxis and the treatment of bipolar disease, depression, and other psychiatric and mood disorders. The histone deacetylase inhibition observed with VPA is responsible for the encouraging experimental and clinical data seen with this drug against certain forms of cancer.[9]

DOSAGE FORMS AND ABSORPTION

VPA is absorbed through the small intestine, and delayed- and extended-release forms are designed to extend the dosage interval and bypass the stomach to reduce dyspepsia. The liquid and tablet forms have a more than 10-fold higher absorption rate constant than the extended-release forms and peak at 1 to 3 hours after ingestion.[10] The delayed-release divalproex sodium (which combines equal amounts of VPA and sodium valproate) has a lag time (Tlag) of 2 hours and then releases quickly for small intestinal absorption at a rapid rate much like the liquid-filled capsule. The extended-release form of divalproex slowly absorbs with time-to-peak of 8 to 16 hours (ka = 0.2) and provides for efficient 24 hours dosing in adolescents and adults. For children, beyond the available liquid (ka = 4), tablet (ka = 4), and capsule (ka = 4) where three to four daily doses are needed to sustain adequate trough levels, the oversized sprinkle capsule (ka = 1.2, Tlag = 1 hour) provides sufficiently slow release to allow twice-daily dosing. Complete bioavailability is evident for all the dosage forms except the extended release where 80% to 90% bioavailability is seen.[10] Co-ingested food moderately lengthens the Tmax for the sprinkle capsule and can double it for the delayed-release tablet. Rectal administration of the syrup or suppositories can provide an alternative route to obtain therapeutic plasma levels.[11]

Male and female adults differ in disposition for sustained-release valproate, because the concentration to dose ratio was observed as higher in adult females than in males.[5] This is likely less to do with differences in intrinsic hepatic clearance than the amount of enterohepatic recirculation, which is twice as high in females than in males. This manifests in a larger area under the curve (AUC) for an equivalent dose and a significant "second peak" in females.[12]

PROTEIN BINDING

Although proportional serum protein binding is present for the great majority of drugs that bind primarily to albumin, VPA exhibits saturable binding within the therapeutic concentration range, because the molar concentration of VPA approaches and exceeds that of its binding protein, albumin.[3,4,6] When evaluated after intravenous (IV) dosing and normal albumin levels, the unbound fraction for VPA was variable with the total serum concentration, demonstrating saturable binding to albumin, as has been consistently reported. Binding percentages ranging from 5% to 19%[13] and 3.9% to 20.6%[14] have been reported in children when normal albumin binding capacity and affinity is present; the latter over a sixfold range of total VPA concentrations.[14] Nonlinear approaches to model protein binding based on a maximum binding site concentration and dissociation constant show VPA binding ranging from 8.5% at total concentrations of 50 mg/L, 11% at 75 mg/L, 15% at 100 mg/L, and 27.2% at 150 mg/L.[15] Likewise, elderly patients showed an unbound fraction of 10%, 13%, and 17.4% at VPA daily doses of 500, 1,000, and 1,500 mg, respectively.[4] In vitro studies show the increase in unbound fraction with lower human serum albumin concentrations, with a threefold increase observed when the albumin concentration was varied from 4 to 2 g/dL.[16] Brain-to-plasma concentration ratios follow similarly to the free fraction of VPA, and the variability is similar to that of the fourfold range of serum protein binding of VPA in humans.[17]

Binding of VPA is also subject to displacement interactions and is, as expected, decreased when hypoalbuminemia exists. Maximum binding capacity is lower at the extremes of age in infants and the elderly, with lower albumin levels more typical in these age groups.[18,19] The elderly can also have reduced affinity for binding,[20] likely because of higher serum-free fatty acid concentrations, and as is seen with correlations of free fatty acid content and unbound fraction of VPA in diabetes.[21] Therefore, unbound concentrations will be higher for a given total concentration in the elderly than that in younger adults and children.[21] The unbound fraction of VPA increases in late pregnancy and in patients with renal disease, chronic liver disease, nephrotic syndrome, protein-losing enteropathy, traumatic brain injury, critical illness, and other conditions associated with low albumin concentrations. There are linear and nonlinear equations to estimate the unbound fraction or free concentration of VPA taking into account hypoalbuminemia, age, concentration dependence, or displacement interactions,[3,6,14,15] but none that account for them together in one multivariate expression.

Displacement interactions of VPA also occur with exogenous administration of fatty acids containing products (e.g., propofol),[22] salicylates, highly protein-bound nonsteroidal anti-inflammatory drugs such as ibuprofen and naproxen,[23] and with uremic compounds disrupting albumin binding in the sera of renal failure patients.[24] Significant renal impairment can more than double the free fraction to 20%.[25] Aspirin and other salicylates create an increased toxicity risk, because they can additionally impair mitochondrial β-oxidation (and the intrinsic clearance) of VPA, while increasing the unbound fraction, leading to elevations of the receptor-available VPA.[26] Risperidone may displace protein binding, leading to increases in valproate-induced encephalopathy.[27] Highly protein-bound drugs with weaker affinity will be displaced by VPA, leading to changes in pharmacokinetics, pharmacodynamics, and serum level interpretation for drugs such as warfarin, oral sulfonylurea agents, carbamazepine, the active mono-hydroxy metabolite of oxcarbazepine, and phenytoin.[28] Equations to determine the degree of displacement of other narrow-therapeutic index agents by VPA can be clinically utilized to "correct" for the protein binding disturbance and assist blood level interpretation.[29,30]

Within numerous population pharmacokinetic modeling studies of VPA, surrogates to saturable protein binding are found in the form clearance estimates taken as a function of fixed effects that include nonlinear additive or multiplicative (exponent less than 1), expressions of the daily VPA dose,[31–34] because as the dose increases, total clearance for this low extraction ratio drug will increase,[35] and the rise in VPA Css will be less than proportional to the increase in daily dose (see metabolism and clearance).

VOLUME OF DISTRIBUTION

Although lipid soluble by chemistry, V is restricted to 0.1 to 0.4 L/kg because of the high plasma protein binding of 90% to 95% and a pKa of 4.8, with the drug being mostly ionized at blood pH. The mean V approximates 0.2 L/kg[3,13] in adults and is higher with decreased protein binding.[6,13,34] When standardized to body weight, V of VPA is higher in infants and young children because of lower protein binding, with reduced albumin content and altered body composition compared to adolescents and young adults.[36]

Higher VPA doses would be expected to increase the unbound fraction for peak plasma levels, and thereby increase the distribution volume because more drug exits the intravascular space. This is supported by data showing higher distribution volume (and disproportionately higher peak-free concentrations) after a 30 mg/kg IV loading dose of VPA compared with a 20 mg/kg dose.[37] Total concentrations after the 30 mg/kg dose were, however, only 20% higher during the first 60 minutes postinfusion despite a 50% higher dose. This is meaningful in the context of the most recent recommendations for the management of status epilepticus during the second phase of therapy that call for loading doses as high as 40 mg/kg (maximum 3,000 mg) as a single dose.[38] Response in status epilepticus with after bolus total concentrations of 103 to 135 mg/L was more prompt than delayed response seen with levels of 85 to 102 mg/L.[39] This is likely owing to higher delivery of free drug to the brain and cerebrospinal fluid.[17]

METABOLISM AND CLEARANCE

Three main routes of metabolism produce about 10 to 20 metabolites for VPA,[7] some purported to have CNS activity during long-term therapy. Glucuronidation to

VPA-glucuronide is responsible for 40% to 50% of the disposition of VPA, predominantly using UGT1A3 and UGT2B7. Mitochondrial β-oxidation accounts for 30% to 40%, and the cytochrome p450 system (mainly CYP2C9) a more minor 10% that produces hydroxylated metabolites and unsaturated moieties.[7] Children have more accentuated CYP2C9 activity compared to adults and utilize this pathway more, with longer time to full maturation of some glucuronidating enzymes.[40] This is one reason why the production of 4-ene VPA via this pathway, and its potential to cause fatal hepatotoxicity, is more selected toward younger children, with additional risks, including mitochondrial diseases, inborn errors of metabolism, and/or with polytherapy with enzyme-inducing antiepileptic drugs (AEDs).[41] Moreover, the therapeutic use of carnitine, in those at greater risk for hyperammonemia and drug-induced liver injury, in part prevents the incorporation of the toxic 4-ene VPA into mitochondria where 2,4-diene-VPA-CoA can be produced, itself a hepatotoxin.[42]

Selected polymorphisms in UGT and CYP2C9 can reduce VPA clearance via these pathways,[7] but phenotypic expression does not always follow genotype, because CYP2C9 expression can downregulate in epilepsy.[43] Therefore, reduced function alleles do not consistently affect population-wide pharmacokinetics. Yet, normal CYP2C9 expressers consistently showed higher dose requirements than low expressers, show a higher VPA,[43] and dose guidance using CYP2C9 genotype and phenotype expression in children more precisely predicted dose, achieved therapeutic range serum concentrations, and reduced hyperammonemia and other metabolic adverse effects.[40] The same impact of CYP2C9 polymorphisms was not seen in adults, where no differences in concentration to dose ratio were observed between patients with wild-type and poor metabolism alleles.[44]

Given the concentration-dependent protein binding and low extraction ratio (i.e., rate limitation is with intrinsic clearance), total VPA clearance increases with increasing unbound fraction:

$$Cl\ hepatic = fu \times Cl\ intrinsic$$
$$Css = Dose\ (F)/Cl\ hepatic$$

Therefore, as the fraction unbound increases with higher doses and total concentrations, so too the total clearance and total steady-state concentration will increase less-than-proportionately with increasing dose.

Because mathematically:

$$C\ unbound = fu \times C\ total$$

The C total decrease and fraction unbound increase will offset each other, leaving a relatively stable unbound VPA concentration, but total levels must be interpreted carefully with recognition that the relationship between free levels and total levels changes when protein binding changes, and any factor altering intrinsic clearance, will alter the accumulation of free VPA concentrations.

Relatively reduced drug metabolic activity is observed in the elderly, with the concentration to dose ratio of VPA higher than that in young adults.[4,19,44] Decreased intrinsic clearance coupled with lower protein binding will often manifest as total drug concentrations being similar to younger adults but with higher free concentrations and clinical effect. Furthermore, the greater likelihood of polytherapy and interacting medications in this age group makes the elderly of specific concern for VPA toxicity, with needs for closer clinical and therapeutic drug monitoring. Similar considerations are present for patients with hepatic and renal impairment with reduced clearance and altered protein binding.

Clearances of VPA on monotherapy are within typical ranges of 12 to 25 mL/hr/kg in children and 6 to 12 mL/kg/hr in adults with elimination half-lives ranging from 6 to 12 hours and 8 to 20 hours, respectively. The half-life may be shorter when protein binding is lower, depending on whether expansion of V offsets the increase in total Cl. Larger clearance and shorter half-life are expected when enzyme-inducing co-medications are prescribed. Increased intrinsic clearance of VPA is also recognized in traumatic brain injury.[45]

INTERACTIONS

Comprehensive review of all VPA drug interactions is beyond the scope of this chapter, but thorough reviews are available in the literature.[28,46,47] Selected examples are given in the cases at the end of the chapter.

Most interactions involving VPA are pharmacokinetically based. VPA is an inhibitor of the enzymes CYP2C9, epoxide-hydroxylase, and UDP-glucuronosyltransferases, thereby slowing the metabolism of AEDs such as phenytoin, phenobarbital, clobazam, carbamazepine (to its 10,11-epoxide), and lamotrigine to varying degrees.[46] At high serum concentrations, VPA may decrease its own intrinsic clearance,[4] further complicating its kinetics and level interpretation. Enzyme-inducing AEDs (e.g., phenobarbital, phenytoin, carbamazepine) and non-AEDs (e.g., rifampin) can accelerate VPA metabolism to varying degrees and motivate increase in VPA doses necessary to sustain therapeutic levels. Therefore, the nature of the complex induction and inhibition of the AEDs involved in polytherapy with VPA commands attention to measuring serum levels of all interacting narrow-therapeutic index AEDs during therapy, even when the dose is adjusted for a single agent within the regimen.

Potent inhibitors of VPA p450 enzyme metabolism, such as isoniazid, serotonin reuptake inhibitors (e.g., fluoxetine, paroxetine),[48] and imidazoles (e.g., voriconazole) can increase serum levels and AUC of VPA, and increase its toxicity profile.[47] When combined, competitive inhibition by VPA of UGT2B7-mediated glucuronidation of lamotrigine can double the latter's elimination half-life, increase its levels two- to threefold,[49] and potentiate its toxicity, including the risk of Stevens–Johnson syndrome and toxic epidermal necrolysis. This can be furthered by specific polymorphisms in UGT2B7 and UGT1A4 in the presence of higher VPA concentrations.[50] Therefore, slow titration with small incremental doses of lamotrigine is necessary when added to VPA. In parallel, specific polymorphisms in UTG2B7 may also heighten VPA serum concentrations and is amplified by concomitant lamotrigine competition for glucuronidation, enhancing VPA toxicity risk.[51]

VPA can show different interactions within the same class of medications. For instance, VPA raises the AUC of injectable paliperidone by 50%, yet has a mostly neutral effect on risperidone levels, and lowers those of olanzapine, resulting in breakthrough psychiatric symptoms.[48,52] Inhibition of CYP2C9 and CYP3A4 by VPA leads to increased CNS side effects of amitriptyline, with the mean concentration to dose ratio for amitriptyline 67% higher than for those patients not concomitantly taking VPA, and a 228% higher value for the active nortriptyline metabolite.[53]

Important functional and pharmacokinetic interactions involve females of child-bearing age.[1] Attempts to mitigate the known teratogenic effects of VPA in early-stage pregnancy embody pregnancy avoidance via contraception or choosing other AEDs that can provide similar clinical response patient. Withdrawal of VPA in an attempt to avoid pregnancy complications engenders its own risk of increased seizure activity.[54]

Among AED monotherapies, VPA had the largest differential effect on hormonal contraception versus nonhormonal contraception. When VPA was combined with hormonal contraception, 32% of patients had an increase in seizures compared with those on nonhormonal methods.[55] Notably, VPA has significantly lower serum levels while women take active combined oral contraceptives as compared to inactive pills, with a 21% and 45% increase in total and intrinsic VPA clearance, respectively, likely because of induction of glucuronosyltransferase by ethinylestradiol.[56] Understanding among the clinicians of these drug interactions is lacking and adds to the potential risks of combined oral contraceptive and VPA use,[57] and the need for pharmacist input.

DOSING AND THERAPEUTIC DRUG MONITORING

Doses of VPA vary somewhat by the indication. Low doses of 500 to 1,500 mg/day in adolescents and adults may be sufficient for prophylaxis of migraine headaches,[58] with low levels also providing adjunctive benefit to alcohol withdrawal treatment,[59] and in the primary management of juvenile myoclonic epilepsy.[60] Higher doses with blood level monitoring may be necessary for other seizure types, particularly of focal origin, and where enzyme-inducing co-medications are in use. VPA dose ranges of 10 to 30 mg/kg/day for adults and 15 to 60 mg/kg/day in pediatric patients are most common for the drug's indications. The generally accepted therapeutic range for epilepsy is 50 to 100 mg/L,[61] with some patients requiring higher levels if only partial response is obtained within the stated range. Further validation of the therapeutic range has been documented in a population pharmacokinetics/pharmacodynamic evaluation with probit analysis for the concentrations associated with diminished seizure activity in patients on mono- and polytherapy. Highest probability of anti-seizure response to VPA was in the range of 50 to 70 mg/L,[34] so it is sensible that the lower end of the therapeutic range should be the first target to evaluate efficacy in individuals. In mania and bipolar disease, VPA levels of 50 to 125 mg/L have established efficacy.[62]

There are a number of adverse effects of VPA that are dose or concentration related.[63] Hyperammonemia and associated encephalopathy have been related to VPA serum concentrations, free levels in particular,[64] although not in all cases, because other comorbid factors with VPA use exist.[65] This CNS adverse effect is particularly concerning for confusion with, or adding to, the CNS conditions that VPA is used to treat. Topiramate increases the risk of VPA-induced encephalopathy, although VPA may lower topiramate concentrations by 10% to 15%.[66]

Thrombocytopenia and other blood dyscrasias of drugs are typically idiosyncratic and irrespective of concentration exposure. This is not the case for VPA, where platelet counts may decrease to less than 100,000/μL when VPA concentrations exceed 100 mg/L for females and 130 mg/L for males.[67] Dangerously low platelet counts are not observed

KEY PARAMETERS: Valproic Acid

THERAPEUTIC PLASMA CONCENTRATION	50–100 mg/L (UP TO 125 mg/L FOR BPD/MANIA)
F	
Extended-release tablets	0.8–0.9
All other forms	1.0
S	1.0
V_d[a]	0.2 (range: 0.1–0.4) L/kg
Cl[b,c]	
Children	10–25 mL/kg/hr
Adults	6–12 mL/kg/hr
t½	
Children	6–12 hr
Adults	10–20 hr
fu[d] (fraction unbound in plasma)	0.1–0.5, typical value = 0.1

[a]Volume of distribution may be increased in infants, elderly, liver and renal disease, hypoalbuminemia, or with displacers of VPA binding.
[b]Clearance is decreased in the elderly, neonates and infants, functional liver disease, drugs that impair intrinsic clearance, or compete for glucuronidation; presence of poor function allelic polymorphisms of CYP2C9 or UGT.
[c]Clearance may be increased in patients receiving co-therapy with enzyme-inducing antiepileptic agents or other drugs that induce p450 or glucuronidation, or in patients with polymorphisms imparting higher than normal metabolic enzymatic function. Free drug clearance may be decreased at higher VPA concentrations. Higher clearance is seen in patients with traumatic brain injury in the absence of liver impairment.
[d]Protein binding is concentration dependent within the therapeutic range; the fraction unbound increases with higher VPA levels and with drugs and free fatty acids that displace VPA from albumin binding sites. Protein binding will be lower in disease states where poor synthesis (liver disease, malnutrition, elderly, critical illness) or increased losses (nephrotic syndrome, other renal diseases, protein-losing enteropathy, critical illness) of albumin exist.
VPA, valproic acid.

if this cell line is solely involved, clotting is not usually compromised, and recovery to normal platelet counts occurs with either temporarily suspending VPA or reducing VPA dosage and concentration. The more rare neutropenia can also be dose related.[68]

Quality of life measures in patients with epilepsy can be affected by the disease itself, comorbidities, and co-medications. While VPA affects psychomotor functions and mental acuity less than some other AEDs, overall quality of life measures are observed to be inversely proportional to serum VPA levels.[69]

Along with the indirect relationship of VPA fatal hepatoxicity to concentration (via toxic metabolite formation/accumulation) described above, γ-glutamyltransferase elevations, an indicator of hepatobiliary disease has been correlated with VPA concentrations,[70] and is not from induction of enzyme production as for phenytoin and phenobarbital. Other serious abdominal adverse effects such a VPA-induced pancreatitis are not concentration or dose related.[71] Weight gain, low thyroid levels, tremors, and teratogenicity have all been linked to some extent with dose exposure or serum VPA levels.[72–74]

VPA levels are best obtained at steady state for patients on maintenance therapy for epilepsy, to assure compliance and correlation with clinical benefit, and avoid potential concentration-related toxicities.[61] This is less necessary with use in migraine headaches, because low doses are usually sufficient for prophylaxis, and may be useful for mania or bipolar disease treatment if therapeutic endpoints are not met. Repeat measurements of VPA levels should be done when toxicity occurs, when the dose is changed, when anticipated pharmacokinetic drug interactions exist, and when efficacy is lost.[61] Levels may also be obtained upon admission to the hospital for recurrence or breakthrough seizures, and after loading doses are given to assure achievement of the target concentration. Predose levels taken with rapidly absorbed syrup and tablet, and IV preparations may overestimate Cl when Cl is calculated as Dose * F/Css, because the steady-state trough level is higher than the average Css, especially those with faster clearances, such as children or those taking metabolism-inducing drugs. The Css is better represented with trough level sampling for extended- and delayed-release preparations. For practical purposes, if trough concentrations are monitored consistently in the individual patient, then the concentration to dose ratio is useful and can be compared on different doses, and the relationship between serum concentration and effectiveness can be accurately evaluated. Unbound drug concentration measurement of VPA, using ultrafiltration methods, may be needed when correlation to effect or toxicity is elusive, or if liver or renal disease, traumatic brain injury, hypoalbuminemia, or protein binding displacement is present, and especially if a combination of binding-altering factors exists.[61] Elevated unbound VPA Css may better reflect and predict neurotoxicity symptoms in patients with hypoalbuminemia when total VPA Css is within the therapeutic range.[61a]

Question #1   *B.I. is a 46-year-old, 82-kg man admitted to the neurointensive care unit after having serial tonic–clonic seizures emanating from a newly diagnosed glioblastoma. Repeated bolus doses of levetiracetam were not useful in suppressing the seizure activity, and it is decided to administered VPA IV. He has normal liver enzymes and function tests, and his albumin is 4.2 g/dL. A 1,500 mg loading dose given over 30 minutes is prescribed, with a 30-minute postinfusion serum level to be obtained. What peak concentration might be expected?*

Because the typical half-life of valproate in adults is ranges between 10 and 20 hours, no significant drug loss would occur between the time to load dose and the time to peak concentration. Therefore, the peak concentration can be estimated using the single-dose bolus model (Equation 15.1) assuming the average V for an adult is 0.2 L/kg.

$$V = 0.2 \text{ L/kg (82 kg)}$$
$$= 16.4 \text{ L}$$

$$C \text{ peak} = \frac{(S)(F)(D)}{V} \qquad \textbf{(Eq. 15.1)}$$

$$= \frac{(1)(1)(1,500 \text{ mg})}{16.4 \text{ L}}$$
$$= 91.5 \text{ mg/L}$$

Question #2 *What is an appropriate maintenance dose to be administered by continuous IV infusion to achieve an average steady-state concentration of 70 mg/L? If the drug is administered through a nasogastric (NG) tube, what would be an appropriate dosing regimen?*

Using the population Cl = 10 mL/hr/kg, the maintenance dose to achieve the average steady-state concentration of 70 mg/L can be calculated using the continuous infusion model.

$$Cl = 10 \text{ mL/hr/kg } (82 \text{ kg})(1 \text{ L/1,000 mL})$$
$$= 0.82 \text{ L/hr}$$

$$D/\tau = \frac{(Css \text{ ave } [mg/L])(Cl \text{ } [L/hr])}{(S)(F)}$$ **(Eq. 15.2)**

$$= \frac{(70 \text{ mg/L})(0.82 \text{ L/hr})}{(1)(1)}$$
$$= 57.4 \text{ mg/hr}$$

This can also be given by syrup if the gastrointestinal tract is used and access (e.g., NG tube) is gained. Based on the population values of Cl and V, the elimination rate constant (K) and half-life (t½) can be calculated as follows:

$$K = \frac{Cl}{V}$$ **(Eq. 15.3)**

$$= \frac{0.82 \text{ L/hr}}{16.4 \text{ L}}$$
$$= 0.05 \text{ hr}^{-1}$$

$$t\tfrac{1}{2} = \frac{0.693}{K}$$ **(Eq. 15.4)**

$$= \frac{0.693}{0.05 \text{ hr}^{-1}}$$
$$= 13.9 \text{ hr}$$

In order to minimize peak to trough fluctuation in plasma concentrations, the dosing interval for a rapid-release product should be much less than the half-life. Using an interval of every 6 hours, the dose can be calculated using Equation 15.2 as:

$$= \frac{(70 \text{ mg/L})(0.82 \text{ L/hr})(6 \text{ hr})}{(1)(1)}$$

$$= 344, \text{ or } \sim 350 \text{ mg}$$

Question #3 *B.I. was receiving an emergent* computed tomography *scan immediately after receiving his IV load of VPA. Instead of the planned postbolus level, a serum level is obtained 8 hours after completed infusion and measures 55 mg/L. What maintenance dose would be recommended to maintain an average steady-state concentration of 70 mg/L? What are the estimated steady-state Cmax and Cmin concentrations on this prescribed dose?*

The estimated peak and the 8-hour postinfusion measured concentrations can be used to determine the revised VPA clearance.

$$K = \frac{\ln\left(\dfrac{C_1}{C_2}\right)}{\Delta t}$$

(Eq. 15.5)

$$= \frac{\ln\left(\dfrac{91.5 \text{ mg/L}}{55 \text{ mg/L}}\right)}{7 \text{ hr}}$$

$$= 0.073 \text{ hr}^{-1}$$

$$t\tfrac{1}{2} = \frac{0.693}{K}$$

$$= \frac{0.693}{0.073 \text{ hr}^{-1}}$$

$$= 9.5 \text{ hr}$$

The revised Cl can be calculated using the population V and revised K.

$$Cl = (K)(V)$$

$$= (0.073 \text{ hr}^{-1})(16.4 \text{ L})$$

$$= 1.2 \text{ L/hr}$$

The revised dose can then be calculated using Equation 15.2 to achieve the desired average steady-state concentration of 70 mg/L.

$$= \frac{(70 \text{ mg/L})(1.2 \text{ L/hr})(6 \text{ hr})}{(1)(1)}$$

$$= 504, \text{ or } \sim 500 \text{ mg IV or syrup q6h}$$

We can use the parameters determined above to calculate the steady-state peak and trough (predose) concentrations of the 500 mg IV every 6-hour regimen using the steady-state bolus Equation 15.6. Because t½ is 9.5 hours, we consider the drug lost and gained during the short infusion negligible.

The steady-state Cmax can also be calculated using Equation 15.6.

$$\text{Css max} = \frac{\dfrac{(S)(F)(D)}{V}}{1 - e^{-(K)(\tau)}} \qquad \textbf{(Eq. 15.6)}$$

$$= \frac{\dfrac{(1)(1)(500 \text{ mg})}{16.4}}{1 - e^{-(0.073)(6)}}$$

$$= 85.96, \text{ or } \sim 86 \text{ mg/L}$$

The steady-state Cmin can then be calculated using the Cmax and revised K with Equation 15.7 as follows:

$$\text{Css min} = (\text{Css max})e^{-(K)(\tau)} \qquad \textbf{(Eq. 15.7)}$$

$$= (86 \text{ mg/L})e^{-(0.073 \text{ hr}^{-1})(6 \text{ hr})}$$

$$= 55.5 \text{ mg/L}$$

Question #4 *B.I. has his seizures controlled while in the intensive care unit on a dose of VPA of 500 mg every 8 hours, but spikes a fever and has an elevated neutrophil count. He has a history of documented urinary tract infections, with extended-spectrum β-lactamases producing Escherichia coli is placed on meropenem 1,000 mg every 8 hours on suspicion of recurrence. Two days later, he has a breakthrough tonic–clonic seizure, and a stat mid-interval VPA level comes back at 25 mg/L. All of the doses are checked, and another serum sample is sent for verification, and it results as 19 mg/L. A 1,000 mg loading dose is given, and the maintenance dose is increased to 750 mg every 8 hours. The next morning, B.I. has another brief breakthrough seizure, and the VPA level sent is 25 mg/L. Rapid calculation demonstrates a clearance value that is not physiologically plausible. What accounts for the repeated low levels?*

A major pathway of VPA metabolism is via glucuronidation, and deglucuronidation by hydrolysis may contribute active drug back into the circulation. The carbapenem antibiotics (e.g., imipenem, doripenem, meropenem) all feature inhibition of the VPA-glucuronidase enzyme acylpeptide hydrolase, located in the cytosol of the liver and kidney, which blocks the deglucuronidation of VPA and enhances the urinary elimination of VPA-glucuronide.[75,76] This increases the apparent clearance dramatically, and VPA levels fall more than 50%, even for increased dosing,[76,77] hence precipitating seizures in those vulnerable to breakthrough. Even increases in dose may not sustain a therapeutic level or outcome, and other antimicrobials, susceptibility permitting, or additional AEDs may be required. Despite the relatively short half-lives of the carbapenems, the effect on blocking deglucuronidation lasts for several days[76,77], and levels may take a week or more to return to pre-carbapenem values. Meropenem and ertapenem show greater decreases in VPA levels in patients than with imipenem.[77] Care must be taken to reduce the dose of VPA back to the baseline VPA doses that had been significantly raised in an attempt to obtain therapeutic concentrations, because once the interaction reverses, the VPA levels may rise dramatically to levels promoting toxicity. Perhaps more concerning is the convenient use of parenteral meropenem to treat various community infections in the nonhospital setting, thereby increasing the risk of breakthrough seizure activity in a less monitored location.

Question #5   *B.I.'s seizures are eventually controlled on a regimen of depakote delayed-release tablets of 500 mg orally every 8 hours, with a steady-state trough concentration of 50 mg/L. He is diagnosed with depression, and fluoxetine is added to his regimen. He is seen in clinic a month later, and it is noted that his nutrition has been poor and that he has lost 7 kg. His depression is slightly improved, but a noticeable tremor of his right hand is present, and he is sleepy during the day. His labs show that his albumin is low at 2.8 g/dL, his ammonia level has risen to 98 μmol/L, and his follow-up trough VPA level is now 70 mg/L. What assessment can be made regarding any changes in the pharmacokinetics of VPA and associated toxicity findings?*

B.I.'s VPA revised Cl can be calculated from the trough level. Because the time to maximum concentrations (Tmax) with the delayed-release tablets is approximately 8 hours, the fluctuation in between peak and trough concentrations with every 8-hour dosing is minimal, and, therefore, the trough concentration can be considered an average steady state. The revised Cl can then be calculated using Equation 15.8.

$$Cl\ (L/hr) = \frac{(S)(F)(D)}{Css\ ave\ (\tau)} \qquad \text{(Eq. 15.8)}$$

$$= \frac{(1)(1)(500\ mg)}{(50\ mg/L)\ (8\ hr)}$$

$$= 1.25\ L/hr\ or\ 16.67\ mL/hr/kg$$

After adding fluoxetine, we have

$$= \frac{(1)(1)(500 \text{ mg})}{(70 \text{ mg/L})(8 \text{ hr})}$$
$$= 0.89 \text{ L/hr}$$

With the 40% increase in steady-state blood level to 70 mg/L, B.I.'s VPA clearance is reduced to 0.893 L/hr, or 11.90 mL/hr/kg, a decrease of 28.6%. Fluoxetine can moderately inhibit CYP2C9 metabolism, an important pathway in the metabolism of VPA, thus limiting its intrinsic clearance.[28,47,48]

However, the total concentration measured is not outside the therapeutic range, or consistent with levels that dose-related toxicities, although individual sensitivities should be clinically considered.

Concentration-dependent protein binding is evident within the therapeutic range, and considering that the hypoalbuminemia is present in BI, an assessment of the free concentration given reduced binding capacity may be useful in sorting out these apparent concentration-related toxicities. There are a number of equations and graphic relationships that illustrate the nonlinearity of the relationship between free and total (free + bound) concentrations. A simple linearized version of this nonlinear relationship is given in the following equation[78]:

$$\text{fraction unbound (fu)} = 0.0015 \text{ Cp total} \qquad \textbf{(Eq. 15.9)}$$

$$\text{For B.I., fu} = 0.0015 (70)$$
$$= 0.105 \text{ or } 10.5\%$$

The free concentration can be calculated from the total (measured) concentration and the estimated fraction unbound (fu) as:

$$\text{Free Concentration} = \text{Total Concentration (fu)} \qquad \textbf{(Eq. 15.10)}$$

$$= 70 \text{ mg/L } (0.105)$$
$$= 7.35 \text{ mg/L}$$

The therapeutic range of free VPA is 2.5 to 10 mg/L (based on the normal fu of 0.05 to 0.1).

With B.I.'s hypoalbuminemia, the free fraction is increased when the binding capacity (i.e., albumin concentration) diminishes. For total VPA concentrations less that 75 mg/L, an accurate corrected level can be calculated using Equation 15.11, where ALB is the albumin concentration in g/dL.[79]

$$\text{Percent Free} = 130.2 \times e^{-(0.72)(\text{ALB})} \qquad \textbf{(Eq. 15.11)}$$

For B.I. at an albumin concentration of 2.8 g/dL, the percent free is estimated to be 17.34%, and, therefore, the free concentration = 0.1734 × 70 mg/L = 12.14 mg/L, which exceeds the therapeutic range for free drug, and can explain the adverse effects seen in this patient.

$$\text{Percent Free} = 130.2 \times e^{-(0.72)(2.8)}$$

$$= 17.34\%$$

$$\text{Free Concentration} = \text{Total Concentration (fu)}$$

$$= 70 \text{ mg/L } (0.1734)$$

$$= 12.14 \text{ mg/L}$$

Question #6   *B.I. is receiving treatment for his brain tumor and has a breakthrough seizure during a clinic visit despite adequate VPA serum concentrations. Phenytoin is added at a dose of 400 mg/day, and B.I.'s seizures are controlled. The phenytoin steady-state concentration is 6.6 mg/L, and the physician is contemplating increasing the phenytoin dose to achieve the therapeutic range of 10 to 20 mg/L. B.I. still has an albumin concentration of 2.8 g/dL. Should the phenytoin dose be increased?*

We can anticipate that VPA will competitively displace phenytoin from protein binding sites on albumin, and combined with the lower binding capacity, the phenytoin unbound fraction will be markedly elevated above normal.

A calculation of the free fraction of phenytoin can be made using an equation derived from the literature[29]:

$$\text{Phenytoin fu} = 0.1 + [0.0151 \times (4.08 - \text{ALB})] + (0.0525 \times \text{VPA})$$
$$+ (0.0385 \times \text{CBZ}) \qquad \textbf{(Eq. 15.12)}$$

where ALB is the albumin concentration in g/dL, and VPA and CBZ are 1 if the patient is on those co-medications (which raise the free fraction of phenytoin by 52.5 and 38.5%, respectively), otherwise it is 0. The 0.1 is the normal free fraction of phenytoin.

Therefore, for B.I.:

$$\text{Phenytoin fu} = 0.1 + [0.0151 \times (4.08 - \text{ALB})] + (0.0525 \times \text{PA}) + (0.0385 \times \text{CBZ})$$
$$= 0.1718 \text{ (or 17.2\%)}$$

$$\text{Phenytoin free concentration} = (\text{fu})(\text{Css})$$
$$= (0.1718)(6.6 \text{ mg/L})$$
$$= 1.14 \text{ mg/L}$$

The estimated free phenytoin concentration would be in the stated therapeutic range for unbound phenytoin concentrations of 1 to 2 mg/L.

Alternatively, the corrected total phenytoin concentration can be calculated as:

$$\text{Css corrected} = \text{Css measured}\left(\frac{\text{fu calculated}}{\text{fu normal}}\right) \qquad \text{(Eq. 15.13)}$$

$$= 6.6 \text{ mg/L}\left(\frac{0.1718}{0.1}\right)$$

$$= 11.4 \text{ mg/L}$$

Therefore, B.I. should not require a dose change, given the free phenytoin level estimate and corrected total phenytoin level are within their respective therapeutic ranges, and B.I. is sustaining good anti-seizure response from the combination.

Question #7 *M.Z. is an 11-year-old, 42 kg prepubescent female with a history of focal convulsive epilepsy that is incompletely controlled by high therapeutic doses of carbamazepine, and VPA will be added. To accommodate her school schedule, she is prescribed 500 mg of depakote to be taken at 800 and 2,000 daily (23.8 mg/kg/day). What would be her estimated average steady-state serum level?*

Concomitant use of other antiepileptic agents is known to increase the metabolic clearance of VPA. Carbamazepine induces CYP4503A4 metabolism of VPA, which requires increased doses of VPA to maintain therapeutic concentrations. In addition, as stated previously, VPA exhibits dose-dependent changes in clearance as a function of saturable protein binding. Several population pharmacokinetic models have been published that relate dose-dependent changes in VPA clearance as a surrogate to saturable protein binding, as well as incorporating adjustments for common drug interactions. One such model developed from a pediatric population is represented in Equation 15.14.

$$\text{Cl (L/hr)} = 0.012\left(\text{wt in kg}\right)^{0.715} \times \text{Dose(mg/kg} \cdot \text{hr)}^{0.306} \times (1 + 0.359 \times \text{CBZ})$$

$$\text{(Eq. 15.14)}$$

where CBZ is 1 if co-medicated with carbamazepine, otherwise it is 0 (indicating an increase in VPA clearance by 35.9% when carbamazepine is present).[32]

$$= 0.012 \times (42 \text{ kg})^{0.715} \times (23.8 \text{ mg/kg} \cdot \text{hr})^{0.306} \times (1 + 0.359 \times 1)$$

$$= 0.012 \times 14.475 \times 2.638 \times 1.359$$

$$= 0.6226 \text{ L/hr}$$

$$= 14.83 \text{ mL/hr/kg}$$

The average steady-state concentration can be calculated using Equation 15.15 as:

$$\text{Css ave} = \frac{(S)(F)(D)}{(Cl)(\tau)} \qquad \textbf{(Eq. 15.15)}$$

$$= \frac{(1)(1)(500\ \text{mg})}{(0.62\ \text{L/hr})(12\ \text{hr})}$$

$$= 67\ \text{mg/L}$$

A model constructed and tested in adults from the same investigators[31] has similar structure, including clearance induction terms for phenytoin (PHT) and phenobarbital (PB):

$$Cl\ (\text{L/hr}) = 0.004\ \big(\text{wt in kg}\big) \times \text{Dose}(\text{mg/kg} \cdot \text{hr})^{0.304} \times (1 + 0.359 \times CBZ)$$
$$\times \big(1 + 0.541 \times PHT\big) \times (1 + 0.397 \times PB)$$

Other mathematical expressions encompassing the same and other covariates in ethnically and pharmacogenetically diverse populations have been published, with lower and higher magnitudes of effect of co-medications on clearance.[33,34,80–82,82a] Conversely, the statistical magnitude of VPA effect on the clearance of other AEDs and non-AEDs has been captured in population pharmacokinetic models of those agents.[83,84]

ACKNOWLEDGMENT

The important work of Michelle Wheeler to a previous version of this chapter is acknowledged.

REFERENCES

1.   Tomson T, Battino D, Perucca E. Valproic acid after five decades of use in epilepsy: time to reconsider the indications of a time-honored drug. *Lancet Neurol.* 2016;15(2):210–218.

2.   Guerrini R. Valproate as a mainstay of therapy for pediatric epilepsy. *Pediatr Drugs.* 2006;8(2):113–129.

3.   Panomvana N, Ayudhya D, Suwanmanee J, et al. Pharmacokinetic parameters of total and unbound valproic acid and their relationships to seizure control in epileptic children. *Am J Ther.* 2006;13(3):211–217.

4.   Felix S, Sproule BA, Hardy BG, et al. Dose-related pharmacokinetics and pharmacodynamics of valproate in the elderly. *J Clin Psychopharmacol.* 2003;23(5):471–478.

5.   Smith RL, Haslemo T, Refsum H, et al. Impact of age, gender and CYP2C9/2C19 genotypes on dose-adjusted steady-state serum concentrations of valproic acid—a large-scale study based on naturalistic therapeutic drug monitoring data. *Eur J Clin Pharmacol.* 2016;72(9):1099–1104.

6.   Cloyd JC, Fischer JH, Kriel RL, et al. Valproic acid pharmacokinetics in children. IV. Effects of age and antiepileptic drugs on protein binding and intrinsic clearance. *Clin Pharmacol Ther.* 1993;53(1):22–29.

7.   Ghodke-Puranik Y, Thorn CF, Lamba JK, et al. Valproic acid pathway: pharmacokinetics and pharmacodynamics. *Pharmacogenet Genomics.* 2013;23(4):236–241.

8.   Schmidt D, Schachter SC. Drug treatment of epilepsy in adults. *BMJ.* 2014;348:g254.

9.   Salminen JK, Tammela TL, Auvinen A, et al. Antiepileptic drugs with histone deacetylase inhibition activity and prostate cancer risk: a population-based case-control study. *Cancer Causes Control.* 2016;27(5):637–645.

10. Dutta S, Reed RC. Distinct absorption characteristics of oral formulations of valproic acid/divalproex available in the United States. *Epilepsy Res.* 2007;73(3):275–283.

11. DiScala SL, Nhi N, Tran NN, et al. Valproic acid suppositories for management of seizures for geriatric patients in palliative care. *Consult Pharm.* 2016;31(6):313–319.

12. Ibarra M, Marta Vázquez M, Fagiolino P, et al. Sex related differences on valproic acid pharmacokinetics after oral single dose. *J Pharmacokinet Pharmacodyn.* 2013;40(4):479–486.

13. Cloyd JC, Dutta S, Cao G, et al; Depacon Study Group. Valproate unbound fraction and distribution volume following rapid infusions in patients with epilepsy. *Epilepsy Res.* 2003;53(1–2):19–27.

14. Otten N, Hall K, Irvine-Meek J, et al. Free valproic acid: steady-state pharmacokinetics in patients with intractable epilepsy. *Can J Neurol Sci.* 1984;11(4):457–460.

15. Ueshima S, Aiba T, Makita T, et al. Characterization of non-linear relationship between total and unbound serum concentrations of valproic acid in epileptic children. *J Clin Pharm Ther.* 2008;33(1):31–38.

16. Bailey DN, Briggs JS. The binding of selected therapeutic drugs to human serum alpha-1 acid glycoprotein and to human serum albumin in vitro. *Ther Drug Monitor.* 2004;26(1):40–43.

17. Shen DD, Ojemann GA, Rapport RL, et al. Low and variable presence of valproic acid in human brain. *Neurology.* 1992;42(3 Pt 1):582–585.

18. Ueshima S, Aiba T, Ishikawa N, et al. Poor applicability of estimation method for adults to calculate unbound serum concentrations of valproic acid in epileptic neonates and infants. *J Clin Pharm Ther.* 2009;34(4):415–422.

19. Lampon N, Tutor JC. Apparent clearance of valproic acid in elderly epileptic patients: estimation of the confounding effect of albumin concentration. *Ups J Med Sci.* 2012;117(1):41–46.

20. Butler JM, Begg EJ. Free drug clearance in elderly people. *Clin Pharmacokinet.* 2008;47(5):297–321.

21. Gatti G, Crema F, Attardo-Parrinello G, et al. Serum protein binding of phenytoin and valproic acid in insulin-dependent diabetes mellitus. *Ther Drug Monit.* 1987;9(4):389–391.

22. Hatton C, Riker R, Gagnon DJ, et al. Free serum valproate concentration more reliable than total concentration in critically ill patients. *Resuscitation.* 2016;105:e15–e16.

23. Christensen H, Baker M, Tucker GT, et al. Prediction of plasma protein binding displacement and its implications for quantitative assessment of metabolic drug-drug interactions from in vitro data. *J Pharm Sci.* 2006;95(12):2778–2787.

24. Dasgupta A, Jacques M, Malhotra D. Diminished protein binding capacity of uremic sera for valproate following hemodialysis: role of free fatty acids and uremic compounds. *Am J Nephrol.* 1996;16(4):327–333.

25. Gugler R, Mueller G. Plasma protein binding of valproic acid in healthy subjects and in patients with renal disease. *Br J Clin Pharmacol.* 1978;5(5):441–446.

26. Sandson NB, Marcucci C, Bourke DL, et al. An interaction between aspirin and valproate: the relevance of plasma protein displacement drug-drug interactions. *Am J Psychiatry.* 2006;163(11):1891–1896.

27. Rodrigues-Silva N, Venancio A, Bouça J. Risperidone, a risk factor for valproate-induced encephalopathy? *Gen Hosp Psychiatry.* 2013;35(4):452–e5–452–e6.

28. Zaccara G, Perucca E. Interactions between antiepileptic drugs, and between antiepileptic drugs and other drugs. *Epileptic Disord.* 2014;16(4):409–432.

29. Joerger M, Huitema AD, Boogerd W, et al. Interactions of serum albumin, valproic acid and carbamazepine with the pharmacokinetics of phenytoin in cancer patients. *Basic Clin Pharmacol Toxicol.* 2006;99(2):133–140.

30. Ratnaraj N, Hjelm M. Prediction of free levels of phenytoin and carbamazepine in patients comedicated with valproic acid. *Ther Drug Monit.* 1995;17(4):327–332.

31. Blanco-Serrano B, Otero MJ, Santos-Buelga D, et al. Population estimation of valproic acid clearance in adult patients using routine clinical pharmacokinetic data. *Biopharm Drug Dispos.* 1999;20(5):233–240.

32. Serrano BB, García-Sánchez MJ, Otero MJ, et al. Valproate population pharmacokinetics in children. *J Clin Pharm Ther.* 1999;24(1):73–80.

33. Lin WW, Jiao Z, Wang CL, et al. Population pharmacokinetics of valproic acid in adult Chinese epileptic patients and its application in an individualized dosage regimen. *Ther Drug Monit.* 2015;37(1):76–83.

34.   Nakashima H, Oniki K, Nishimura M, et al. Determination of the optimal concentration of valproic acid in patients with epilepsy: a population pharmacokinetic-pharmacodynamic analysis. *PLoS One*. 2015;10(10):e0141266.

35.   Gidal BE, Pitterle ME, Spencer NW, et al. Relationship between valproic acid dosage, plasma concentration and clearance in adult monotherapy patients with epilepsy. *J Clin Pharm Ther*. 1995;20(4):215–219.

36.   Chiba K, Suganuma T, Ishizaki T, et al. Comparison of steady-state pharmacokinetics of valproic acid in children between monotherapy and multiple antiepileptic drug treatment. *J Pediatr*. 1985;106(4):653–658.

37.   Limdi NA, Knowlton RK, Cofield SS, et al. Safety of rapid intravenous loading of valproate. *Epilepsia*. 2007;48(3):478–483.

38.   Glauser T, Shinnar S, Gloss D, et al. Evidence-based guideline: treatment of convulsive status epilepticus in children and adults: report of the Guideline Committee of the American Epilepsy Society. *Epilepsy Curr*. 2016;16(1):48–61.

39.   Uberall MA, Trollmann R, Wunsiedler U, et al. Intravenous valproate in pediatric epilepsy patients with refractory status epilepticus. *Neurology*. 2000;54(11):2188, 2189.

40.   Bűdi T, Tóth K, Nagy A, et al. Clinical significance of CYP2C9-status guided valproic acid therapy in children. *Epilepsia*. 2015;56(6):849–855.

41.   Star K, Edwards IR, Choonara I. Valproic acid and fatalities in children: a review of individual case safety reports in VigiBase. *PLoS One*. 2014;9(10):e108970.

42.   Lheureux PE, Hantson P. Carnitine in the treatment of valproic acid-induced toxicity. *Clin Toxicol (Phila)*. 2009;47(2):101, 111.

43.   Tóth K, Bűdi T, Kiss Á, et al. Phenoconversion of CYP2C9 in epilepsy limits the predictive value of CYP2C9 genotype in optimizing valproate therapy. *Personal Med*. 2015;12(3):199–207.

44.   Smith RL, Haslemo T, Refsum H, et al. Impact of age, gender and CYP2C9/2C19 genotypes on dose-adjusted steady-state serum concentrations of valproic acid: a large-scale study based on naturalistic therapeutic drug monitoring data. *Eur J Clin Pharmacol*. 2016;72(9):1099–1104.

45.   Anderson GD, Temkin NR, Awan AB, et al. Effect of time, injury, age and ethanol on interpatient variability in valproic acid pharmacokinetics after traumatic brain injury. *Clin Pharmacokinet*. 2007;46(4):307–318.

46.   Patsalos PN. Drug interactions with the newer antiepileptic drugs (AEDs)—Part 1: Pharmacokinetic and pharmacodynamic interactions between AEDs. *Clin Pharmacokinet*. 2013;52:927–966.

47.   Patsalos PN. Drug interactions with the newer antiepileptic drugs (AEDs)—Part 2: Pharmacokinetic and pharmacodynamic interactions between AEDs and drugs used to treat non-epilepsy disorders. *Clin Pharmacokinet*. 2013;52(12):1045–1061.

48.   Spina E, Pisani F, de Leon J. Clinically significant pharmacokinetic drug interactions of antiepileptic drugs with new antidepressants and new antipsychotics. *Pharmacol Res*. 2016;106:72–86.

49.   Lalic M, Cvejic J, Popovic J, et al. Lamotrigine and valproate pharmacokinetics interactions in epileptic patients. *Eur J Drug Metab Pharmacokinet*. 2009;34(2):93–99.

50.   Liu L, Zhao L, Wang Q, et al. Influence of valproic acid concentration and polymorphism of UGT1A4*3, UGT2B7 -161C>T and UGT2B7*2 on serum concentration of lamotrigine in Chinese epileptic children. *Eur J Clin Pharmacol*. 2015;71(11):1341–1347.

51.   Wang Q, Zhao L, Liang M, et al. Effects of UGT2B7 genetic polymorphisms on serum concentrations of valproic acid in Chinese children with epilepsy comedicated with lamotrigine. *Ther Drug Monit*. 2016;38(3):343–349.

52.   Habibi M, Hart F, Bainbridge J. The impact of psychoactive drugs on seizures and antiepileptic drugs. *Curr Neurol Neurosci Rep*. 2016;16(8):71.

53.   Unterecker S, Burger R, Hohage A, et al. Interaction of valproic acid and amitriptyline: analysis of therapeutic drug monitoring data under naturalistic conditions. *J Clin Psychopharmacol*. 2013;33(4):561–564.

54.   Tomson T, Battino D, Bonizzoni E, et al; EURAP Study Group. Withdrawal of valproic acid treatment during pregnancy and seizure outcome: observations from EURAP. *Epilepsia*. 2016;57(8):e173–e177.

55.   Herzog AG, Mandle HB, Cahill KE, et al. Differential impact of contraceptive methods on seizures varies by antiepileptic drug category: Findings of the Epilepsy Birth Control Registry. *Epilepsy Behav*. 2016;60:112–117.

56. Galimberti CA, Mazzucchelli I, Arbasino C, et al. Increased apparent oral clearance of valproic acid during intake of combined contraceptive steroids in women with epilepsy. *Epilepsia*. 2006;47(9):1569–1572.

57. Suto HS, Braga GC, Scarpellini GR, et al. Neurologist knowledge about interactions between antiepileptic drugs and contraceptive methods. *Int J Gynaecol Obstet*. 2016;134(3):264–267.

58. Kinze S, Clauss M, Reuter U, et al. Valproic acid is effective in migraine prophylaxis at low serum levels: a prospective open-label study. *Headache*. 2001;41(8):774–778.

59. De Iuliis V, Gelormini R, Flacco M, et al. Comparison of serum total valproic acid levels and %CDT Values in chronic alcohol addictive patients in an Italian clinic: a Retrospective study. *Drugs Real World Outcomes*. 2016;3:7–12.

60. Hernández-Vanegas LE, Jara-Prado A, Ochoa A, et al. High-dose versus low-dose valproate for the treatment of juvenile myoclonic epilepsy: going from low to high. *Epilepsy Behav*. 2016;61:34–40.

61. Patsalos PN, Berry DJ, Bourgeois BF, et al. Antiepileptic drugs—best practice guidelines for therapeutic drug monitoring: a position paper by the subcommission on therapeutic drug monitoring, ILAE Commission on Therapeutic Strategies. *Epilepsia*. 2008;49(7):1239–1276.

61a. Wallenburg E, Klok B, de Jong K, et al. Monitoring protein-unbound valproic acid serum concentrations in clinical practice. *Ther Drug Monit*. 2017;39(3):269–272.

62. Bowden CL, Janicak PG, Orsulak P, et al. Relation of serum valproate concentration to response in mania. *Am J Psychiatry*. 1996;153:765–770.

63. Nanau RM, Neuman MG. Adverse drug reactions induced by valproic acid. *Clin Biochem*. 2013;46(15):1323–1338.

64. Itoh H, Suzuki Y, Fujisaki K, et al. Correlation between plasma ammonia level and serum trough concentration of free valproic acid in patients with epilepsy. *Biol Pharm Bull*. 2012;35(6):971–974.

65. Chopra A, Kolla BP, Mansukhani MP, et al. Valproate-induced hyperammonemic encephalopathy: an update on risk factors, clinical correlates and management. *Gen Hosp Psychiatry*. 2012;34(3):290–298.

66. Blackford MG, Do ST, Enlow TC, et al. Valproic acid and topiramate induced hyperammonemic encephalopathy in a patient with normal serum carnitine. *J Pediatr Pharmacol Ther*. 2013;18(2):128–136.

67. Nasreddine W, Beydoun A. Valproate-induced thrombocytopenia: a prospective monotherapy study. *Epilepsia*. 2008;49(3):438–445.

68. Stoner SC, Deal E, Lurk JT. Delayed-onset neutropenia with divalproex sodium. *Ann Pharmacother*. 2008;42(10):1507–1510.

69. Jakovljevic MB, Jankovic SM, Jankovic SV, et al. Inverse correlation of valproic acid serum concentrations and quality of life in adolescents with epilepsy. *Epilepsy Res*. 2008;80(2–3):180–183.

70. Ogusu N, Saruwatari J, Nakashima H, et al. Impact of the superoxide dismutase 2 Val16Ala polymorphism on the relationship between valproic acid exposure and elevation of γ-glutamyltransferase in patients with epilepsy: a population pharmacokinetic-pharmacodynamic analysis. *PLoS One*. 2014;9(11):e111066.

71. Cofini M, Quadrozzi F, Favoriti P, et al. Valproic acid-induced acute pancreatitis in pediatric age: case series and review of literature. *G Chir*. 2015;36(4):158–160.

72. Kim SH, Chung HR, Kim SH, et al. Subclinical hypothyroidism during valproic acid therapy in children and adolescents with epilepsy. *Neuropediatrics*. 2012;43(3):135–139.

73. Hamed SA, Abdellah MM. The relationship between valproate induced tremors and circulating neurotransmitters: a preliminary study. *Int J Neurosci*. 2017;127(3):236–242.

74. Tomson T, Marson A, Boon P, et al. Valproate in the treatment of epilepsy in girls and women of childbearing potential. *Epilepsia*. 2015;56(7):1006–1019.

75. Suzuki E, Yamamura N, Ogura Y, et al. Identification of valproic acid glucuronide hydrolase as a key enzyme for the interaction of valproic acid with carbapenem antibiotics. *Drug Metab Dispos*. 2010;38(9):1538–1544.

76. Suzuki E, Nakai D, Ikenaga H, et al. In vivo inhibition of acylpeptide hydrolase by carbapenem antibiotics causes the decrease of plasma concentration of valproic acid in dogs. *Xenobiotica*. 2016;46(2):126–131.

77. Wu CC, Pai TY, Hsiao FY, et al. The effect of different carbapenem antibiotics (ertapenem, imipenem/cilastatin and meropenem) on serum valproic acid concentrations. *Ther Drug Monit*. 2016;38(5):587–592.

78. Dutta S, Faught E, Limdi NA. Valproate protein binding following rapid intravenous administration of high doses of valproic acid in patients with epilepsy. *J Clin Pharm Ther.* 2007;32(4):365–371.

79. Hermida J, Tutor JC. A theoretical method for normalizing total serum valproic acid concentration in hypoalbuminemic patients. *J Pharmacol Sci.* 2005;97(4):489–493.

80. Correa T, Rodríguez I, Romano S. Population pharmacokinetics of valproate in Mexican children with epilepsy. *Biopharm Drug Dispos.* 2008;29(9):511–520.

81. EL Desoky ES, Fuseau E, EL Din Amry S, et al. Pharmacokinetic modelling of valproic acid from routine clinical data in Egyptian epileptic patients. *Eur J Clin Pharmacol.* 2004;59(11):783–790.

82. Ding J, Wang Y, Lin W, et al. A population pharmacokinetic model of valproic acid in pediatric patients with epilepsy: a non-linear pharmacokinetic model based on protein-binding saturation. *Clin Pharmacokinet.* 2015;54(3):305–317.

82a. Methaneethorn J. Population pharmacokinetics of valproic acid in patients with mania: implication for individualized dosing regimens. *Clin Ther.* 2017;39(6):1171–1181.

83. Arzimanoglou A, Ferreira JA, Satlin A, et al. Safety and pharmacokinetic profile of rufinamide in pediatric patients aged less than 4 years with Lennox-Gastaut syndrome: an interim analysis from a multicenter, randomized, active-controlled, open-label study. *Eur J Paediatr Neurol.* 2016;20(3):393–402.

84. Vučićević K, Jovanović M, Golubović B, et al. Nonlinear mixed effects modelling approach in investigating phenobarbital pharmacokinetic interactions in epileptic patients. *Eur J Clin Pharmacol.* 2015;71(2):183–190.

16

VANCOMYCIN

Timothy J. Bensman and Paul M. Beringer

By the end of the vancomycin chapter, the learner should be able to:

1. Describe the relationship between plasma vancomycin concentration and its bactericidal and postantibiotic effects.
2. Describe the rationale for monitoring AUC_{24hr} to maximize the efficacy and safety of vancomycin.
3. Devise a plasma sampling strategy to obtain an accurate estimate of the individuals AUC_{24hr}.
4. Devise dosing schemes for patients on standard hemodialysis, high-flux hemodialysis, continuous ambulatory peritoneal dialysis (CAPD), and continuous renal replacement therapy (CRRT).
5. Describe the effect of obesity on the pharmacokinetic parameters for vancomycin.
6. Describe appropriate monitoring parameters to minimize dose-related adverse effects

Vancomycin is a glycopeptide antibiotic with a gram-positive spectrum of activity that is effective in the treatment of infections involving methicillin-resistant *Staphylococcus aureus* (MRSA). It is also an alternative to penicillin in patients who have a history of serious penicillin allergy.[1–6] Vancomycin is bactericidal for most gram-positive organisms, except against enterococci, and it is synergistic with gentamicin against most strains of *S. aureus* and enterococci.[5,7] There has been a resurgence in the use of vancomycin because of the increased prevalence of MRSA.

Vancomycin is poorly absorbed orally and has been used to treat gastrointestinal overgrowths of gram-positive bacteria. When used to treat systemic infections, vancomycin must be given by the intravenous route or intraperitoneally for those patients receiving continuous ambulatory peritoneal dialysis (CAPD). The usual adult dose, in patients with normal renal function, is 1 g (10 to 15 mg/kg) administered intravenously over 60 minutes every 8 to 12 hours.[4–6] Vancomycin is eliminated by renal excretion and requires dosage adjustment, particularly in the elderly and in patients with diminished renal function.

Vancomycin use is associated with several dose-related adverse effects, including a pseudoallergic reaction, nephrotoxicity, and ototoxicity. The pseudoallergic reaction (Red man syndrome) is characterized by flushing around the head and neck region and puritis and is mediated by histamine release. The reaction can be mitigated by administering by a slower infusion rate and/or adding an antihistamine. Therapeutic drug monitoring is employed to reduce the risk for development of nephrotoxicity and ototoxicity. The ideal vancomycin dosing regimen is one that results in trough concentrations that are in the range of 5 to 15 and peak concentrations less than 50 mg/L.[1,2,5,6,8–15] Patients most likely to benefit from vancomycin plasma concentration monitoring are those at highest risk for therapeutic failure or potential drug toxicity. These include pediatrics, burn, and cystic fibrosis patients owing to high clearances and short half-lives. In addition, it is important to monitor plasma vancomycin concentrations in patients with poor renal function who are receiving empiric dosages, because they are at greater risk of toxicity.

THERAPEUTIC AND TOXIC PLASMA CONCENTRATIONS

Efficacy

The efficacy of vancomycin therapy has been associated with attainment of target steady-state trough concentrations, although accumulating clinical evidence indicates a stronger association with achievement of a 24-hour area under the curve/minimum inhibitory concentration (AUC_{24hr}/MIC) >400.[16,17] The Clinical Laboratory Standards Institute susceptibility breakpoint for vancomycin is 2 mcg/mL for *S. aureus* and typically ranges from 0.5 to 2 mcg/mL.[18] It has been demonstrated that serum unbound trough concentrations five times the MIC are optimal for bacterial eradication and clinical success.[15] Considering plasma protein binding of 50%, the target trough concentrations for efficacy range from 5 to 20 mg/L (0.5 to 2 mcg/mL times 5 divided by 50%). High-dose regimens achieving 10 to 20 mcg/mL are favored in patients with endocarditis, nosocomial infections, pneumonia, and other systemic infections who are at greater risk of therapeutic failure.[8,10,11,15,19–21] However, the high dose regimens need to be evaluated in the context of the patients risk for nephrotoxicity (see safety below).

A growing body of evidence supports the AUC_{24hr}/MIC ratio of 400 as the clinically relevant therapeutic target, where AUC_{24hr} is expressed as mg/L · hr and MIC is expressed as mg/L.[14,15,22,23] The rationale for targeting an AUC_{24hr}/MIC for vancomycin is based on the pharmacodynamic properties of concentration-independent killing and a modest dose-dependent postantibiotic effect of 0.5 to 3 hours.[5,24] Alternative antibiotic agents should be considered in patients with infections involving MRSA strains with MICs ≥2 mcg/mL because of the inability to achieve an AUC_{24hr}/MIC >400 without significantly increasing the risk for development of nephrotoxicity.[25]

Safety

A relatively high incidence of adverse effects was initially associated with vancomycin. However, it is believed that some of these adverse reactions were caused by impurities in the original products; the current formulations are more pure.[1] Phlebitis and a histamine reaction that presents as flushing, tachycardia, and hypotension are known side effects associated with vancomycin therapy. To minimize the histamine response, vancomycin should be infused slowly over 60 to 120 minutes, and/or premedication with an antihistamine should be considered.[26,27] In addition, vancomycin therapy is associated with dose-related nephrotoxicity and ototoxicity. As a single agent, vancomycin is associated with a low incidence of nephrotoxicity (5%); however, when it is combined with aminoglycoside antibiotics, the incidence may be as high as 30%.[28] Higher rates of nephrotoxicity (11% to 20%) have been observed when trough vancomycin concentrations of 15 to 20 mg/L are targeted,[18,22,26] and more so (30% to 45%) when high-dose therapy is maintained for 2 weeks or longer.[15,29,30] At the present time, research on the association between vancomycin AUC_{24hr} and nephrotoxicity is limited. However, in two retrospective studies, similar breakpoint AUC_{24hr} were found at $\geq$1,300 and >1,063 mg · hr/L.[20,31] While, additional studies are needed, an AUC_{24} of 800 represents a conservative threshold with minimal risk of toxicity while achieving microbiologic efficacy with MICs up to 2 mg/L (i.e., $AUC_{24hr}/MIC = 400$). In terms of

KEY PARAMETERS: Vancomycin

	ADULT	PEDIATRIC
Therapeutic plasma concentration[a]		
Peak	<40–50 mg/L	<40–50
Trough	5–15 mg/L	5–15
F (oral)	<5%	<5%
V[b]	V = 0.72 L/kg if Cl_{Cr} is $\geq$60 mL/min V = 0.9 L/kg if Cl_{Cr} is <60 mL/min	V (L) = 0.636 × Wt
Cl[c]	Cl (mL/min) = (Cl_{Cr} × 0.689) + 3.66	Cl (L/hr) = 0.248 × $Wt^{0.75}$ × $(0.48/SCr)^{0.361}$ × $(\ln(age)/7.8)^{0.995}$
t½	6–7 hr	2–4 hr
fu[d] (fraction unbound in plasma)	0.45–0.7	0.61–0.95

[a]A total drug peak concentration of approximately 30 mg/L is a reasonable target; however, to ensure efficacy, trough concentrations should be maintained at or above 5 mg/L.
[b]Actual body weight (ABW).
[c]ABW and age in days.
[d]The fraction unbound in plasma may be as high as 0.8 to 0.9 in patients with end-stage renal disease.

ototoxicity, peak concentrations greater than 50 mg/L have been associated with hearing loss; with the majority of cases reported at concentrations >80 mg/L.[1,3,28]

With respect to determining patient-specific dosages, a variety of methods have been developed and proposed to estimate the pharmacokinetic parameters.[32-34] While most of the methods yield reasonable estimates of plasma vancomycin concentrations from a given dosage, the parameters used are based on population averages with sufficient variability such that therapeutic drug monitoring is still necessary when indicated.

BIOAVAILABILITY (F)

Vancomycin is poorly absorbed following oral administration (i.e., <5%); as a result, parenteral or intraperitoneal administration is necessary for the treatment of systemic infections. Vancomycin's limited oral bioavailability has been used advantageously to treat enterocolitis.[1,4-6]

VOLUME OF DISTRIBUTION (V)

The volume of distribution for vancomycin ranges between 0.5 and 1 L/kg.[32,35,36] In clinical practice, an average value of 0.7 L/kg is often used; however, the method described by Matzke et al. for estimating V for vancomycin in adults (i.e., those older than 18 years) splits population estimates by Cl_{Cr} and has the highest precision and least bias.[34,37] In Pediatrics, weight has been shown to influence volume of distribution.[38]

Adults:

$$V = 0.72 \text{ L/kg if } Cl_{Cr} \text{ is } \geq 60 \text{ mL/min} \qquad \textbf{(Eq. 16.1)}$$

$$V = 0.9 \text{ L/kg if } Cl_{Cr} \text{ is } < 60 \text{ mL/min} \qquad \textbf{(Eq. 16.2)}$$

Pediatrics:

$$V \text{ (L)} = 0.636 \times \text{Weight} \qquad \textbf{(Eq. 16.3)}$$

A two- or three-compartment model best describes the distribution of vancomycin. The complexity of this model can be problematic when peak plasma samples are obtained during the distribution phase. In clinical practice, a one-compartment model is frequently used.[13,32,39] Vancomycin has moderate plasma protein binding. The percentage unbound in plasma is approximately 60%, with a reported range of 45% to 70%.[35,40-42] Data in patients with end-stage renal disease suggest that the fraction unbound (fu) in plasma may be as high as 0.8 to 0.9.[43,44]

CLEARANCE (Cl)

Vancomycin is eliminated primarily by the renal route; approximately 5% of the dose is metabolized.[35,45] The clearance of vancomycin is highly correlated with creatinine clearance[32,36,39]:

$$\text{Cl}_{Cr} \text{ for Males (mL/min)} = \frac{(140 - \text{Age in years})(\text{Weight in kg})}{(72)(\text{SCr}_{ss})} \tag{Eq. 16.4}$$

$$\text{Cl}_{Cr} \text{ for Females (mL/min)} = (0.85)\frac{(140 - \text{Age in years})(\text{Weight in kg})}{(72)(\text{SCr}_{ss})} \tag{Eq. 16.5}$$

For issues that should be considered when estimating creatinine clearance, see Chapter 3.

Vancomycin clearance in adults:

$$\text{Cl (mL/min)} = (\text{Cl}_{Cr} \times 0.689) + 3.66 \tag{Eq. 16.6}$$

Vancomycin clearance in pediatrics:

$$\text{Cl (L/hr)} = 0.248 \times \text{Wt}^{0.75} \times (0.48/\text{SCr})^{0.361} \times (\ln (\text{Age in days})/7.8)^{0.995} \tag{Eq. 16.7}$$

Very little vancomycin is cleared by standard hemodialysis or peritoneal dialysis.[10,46,47] In patients undergoing CAPD, the small but continuous drug loss caused by peritoneal dialysis exchanges is significant. The usual approach is to replace vancomycin with intermittent intravenous injections on a somewhat more frequent basis than is usually done for patients with end-stage renal disease (in some cases, as often as every 3 to 5 days), or to instill vancomycin directly into the peritoneal space to treat peritonitis and achieve systemic concentrations of vancomycin.[48,49] Some caution should be used in evaluating plasma concentrations in patients with end-stage renal disease. Some immunoassays that use polyclonal antibodies overestimate actual vancomycin concentrations owing to an accumulation of pseudometabolites (crystalline degradation products) that cross-react with the assay.[49,50] In patients undergoing high-flux or high-efficiency hemodialysis, a significant amount of vancomycin can be removed. Early studies estimated that as much as 30% of vancomycin was removed during high-flux hemodialysis; recent reports indicate that only 17% of vancomycin is removed during these procedures. Early investigators did not recognize that a redistribution of vancomycin occurs after the completion of dialysis.[51,52] Owing to wide interpatient variability, monitoring plasma vancomycin concentrations to determine individual dosing requirements is often required.

HALF-LIFE (t½)

The usual serum half-life of vancomycin in adults is 6 to 7 hours; in patients with end-stage renal disease, the half-life may approach 7 days.[10,32,35,44] This wide range in the serum half-life partially explains the variability in the dose and dosing intervals used for vancomycin. Adult patients with normal renal function may receive the drug every 8 to 12 hours, whereas those with end-stage renal disease may receive a dose once a week.[10,46]

NOMOGRAMS

Dosing nomograms for vancomycin are available.[10,53] However, an understanding of the desired therapeutic range and the pharmacokinetic parameters of vancomycin provides the clinician more flexibility to tailor doses and dosing intervals that meet the specific needs of the patient. For example, using pharmacokinetic parameters allows targeting plasma vancomycin AUC_{24hr}/MIC which is particularly advantageous when treating infections with vancomycin-intermediate–sensitive bacteria.

TIME TO SAMPLE

Steady-state trough concentration monitoring is currently the standard of care[25]; however, given the discordance between trough levels and AUC_{24hr}, it is advisable to measure both peak and trough concentrations to more accurately estimate the AUC_{24hr}.[54] Measurement of both peak and trough concentrations may also be helpful in patients in whom the pharmacokinetic parameters may be difficult to estimate with confidence (e.g., very overweight or underweight patients).

   If only a steady-state trough concentration is available, peak concentrations can be estimated with reasonable accuracy based on the dose administered, an estimate of the volume of distribution, and a measured trough concentration. This is especially true in patients with diminished renal function and a long vancomycin half-life.

   If the trough concentration is known, the peak concentration (Css max) can be approximated using Equation 16.8.

$$Css\ max = \left[Css\ min\right] + \left[\frac{(S)(F)(Dose)}{V}\right] \qquad \textbf{(Eq. 16.8)}$$

The (S)(F)(D)/V represents the change in concentration (ΔC) following a dose.

   As described in Part I (see Chapter 2), the use of the above equation requires that several conditions be met. They are as follows:

1. Steady state has been achieved.
2. The measured plasma concentration is a trough concentration.
3. The bolus dose is an acceptable model.

   In the clinical setting, trough concentrations are often obtained slightly before the true trough. Because vancomycin has a relatively long half-life, most plasma concentrations obtained within 1 hour of the true trough can be assumed to have met condition 2 above.

Because vancomycin follows a multicompartmental model, it is difficult to avoid the distribution phase when obtaining peak plasma concentrations.[55] If a 1-compartment model is to be applied, samples should be obtained at least 1 or possibly 2 hours after the end of the infusion period. It is difficult to evaluate the appropriateness of a dosing regimen that is based on plasma samples obtained before steady state. Additional plasma concentrations are required to more accurately estimate a patient's apparent clearance and half-life, and to ensure that any dosing adjustments based on a non–steady-state trough concentration actually achieve the targeted steady-state concentrations.

Question #1   *B.C., a 65-year-old, 45-kg man with a serum creatinine concentration of 2.2 mg/dL, is being treated for a presumed hospital-acquired, MRSA infection. Design a dosing regimen that will produce peak concentrations less than 50 mg/L and trough concentrations of 5 to 15 mg/L.*

The first step in calculating an appropriate dosing regimen for B.C. is to estimate his pharmacokinetic parameters (i.e., clearance, volume of distribution, elimination rate constant, and half-life).

B.C.'s creatinine clearance is estimated to be approximately 21.3 mL/min, as shown using Equation 16.4:

$$\text{Cl}_{\text{Cr}} \text{ for Males (mL/min)} = \frac{(140 - \text{Age in years})(\text{Weight in kg})}{(72)(\text{SCr}_{ss})}$$

$$= \frac{(140 - 65)(45 \text{ kg})}{(72)(2.2 \text{ mg/dL})}$$

$$= 21.3 \text{ mL/min}$$

Using Equation 16.6, the corresponding vancomycin clearance for B.C. is 1.1 L/hr.

$$\text{Cl (mL/min)} = (\text{Cl}_{\text{Cr}} \times 0.689) + 3.66$$

$$= 21.3 \text{ mL/min } (0.689) + 3.66$$

$$= 18.3 \text{ mL/min}$$

or

$$= 18.3 \text{ mL/min} \times \frac{60 \text{ min/hr}}{1,000 \text{ mL/L}}$$

$$= 1.1 \text{ L/hr}$$

The volume of distribution for B.C. can be calculated using Equation 16.2 (see Key Parameters, this chapter). According to the following calculations, B.C.'s expected volume of distribution would be 40.5 L.

$$V(L) = 0.9 \text{ L/kg (45 kg)} = 40.5 \text{ L}$$

The calculated vancomycin clearance of 1.1 L/hr and the volume of distribution of 40.5 L can then be used to estimate the elimination rate constant of 0.027 hr^{-1} using Equation 16.9.

$$K = \frac{Cl}{V} \qquad \text{(Eq. 16.9)}$$

$$= \frac{1.1 \text{ L/hr}}{40.5 \text{ L}}$$

$$= 0.027 \text{ hr}^{-1}$$

and the corresponding vancomycin half-life can be calculated using Equation 16.10:

$$t\tfrac{1}{2} = \frac{(0.693)(V)}{Cl} \qquad \text{(Eq. 16.10)}$$

$$= \frac{(0.693)(V)}{Cl}$$

$$= \frac{(0.693)(40.5 \text{ L})}{1.1 \text{ L/hr}}$$

$$= 25.5 \text{ hr}$$

Using Equation 16.11, with the patient's weight, and the volume of distribution of 40.5 L that we calculated above, and substituting the usual maintenance dose as 15 mg/kg for the dose, it can be seen that the initial plasma concentration should be approximately 17 mg/L.

$$C_0 = \frac{(S)(F)(\text{Loading Dose})}{V} \qquad \text{(Eq. 16.11)}$$

$$C_0 = \frac{(1)(1)(15 \text{ mg/kg} \times 45 \text{ kg})}{40.5}$$

$$= 16.7 \text{ mg/L}$$

This value is below the usual targeted peak concentration of about 30 mg/L. The initial dose (i.e., loading dose) can be calculated using the assumed volume of distribution of 40.5 L using Equation 16.12. The salt form and bioavailability are assumed to be

1.0 when vancomycin is administered intravenously. Using an initial target of 30 mg/L, the loading dose would be approximately 1250 mg.

$$\text{Loading Dose} = \frac{(V)(C)}{(S)(F)} \qquad \text{(Eq. 16.12)}$$

$$= \frac{(40.5)(30 \text{ mg/L})}{(1)(1)}$$
$$= 1{,}215 \sim 1{,}250 \text{ mg}$$

There are no known renal or ototoxicities associated with elevated vancomycin levels that occur during the distribution phase. However, to minimize the cardiovascular effects associated with rapid administration, the initial and subsequent doses should be administered over approximately 60 minutes. In addition, if peak concentrations are measured, samples should be drawn at least 1 to 2 hours after completion of the infusion period to avoid the distribution phase (if using a one-compartment model as demonstrated here).

The maintenance dose can be calculated by a number of methods. One approach might be to first approximate the hourly infusion rate required to maintain the desired average concentration. Then, the hourly infusion rate can be multiplied by an appropriate dosing interval to calculate a reasonable dose to be given on an intermittent basis. For example, if an average concentration of 20 mg/L is selected (approximately halfway between the desired peak concentration of $\approx$30 mg/L and trough concentration of $\approx$10 mg/L), the hourly administration rate would be 22 mg/hr (Equation 16.13).

$$\text{Maintenance Dose} = \frac{(Cl)(Css \text{ ave})(\tau)}{(S)(F)} \qquad \text{(Eq. 16.13)}$$

$$= \frac{(1.1 \text{ L/hr})(20 \text{ mg/L})(1 \text{ hr})}{(1)(1)}$$
$$= 22 \text{ mg/hr}$$

Although a number of dosing intervals could be selected, 24 hours is reasonable because it is a convenient interval and approximates B.C.'s half-life for vancomycin of 25.5 hours. A dosing interval of approximately 1 half-life should result in peak concentrations of 30 mg/L and trough concentrations that are within the 5 to 15 mg/L range, in this case. If an interval of 24 hours is selected, the dose would be approximately 500 mg.

$$\text{Maintenance Dose} = \frac{(1.1 \text{ L/hr})(20 \text{ mg/L})(24 \text{ hr})}{(1)(1)}$$
$$= 528 \sim 500 \text{ mg}$$

This method assumes that the average concentration is halfway between the peak and trough. As mentioned in Part I (see Chapter 2), this is approximately correct as long as the dosing interval is less than or approximately equal to the drug's half-life. When dosing intervals greatly exceed the half-life, the true average concentration is much lower than halfway between the peak and trough levels.

A second approach that can be used to calculate the maintenance dose is to select a desired peak and trough concentration that is consistent with the therapeutic range and B.C.'s vancomycin half-life. For example, if steady-state peak concentrations of 30 mg/L are desired, it would take approximately two half-lives for that peak level to fall to 7.5 mg/L (a level of 30 mg/L declines to 15 mg/L in one half-life and to 7.5 mg/L in another half-life). Because the vancomycin half-life in B.C. is approximately 1 day, the dosing interval would be 48 hours. The dose to be administered every 48 hours can be calculated using Equation 16.14.

$$\text{Dose} = \frac{(V)(Css\ max - Css\ min)}{(S)(F)} \tag{Eq. 16.14}$$

$$= \frac{(40.5\ L)(30\ mg/L - 7.5\ mg/L)}{(1)(1)}$$

$$= 911 \sim 900\ mg$$

The peak and trough concentrations that are expected using this dosing regimen can be calculated using Equations 16.15 and 16.17 respectively.

$$Css\ max = \frac{\dfrac{(S)(F)(Dose)}{V}}{1 - e^{-K\tau}} \tag{Eq. 16.15}$$

$$= \frac{\dfrac{(1)(1)(900\ mg)}{40.5\ L}}{(1 - e^{-(0.027\ hr^{-1})(48\ hr)})}$$

$$= 30.6\ mg/L$$

Note that although 30.6 mg/L is an acceptable peak, the actual clinical peak would normally be obtained approximately 1 hour after the end of a 1-hour infusion, or 2 hours after this calculated peak concentration, and would be about 29 mg/L, as calculated by Equation 16.16.

$$C_2 = C_1(e^{-Kt}) \tag{Eq. 16.16}$$

$$= 30.6\ mg/L(e^{-(0.027\ hr^{-1})(2\ hr)})$$

$$= 29\ mg/L$$

The calculated trough concentration would be about 8 mg/L (Equations 16.17 and 16.18).

$$\text{Css min} = \frac{\dfrac{(S)(F)(\text{Dose})}{V}}{1 - e^{-K\tau}}(e^{-K\tau}) \qquad \text{(Eq. 16.17)}$$

$$\text{Css min} = (\text{Css max})(e^{-K\tau}) \qquad \text{(Eq. 16.18)}$$

$$= (30.6 \text{ mg/L})(e^{-(0.027 \text{ hr}^{-1})(48 \text{ hr})})$$
$$= 8.4 \text{ mg/L}$$

This process of checking the expected peak and trough concentrations is most appropriate when the dose or the dosing interval has been changed from a calculated value (e.g., twice the half-life) to a practical value (e.g., 8, 12, 18, 24, 36, or 48 hours). If different plasma vancomycin concentrations are desired, Equations 16.15 and 16.17 can be used to target specific vancomycin concentrations by adjusting the dose and/or the dosing interval. For example, a dosage regimen of 1,000 mg every 48 hours would result in calculated peak and trough concentrations of 34 and 9.3 mg/L, respectively. Alternatively, 800 mg every 36 hours would result in an expected peak concentration of 31.7 mg/L and a trough concentration of 12.0 mg/L, at steady state.

A third alternative is to rearrange Equation 16.17:

$$\text{Css min} = \frac{\dfrac{(S)(F)(\text{Dose})}{V}}{1 - e^{-K\tau}}(e^{-K\tau})$$

such that the dose can be calculated.

$$\text{Dose} = \frac{(\text{Css min})(V)\left(1 - e^{-K\tau}\right)}{(S)(F)\left(e^{-K\tau}\right)} \qquad \text{(Eq. 16.19)}$$

Note that it is the Css min or trough concentration that is used to solve for dose. Making the appropriate substitutions for the parameters indicated in Equation 16.19 and choosing a target trough concentration of 10 mg/L and a dosing interval of 24 hours, a dose of approximately 369 ~ 400 mg is calculated.

$$\text{Dose} = \frac{(\text{Trough})(1 - e^{-K\tau}(V))}{e^{-K\tau}}$$
$$= \frac{(10 \text{ mg/L})(1 - e^{-(0.027 \text{ hr}^{-1})(24 \text{ hr})})(40.5 \text{ L})}{e^{-(0.027 \text{ hr}^{-1})(24 \text{ hr})}}$$
$$= 369 \sim 400 \text{ mg}$$

Alternatively, doses could have been calculated for dosing intervals of 36 or 48 hours if those intervals were deemed to be appropriate.

Question #2   *E.K., a 60-year-old, 50-kg woman with a serum creatinine of 1.0 mg/dL, has been empirically started on 750 mg of vancomycin every 12 hours for treatment of a hospital-acquired staphylococcal infection. What are the expected peak and trough vancomycin concentrations for E.K.?*

To calculate the peak and trough concentrations, E.K.'s, clearance, volume of distribution, and elimination rate constant (or half-life) need to be estimated.

E.K.'s creatinine clearance can be calculated using Equation 16.5, and Equation 16.6 can be used to calculate her vancomycin clearance of 2.2 L/hr, as shown in the following:

$$Cl_{Cr} \text{ for Females } (mL/min) = (0.85)\frac{(140 - \text{Age in years})(\text{Weight in kg})}{(72)(SCr_{ss})}$$

$$= (0.85)\frac{(140 - 60)(50 \text{ kg})}{(72)(1.0 \text{ mg/dL})}$$

$$= 47.2 \text{ mL/min}$$

Using Equation 16.6 to calculate vancomycin clearance:

$$Cl \text{ (mL/min)} = (Cl_{Cr} \times 0.689) + 3.66$$

$$= 47.2 \text{ mL/min } (0.689) + 3.66$$

$$= 36.2 \text{ mL/min}$$

or

$$= 36.2 \text{ mL/min} \times \frac{60 \text{ min/hr}}{1,000 \text{ mL/L}}$$

$$= 2.2 \text{ L/hr}$$

Using Equation 16.2, the expected volume of distribution for E.K. is 45 L.

$$V(L) = 0.9 \text{ L/kg } (50 \text{ kg})$$

$$= 45 \text{ L}$$

Equation 16.9 can now be used to calculate E.K.'s elimination rate constant and Equation 16.10 to calculate the corresponding half-life.

$$K = \frac{Cl}{V}$$

$$= \frac{2.2 \text{ L/hr}}{45 \text{ L}}$$

$$= 0.049 \text{ hr}^{-1}$$

and the corresponding vancomycin half-life can be calculated as follows:

$$t\frac{1}{2} = \frac{(0.693)(V)}{Cl}$$

$$= \frac{(0.693)(V)}{Cl}$$

$$= \frac{(0.693)(45 \text{ L})}{2.2 \text{ L/hr}}$$

$$= 14.2 \text{ hr}$$

Equations 16.15 and 16.17 can be used to calculate the expected peak and trough concentrations for E.K.

$$Css \text{ max} = \frac{\frac{(S)(F)(Dose)}{V}}{1 - e^{-K\tau}}$$

$$= \frac{\frac{(1)(1)(750 \text{ mg})}{45 \text{ L}}}{(1 - e^{-(0.049 \text{ hr}^{-1})(12)})}$$

$$= 37.6 \text{ mg/L}$$

To calculate the clinical peak concentration, which is usually sampled 2 hours after the start of a vancomycin infusion (1 hour after the end of a 1-hour infusion), the Css max could be decayed for 2 hours using Equation 16.16.

$$= 37.6 \text{ mg/L}(e^{-(0.049 \text{ hr}^{-1})(2 \text{ hr})})$$

$$= 34.1 \text{ mg/L}$$

Css min can be calculated using Equation 16.17 and the dosing interval of 12 hours.

$$\text{Css min} = \text{Css max} \times (e^{-K\tau})$$

$$= 37.6 \text{ mg/L}(e^{-(0.049 \text{ hr}^{-1})(12 \text{ hr})})$$

$$= 20.9 \text{ mg/L}$$

Although the expected peak concentration of ≈ 34 mg/L is not above the usually accepted range for peak concentrations, the trough concentration of 20.9 mg/L is above the usual targeted range of 5 to 15 mg/L, which is targeted for efficacy/safety. This suggests that decreasing the dose and/or increasing the dosing interval, as well as monitoring plasma concentrations of vancomycin, would be appropriate.

Question #3   *A culture indicates that the infection is caused by MRSA with an MIC of 1.0 mg/L. A steady-state trough concentration of 25 mg/L was obtained for E.K. Design a dosing regimen that will produce therapeutic vancomycin concentrations and an $AUC_{24}/MIC \geq 400$ for E.K.*

To design such a regimen, E.K.'s pharmacokinetic parameters should first be revised so that they are consistent with the observed trough concentration of 25 mg/L. Some assumptions will have to be made. Because the measured trough concentration is higher than predicted, her half-life is longer than the estimate of 14.2 hours. For E.K., the percentage fluctuation between peak and trough concentrations should be relatively small at steady state because her dosing interval of 12 hours is shorter than her apparent half-life. Therefore, the best approach is to use the literature estimate for volume of distribution and then calculate the corresponding elimination rate constant and clearance values.

If E.K.'s volume of distribution is assumed to be 45 L (see calculation above using Equation 16.1) and the observed trough concentration of 25 mg/L is used, a peak concentration of approximately 42 mg/L can be calculated by using Equation 16.8, as follows:

$$\text{Css max} = [25 \text{ mg/L}] + \left[\frac{(1)(1)(750 \text{ mg})}{45.0 \text{ L}} \right]$$

$$= 41.7 \text{ mg/L}$$

Using the observed trough concentration of 25 mg/L and the predicted peak concentration of 42 mg/L, an elimination rate constant (K) can be calculated using Equation 16.20, where C_1 is the peak concentration of 42 mg/L, C_2 is the trough concentration of 25 mg/L, and the interval between those two concentrations, t, is the dosing interval of 12 hours.

$$K = \frac{\ln\left(\dfrac{C_1}{C_2}\right)}{t}$$ (Eq. 16.20)

$$= \frac{\ln\left(\dfrac{42 \text{ mg/L}}{25 \text{ mg/L}}\right)}{12 \text{ hr}}$$

$$= 0.043 \text{ hr}^{-1}$$

This apparent elimination rate constant of 0.043 hr^{-1} corresponds to a half-life of approximately 16 hours (Equation 16.21).

$$t\tfrac{1}{2} = \frac{0.693}{K}$$ (Eq. 16.21)

$$= \frac{0.693}{0.043 \text{ hr}^{-1}}$$

$$= 16 \text{ hr}$$

The apparent elimination rate constant of 0.043 hr^{-1} and the assumed volume of distribution of 45 L can be used in Equation 16.22 to calculate E.K.'s vancomycin clearance.

$$Cl = (K)(V)$$ (Eq. 16.22)

$$= (0.043 \text{ hr}^{-1})(45 \text{ L})$$

$$= 1.94 \text{ L/hr}$$

Because the revised t½ is ≥τ, we expect Css ave to be halfway between Css max and Css min. Therefore, clearance could have been approximated by assuming Css ave is approximately equal to:

$$\text{Css ave} = \text{Css min} + \left(\frac{1}{2}\right)\frac{(S)(F)(\text{Dose})}{V}$$ (Eq. 16.23)

and then calculating clearance by using Equation 16.24 (see Chapter 2):

$$Cl = \frac{(S)(F)(Dose/\tau)}{Css\ ave} \hspace{2cm} \textbf{(Eq. 16.24)}$$

The maintenance dose can then be calculated using Equation 16.17. Because the apparent half-life is approximately 16 hours, the most logical dosing interval and Css min would be 24 hours and 10 to 15 mg/L, respectively.

$$Dose = \frac{(Css\ min)(V)(1 - e^{-K\tau})}{(S)(F)(e^{-K\tau})}$$

$$Dose = \frac{(12.5\ mg/L)(45\ L)\left(1 - e^{-(0.043\ hr^{-1})(24\ hr)}\right)}{(1)(1)\left(e^{-(0.043\ hr^{-1})(24\ hr)}\right)}$$

$$= 1,016 \sim 1,000\ mg$$

We can round the dose to 1,000 mg every 24 hours, which should result in a steady-state Cmax concentration of approximately 35 mg/L by using Equations 16.15.

$$Css\ max = \frac{\dfrac{(S)(F)(Dose)}{V}}{1 - e^{-K\tau}}$$

$$= \frac{\dfrac{(1)(1)(1,000\ mg)}{45\ L}}{\left(1 - e^{-(0.043\ hr^{-1})(24\ hr)}\right)}$$

$$= 34.5\ mg/L$$

A trough concentration of approximately 12 mg/L can be calculated using Equation 16.18.

$$Css\ min = (Css\ max)(e^{-K\tau})$$

$$= (34.5\ mg/L)\left(e^{-(0.043\ hr^{-1})(24\ hr)}\right)$$

$$= 12.3\ mg/L$$

This trough concentration of approximately 12 mg/L is within the usual therapeutic range (5 to 15 mg/L).

The AUC_{24}/MIC for this case can be determined by employing Equation 16.25:

$$AUC_{24}/MIC = \frac{Dose_{24}\ (mg)}{Cl(L/hr) \times MIC(mg/L)} \hspace{1.5cm} \textbf{(Eq. 16.25)}$$

$$= \frac{1,000\ mg}{(1.94\ L/hr)(1\ mg/L)}$$

$$= 515$$

Hence, the dose of 1,000 mg every 24 hours produces peak and trough vancomycin concentrations within the usual therapeutic range, and also yields a desirable $AUC_{24}/MIC > 400$.

If a peak (2 hours after a 1 hour infusion) and trough (40 mg/L) were available, then one could use the peak–trough approach to revise patient-specific parameters and to calculate the dose required to achieve an AUC_{24}/MIC of around 400. Assuming that the trough was drawn right before the start of infusion and using Equation 16.20, we have

$$K = \frac{\ln\left(\dfrac{C_1}{C_2}\right)}{t}$$

$$= \frac{\ln\left(\dfrac{40}{25}\right)}{9}$$

$$= 0.052$$

This apparent elimination rate constant of $0.052\ hr^{-1}$ corresponds to a half-life of approximately 13.3 hours (Equation 16.21).

$$t\tfrac{1}{2} = \frac{0.693}{K}$$

$$= \frac{0.693}{0.052\ hr^{-1}}$$

$$= 13.3\ hr$$

Because the infusion time (1 hour) is short relative to the half-life (13 hours), the bolus model is appropriate to determine the revised V.

$$V = \frac{\dfrac{Dose}{Css\ peak}}{1 - e^{-(K)(\tau)}} e^{-(K)(t)}$$

$$= \frac{\dfrac{750\ mg}{40\ mg/L}}{1 - e^{-(0.052)(12)}} e^{-(0.052)(3)}$$

$$= 34.6\ L$$

The revised clearance can be calculated using the revised K and V and Equation 16.22:

$$Cl\ (L/hr) = (K)(V)$$

$$= 0.052\ hr^{-1}\ (34.6\ L)$$

$$= 1.8\ L/hr$$

Now, we can calculate a dose to achieve a target AUC_{24hr}/MIC of 400 using Equation 16.25.

$$AUC_{24hr}/MIC = \frac{Dose_{24}}{Cl \times MIC}$$

$$Dose_{24hr} = AUC_{24hr}/MIC \times Cl \times MIC$$

$$= 400 \times 1.8 \times 1$$

$$= 720 \text{ mg}$$

We can round this dose to 750 mg every 24 hours and check the steady-state Css max concentration using Equation 16.15

$$Css\ max = \frac{\dfrac{(S)(F)(Dose)}{V}}{1 - e^{-K\tau}}$$

$$= \frac{\dfrac{(1)(1)(750 \text{ mg})}{34.6 \text{ L}}}{1 - e^{-(0.052)(24)}}$$

$$= 30.4 \approx 30 \text{ mg/L}$$

A steady-state trough concentration can be calculated using Equation 16.18.

$$Css\ min = (Css\ max)(e^{-K\tau})$$

$$= (30)\left(e^{-(0.052 \text{ hr}^{-1})(24 \text{ hr})}\right)$$

$$= 8.6 \approx 9 \text{ mg/L}$$

Here, we then see that the target AUC_{24}/MIC of >400 is achieved while also maintaining a therapeutic trough concentration. The peak concentration minimizes ototoxicity risks.

It should be noted that without the peak level, we would have to assume the population average for volume of 45 L compared with our revised estimate of 35 L. Using the peak–trough approach, a dose reduction of 250 mg was observed. This example illustrates that measuring both peak and trough concentrations provides a more precise means to determine individualized pharmacokinetic parameters (i.e., Cl, V) to achieve therapeutic success and minimize toxicities (i.e., nephrotoxicity).

Question #4   *A.C., a 50-year-old, 60-kg woman with end-stage renal disease and a serum creatinine of 9 mg/dL, is undergoing standard intermittent hemodialysis treatments three times a week and, currently, has an apparent shunt infection that is to be treated with vancomycin. Calculate an appropriate dose for A.C.*

Vancomycin is extensively cleared by the kidneys; consequently, patients with end-stage renal disease have prolonged half-lives that average 5 to 7 days. This extended half-life is consistent with a residual vancomycin clearance of 3 to 4 mL/70 kg/min (0.18 to 0.24 L/70 kg/hr) and an average volume of distribution. Depending on A.C.'s residual renal function, the half-life may be shorter or longer than this general range. Note that for dialysis patients, it is not appropriate to use their SCr to estimate creatinine clearance with Equation 16.9 or 16.21 because the SCr is not at steady state. The duration and frequency of A.C.'s hemodialysis is not a factor in vancomycin dosing because the amount of vancomycin cleared during standard hemodialysis is negligible.

The usual approach to the use of vancomycin in patients receiving intermittent hemodialysis is to administer 1 g every 5 days to 2 weeks. Using Equation 16.2 to estimate the volume of distribution gives:

$$V = 0.9 \text{ L/kg if Cl}_{Cr} \text{ is } <60 \text{ mL/min}$$
$$= 0.9 \text{ L/kg (60 kg)}$$
$$= 54 \text{ L}$$

Then, one can see from Equation 16.26 that the first 1-g dose should result in an initial peak concentration of 18.5 mg/L.

$$C_0 = \frac{(S)(F)(\text{Loading Dose})}{V} \qquad \textbf{(Eq. 16.26)}$$

$$= \frac{(1)(1)(1,000 \text{ mg})}{54 \text{ L}}$$

$$= 18.5 \text{ mg/L}$$

For a dose of 1 g administered weekly, steady-state peak and trough levels of approximately 38.5 and 20 mg/L, respectively, can be calculated using an average vancomycin clearance of 3.5 mL/min (0.21 L/hr), a volume of distribution of 54 L, and a corresponding elimination rate constant of 0.0039 hr^{-1} (Equations 16.15 and 16.18).

$$\text{Css max} = \frac{(S)(F)(\text{Dose})}{V} \frac{1}{1 - e^{-K\tau}}$$

$$= \frac{\dfrac{(1)(1)(1,000 \text{ mg})}{54 \text{ L}}}{1 - e^{-(0.0039 \text{ hr}^{-1})(24 \text{ hr/day})(7 \text{ days})}}$$

$$= 38.5 \text{ mg/L}$$

$$\text{Css min} = (\text{Css max})(e^{-K\tau})$$

$$= (38.5)\left(e^{-(0.0039)(24 \text{ hr/day})(7 \text{ days})}\right)$$

$$= 20 \text{ mg/L}$$

If the 1-g dose had been administered every 2 weeks, the expected peak and trough vancomycin concentrations would have been approximately 25 and 7 mg/L, respectively.

However, because of the long half-life of vancomycin in renal failure (approximately 1 week) and a usual course of therapy of 2 weeks, steady state would not be achieved. Alternatively, if a dose of 500 mg was given weekly for a prolonged period, the expected steady-state peak and trough concentrations would have been approximately 19 and 10 mg/L, respectively. When the same average dosing rate $[(S)(F)(Dose/\tau)]$ is administered as a smaller dose given more frequently, the steady-state peak concentration is lower and the steady-state trough concentration is higher, but the average steady-state concentration is the same, as demonstrated by Equation 16.27 (also see Interpretation of Plasma Drug Concentrations in Chapter 2).

$$Css\ ave = \frac{(S)(F)(Dose/\tau)}{Cl} \qquad \textbf{(Eq. 16.27)}$$

$$= \frac{(1)(1)(1,000\ mg)/(14\ days)(24\ hr/day)}{0.21\ L/hr}$$

$$= 14.2\ mg/L$$

vs.

$$= \frac{(1)(1)(500\ mg)/(7\ days)(24\ hr/day)}{0.21\ L/hr}$$

$$= 14.2\ mg/L$$

If an extended course of therapy is anticipated, it is probably advisable to obtain vancomycin plasma levels to make certain that A.C.'s actual plasma levels are within an acceptable range. In seriously ill patients, it might be appropriate to obtain an initial vancomycin level 3 to 5 days after the initiation of therapy. The purpose is to ensure that the patient's actual clearance is not unusually large, resulting in vancomycin levels that are below the desired therapeutic range.

If A.C. had been receiving CAPD as her method of dialysis, it is probable that the vancomycin would be administered via her peritoneal dialysis fluid. The usual approach is to place 15 to 30 mg/kg of vancomycin (~1 to 2 g for A.C.) into an initial dialysate exchange, which should result in approximately 50% of that dose being absorbed during the usual 4- to 6-hour dwell time. Her maintenance dose would then be administered in one of two ways. An additional 15 to 30 mg/kg dose could be administered in single exchanges every 3 to 5 days such that her predose trough vancomycin concentration would be maintained at ≈10 mg/L. A less common, alternative method for maintenance therapy is to place in each dialysis exchange enough vancomycin to achieve a dialysate concentration of 15 to 20 mg/L (30 to 40 mg in a 2-L exchange). This technique of placing vancomycin in each exchange results in an average steady-state plasma concentration approximately equal to the concentration of vancomycin in the dialysate fluid, after multiple exchanges (i.e., 15 to 20 mg/L).[42,43]

Question #5 *Suppose A.C. was given an initial 1-g dose and 3 days later, she underwent high-flux hemodialysis for 2 hours. Calculate a replacement dose after the dialysis session.*

Although the amount of vancomycin removed by standard hemodialysis is negligible, high-flux hemodialysis has been reported to remove approximately 17% over 2 hours.[47] Assuming the initial plasma concentration is 18.5 mg/L and using the estimated K of 0.0039 hr^{-1}, as calculated above for A.C, the predialysis concentration can be determined using Equation 16.16.

$$C_2 = C_1(e^{-Kt})$$

$$= 18.5 \text{ mg/L}\left(e^{-(0.0039 \text{ hr}^{-1})(72 \text{ hr})}\right)$$

$$= 14 \text{ mg/L}$$

If the plasma concentration declines by approximately 17% because of high-flux hemodialysis, then the postdialysis plasma concentration will be 83% of the predialysis concentration. This ignores any additional elimination from the intrinsic clearance during the 2-hour dialysis period, because it is negligible.

$$C \text{ postdialysis} = 14 \text{ mg/L}(0.83)$$

$$= 11.6 \text{ mg/L}$$

If a replacement dose is desired at this point, the dose can be calculated using Equation 16.28.

$$\text{Dose} = \frac{(V)(\Delta C)}{(S)(F)} \qquad \textbf{(Eq. 16.28)}$$

$$= \frac{(54 \text{ L})(18.5 \text{ mg/L} - 11.6 \text{mg/L})}{(1)(1)}$$

$$= 373 \sim 375 \text{ mg}$$

A similar approach can be used in a stepwise fashion to determine dosing needs on any particular day and dialysis schedule. The amount of actual drug loss will depend on the intrinsic Cl, V, time of decay (t), duration of hemodialysis, and efficiency of the dialysis treatment.

Question #6   *A.C. became hemodynamically unstable. Therefore, hemodialysis was discontinued, and continuous renal replacement therapy (CRRT) was initiated with an ultrafiltration rate of 1 L/hr. How should the vancomycin dosage be changed?*

In this case, it would be advisable to monitor vancomycin concentrations until the level declines to a point where therapy can be reinstituted (e.g., 5 to 15 mg/L). Recall from chapter 3 that not all CRRT is the same. Here the patient is undergoing CVVH given the reported ultrafiltration rate. Since no sieve coefficient is reported a good approximation is the fraction of unbound drug. Using the population average (fu = 0.6), we can estimate the clearance owing to CRRT as follows:

$$Cl_{CRRT}\text{Maximum} = (fu)(CRRT \text{ Flow Rate})$$

$$= (0.6)(1 \text{ L/hr})$$

The total vancomycin clearance would be the sum of the clearance owing to CRRT, and the estimated intrinsic clearance previously estimated as 0.21 L/hr.

$$Cl = Cl_{CRRT} + Cl_{pat}$$

$$= 0.6 \text{ L/hr} + 0.21 \text{ L/hr}$$

$$= 0.81 \text{ L/hr}$$

Now that we have estimated the Cl, using the previously estimated V, we can use Equation 16.9 to calculate the elimination rate constant as 0.015 hr^{-1}, and Equation 16.10 to calculate the half-life of 46 hours. Based on this information, we can employ Equations 16.15 and 16.18 to estimate the steady-state peak and trough concentrations, respectively, for a dose of 750 mg every 48 hours.

$$Css \text{ max} = \frac{\dfrac{(S)(F)(Dose)}{V}}{1 - e^{-K\tau}}$$

$$= \frac{\dfrac{(1)(1)(750 \text{ mg})}{54 \text{ L}}}{\left(1 - e^{-(0.015 \text{ hr}^{-1})(48 \text{ hr})}\right)}$$

$$= 27.1 \text{ mg/L}$$

$$Css \text{ min} = (Css \text{ max})(e^{-K\tau})$$

$$= (27.1 \text{ mg/L})\left(e^{-(0.015 \text{ hr}^{-1})(48 \text{ hr})}\right)$$

$$= 13.2 \text{ mg/L}$$

Question #7   *K.G., a 10-year-old, 45-kg female with a serum creatinine of 0.6 mg/dL, requires vancomycin for an MRSA infection with MIC = 1. Based on this information, estimate K.G.'s vancomycin maintenance regimen to achieve a trough of 10 to 15 mg/L and AUC$_{24}$/MIC > 400.*

The V and Cl can be estimated using the pediatric population parameters described in the Key Parameters table and using Equation 16.3.

$$V = 0.636 \times Wt$$

$$= 28.62 \text{ L}$$

and Equation 16.7

$$Cl = 0.248 \times Wt^{0.75} \times \left(\frac{0.48}{Scr}\right)^{0.361} \times (\ln(Age \text{ in days})/7.8)^{0.995}$$

Recall from the Key Parameters table that Age should be days and Weight as actual Kg.

$$Cl = 0.248 \times 45^{0.75} \times \left(\frac{0.48}{0.6} \right)^{0.361} \times (\ln(3,650)/7.8)^{0.995}$$

$$= 4.31 \times 0.923 \times 1.05$$

$$= 4.18 \text{ L/hr}$$

To determine the dosing interval, we can calculate the half-life using the above parameters with Equation 16.10.

$$t\frac{1}{2} = \frac{(0.693)(V)}{Cl}$$

$$= \frac{(0.693)(28.62 \text{ L})}{(4.18 \text{ L/hr})}$$

$$= 4.7 \text{ hr}$$

Given the above half-life, we dose every 6 hours which is within the recommended one to two half-lives. Now, we are left to determine what dose to administer at each 6-hour interval. Because AUC_{24}/MIC of 400 is associated with efficacy and, therefore, the primary target for dosing is calculated using Equation 16.24.

$$Dose_{24} = AUC_{24}/MIC \times Cl \times MIC$$

$$= 400 \times 4.18 \times 1$$

$$= 1,672 \text{ mg}$$

We round the daily dose to 1,600 mg for ease of dosing. Based on the half-life of 5 hours, a dosing frequency of every 6 hours is appropriate (e.g., 400 mg intravenously every 6 hours). Vancomycin is commonly dosed at every 6 hours in pediatrics owing to the short half-life. Alternatively, since the AUC_{24hr}/MIC is the pharmacodynamic driver, another option is to dose 500 mg every 8 hours. However, higher doses administered less frequently increases the chance for Red man syndrome. Now that we have a proposed plan that hits the AUC goal, let us also ensure that it achieves a safe and effective trough between 10 and 15 mg/L. Before, we do that however, we need to calculate the elimination rate constant by rearranging Equation 16.20.

$$K = 0.693/t\frac{1}{2}$$

$$= 0.693/4.7$$

$$= 0.147$$

Now, using Equation 16.17, we can calculate the expected trough level.

$$\text{Css min} = \frac{\dfrac{(S)(F)(\text{Dose})}{V}}{1 - e^{-K\tau}}(e^{-K\tau})$$

$$= \frac{\dfrac{(1)(1)(400)}{28.6}}{1 - e^{-(0.147)(6)}}\left(e^{-(0.147)(6)}\right)$$

$$= 9.9 \sim 10 \text{ mg/L}$$

The trough estimate is both within efficacy and safety parameters. Finally, we should ensure that the estimated peak is also within safety limits for ototoxicity. Following Equation 16.15,

$$\text{Css max} = \frac{\dfrac{(S)(F)(\text{Dose})}{V}}{1 - e^{-K\tau}}$$

$$= \frac{\dfrac{(1)(1)(400)}{28.6}}{1 - e^{-0.147(6)}}$$

$$= 23.9 \text{ mg/L}$$

A peak of 24 mg/L is far below 50 mg/L associated with an increased risk for ototoxicity.

Therefore, 400 mg every 6 hours is an appropriate initial dosing regimen.

Question #8   *C.U. is a 40-year-old, 5-foot 7-inch, 105-kg man with a serum creatinine of 1.2 mg/dL. He has a penicillin allergy history, and, for that reason, vancomycin is being considered for empiric therapy. What size descriptor (e.g., ideal body weight, actual body weight [ABW], ABW$_{adj}$) should the dosing regimen of vancomycin be based on for C.U.?*

The volume of distribution of vancomycin is greater in obese subjects than that in nonobese subjects. The apparent volume of distribution for vancomycin tends to correlate best with actual (total) body weight, although there is a fair degree of variability.[9,32,36,56–58] For clearance, some investigators have reported higher vancomycin clearances in obese patients, whereas others have observed that vancomycin clearance is still essentially equivalent to creatinine clearance.[9,32,36,56–58] Use of ABW or ABW$_{adj}$ in the creatinine clearance equation is recommended for patients with a body mass index (BMI) between 30 and 40 and lean body weight (LBW$_{2005}$) for those with BMI > 40 (see Chapter 3).[59–61] Using the Matzke method to estimate clearance with ABW was shown to be the most precise and least biased among seven published methods where 61% (116 of 189) of subjects were obese.[34] Owing to the wide variability in the pharmacokinetic parameters, monitoring serum vancomycin concentrations in very obese patients is advisable. To calculate the expected pharmacokinetic parameters for C.U., first estimate the patients BMI using Equation 16.29.

$$\text{BMI (kg/m}^2) = \frac{\text{Weight (kg)}}{\text{Height in m}^2} \qquad \textbf{(Eq. 16.29)}$$

$$= \frac{105}{1.7^2}$$

$$= 36.3$$

Because BMI < 40, we use ABW.

If C.U. had a BMI ≥ 40, then Equation 16.30 (male) or 16.31 (female) for LBW would have been used as calculated by Janmahasatian et al.[62] and Cl_{Cr} estimated using this body size descriptor to calculate vancomycin Cl using the Matzke method. This approach is supported by the observation that at extreme, BMI's ABW does not scale proportionally, thus lower mg/kg doses can be used.[63]

$$\text{LBW}_{\text{Male}}: (9{,}270 \times \text{TBW})/(6{,}680 + 216 \times \text{BMI}) \qquad \textbf{(Eq. 16.30)}$$

$$\text{LBW}_{\text{Female}}: (9{,}270 \times \text{TBW})/(8{,}780 + 244 \times \text{BMI}) \qquad \textbf{(Eq. 16.31)}$$

Next, creatinine clearance can be obtained using Equation 16.9.

$$\text{Cl}_{Cr} \text{ for Males} = \frac{(140 - \text{Age in years})(\text{Weight}}{72 \times \text{SCr}_{ss} \text{ (mg/dL)}}$$

$$= \frac{(140 - 40)(105 \text{ kg})}{72(1.2 \text{ mg/dL})}$$

$$= 121.5 \text{ mL/min}$$

We can then calculate vancomycin clearance using Equation 16.6:

$$\text{Cl (mL/min)} = (\text{Cl}_{Cr} \times 0.689) + 3.66$$

$$= (121.5 \text{ mL/min} \times 0.689) + 3.66$$

$$= 87.4 \text{ mL/min}$$

To convert to L/hr:

$$\text{Cl (L/hr)} = 87.4 \text{ mL/min} \times \left(\frac{60 \text{ min/hr}}{1{,}000 \text{ mL/L}} \right)$$

$$= 5.2$$

Equation 16.1 can be used to calculate C.U.'s volume of distribution:

$$V = 0.72 \text{ L/kg if Cl}_{Cr} \text{ is} > 60 \text{ mL/min}$$

$$= 0.72 \text{ L/kg (105 kg)}$$

$$= 75.6 \text{ L}$$

and Equation 16.9 can be used with the clearance of 5.2 L/hr and the volume of distribution of 75.6 L to calculate an elimination rate constant of 0.036 hr^{-1}.

$$K = \frac{Cl}{V}$$

$$= \frac{5.2}{75.6}$$

$$= 0.069 \text{ hr}^{-1}$$

Finally, using Equation 16.10, the vancomycin t½ can be estimated to be 10 hours.

$$t\frac{1}{2} = \frac{0.693}{K}$$

$$= \frac{0.693}{0.069}$$

$$= 10.04 \text{ hr}$$

Given the half-life and the desire to choose a dosing interval that is between one and two half-lives for vancomycin, a logical approach would be to use a convenient dosing interval of 12 hours, a AUC$_{24}$/MIC ratio ≥400, and trough concentration between 10 and 15 mg/L. If we assume an MIC = 1, use Equation 16.24 to solve for a dose.

$$\text{Dose}_{24} = \text{AUC}_{24}/\text{MIC} \times Cl \times \text{MIC}$$

$$= 400 \times 5.2 \times 1$$

$$= 2,080 \text{ mg}$$

This dose would usually be rounded off to a reasonable amount (closest 250 interval). Based on the half-life of 10 hours, a dosing interval of every 12 hours is appropriate (e.g., 1,000 mg given every 12 hours). The steady-state peak and trough concentrations on this new dose could be confirmed by using Equations 16.17 and 16.15.

$$\text{Css min} = \frac{\dfrac{(S)(F)(Dose)}{V}}{1 - e^{-K\tau}}(e^{-K\tau})$$

$$= \frac{\dfrac{(1)(1)(1,000)}{75.6}}{1 - e^{-(0.069)(12)}}\left(e^{-(0.069)(12)}\right)$$

$$= 10.3 \text{ mg/L}$$

$$\text{Css max} = \frac{\dfrac{(S)(F)(Dose)}{V_d}}{1 - e^{-K\tau}}$$

$$= \frac{\dfrac{(1)(1)(1,000)}{75.6}}{1 - e^{-0.069(12)}}$$

$$= 23.5 \text{ mg/L}$$

If an alternative trough is desired (e.g., 15 mg/L), the new dose can be calculated by simply using a ratio of the new target concentration to the current concentration. At a dose of 1,000 mg, the vancomycin Css min = 10 mg/L and will be labeled as (Css min current).

$$\text{New Dose} = \text{Current Dose}\left(\frac{\text{New Trough}}{\text{Current Trough}}\right)$$

$$= (1,000 \text{ mg})\left(\frac{15 \text{ mg/L}}{10 \text{ mg/L}}\right)$$

$$= 1,500 \text{ mg q12h}$$

This technique of using a ratio of concentrations to calculate the new dose is appropriate as long as the dosing interval and time of sampling have not changed for a drug that exhibits stable linear pharmacokinetics. Note that any difference between the plasma concentrations calculated by the two methods is because of rounding-off errors and not to any other assumptions. Finally, therapeutic monitoring and revision with two-sample measurement approach (peak and trough) was shown to significantly improve target trough concentration attainment in the obese population and is, therefore, strongly advocated for revision of initial dosing regimens.[64]

REFERENCES

1. Alexander MR. A review of vancomycin: after 15 years of use. *Ann Pharmacother*. 1974;8(9):520–525.

2. Kirby WM, Perry DM, Bauer AW. Treatment of staphylococcal septicemia with vancomycin: report of thirty-three cases. *N Eng J Med*. 1960;262:49–55.

3. Banner W Jr, Ray CG. Vancomycin in perspective. *Am J Dis Child*. 1984;138(1):14–16.

4. Cunha BA, Ristuccia AM. Clinical usefulness of vancomycin. *Clin Pharm*. 1983;2(5):417–424.

5. Wilhelm MP. Vancomycin. *Mayo Clin Proc*. 1991;66(11):1165–1170.

6. Lundstrom TS, Sobel JD. Antibiotics for gram-positive bacterial infections: vancomycin, teicoplanin, quinupristin/dalfopristin, and linezolid. *Infect Dis Clin North Am*. 2000;14(2):463–474.

7. Watanakunakorn C, Tisone JC. Synergism between vancomycin and gentamicin or tobramycin for methicillin-susceptible and methicillin-resistant *Staphylococcus aureus* strains. *Antimicrob Agents Chemother*. 1982;22(5):903–905.

8. Rotschafer JC, Crossley K, Zaske DE, et al. Pharmacokinetics of vancomycin: observations in 28 patients and dosage recommendations. *Antimicrob Agents Chemother*. 1982;22(3):391–394.

9. Blouin RA, Bauer LA, Miller DD, et al. Vancomycin pharmacokinetics in normal and morbidly obese subjects. *Antimicrob Agents Chemother*. 1982;21(4):575–580.

10. Moellering RC Jr, Krogstad DJ, Greenblatt DJ. Vancomycin therapy in patients with impaired renal function: a nomogram for dosage. *Ann Intern Med*. 1981;94(3):343–346.

11. Zimmermann AE, Katona BG, Plaisance KI. Association of vancomycin serum concentrations with outcomes in patients with gram-positive bacteremia. *Pharmacotherapy*. 1995;15(1):85–91.

12. Mulhern JG, Braden GL, O'Shea MH, et al. Trough serum vancomycin levels predict the relapse of gram-positive peritonitis in peritoneal dialysis patients. *Am J Kidney Dis*. 1995;25(4):611–615.

13. Welty TE, Copa AK. Impact of vancomycin therapeutic drug monitoring on patient care. *Ann Pharmacother*. 1994;28(12):1335–1339.

14. American Thoracic Society; Infectious Diseases Society of America. Guidelines for the management of adults with hospital-acquired, ventilator-associated, and healthcare-associated pneumonia. *Am J Respir Crit Care Med*. 2005;171(4):388–416.

15. Hidayat LK, Hsu DI, Quist R, et al. High-dose vancomycin therapy for methicillin-resistant *Staphylococcus aureus* infections: efficacy and toxicity. *Arch Intern Med*. 2006;166(19):2138–2144.

16. Men P, Li HB, Zhai SD, et al. Association between the AUC0-24/MIC ratio of vancomycin and its clinical effectiveness: a systematic review and meta-analysis. *PLoS One*. 2016;11(1):e0146224.

17. Prybylski JP. Vancomycin trough concentration as a predictor of clinical outcomes in patients with *Staphylococcus aureus* Bacteremia: a meta-analysis of observational studies. *Pharmacotherapy*. 2015;35(10):889–898.

18. Clinical and Laboratory Standards Institute (CLSI). Performance standards for antimicrobial susceptibility testing, 16th informational supplement. Wayne, PA: Clinical and Laboratory Standards Institute; 2006.

19. Karchmer AW. Staphylococcal endocarditis. Laboratory and clinical basis for antibiotic therapy. *Am J Med*. 1985;78(6b):116–127.

20. Lodise TP, Patel N, Lomaestro BM, et al. Relationship between initial vancomycin concentration-time profile and nephrotoxicity among hospitalized patients. *Clin Infect Dis*. 2009;49(4):507–514.

21. Wong-Beringer A, Joo J, Tse E, et al. Vancomycin-associated nephrotoxicity: a critical appraisal of risk with high-dose therapy. *Int J Antimicrob Agents*. 2011;37(2):95–101.

22. Mohr JF, Murray BE. Point: vancomycin is not obsolete for the treatment of infection caused by methicillin-resistant *Staphylococcus aureus*. *Clin Infect Dis*. 2007;44(12):1536–1542.

23. Moise-Broder PA, Forrest A, Birmingham MC, et al. Pharmacodynamics of vancomycin and other antimicrobials in patients with *Staphylococcus aureus* lower respiratory tract infections. *Clin Pharmacokinet*. 2004;43(13):925–942.

24. Aeschlimann JR, Hershberger E, Rybak MJ. Analysis of vancomycin population susceptibility profiles, killing activity, and postantibiotic effect against vancomycin-intermediate *Staphylococcus aureus*. *Antimicrob Agents Chemother*. 1999;43(8):1914–1918.

25. Liu C, Bayer A, Cosgrove SE, et al. Clinical practice guidelines by the infectious diseases society of america for the treatment of methicillin-resistant *Staphylococcus aureus* infections in adults and children: executive summary. *Clin Infect Dis*. 2011;52(3):285–292.

26. Newfield P, Roizen MF. Hazards of rapid administration of vancomycin. *Ann Intern Med*. 1979;91(4):581.

27. Cook FV, Farrar WE Jr. Vancomycin revisited. *Ann Intern Med*. 1978;88(6):813–818.

28. Farber BF, Moellering RC Jr. Retrospective study of the toxicity of preparations of vancomycin from 1974 to 1981. *Antimicrob Agents Chemother*. 1983;23(1):138–141.

29. Jeffres MN, Isakow W, Doherty JA, et al. A retrospective analysis of possible renal toxicity associated with vancomycin in patients with health care-associated methicillin-resistant *Staphylococcus aureus* pneumonia. *Clin Ther*. 2007;29(6):1107–1115.

30. Lodise TP, Lomaestro B, Graves J, et al. Larger vancomycin doses (at least four grams per day) are associated with an increased incidence of nephrotoxicity. *Antimicrob Agents Chemother*. 2008;52(4):1330–1336.

31. Le J, Ny P, Capparelli E, et al. Pharmacodynamic characteristics of nephrotoxicity associated with vancomycin use in children. *J Pediatric Infect Dis Soc*. 2015;4(4):e109–e116.

32. Rushing TA, Ambrose PJ. Clinical application and evaluation of vancomycin dosing in adults. *J Pharm Technol*. 2001;17(2):33–38.

33. Lee E, Winter ME, Boro MS. Comparing two predictive methods for determining serum vancomycin concentrations at a Veterans Affairs Medical Center. *Am J Health Syst Pharm*. 2006;63(19):1872–1875.

34. Murphy JE, Gillespie DE, Bateman CV. Predictability of vancomycin trough concentrations using seven approaches for estimating pharmacokinetic parameters. *Am J Health Syst Pharm*. 2006;63(23):2365–2370.

35. Krogstad DJ, Moellering RC Jr, Greenblatt DJ. Single-dose kinetics of intravenous vancomycin. *J Clin Pharmacol*. 1980;20(4 Pt 1):197–201.

36. Ducharme MP, Slaughter RL, Edwards DJ. Vancomycin pharmacokinetics in a patient population: effect of age, gender, and body weight. *Ther Drug Monit*. 1994;16(5):513–518.

37. Matzke GR, McGory RW, Halstenson CE, et al. Pharmacokinetics of vancomycin in patients with various degrees of renal function. *Antimicrob Agents Chemother*. 1984;25(4):433–437.

38. Le J, Bradley JS, Murray W, et al. Improved vancomycin dosing in children using area under the curve exposure. *Pediatr Infect Dis J*. 2013;32(4):e155–e163.

39. Leonard AE, Boro MS. Vancomycin pharmacokinetics in middle-aged and elderly men. *Am J Hosp Pharm*. 1994;51(6):798–800.

40. Ackerman BH, Taylor EH, Olsen KM, et al. Vancomycin serum protein binding determination by ultrafiltration. *Drug Intell Clin Pharm*. 1988;22(4):300–303.

41. Rodvold KA, Blum RA, Fischer JH, et al. Vancomycin pharmacokinetics in patients with various degrees of renal function. *Antimicrob Agents Chemother*. 1988;32(6):848–852.

42. Rybak MJ, Albrecht LM, Berman JR, et al. Vancomycin pharmacokinetics in burn patients and intravenous drug abusers. *Antimicrob Agents Chemother*. 1990;34(5):792–795.

43. Bickley SK. Drug dosing during continuous arteriovenous hemofiltration. *Clin Pharm*. 1988;7(3):198–206.

44. Dupuis RE, Matzke GR, Maddux FW, et al. Vancomycin disposition during continuous arteriovenous hemofiltration. *Clin Pharm*. 1989;8(5):371–374.

45. Nielsen HE, Hansen HE, Korsager B, et al. Renal excretion of vancomycin in kidney disease. *Acta Medica Scandinavica*. 1975;197(4):261–264.

46. Lindholm DD, Murray JS. Persistence of vancomycin in the blood during renal failure and its treatment by hemodialysis. *N Engl J Med*. 1966;274(19):1047–1051.

47. Ayus JC, Eneas JF, Tong TG, et al. Peritoneal clearance and total body elimination of vancomycin during chronic intermittent peritoneal dialysis. *Clin Nephrol*. 1979;11(3):129–132.

48. Paton TW, Cornish WR, Manuel MA, et al. Drug therapy in patients undergoing peritoneal dialysis. Clinical pharmacokinetic considerations. *Clin Pharmacokinet*. 1985;10(5):404–425.

49. Morse GD, Farolino DF, Apicella MA, et al. Comparative study of intraperitoneal and intravenous vancomycin pharmacokinetics during continuous ambulatory peritoneal dialysis. *Antimicrob Agents Chemother*. 1987;31(2):173–177.

50. Smith PF, Morse GD. Accuracy of measured vancomycin serum concentrations in patients with end-stage renal disease. *Ann Pharmacother.* 1999;33(12):1329–1335.

51. Lanese DM, Alfrey PS, Molitoris BA. Markedly increased clearance of vancomycin during hemodialysis using polysulfone dialyzers. *Kidney Int.* 1989;35(6):1409–1412.

52. Pollard TA, Lampasona V, Akkerman S, et al. Vancomycin redistribution: dosing recommendations following high-flux hemodialysis. *Kidney Int.* 1994;45(1):232–237.

53. Karam CM, McKinnon PS, Neuhauser MM, et al. Outcome assessment of minimizing vancomycin monitoring and dosing adjustments. *Pharmacotherapy.* 1999;19(3):257–266.

54. Neely MN, Youn G, Jones B, et al. Are vancomycin trough concentrations adequate for optimal dosing? *Antimicrob Agents Chemother.* 2014;58(1):309–316.

55. Schaad UB, McCracken GH Jr, Nelson JD. Clinical pharmacology and efficacy of vancomycin in pediatric patients. *J Pediatr.* 1980;96(1):119–126.

56. Vance-Bryan K, Guay DR, Gilliland SS, et al. Effect of obesity on vancomycin pharmacokinetic parameters as determined by using a Bayesian forecasting technique. *Antimicrob Agents Chemother.* 1993;37(3):436–440.

57. Bearden DT, Rodvold KA. Dosage adjustments for antibacterials in obese patients: applying clinical pharmacokinetics. *Clin Pharmacokinet.* 2000;38(5):415–426.

58. Grace E. Altered vancomycin pharmacokinetics in obese and morbidly obese patients: what we have learned over the past 30 years. *J Antimicrob Chemother.* 2012. doi:10.1093/jac/dks066.

59. Winter MA, Guhr KN, Berg GM. Impact of various body weights and serum creatinine concentrations on the bias and accuracy of the Cockcroft-Gault equation. *Pharmacotherapy.* 2012;32(7):604–612.

60. Bouquegneau A, Vidal-Petiot E, Moranne O, et al. Creatinine-based equations for the adjustment of drug dosage in an obese population. *Br J Clin Pharmacol.* 2016;81(2):349–361.

61. Park EJ, Pai MP, Dong T, et al. The influence of body size descriptors on the estimation of kidney function in normal weight, overweight, obese, and morbidly obese adults. *Ann Pharmacother.* 2012;46(3):317–328.

62. Janmahasatian S, Duffull SB, Ash S, eta l. Quantification of lean bodyweight. *Clin Pharmacokinet.* 2005;44(10):1051–1065.

63. Morrill HJ, Caffrey AR, Noh E, et al. Vancomycin dosing considerations in a real-world Cohort of obese and extremely obese patients. *Pharmacotherapy.* 2015;35(9):869–875.

64. Hong J, Krop LC, Johns T, et al. Individualized vancomycin dosing in obese patients: a two-sample measurement approach improves target attainment. *Pharmacotherapy.* 2015;35(5):455–463.

NOMOGRAMS FOR CALCULATING BODY SURFACE AREA

Nomogram for Calculating the Body Surface Area of Children[a]

[a]From the formula of DuBois and DuBois. *Arch Intern Med*. 1916;17:863: $S = W^{0.425} \times H^{0.725} \times 71.84$, or log $S = 0.425$ log W + 0.725 log H + 1.8564, where S is body surface area in cm^2, W is weight in kg, and H is height in cm. (Reprinted with permission from the publisher. Lontmer C, ed. *Geigy Scientific Tables*. Vol 1. 8th ed. Base: Ciba-Geigy; 1981:226–227.)

Nomogram for Calculating the Body Surface Area of Adults[a]

Height	Surface area	Weight

Height (cm | in):
0 — 79 in
195 — 78, 77
190 — 76, 75, 74
185 — 73, 72
180 — 71, 70
175 — 69, 68
170 — 67, 66
165 — 65, 64
160 — 63, 62
155 — 61, 60
150 — 59, 58
145 — 57, 56
140 — 55, 54
135 — 53, 52
130 — 51, 50
125 — 49, 48
120 — 47, 46
115 — 45, 44
110 — 43, 42
105 — 41, 40
cm 100 — 39 in

Surface area (m²):
2.80 m²
2.70
2.60
2.50
2.40
2.30
2.20
2.10
2.00
1.95
1.90
1.85
1.80
1.75
1.70
1.65
1.60
1.55
1.50
1.45
1.40
1.35
1.30
1.25
1.20
1.15
1.10
1.05
1.00
0.95
0.90
0.90 m²

Weight (kg | lb):
kg 150 — 330 lb
145 — 320
140 — 310
135 — 300
130 — 290
125 — 280
120 — 270, 260
115 — 250
110 — 240
105 — 230
100 — 220
95 — 210
90 — 200
85 — 190
80 — 180, 170
75 — 160
70 — 150
65 — 140
60 — 130
55 — 120
50 — 110, 105
45 — 100, 95
40 — 90, 85
35 — 80, 75
kg 30 — 70, 66 lb

[a]From the formula of DuBois and DuBois. *Arch Intern Med.* 1916;17:863: $S = W^{0.425} \times H^{0.725} \times 71.84$, or log $S = 0.425$ log $W + 0.725$ log $H + 1.8564$, where S is body surface area in cm², W is weight in kg, and H is height in cm. (Reprinted with permission from the publisher. Lontmer C, ed. *Geigy Scientific Tables.* Vol 1. 8th ed. Base: Ciba-Geigy; 1981:226–227.)

COMMON EQUATIONS USED THROUGHOUT THE TEXT

The following is a list of equations that are frequently used in pharmacokinetic calculations. They are grouped together according to specific dosing situations. For a complete discussion, refer to the text and figures cited next to each equation. Although some of the equations may appear complicated, most are simple rearrangements of basic equations that can be broken down into one or more of the following components:

$\dfrac{(S)(F)(Dose)}{V}$	The change in plasma concentration following a dose (ΔCp).
$\dfrac{(S)(F)(Dose/t)}{Cl}$	Average steady-state concentration.
(e^{-Kt})	Fraction remaining after time of decay (t).
$(1 - e^{-Kt})$	Fraction lost during decay phase *or* fraction of steady state achieved during infusion.

SINGLE DOSE (ABSORPTION TIME OR $t_{in} \leq \frac{1}{6} t\frac{1}{2}$)

$\text{Loading Dose} = \dfrac{(V)(C)}{(S)(F)}$	Part I: Chapter 1: Basic Principles, Equation 1.11; Part I: Chapter 2: Selecting the Appropriate Equation and Interpretation of Measured Drug Concentrations, Figure 2.1
$\dfrac{\text{Incremental}}{\text{Loading Dose}} = \dfrac{(V)(C_{desired} - C_{initial})}{(S)(F)}$	Part I: Chapter 1: Basic Principles, Equation 1.12
$C = \dfrac{(S)(F)(\text{Loading Dose})}{(V)}$ $= (\text{Change in Concentration})$	Part I: Chapter 2: Selecting the Appropriate Equation and Interpretation of Measured Drug Concentrations, Equation 2.1; Figure 2.1

$$C_1 = \frac{(S)(F)(\text{Loading Dose})}{V}(e^{-Kt_1})$$

$$= \begin{pmatrix} \text{Change in} \\ \text{Concentration} \end{pmatrix} \begin{pmatrix} \text{Fraction Remaining} \\ \text{after Time of Decay } t_1 \end{pmatrix}$$

Part I: Chapter 2: Selecting the Appropriate Equation and Interpretation of Measured Drug Concentrations, Equation 2.2; Figure 2.1

HALF-LIFE (t½) AND ELIMINATION RATE CONSTANT (K)

$$K = \frac{Cl}{V}$$

Part I: Chapter 1: Basic Principles, Equation 1.27

$$t\frac{1}{2} = \frac{(0.693)(V)}{Cl}$$

Part I: Chapter 1: Basic Principles, Equation 1.30

$$K = \frac{0.693}{t\frac{1}{2}}$$

Part II: Chapter 9: Cytotoxic Anticancer Drugs: Methotrexate and Busulfan, Equation 9.7

$$t\frac{1}{2} = \frac{0.693}{K}$$

Part I: Chapter 1: Basic Principles, Equation 1.29

$$K = \frac{\ln\left(\dfrac{C_1}{C_2}\right)}{t}$$

Part I: Chapter 1: Basic Principles, Equation 1.28

SINGLE DOSE (ABSORPTION OR $t_{in} > \frac{1}{6} t\frac{1}{2}$)

$$C_2 = \frac{(S)(F)(\text{Dose}/t_{in})}{Cl}\left(1 - e^{-Kt_{in}}\right)\left(e^{-Kt_2}\right)$$

Part I: Chapter 2: Selecting the Appropriate Equation and Interpretation of Measured Drug Concentrations, Equation 2.6; Figure 2.4

$$= \begin{pmatrix} \text{Average} \\ \text{Steady-State} \\ \text{Concentration} \end{pmatrix} \begin{pmatrix} \text{Fraction of} \\ \text{Steady State} \\ \text{Achieved after} \\ \text{Time of Infusion } t_{in} \end{pmatrix} \begin{pmatrix} \text{Fraction Remaining} \\ \text{after } t_2 \\ \text{Time of Decay} \end{pmatrix}$$

$$= \begin{pmatrix} \text{Change in} \\ \text{Concentration} \\ \text{at the End of a} \\ \text{Short Infusion} \end{pmatrix} \begin{pmatrix} \text{Fraction Remaining} \\ \text{after } t_2 \\ \text{Time of Decay} \end{pmatrix}$$

CONTINUOUS INFUSION

At Steady State

$$\text{Maintenance Dose} = \frac{(Cl)(Css\ ave)(\tau)}{(S)(F)}$$

Part I: Chapter 1: Basic Principles, Equation 1.16

$$Css\ ave = \frac{(S)(F)(Dose/\tau)}{Cl}$$
$$= \text{Average Steady-State Concentration}$$

Part I: Chapter 1: Basic Principles, Equation 1.33; Part I: Chapter 2: Selecting the Appropriate Equation and Interpretation of Measured Drug Concentrations, Figure 2.2

Decay from Steady State

$$C_2 = \frac{(S)(F)(Dose/\tau)}{Cl}\left(e^{-Kt_2}\right)$$

$$= \begin{pmatrix} \text{Average} \\ \text{Steady-State} \\ \text{Concentration} \end{pmatrix} \begin{pmatrix} \text{Fraction Remaining} \\ \text{after } t_2 \\ \text{Time of Decay} \end{pmatrix}$$

Part I: Chapter 2: Selecting the Appropriate Equation and Interpretation of Measured Drug Concentrations, Equation 2.4; Figure 2.2

Non–Steady State

$$C_1 = \frac{(S)(F)(Dose/\tau)}{Cl}\left(1 - e^{-Kt_1}\right)$$

Part I: Chapter 1: Basic Principles, Equation 1.35; Figure 1.19

$$= \begin{pmatrix} \text{Average} \\ \text{Steady-State} \\ \text{Concentration} \end{pmatrix} \begin{pmatrix} \text{Fraction of} \\ \text{Steady State} \\ \text{Achieved } t_1 \text{Time} \\ \text{after Starting Infusion} \end{pmatrix}$$

Decay from Non–Steady State

$$C_2 = \frac{(S)(F)(Dose/\tau)}{Cl}\left(1 - e^{-Kt_1}\right)\left(e^{-Kt_2}\right)$$

Part I: Chapter 1: Basic Principles, Equation 1.39; Figure 1.19

$$= \begin{pmatrix} \text{Average} \\ \text{Steady-State} \\ \text{Concentration} \end{pmatrix} \begin{pmatrix} \text{Fraction of} \\ \text{Steady State} \\ \text{Achieved } t_1 \\ \text{Time after} \\ \text{Starting Infusion} \end{pmatrix} \begin{pmatrix} \text{Fraction} \\ \text{Remaining} \\ \text{after } t_2 \\ \text{Time of Decay} \end{pmatrix}$$

MULTIPLE DOSE
(CONSISTENT τ AND DOSE): STEADY STATE
Absorption or $t_{in} \leq \frac{1}{6} t\frac{1}{2}$

$$Css_1 = \frac{\frac{(S)(F)(Dose)}{V}}{\left(1 - e^{-Kt}\right)}\left(e^{-K\tau_1}\right)$$

Part I: Chapter 1: Basic Principles, Equation 1.46;
Part I: Chapter 2: Selecting the Appropriate Equation and Interpretation of Measured Drug Concentrations, Figure 2.6

$$= \frac{\left(\begin{array}{c} \text{Change in} \\ \text{Concentration} \end{array}\right)}{\left(\begin{array}{c} \text{Fraction Lost in} \\ \text{Dosing Interval} \end{array}\right)}\left(\begin{array}{c} \text{Fraction} \\ \text{Remaining} \\ \text{after } t_1 \\ \text{Time of Decay} \end{array}\right)$$

$$= \left(\begin{array}{c} \text{Steady-State} \\ \text{Peak} \\ \text{Concentration} \end{array}\right)\left(\begin{array}{c} \text{Fraction Remaining} \\ \text{after } t_1 \\ \text{Time of Decay} \end{array}\right)$$

Absorption or $t_{in} > \frac{1}{6} t\frac{1}{2}$

$$Css_2 = \frac{\frac{(S)(F)(Dose/t_{in})}{Cl}\left(1 - e^{-Kt_{in}}\right)}{1 - e^{-K\tau}}\left(e^{-Kt_2}\right)$$

Part I: Chapter 2: Selecting the Appropriate Equation and Interpretation of Measured Drug Concentrations, Equation 2.10
Part II: Chapter 6: Aminoglycoside Antibiotics, Equation 6.21; Figure 6.2

$$= \frac{\left(\begin{array}{c} \text{Average} \\ \text{Steady-State} \\ \text{Concentration} \end{array}\right)\left(\begin{array}{c} \text{Fraction of} \\ \text{Steady State} \\ \text{Achieved after } t_{in} \\ \text{Time of Infusion} \end{array}\right)\left(\begin{array}{c} \text{Fraction} \\ \text{Remaining} \\ \text{after } t_2 \\ \text{Time of Decay} \end{array}\right)}{\left(\begin{array}{c} \text{Fraction} \\ \text{Lost in a} \\ \text{Dosing Interval} \end{array}\right)}$$

$$= \left(\begin{array}{c} \text{Steady-State} \\ \text{Peak Concentration} \\ \text{at End of Short Infusion} \end{array}\right)\left(\begin{array}{c} \text{Fraction Remaining} \\ \text{after } t_2 \text{ Time of Decay} \end{array}\right)$$

MULTIPLE DOSE (CONSISTENT τ AND DOSE): NON–STEADY STATE

Absorption or $t_{in} \leq \frac{1}{6} t\frac{1}{2}$

$$Css_2 = \frac{\frac{(S)(F)(Dose)}{V}}{1 - e^{-K\tau}}\left(1 - e^{-K(N)\tau}\right)\left(e^{-Kt_2}\right)$$

Part I: Chapter 2: Selecting the Appropriate Equation and Interpretation of Measured Drug Concentrations, Equation 2.8

$$= \left(\frac{\text{Change in Concentration}}{\text{Fraction Lost in Dosing Interval}}\right)\left(\begin{array}{c}\text{Fraction of}\\\text{Steady State}\\\text{Achieved}\\\text{after N Doses}\end{array}\right)\left(\begin{array}{c}\text{Fraction}\\\text{Remaining}\\\text{after } t_2 \text{ Time}\\\text{of Decay}\end{array}\right)$$

$$= \left(\begin{array}{c}\text{Steady-State}\\\text{Peak}\\\text{Concentration}\end{array}\right)\left(\begin{array}{c}\text{Fraction of}\\\text{Steady State}\\\text{Achieved}\\\text{after N Doses}\end{array}\right)\left(\begin{array}{c}\text{Fraction}\\\text{Remaining}\\\text{after } t_2 \text{ Time}\\\text{of Decay}\end{array}\right)$$

MASS BALANCE

$$\frac{(S)(F)(Dose/\tau) - \frac{(C_2 - C_1)V}{t}}{C\,ave} = Cl$$

Part I: Chapter 2: Selecting the Appropriate Equation and Interpretation of Measured Drug Concentrations, Equation 2.17

CREATININE CLEARANCE (Cl_{Cr})

$$\begin{array}{c}Cl_{Cr} \text{ for Males}\\(mL/min)\end{array} = \frac{(140 - Age)(Weight)}{(72)(SCr_{ss})}$$

Part I: Chapter 3: Drug Dosing in Kidney Disease and Dialysis, Equation 3.4

$$\begin{array}{c}Cl_{Cr} \text{ for Females}\\(mL/min)\end{array} = (0.85)\frac{(140 - Age)(Weight)}{(72)(SCr_{ss})}$$

Part I: Chapter 3: Drug Dosing in Kidney Disease and Dialysis, Equation 3.5

where age in years, weight in kg, and SCr_{ss} in mg/dL

$$\begin{array}{c}GFR\\(mL/min/1.73\,m^2)\end{array} = \frac{(0.41)(Height\ in\ cm)}{SCr_{ss}}$$

Part I: Chapter 3: Drug Dosing in Kidney Disease and Dialysis, Equation 3.13

where SCr_{ss} in mg/dL

$$BSA\ in\ m^2 = \left(\frac{Patients\ Weight\ in\ kg}{70\,kg}\right)^{0.7}\left(1.73\,m^2\right)$$

Part I: Chapter 1: Basic Principles, Equation 1.17

NONLINEAR EQUATIONS (PHENYTOIN)

$$(S)(F)(Dose/\tau) = \frac{(Vm)(Css\ ave)}{Km + Css\ ave}$$

Part II: Chapter 14: Phenytoin,
Equation 14.14

$$Css = \frac{(Km)\left[(S)(F)(Dose/\tau)\right]}{Vm - \left[(S)(F)(Dose/\tau)\right]}$$

Part II:
Chapter 14: Phenytoin,
Equation 14.15

Time Required to Achieve 90% of Steady State ($t_{90\%}$)

$$t_{90\%} = \frac{(Km)(V)}{\left[Vm - (S)(F)(Dose/day)\right]^{2}}[(2.3\ Vm)}{-(0.9)(S)(F)(Dose/day)]$$

Part II: Chapter 14: Phenytoin,
Equation 14.23

Has Steady State Been Achieved?

$$90\%t = \frac{\left[115 + (35)(C)\right]\left[C\right]}{(S)(F)(Dose/day)}$$

Part II: Chapter 14: Phenytoin,
Equation 14.24

Days on current maintenance regimen must exceed 90% t value to assure that steady state has been achieved. Dose is in mg/day normalized to 70 kg.

ADJUSTMENT FOR PLASMA PROTEIN BINDING (PHENYTOIN)

Adjustment for Serum Albumin if $Cl_{cr} > 25$ mL/min

$$\frac{\text{Phenytoin Concentration}}{\text{Normal Plasma Binding}} = \frac{\text{Patient's Phenytoin Concentration with Altered Plasma Binding}}{\left[0.9 \times \dfrac{\text{Patient's Serum Albumin}}{4.4\,\text{gm/dL}}\right] + 0.1}$$

Part II: Chapter 14: Phenytoin,
Equation 14.2

Adjustment for Serum Albumin if Patient Receiving Dialysis

$$\frac{\text{Phenytoin Concentration}}{\text{Normal Plasma Binding}} = \frac{\text{Dialysis Patient's Phenytoin Concentration with Altered Plasma Binding}}{\left[(0.9)(0.48)\left(\dfrac{\text{Patient's Serum Albumin}}{4.4\,\text{gm/dL}}\right)\right] + 0.1}$$

Part II:
Chapter 14:
Phenytoin,
Equation 14.3

ALGORITHM FOR EVALUATING AND INTERPRETING PLASMA CONCENTRATIONS

Step 1. Initial Data Collection

Before one can interpret the patient's pharmacokinetic parameters or plasma drug concentrations, appropriate information must be collected so that factors which may influence drug absorption and disposition can be considered.

Relevant Physical Data, Medical and Surgical History:

Height, weight, age, sex, race, current diseases, and symptoms.

Relevant Laboratory Data:

Renal Function: SCr, BUN, Cl_{Cr} (Is the collection complete?)

Hepatic Function: Serum albumin, bilirubin, prothrombin time, serum enzymes.

Protein Binding: Plasma protein concentration. Acidic drugs—Albumin. Basic drugs—Globulins. Evaluate displacing factors such as other drugs or presence of uremia

Thyroid Function

Drug Administration History:

Collect dosing data (dose, frequency, and route) for 3–5 half-lives. In acute care settings consider history prior to admissions as well as during hospital stay.

It is critical to determine the exact time of administration for those doses taken just prior to drug level sampling.

Time of Sampling Relative to the Last Dose:

The best time to sample is usually just prior to the next dose. For drugs with a short half-life, peak and trough levels may be appropriate. Avoid absorption and distribution phase when peak levels are obtained.

(Continued on next page)

Step 2. Evaluation of Reported Plasma Concentrations

Has the patient been receiving constant dosing for more than 3–4 half-lives prior to obtaining the plasma sample?

Yes

No

Non–Steady State Plasma Concentration

The plasma concentration must be evaluated by considering the contribution of each dose at the time the plasma sample was obtained. Use Equation 2.2 for each bolus dose or Equation 2.6 for each "short infusion." If several different sustained infusion rates have been used during the accumulation period, Equations 1.35 or 1.39 should be used for each infusion rate.

C Is Greater Than Expected:

See List A.

V may be less than expected.

Sample may have been obtained during distribution phase.

C Is Less Than Expected:

See List B.

V may be greater than expected.

Sample may have been obtained too soon after the dose was administered and absorption was not yet complete.

List A

When drug concentrations are greater than expected, consider:

1. Increased bioavailability. This is only important if the drug's bioavailability is usually low.
2. Nonadherence. Intake is greater than prescribed.
3. Decreased clearance.
4. Increased plasma protein binding. Changes in plasma protein binding will be most important if fu is ≤0.1 and are unlikely to be significant if fu is >0.5. Increased plasma protein binding will also decrease the volume of distribution and clearance of most drugs.

List B

When drug concentrations are less than expected, consider:

1. Decreased bioavailability.
2. Nonadherence. Intake is less than prescribed.
3. Increased clearance.
4. Decreased plasma protein binding. Changes in plasma protein binding will be most important if fu is ≤0.1. It is unlikely to be significant if fu is >0.5. Decreased plasma protein binding will also increase the volume of distribution and the clearance of most drugs.

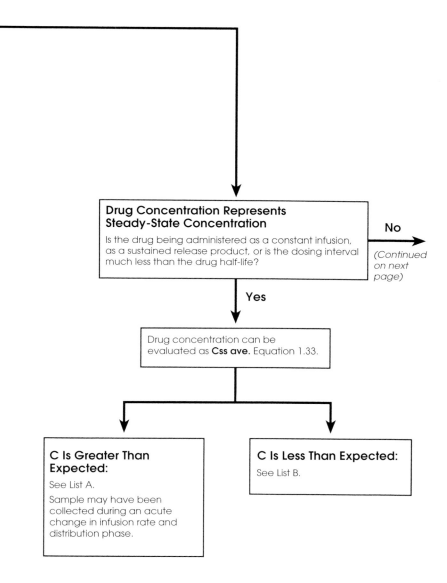

Drug Concentration Represents Steady-State Concentration

Is the drug being administered as a constant infusion, as a sustained release product, or is the dosing interval much less than the drug half-life?

No

(Continued on next page)

Yes

Drug concentration can be evaluated as **Css ave.** Equation 1.33.

C Is Greater Than Expected:

See List A.

Sample may have been collected during an acute change in infusion rate and distribution phase.

C Is Less Than Expected:

See List B.

Step 2. Evaluation of Reported Plasma Concentrations
(Continued)

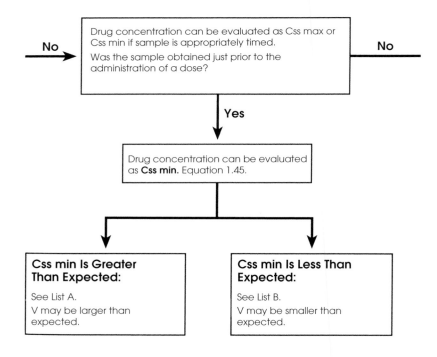

No →

Drug concentration can be evaluated as Css max or Css min if sample is appropriately timed.

Was the sample obtained just prior to the administration of a dose?

No

Yes ↓

Drug concentration can be evaluated as **Css min**. Equation 1.45.

Css min Is Greater Than Expected:

See List A.
V may be larger than expected.

Css min Is Less Than Expected:

See List B.
V may be smaller than expected.

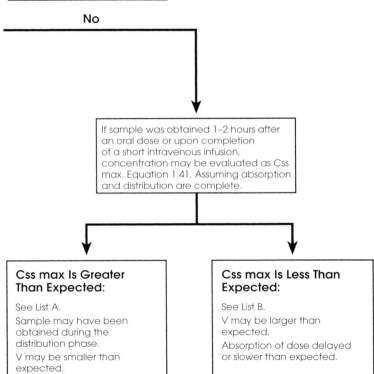

List A

When drug concentrations are greater than expected, consider:

1. Increased bioavailability. This is only important if the drug's bioavailability is usually low.
2. Nonadherence. Intake is greater than prescribed.
3. Decreased clearance.
4. Increased plasma protein binding. Changes in plasma protein binding will be most important if fu is ≤0.1 and are unlikely to be significant if fu is >0.5. Increased plasma protein binding will also decrease the volume of distribution and clearance of most drugs.

List B

When drug concentrations are less than expected, consider:

1. Decreased bioavailability.
2. Nonadherence. Intake is less than prescribed.
3. Increased clearance.
4. Decreased plasma protein binding. Changes in plasma protein binding will be most important if fu is ≤0.1. It is unlikely to be significant if fu is >0.5. Decreased plasma protein binding will also increase the volume of distribution and the clearance of most drugs.

No

If sample was obtained 1–2 hours after an oral dose or upon completion of a short intravenous infusion, concentration may be evaluated as Css max. Equation 1.41. Assuming absorption and distribution are complete.

Css max Is Greater Than Expected:

See List A.

Sample may have been obtained during the distribution phase.

V may be smaller than expected.

Css max Is Less Than Expected:

See List B.

V may be larger than expected.

Absorption of dose delayed or slower than expected.

GLOSSARY OF TERMS AND ABBREVIATIONS

Accumulation Factor: $1/1 - e^{-K\tau}$ or the degree to which a maintenance dose will accumulate when steady state is achieved.

Adjusted Body Weight: A weight for dosing drugs in obese patients that is between ideal body weight and total body weight.

Administration Rate (R_A): The average rate at which a drug is administered to the patient.

Alpha (α): The initial half-life in a two-compartment model, usually representing distribution (see Fig. 1.9).

Amount of Drug in the Body (Ab): The total amount of active drug that is in the body at any given time.

Area Under the Curve (AUC_{24}): The concentration area in units of concentration $\times$ time. A measure of drug exposure that, in some cases, can be a measure of efficacy. See Chapters 6 and 16.

Average Steady-State Concentration (Css ave): The average plasma drug concentration at steady state.

Beta (β): Second decay half-life in a two-compartment model, usually representing elimination.

Bioavailability (F): The fraction of an administered dose that reaches the systemic circulation.

Body Surface Area (BSA): The surface area of a patient, as determined by weight and height (see Appendix I).

Bolus Dose: A model for rapid input of a dose into the body or an individual dose, usually given by intravenous injection.

CAPD: Continuous Ambulatory Peritoneal Dialysis.

$Cl_{adjusted}$: Clearance of a patient that has been adjusted or altered for the presence of a disease state such as renal failure or heart failure.

Cl_{CAPD}: Drug clearance by peritoneal dialysis.

Cl_{CRRT}: Drug clearance by CRRT (see CRRT).

Cl_{dial}: Drug clearance by dialysis.

Cl_{pat}: Drug clearance of a patient, usually associated with decreased renal function.

Clearance (Cl$_t$ or Cl): Total body clearance is a measure of how well a patient can metabolize or eliminate drug. It is used to calculate maintenance doses or average steady-state plasma concentrations.

Clearance, Metabolic (Cl$_m$): A measure of how well the body can metabolize drugs. The major metabolic organ is usually the liver.

Clearance, Renal (Cl$_r$): A measure of how well the kidneys can excrete unchanged or unmetabolized drug. It is usually assumed to be proportional to creatinine clearance.

C′: Plasma concentration measured in the patients with altered plasma protein binding.

C$_1$: The initial plasma concentration at the beginning of a decay phase, usually following a loading dose.

C$_2$: The drug concentration at the end of a decay phase.

C$_{desired}$: Plasma concentration desired following an incremental loading dose.

C free: Unbound or free plasma concentration.

C Normal Binding: Plasma concentration that would be observed or measured if a patient's plasma protein binding is normal.

C$_{initial}$: Plasma concentration present in a patient before an incremental loading dose.

C$_{tin}$: Plasma concentration at the end of a short infusion or at the end of absorption.

Css ave: Average plasma concentration at steady state.

Css max: The maximum or peak concentration at steady state, when a constant dose is administered at a constant dosing interval.

Css min: The minimum or trough concentration at steady state, when a constant dose is administered at a constant dosing interval.

Continuous Renal Replacement Therapy: A type of hemodialysis that is continuous versus intermittent.

Creatinine Clearance (Cl$_{Cr}$): A measure of the kidney's ability to eliminate creatinine from the body. Total renal function is usually assumed to be proportional to creatinine clearance.

CRRT: See Continuous Renal Replacement Therapy.

ΔC: Change in plasma concentration resulting from a single dose.

Dosing Interval (τ): The time interval between doses when a drug is given intermittently.

Dry Weight: Weight of a patient before excessive third-space fluid weight gain.

Dwell Time (T$_D$): The time between instillation and removal of a peritoneal dialysis exchange volume.

e^{-Kt}: Fraction remaining at the end of a time interval.

1 – e^{-Kt}: (a) Fraction lost during a dosing interval at steady state, if t = τ; (b) Fraction of steady state achieved during a constant infusion "t" hours after starting the infusion.

Elimination Rate Constant (K): The fractional rate of drug loss from the body or the fraction of the volume of distribution that is cleared of drug during a time interval.

Elimination Rate (R$_E$): The amount of drug eliminated from the body during a time interval.

Extraction Ratio: Fraction of drug that is removed from the blood or plasma as it passes through the eliminating organ.

First-Pass: Drug removed from the blood or plasma, following absorption from the gastrointestinal tract, before reaching the systemic circulation.

First-Order Elimination: A process whereby the amount or concentration of drug in the body diminishes logarithmically over time. The rate of elimination is proportional to the drug concentration.

fu: Fraction of total plasma concentration that is free or unbound.

Half-Life (t½): Time required for the plasma concentration to be reduced to one-half of the original value.

Half-Life, Alpha (α t½): Initial decay half-life, usually representing distribution of drug into the tissue or slowly equilibrating second compartment in a two-compartmental model.

Half-Life, Beta (β t½): Second decay half-life, usually representing the elimination half-life. Half-life, beta for most drugs can be calculated using the elimination rate constant.

Ideal Body Weight (IBW): Body weight used as an estimate of nonobese weight.

Incremental Loading Dose: An adjusted loading dose required to achieve a desired plasma concentration (C desired) when a preexisting plasma concentration (C observed) is present.

Initial Volume of Distribution (V_i): Initial volume into which the drug rapidly equilibrates following an intravenous bolus dose injection.

Iterative Search: A trial and error process to determine patient-specific pharmacokinetic parameters when direct solutions are not possible owing to the nature of the pharmacokinetic model.

$K_{adjusted}$: Elimination rate constant that has been adjusted or altered for the presence of a disease state such as renal failure.

K_{dial}: Elimination rate constant representing both the patient's drug clearance and the drug clearance by dialysis.

Km (Michaelis–Menten Constant): Plasma concentration at which the rate of metabolism is half the maximum rate.

$K_{metabolic}$ (K_m): The elimination rate constant calculated from the metabolic clearance and the volume of distribution (Cl_m/V).

K_{renal} (K_r): The elimination rate constant calculated from the renal clearance and the volume of distribution (Cl_r/V).

Linear Pharmacokinetics: Assumes the elimination rate constant is not affected by plasma drug concentration and that the rate of drug elimination is directly proportional to the concentration of drug in plasma.

ln: Natural logarithm using the base 2.718 rather than 10, which is used for the common logarithm or log.

Loading Dose: Initial total dose required to rapidly achieve a desired plasma concentration.

Maintenance Dose: The dose required to replace the amount of drug lost from the body so that a desired plasma concentration can be maintained.

Mass Balance: The process of comparing drug administration rate (R_A) to the rate of change of drug in the body (($\Delta C)(V)/t$) in order to estimate drug elimination rate (R_E).

Modified Diet in Renal Disease (MDRD): Equation used for estimating glomerular filtration rate (GFR).

N: The number of doses that have been administered at a fixed-dosing interval.

One-Compartment Model: Assumes that drug distributes rapidly and equally to all areas of the body. Most drugs can be modeled this way if sampling during the initial distribution phase is avoided.

P_{NL} or P′: Plasma protein concentration. P_{NL} refers to the normal plasma protein concentration and P′ refers to the plasma protein concentration of the specific patient.

Pharmacokinetics: Study of the absorption, distribution, metabolism, and excretion of a drug and its metabolites in the body.

Plasma Concentration (C): Concentration of drug in plasma. Usually refers to the total drug concentration and includes both the bound and unbound or free drug concentration.

Salt Form (S): Fraction of administered salt or ester form of the drug that is the active moiety.

Sensitivity Analysis: The practice of examining the relationship between a change in either clearance or volume of distribution and the corresponding change in the calculated plasma concentration (see Chapter 2: Interpretation of Plasma Drug Concentrations: Sensitivity Analysis).

SCr: Serum Creatinine Concentration.

Steady State: Steady state is achieved when the rate of drug administration is equal to the rate of drug elimination.

$t_{90\%}$: Time required to achieve 90% of steady state for phenytoin on a fixed-dosing regimen in a patient with known values of V, Vm, and Km.

Tau (τ): See Dosing Interval.

$\tau - t_{in}$: Time from end of infusion to trough concentration when using a short infusion model.

T_d: Time of dialysis for intermittent hemodialysis.

T_{in}: Time required for drug to be infused or absorbed.

Tissue Concentration (C_t): Concentration of drug in the tissue.

Tissue Volume of Distribution (V_t): Apparent volume into which the drug appears to distribute following rapid equilibration with the initial volume of distribution.

Total Body Weight (TBW): Total weight of a patient usually used for obese patients.

Two-Compartment Model: Comprised of an initial, rapidly equilibrating volume of distribution (V_i) and an apparent second, more slowly equilibrating volume of distribution (V_t).

Unbound V: Volume of distribution based on the free or unbound plasma concentration.

Vm: Maximum rate at which metabolism can occur.

Volume of Distribution (V): The apparent volume required to account for all the drug in the body if it was present throughout the body in the same concentration as in the sample obtained from the plasma.

90% t: Duration of therapy on a fixed-dosing regimen that must be exceeded to assure that a measured phenytoin concentration represents steady state.

Index

Page numbers in *italics* denote figures; those followed by t denote tables

A

AAG (alpha 1-acid glycoprotein), 17, 133
Absorption, 131–132
  drug, 2
  valproic acid, 447–448
Accumulation factor, 52
Acetaminophen, 136
Acetylation capacity, 136
Acidic drugs, binding affinity of, 15
Active drug form, and bioavailability, 7–8
Acute lymphoblastic leukemia, 264–269
Adjusted body weight, 102–105
Administration rate (RA), 10–12
  average, 12
  calculating, 10–11
  and clearance, in steady state, 28–29, *29*
  at fixed dosing intervals, 12
Adverse effects, 218
  of carbamazepine, 243–244
  isavuconazole, 238
  itraconazole, 224
  mycophenolate, 348–349
  posaconazole, 233
  voriconazole, 228
Albumin, 335
  binding affinity of, 13, 15
  binding capacity, 133
  concentration, average normal, 15
Allergic bronchopulmonary aspergillosis, 224
Allograft rejection in solid organ, 321
Alpha 1-acid glycoprotein (AAG), 17, 133
Alpha (α) half-life, 25, 43
Alpha phase drug elimination, 27
Alternative antibiotic agents, 468

Amikacin
  clearance, 138, *139*
  plasma concentrations of peak, 164
  therapeutic, and key parameters, 165t
Aminoglycosides antibiotics, 163–208
  administration of, 164–165
    intramuscular, 175
  bioavailability of, 166
  clearance of
    expected, 186–188, *187*
    non-renal, 169–170
    in obese patients, 169
    penicillin interaction, 170–171
    third compartment pharmacokinetics of,
      188–190
  compartmental modeling of, 188–190
  dialysis of, 194–195
  dosing nomograms for, 172–173, *173*
  dosing regimens of
    adjusting, key parameters in, 186–188, *187*
    in anephric patient, 194–196
    computer programs for, 173
    in CRRT patients with multiple organ failure,
      204–208
    determine appropriateness of, 197–199
    in hemodialysis, 194–196
    in low clearance, 192–194
    for peak plasma concentration, 184–186,
      188–190
    in peritoneal dialysis, 197
    in post dialysis replacement dosing, 195
    third compartment modeling and, 188–190
  elimination half-life of, 172
  elimination rate constant of, 170

Aminoglycosides antibiotics (*continued*)
   apparent, estimating, 183–184
    in drug accumulation, 191–192
    expected, 183–184
   key parameters of, 164–172, 165t
   loading dose of, 175–177
    computer programs for, 173
    in hemodialysis, 194–196
    in patient with multiple organ failure
     receiving CRRT, 204–208
   maintenance dose of, adjusting, 186–188
    in hemodialysis, 194–196
    in low clearance, 192–194
   nephrotoxicity of, 164
   ototoxicity of, 164
   patient specific, estimation, 186–190,
    192–194
   peritoneal dialysis of, 197
   pharmacodynamics of, 164
   plasma concentrations of
    creatinine clearance in estimating,
     176–177, 190
    expected, short infusion modeling *vs.* bolus
     dose modeling, 175–181
    expected steady-state, intermittent infusion
     modeling, 181–183, 197–201
    peak and trough, in low clearance, 192–194
    peak and trough, in steady-state, 175–181,
     197–201
    peak, estimating patient specific, 188–190
    therapeutic, 164–167
    toxic, 164–167
   post dialysis replacement dosing of, 195
   sampling timing, 174–175
   third compartment pharmacokinetics in,
    168, 188–190
   toxicity of, 164
   volume of distribution of, 166–168
    drug accumulation and patient specific,
     191–192
    expected, 183–184
    in obese patients, 166, 167
    in pediatric patients, 167–168
Aminophylline, 8
Amiodarone, 288
  interaction with digoxin, 303–304
Amitriptyline, 451–452
  fu value of, 16t
Amlodipine, 339, 350–352
Amoxicillin-clavulanic acid, 138
Amphotericin B-deoxycholate, 213
Antibiotics
  aminoglycosides, 163–208
  intraperitoneal administration of, 125, 126
  maintenance dose of, calculating, 49

Antifungal agents, 213–215
  mortality rates, 213
  systemic antifungals, 214t
Antithymocyte globulin (ATG), 330
Area under curve (AUC), 272
  aminoglycoside dosing based on, 165t
  busulfan, 273, 276–279
Aspergillus spp., 221
Assays
  busulfan, 272–273
  specificity, 95–96
Ataxia, 373
ATG (antithymocyte globulin), 330
AUC (area under curve), 272, 273, 276–279
Average steady-state plasma concentration, 28–29
Azathioprine, 321

B
Bactericidal activity of aminoglycosides, 163–164
Basic drugs, binding affinity of, 15
Bayesian analysis, of plasma drug concentration,
  92–95
Beta (β) half-life, 25, 43
Bilirubin conjugation, 136
Binding affinity, of plasma proteins, 17–20
Bioavailability
  of aminoglycosides antibiotics, 166
  of busulfan, 273–275
  of carbamazepine, 244
  chemical form of, 8–10
  clearance of, 336
  for cyclosporine, 325–326
  definition of, 6–7
  of digoxin, 282–283
    coadministration of cholestyramine, 282, 283
    intravenous doses and, 295
    product variability, 300
  dosage form, 7–8
  effect of the chemical drug from, 9
  first-pass effect, 10, 11
  of fluconazole, 215
  of isavuconazole, 236
  of itraconazole, 222
  of lithium, 360
  of mycophenolate, 349
  of posaconazole, 231–232
  for sirolimus, 344
  for tacrolimus, 336
  of vancomycin, 470
  volume of distribution of, 336
  of voriconazole, 225–226
Blastomyces dermatitidis, 215
BMI (body mass index), 490–491
Body composition, 111, 132
Body habitus, 132, 164, 182, 202, 449

Body mass index (BMI), 490–491
Body surface area (BSA), 138, 142–143
    calculation of, 31
    and creatinine clearance, 102–105
    dosing algorithm, 258
    dosing based on, 258
    and drug clearance, 31–32
        patient specific revisions, 32
    nomograms for calculating, 497–498
Body weight
    and creatine clearance, 102–105
    ideal and adjusted, 104–105
Bolus dose modeling, 61–62, *62*, 63–67, *66*
Brain imaging techniques, 368
BSA. *See* Body surface area
Busulfan, 271
    administration of, 271
    area under curve, 273, 276–279
    assays, 272–273
    bioavailability, 273–275
    clearance, 275
    dose, 27, 276, 278–279
    half-life, 275
    key parameters, 274
    target plasma concentrations, 271–272, *274*
    time to sample, 272
    units, 271
    volume of distribution, 275

C
Calcineurin inhibitors, 341
Candida albicans, 218–220
Candida infections, 215
CAPD. *See* Continuous ambulatory peritoneal
        dialysis
Carbamazepine, 241–253
    adverse effects of, 243–244
    bioavailability of, 244
    clearance of, 245
        increased, in chronic therapy, 245
        patient specific, 251–252
    complex interaction, *253*
    dosage of, 241, 250–253
    drug interactions with, 246–248, 246t, 247t
    formulation of, 241
    fu value, 16t
    half-life of, 248
    key parameters, 242t
    maintenance dose, 250–252
    metabolism of, *245*
        inhibitors and inducers of, 246t
    pharmacodynamics, 241
    plasma concentrations
        average steady-state, 250
        therapeutic, 242–243, 242t

        time to sample, 248–249
        toxic, 242–243
    sampling timing for, 248–249
    volume of distribution for, 244–245
Carboplatin, 258
Central nervous system (CNS), adverse effects of
        carbamazepine on, 243
Cerebral spinal fluid, 222
    concentrations, 226
Chemical form, of bioavailability, 8–10
CHF (congestive heart failure), 36–37, 76, 282,
        284t
Children Act and Pediatric Research Equity Act,
        130
Chlordiazepoxide, fu value of, 16t
Chlorpromazine, fu value of, 16t
Cholestyramine, decrease bioavailability of
        digoxin, 283
Cirrhosis, and variable plasma protein binding, 17
Clark's rule, 139
Clearance
    of aminoglycosides antibiotics, 169–171
        expected, 186–188, *187*
        non-renal, 169–170
        in obese patients, 169
        penicillin interaction, 170–171
        third compartment pharmacokinetics of,
            169–171
    body surface area in calculating, 31–32
    of busulfan, 275
    calculating, 28
    of carbamazepine, 245
        increased, in chronic therapy, 245
        patient specific, 251–252
    cardiac output and, 36–37
    of creatinine, 100–116
    definition of, 28
    in dialysis, pharmacokinetics of, 116–126
    of digoxin, 285–287
        common factors affecting, 284t
        in congestive heart failure, 291, 299, 304–305
        estimating, 295–296
        in obese patients, 285
        patient specific, in non steadystate, 309–312
        renal function, decreased, 291–293
        in thyroid disease, 301–302
    effect of changes in, *37*
    effect of diminished protein binding, *34*
    and elimination rate, 33–35, *34*
    equations, 503
    and extraction ratio, 35–36
    factors altering, 31–37, 33t
    for first-order drugs, 407
    fluconazole, 216–217
    and fraction unbound in plasma, 33–35, *34*

Clearance (*continued*)
  highly protein-bound drug, *34*
  of isavuconazole, 237
  of itraconazole, 222–223
  and maintenance dose, 30–31
  metabolic, 36–37
  of methotrexate, 262–264
  of mycophenolate, 349
  and plasma concentration evaluation
    hepatic function in, 36–37
    iterative search techniques in, 83–87
    mass balance techniques in, 87–92
    in non steady-state, 86–92
    renal function in, 36–37
    sensitivity analysis in, 80–83
    in steady-state, 83–86
  posaconazole, 232–233
  as proportionality constant, 28
  and protein binding in plasma, 33–35, *34*
  renal, 36–37
  revising, 78–79
    in non steady-state plasma concentration,
      86–92
    single-point estimation of, 90–92
    in steady-state plasma concentration,
      83–86
    using iterative search, 83–87
    using mass balance technique, 87–92
  single-point determination of, 90–92
  total, calculating, 36
  units in calculating, consistency of, 30
  in uremic and non-uremic patients, 33–35
  of valproic acid, 449–451
  of vancomycin, 471
  of voriconazole, 226–227
  weight and body surface in calculating, 31–32
Clinical Laboratory Standards Institute, 468
Clinical Pharmacogenetics Implementation
    Consortium (CPIC), 159
Coccidioides immitis, 215
Codeine, 137
Compartments, plasma and tissue, 25
Congestive heart failure (CHF), 36–37, 76, 282,
    284t
Continuous ambulatory peritoneal dialysis
    (CAPD), 124–126, 467–468, 486
  fraction of steady-state equilibrium in, 125
  maximum expected clearance in, 124
  significant plasma protein binding and
    clearance in, 125
Continuous infusion
  equations, 501
  modeling of, 310–311, 388–390
  at non-steady state, and decay, 47–49
  at steady state, 30, 46, 49, 63

Continuous renal replacement therapy (CRRT),
    122–123, 204–208, 487–488
  dosing in, 123
  maximum dialysis clearance in, 122–123
  monitoring in, 123
  patient with multiple organ failure receiving,
    204–208
  in removing digoxin, 303
  vancomycin, 487–488
Continuous venovenous hemodiafiltration
    (CVVHDF), 216–217
Continuous venovenous hemodialysis (CVVHD),
    216–217
Continuous venovenous hemofiltration (CVVH),
    216–217
Creatinine clearance, 100
  in children, 105–106
  distribution, 291–293
  equation for, 103, 106
  in females, 103
  in males, 103, 103t
  and plasma drug concentration, 100
    age considerations, 103
    in emaciated patients, 103, 105
    gender considerations, 103
    given serum creatinine levels, 285, 290–291
    in non steady-steady, 107–109
    in obese patients, 103–104
    in steady-state, 102–105
    weight or body surface area considerations,
      102–106
  urine creatinine evaluation in, 108–111
Creatinine, serum, 101
  expected daily production of, 112t
  pharmacokinetics of, overview, 101
  steady-state
    in evaluating clearance, 102–106
    time to reach, 106–107
  upward adjustment of, 105
CRRT. *See* Continuous renal replacement
    therapy
CVVH (continuous venovenous hemofiltration),
    216–217
CVVHD (continuous venovenous hemodialysis),
    216–217
CVVHDF (continuous venovenous
    hemodiafiltration), 216–217
Cyclosporine
  administration of, 321–322
  adverse effect, 325
  for allograft rejection, 321–323
  bioavailability of, 325–326
  blood concentration of
    adjusting steady state, 332
    assays of, 324–325, 325t

elevated, in thrombocytopenia and leukopenia, 346
increasing steady state, 329–331
monitoring, 325
in patient with biliary drainage, 333
therapeutic, 324–325, 325t
time to sample, 328–329
toxic, 324–325, 332
clearance of, 326–327
patient specific, estimating, 333
clinical application of, 329–333
concentration *vs.* time curve of, 323
formulations of, 322–323, 322t
fu value of, 16t
half-life of, 328
initial dose of, typical, 324
key parameters of, 322t, 323–329
patient specific, estimating, 328–329
maintenance dose
in conversion to modified cyclosporine, 333
in converting to, 333
to increase blood concentration, 329–331
to new steady state blood concentration, 329–332
toxicity, 332
metabolism of, 326–327
inducers and inhibitors of, 326–327, 327t
modified, 323
oral dosing of, 333
pharmacogenomic applications, 353–354
pharmacokinetics of, 329
sampling time for, 328–329
therapeutics for, 324–325, 325t
toxicity of, 324–325, 332
volume of distribution of, 326
CYP2B6 enzyme, 156–157
CYP2C9 enzyme, 157, 217
CYP2C19 enzyme, 157–158, 217
CYP2D6, 156
CYP3A4 enzyme, 157–158, 217
in carbamazepine metabolism, 246–248, 246t, 247t
CYP3A5 enzyme, 158
CYP3A5 polymorphism, 353
CYP enzymes, 155–158
Cystatin c, 169
Cytochrome, 10
Cytochrome P450 enzyme, 155, 214
maturations rates of, *135*
Cytotoxic anticancer drugs
BSA, 258
cytotoxic chemotherapy, 257
pharmacokinetic variability, substantial reduction in, 258
renal function, dosing based on, 258

therapeutic drug monitoring, 259
Cytotoxic chemotherapy, 257

D
Dextromethorphan, 134–135
Dialysis calculations, 119–121
in continuous renal replacement theory, 122–123
in high-flux hemodialysis, 121–122
in intermittent hemodialysis, 119–121
limitations of, 121
Dialysis clearance, 118–119
maximum expected, in continuous ambulatory peritoneal dialysis, 124–126
maximum, in continuous renal replacement therapy, 122–123
Dialysis therapy
blood, 116–118
continuous renal replacement therapy, 122–123
peritoneal, 124–126
Diazepam, fu value of, 16t
Digibind, digoxin and, 315
Digitoxin, fu value of, 16t
Digoxin, 282–315
administration of, 282, 289–290, 293–294
amiodarone, interaction with, 303–304
bioavailability of, 282–283
coadministration of cholestyramine and, 282–283
intravenous doses and, 295
product variability, 300
clearance of, 285–287
common factors affecting, 284t
in congestive heart failure, 291, 299, 304–305, *304*
estimating, 295–296
in obese patients, 287
patient specific, in non steady-state, 309–312
renal function, decreased, 291–293
in thyroid disease, 301–302
in decreased creatinine clearance, 291–293
dialysis, 302–303
displacement by quinidine, 305, *306*
distribution of, 134
division of, 289–290
dosing interval for, 289–290
drug interaction with
amiodarone, 303–304
P-glycoprotein, 282
propafenone, 306
quinidine, 288–289, 303–304
St. John's wort, 282
verapamil, 306
elimination rate constant of, 295–298
formulation, 282, 283t, 289–290, 293–294

Digoxin (*continued*)
  fu value of, 16t
  half-life for, 287, 295, 297, 313–314
  hemodialysis, 302–303
  intravenous dose of, calculating equivalent, 295
  key parameters of, 282–288, 283
    patient specific, estimating, 304–312
  loading dose of, 282, 288–289
    in congestive heart failure, 288–289
  maintenance dose of, 282, 293–294
    adjusting, in toxicity, 295–298
    average steady-state, 290–291, 293–294
    oral, conversion to intravenous dosing, 295
    to therapeutic endpoint, 293
    in thyroid disease, 301–302
  in obese patient, 284
  oral dosage form of, 12, 22–23, 289–290, 293,
    295
  plasma concentration of
    creatinine clearance decline and, 291
    decaying, 297–298, 308–311
    in drug interaction, 304–305
    elevated, 298–299, 300
    expected, 306–312
    in hemodialysis, 302–303
    non steady-state, 309–314
    and product variation in bioavailability, 300
    steady-state, 290–291, 293–294, 301–302
    therapeutic, 282, 283t
    time to sample, 288–289, 299
  and quinidine, interaction, 288–289, 305
  sampling timing for, 288–289, 299
  tablet form of, 12, 22–23, 282, 289–290, 294
  theoretical two-compartment model for, 286
  in thyroid disease, 301–302
  and thyroid function, 301
  toxicity of
    dosing adjustments in, 295–298
    hemodialysis and, 303
  volume of distribution for, 283–285, 295–296
    calculating, 295
    common factors affecting, 284t
    in congestive heart failure, 288–289
    in decreased renal function, 291–293
    in thyroid disease, 283–284, 301–302
    two-compartment model for, 283–284, 286
Diltiazem, 338–339
Distribution half-life, 25, 43
Dosage adjustment, vancomycin, 468
Dosage forms
  and bioavailability, 7–8
  valproic acid, 447–448
Dose dumping, 7
Dosing interval (tau), 10–11, 83–84
  calculating in maintenance therapy, 49–51

  fixed, 12
  and key parameter adjustments, 76–83
  longer than half-life, 49
  shorter than half-life, 49, 82
Dosing, pharmacokinetic model of
  appropriate, selecting, 61–62
  continuous infusion to steady-state, 63
  discontinuation of infusion, after steady-state,
    63
  initiation and discontinuation of infusion,
    before steady-state, 63–67
  intermittent administration, at regular intervals,
    to steady-state, 68, 69
  loading dose, 61–62, 62, 66, 67
  series of individual dose, 68–71
  short infusion, 63–67, 65
  sustained release formulation, 71–72
Dosing rate, and average steady-state plasma
    concentration, 39, 41
Drug absorption
  incomplete, 7
  rate of, 7
Drug clearance, *142*
Drug disposition, 155
  absorption, 131–132
  distribution and protein binding, *123*, 132–134
  metabolism and excretion, 134–139
Drug metabolism, 141t
  development of, 134
Dwell time, 124, 393

E
Echinocandin, 213–214, 214t
Elimination
  distribution and protein binding, *123*, 132–134
  half-life, 25, 43
  rate, 33–35, 34
    proportionality, to drug concentration, 39
Elimination rate constant, 39–41, 44t
  after infusion initiation, 45–47, 46
  of aminoglycosides antibiotics, 171
    apparent, estimating, 183–184
    in drug accumulation, 191–192
    expected, 183–184
  clinical application of, 44t
  definition of, 41
  equations, 500
  and expected plasma concentration after
    infusion discontinuation, 46, 47–49
  first-order accumulation, 45
  first-order elimination, 38, 40, 45
ELISA (enzyme linked immunosorbent assay),
    95, 336
EMIT (enzyme-multiplied immunoassay
    technique), 95

Encephalopathy, 228
Enzyme immunoassay, 95
Enzyme linked immunosorbent assay (ELISA), 95, 336
Enzyme-multiplied immunoassay technique (EMIT), 95
Equations
  adjustment for plasma protein binding, 504
  appropriate, selecting, 61, 72–74
  bolus dose, 61
  clearance, 503
  continuous infusion, 501
    at non-steady state, and decay, 47–49
    at steady state, 30, 46, 49, 63
  creatinine clearance, 103
  discontinuation of infusion, after steady-state, 63
  elimination rate constant, 39–42
  half-life, 43
    and elimination rate constant, 500
  ideal body weight, 103
  individual dose series, 68–71
  infusion model, 64–66
  initiation and discontinuation of infusion, before steady-state, 63–67
  intermittent administration, at regular intervals, to steady-state, 68
  loading dose
    followed by infusion, 67
    incremental, 23
  mass balance, 87–88, 503
  multiple dose, 502–503
    at non steady-state, 70
    at steady-state, 51–52, 68, 71–72
  nonlinear, 71, 504
  series of individual dose, 68–71
  short infusion, 64–66, 65
  single dose, 64–66, 499–500, 500
Equivalent dose, 7
Erythrocyte–plasma lithium concentration ratio, 368
Ethosuximide, fu value of, 16t
Excretion, 134–139
Exocrine function, pediatric diseases of, 131
Extraction ratio, and clearance, 34, 35–36

F
First compartment, 25
First order accumulation, 45
First order drugs, volume of distribution and clearance, 39
First order elimination, 45
  characteristics of, 38
  concentration vs. time in, 38–40
  pharmacokinetics of, 38–39
First-pass effect, and bioavailability, 10, 11, 11

Fixed dosing intervals, and administration rate at, 12
Fluconazole, 346
  adverse effects, 218
  bioavailability of, 215
  clearance, 216–217
  doses of, 217
  key parameters, 217
  pharmacokinetics, 218
    drug interactions, 217
  serum concentrations, 221
  therapeutic range of, 215
  time to sample, 218
  volume of distribution, 215–216
Fluorescence polarization immunoassay (FPIA), 95
Focal epilepsy disorders, 447
Fosphenytoin, 400, 401, 439
FPIA (fluorescence polarization immunoassay), 95
Fraction unbound (fu), 13
  for drugs
    with low plasma protein binding, 19
    with significant plasma protein binding, 18, 19–20
  increased and clearance, 33–36, 34
  monitoring, in clinical practice, 20
  and normal plasma protein binding, 13
  for selected drugs, 16, 16t
Free drugs concentration, calculation of, 17–19

G
Gabapentin, fu value of, 16t
Gas chromatography–mass spectrometric detection (GC–MS), 272–273
Gastric acid production, 131
GC-MS (gas chromatography-mass spectrometric detection), 272–273
Genotype-guided dosing, 158, 159
Gentamicin/tobramycin, 133, 173
  fu value of, 16t
  key parameters, 165t
  plasma concentrations of, 164
    peak, 164–167
    therapeutic, 165t
  usual dose for, 163–164
"Get the dose right" for children, 130
GFR. See Glomerular filtration rate
GI tract, 140t
Globulins, and binding affinity with acidic drugs, 15
Glomerular filtration rate (GFR), 216, 258
  development, 137–138
  MDRD to estimate, 112–116, 169
    adjusting for the patient's size, 114
    longer version, 112
    shorter or modified version, 112
Gram-positive bacteria, 467–468

H

Half-life, 25, 43
  of busulfan, 275
  of carbamazepine, 248
  clinical application of, 44t
  definition of, 43
  for digoxin, 287, 295, 313–314
    estimating, 297
  in dosing interval estimation, 49–51
  in drug distribution, 25
  and elimination time, 45
  equations, 500
  and interpreting steady-state plasma
    concentration, 45
  of lithium, 362
  of methotrexate, 264
  of mycophenolate, 349–350
  of vancomycin, 472
HD. *See* Hemodialysis
Hematopoietic stem cell transplantation (HSCT),
  271
Hemodialysis (HD), 341–342, 367, 485–487
  in digoxin, 302–303
  high-flux, 122
  intermittent, and post dialysis drug
    administration, 116–117
  maintenance dose calculation in, 115
  pharmacokinetic modeling of, 116–117
  plasma concentration
    at beginning and end of, 118
    between procedures, 116–117, 117
  plasma profile for drug, 119
  post dialysis replacement dose calculation,
    116–117
  vancomycin, 486–487
Hepatic function, 36–37
  dosing based on, 259
High-performance liquid chromatography
  (HPLC), 221, 324
High-performance liquid chromatography with
  tandem mass spectrometric detection
  (HPLC/MS/MS), 343
High-performance liquid chromatography with
  ultraviolet detection (HPLC UV), 343
HLA-B*1502 allele, 243
HPLC (high-performance liquid
  chromatography), 221, 324
HSCT (hematopoietic stem cell transplantation),
  271

I

Ideal body weight, 103–104, 166–168, 188–190,
  284, 287, 407
Imipramine, fu value of, 16t
Immunoglobulin A (IgA) concentration, 133

Immunosuppressants
  drug-drug interactions, 327t
  formulations, 322, 323
  therapeutic blood levels of, and allograft
    rejection, 321
  therapy, 321
Incremental loading dose, 23
Indomethacin, 263
Infusion modeling
  bolus *vs.*, 63–67, 66
  continuous, to steady-state, 63
  discontinuation of, 63
  initiation and discontinuation of, before steady
    state, 63–67
  intermittent, at regular intervals, to steady-state,
    68, 69
  loading (bolus), 61
  short, 64–66
Initial volume distribution, 25
  and loading dose estimation, 25–27
  and plasma drug concentration, 25–27
Interactions, valproic acid (VPA), 451–452
Interleukin-2 (IL-2), 321
Intermittent IV infusion, *181*
Intramuscular absorption, 131–132
Isavuconazole
  adverse effects, 238
  bioavailability of, 236
  clearance, 237
  key parameters, 237
  pharmacokinetics, 238
    drug interactions, 237–238
  therapeutic range of, 236
  time to sample, 238
  volume of distribution, 237
Iterative search in clearance adjustment, 83–87
Itraconazole, 220–221
  adverse effects, 224
  bioavailability of, 222
  clearance, 222–223
  key parameters, 223
  pharmacokinetics, 224
    drug interactions, 223
  therapeutic range of, 221
  time to sample, 224
  volume of distribution, 222

K

Ketoprofen, 263
Key parameters
  patient specific, 76
  in plasma concentration interpretation, 75–76
  revising
    assay specificity in, 95–96
    Bayesian analysis in, 92–95

creatinine clearance, 100–116
dialysis of drugs in, 116–126
maximum plasma drug concentration in, 51
minimum plasma drug concentration in, 53–54
sampling timing in, 75–76
sensitivity analysis in, 80–83
revising clearance as
in non steady-state plasma concentration, 86–92
in single point estimation of, 90–92, *90*
in steady-state plasma concentration, 83–86
using iterative search, 83–87
using mass balance technique, 87–92
Kinetic behavior of drugs, 130

L

Lean body weight (LBW), 490–491
Leucovorin rescue, *263*, 264, 267, 271
methotrexate, 260–262
Lidocaine
fu value of, 16t
intravenous, clearance in, 29
loading dose of, estimating, 25
Lithium
bioavailability of, 360
cerebrospinal fluid concentrations of, 362
clearance, 361
commercially available preparation, 359t
concentrations, 368
dosing regimen, 365–366
drug–drug interactions, 361t
fu value of, 16t
half-life, 362
initial dose selection, 363
intentional hand tremors, 367
intermittent vomiting and diarrhea, 367
intoxication, 367
key parameters, 360
obese patient, 367–368
plasma concentration, 363–364, 366
prediction methods, 363
responders, 363
significant two-compartment modeling of, 27
slow tissue distribution of, 26–27
special populations
children, 362
pregnancy, 363
seniors/older adults, 362–363
steady state, 363–364
tablets and capsules, 359
therapeutic actions, 368
therapeutic and toxic plasma concentrations, 359–360
time of sampling, 362

tissue penetration, 362
two-compartment pharmacokinetic model, 362
volume of distribution, 360
Liver function, and drug clearance, 36
Loading dose, 22–23, *23*
and decreased plasma protein binding, 24
and decreased tissue binding, 24
followed by infusion, 67
incremental, 23
initial volume of distribution and, effect of, 24, 25–27
plasma concentration *vs.* time curve for, 67
tissue volume of distribution and, effect of, 24, 27
volume of distribution and, 22–23
factors altering, 24

M

Maintenance dose, 30–31
change in, and steady-state plasma concentration, 39, 41
and dosing interval estimation, using half-life, 49–51
and drug clearance, 30–31
in hemodialysis, 115
Mass balance, 87–90
equation for, 87–88
equations, 503
technique, 313–314, 395–396, 400–402
Maturation model, 143–145
Matzke method, 490–491
Maximum plasma drug concentration, 51–52
Maximum tolerated dose, 257
MDRD. *See* Modification of Diet in Renal Disease
Mechanism of action, 447
MEIA (microparticle enzyme immunoassay), 336
Metabolic clearance, 10, 36–37
Metabolism, 134–139
Metabolites, active
drugs with, 96t
and pharmacologic response, 95–96
Methadone, fu value of, 16t
Methemoglobinemia, 132
Methicillin-resistant *Staphylococcus aureus* (MRSA), 467
Methotrexate (MTX), *263*
acute lymphoblastic leukemia, 264–269
administration of, 259–260
clearance, 262–264
consistency of units in calculating, 31
dosage of, 259–260
fu value of, 16t
half-life, 264
key parameters, 261
rescue therapy, 269–271

Methotrexate (*continued*)
  toxic plasma concentrations, 260
    leucovorin rescue, 260–262
  units, 260
  volume of distribution, 262
MIC. *See* Minimum inhibitory concentration
Microparticle enzyme immunoassay (MEIA), 336
Midazolam, 135
Minimum inhibitory concentration (MIC), 146–
    147, 193, 468, 469, 480–484
  for bacteria and aminoglycosides, 64
Minimum plasma drug concentration, 53–54
  slow absorption rate and, 54
Modification of Diet in Renal Disease (MDRD)
  adjusting for the patient's size, 112
  equation to estimate glomerular filtration rate
    (eGFR), 112–116, 169
  longer version, 112
  shorter or modified version, 112
10-monohydroxy metabolite (MHD), 249
Morphine, 136–137
MTX. *See* Methotrexate
Multiple dose equations, 502–503
Multivariate modeling, 133
Muscle tissue, 140t
Mycophenolate
  administration of, 347–348
  adverse effects, 348–349, 351
  bioavailability of, 349
  cadaveric kidney transplant, 350–351
  clearance, 349
  clinical pharmacogenomics of, 350
  half-life, 349–350
  key parameters, 347–348
  loading dose of, 350–351
  mofetil, 321
  monitoring, 351
  therapeutic and toxic concentrations, 348
  time to sample, 350
  timing of dose, 351–352
  volume of distribution, 349

N

Nafcillin, fu value of, 16t
Nelfinavir, fu value of, 16t
Nephrotoxicity, 164, 339, 468, 469
Neurotoxicity, 339
New dosage form, bioavailability of, 7, 295
Nomograms
  for aminoglycosides antibiotics, 172–173, *173*
  and computers, 172–173, *173*
  for vancomycin, 472
Noncompartmental data analysis, 273
Nonlinear equations, 504
Non significant two-compartmental drugs, 27–28

Nonstandardized drug clearances, 139–140
Non steady-stat e plasma concentrations, 86–92
Nonsteroidal anti-inflammatory drugs (NSAID),
    341–342
Normal binding concentration, 14–15
Normal plasma protein binding, 14–15

O

OATP2B1 expression, 131
Obesity, clinical, definition of, 104–105
Offset of drug effect, evaluating, 26
Orbit graph method, 420, *421*
Ototoxicity, 468, 469
  of aminoglycosides antibiotics, 164
Oxcarbazepine, 249

P

Pantoprazole, 350–351
Parenteral administration, bioavailability in, 7–8
Parenteral administration modeling
  continuous infusion, to steady-state, 63
  discontinuation of infusion, after steady-state,
    63
  infusion, before steady-state, 63–67
  infusion following loading dose, 67
  intermittent infusion, as regular intervals, to
    steady-state, 68
  loading (bolus) infusion, 62, *62*, 66
  short infusion, 64–66, *65*
Patient specific parameters, 76–95
PCAs (postconceptional ages), 131
Pediatrics
  drug disposition and elimination
    absorption, 131–132
    distribution and protein binding, *123*,
      132–134
    metabolism and excretion, 134–139
  pharmacodynamics and pharmacokinetically
    directed dosing, 146–147, *147*
  pharmacokinetic scaling and modeling, 139–145
Peritoneal dialysis, 124–126
  fraction of steady-steady equilibrium in, 124
  maximum clearance calculation in, 124
  significant plasma protein binding and
    clearance in, 125
P-glycoprotein, 282, 325–326, 335
Pharmacodynamics, 146–147, *147*
Pharmacogenetics, 155
  CPIC, 159
  CYP enzymes, 155
    pharmacogenetics of, 156–158
  pharmacogenetics and drug disposition, 155
  pharmacogenomics-informed therapeutic drug
    monitoring, 158–159, *159*
  variability in drug response, 154

Pharmacogenomics-informed therapeutic drug monitoring, 158–159, *159*
Pharmacokinetically directed dosing, 146–147, *147*
Pharmacokinetic alterations in childhood, 139, 140–141t
Pharmacokinetic behavior, 130
Pharmacokinetic models/modeling, 139–145
  selecting appropriate, 63, 72–74
Pharmacokinetic parameters
  desired plasma drug concentration as, 12–21
  revising
    dialysis of drugs in, 116–126
    maximum plasma drug concentration in, 51–52
    minimum plasma drug concentration in, 53–54
  volume of distribution as, 20–28
Pharmacokinetics
  fluconazole, 218
  isavuconazole, 238
  itraconazole, 224
  of most cytotoxic drugs, 257
  posaconazole, 233
  scaling, 139–145
  variability, substantial reduction in, 258
  voriconazole, 228–229
Phenobarbital, 372–396
  administration of, 372–373, 379–380
  bioavailability of, 373
  clearance of, 374
    in children, 374
    in newborn, 375–376
    renal, 390
  concentration–time curve, *389*
  dialysis of, 389–393
  drug interaction with, 439–440
  and effect on phenytoin plasma concentration, 439–440
  formulations of, 373
  fu value of, 16t
  half-life of, 374
  key parameters of, 372, 373
    patient-specific, 385–388, 388–390
  loading dose of, 372–373
    and average plasma concentration, 375–376, 377–378
  maintenance dose of, 373
    adjusting, 377–379, 385–388, 389–393
    administration of, 379–380
    in children, 393–394
    oral, 379–380
    post-dialysis replacements of, 389–393
  plasma concentrations of
    after loading dose increase, 375–376

average, 375–376, 394–396
in continuous ambulatory peritoneal dialysis, 392–393
in decreasing plasma protein binding, 390
in decreasing renal function, 390
in dialysis, 389–393
drug interaction and effect on, 439–440
in hemodialysis, 389–393
in newborn, 375–376, 377–378
non-steady-state continuous infusion modeling of, 388–390
patient-specific, estimating, 385–388, 388–390
steady-state, average, 375–376, 394–396, *408*
therapeutic, 372, 373, 380
time to sample, 374–375
toxic, 373
  plasma concentrations of, steady-state, 394–396
    empirical clinical guideline, 380
    final, 382–383
    mass balance, 395–396
    time to reach, 380
    trough, 384–385
  renal clearance of, 390
  replacements dose of, post-dialysis, 389–393
  sampling timings for, 374–375
  in tablet form, 393–394
  volume of distribution of, 373
Phenobarbital (PB), 461–462
Phenytoin, 398–401
  administration of, 400
    oral *vs.* intramuscular, 439
  bioavailability of, 405–406
  capacity-limited metabolism, 400–402, 407–412, 422–423
  clearance of, concentration dependent, 412
  displacement of, from plasma protein binding sites, 405
    adjustment in, 405
  drug interaction with, *253*, 410, 411t, 439–440
  fu value of, 16t
  half life of
    concentration-dependent, 413–417
    and decaying plasma concentration, 416–417
    individual dosing of, problems of, 400
    limited utility of, 413–415
    and time to reach steady-state, 415
  individual dosing of, problems of, 400
  key parameters of, 401, 405–418
  loading dose of, 400
    in adjusting plasma concentration upward, 420–421
    and administration, 418–419
  maintenance dose of, 400
    in lower plasma concentration, 424–426

Phenytoin (*continued*)
    in new steady-state, 419–420, 423–424,
        427–429, *428*
    in uremic patient, 433–434
    metabolism of, capacity-limited, 400–402,
        407–412, 422–423
    phenobarbital and interaction with, 439–440
    plasma concentrations of
        altered plasma protein binding *vs.* normal
            plasma protein binding, 436–437
        creatinine clearance and effect on, 403–404
        decay of, timing, 426–427, 430
        decay rate of, 416–417
        and effect on, 401, 405, 430–431, 435–436
        expected, and altered plasma binding,
            435–436
        hypoalbuminemia and effect on, 402–403,
            404, 430–431
        increasing, loading dose calculation, 420–421
        maintenance dose adjustment in, 420
        non linear equations for, 408–409
        orbit graph method of calculating, 419–420
        patient specific parameters and, 427–429
        phenobarbitol effect on, 439–440
        in plasmapheresis, 436
        in renal failure, 403–404
        in steady-state, 422–423
        therapeutic, 401–405
        time to reach, 415, 417–418
        time to sample, 417–418
        toxic, 401–405, 424–426
        in uremic patients, 430–431, 433–434
    sampling timing for, 417–418
    toxicity of, 401–405, 424–426
    volume of distribution, 406–407
Phenytoin (PHT), 461–462
Plasma drug concentrations
    administration rate in estimating, 28–29
    after infusion discontinuation, 47–49
    after infusion initiation, 45–47
    algorithm for evaluating and interpreting,
        505–509
    of aminoglycosides antibiotics, 164–167
        creatinine clearance in estimating, 176–177
        expected, short infusion modeling *vs.* bolus
            dose modeling, 175–181
        expected steady-state, intermittent infusion
            modeling, 181–183, 197–201
        peak and trough, in low clearance, 192–194
        peak and trough, in steady-state, 175–181,
            197–201
        peak, estimating patient specific, 188–190
        therapeutic, 164–167
        toxic, 164–167
    assay specificity in evaluating, 95–96

average steady-state, 28–29, 39, 45–49
Bayesian analysis in evaluating, 92–95
bolus dose modeling of, 61, 63–67, *66*
carbamazepine
    average steady-state, 250
    therapeutic, 242–243, 242t
    time to sample, 248–249
    toxic, 242–243
clearance in estimating, 28–37, 78–79, *79*
    in non-steady-state, 86–92
    in steady state, 83–86
in clinical practice, monitoring, 17–19
cyclosporine, 322, 345
decreased binding affinity on, *18*
desired, 12–21
determining parameter in, for given dosage
    regimen, 49–50
of digoxin
    average, 290–291, 293–294
    continuous infusion modeling, 310–311
    creatinine clearance decline and, 291
    in drug interaction, 304–305
    expected, 306–312
    false-positive determinations, 300
    in hemodialysis, 302–303
    individual doses series modeling, 308–309,
        310–311
    interpreting, 298–299
    non steady-state, 309–314
    to predetermined level, 295, 297–298
    and product variation in bioavailability, 300
    therapeutic, 282, 283t
    time to reach, in thyroid disease, 301–302
    time to sample, 287–288, 299
dosing interval in estimating, 49–52
dosing rate in estimating, 39, 41
elimination rate constant in estimating, 39–42
evaluating and interpreting, 75–96
expected, 83
fraction unbound in estimating, 14–15, 16t
free (effective) drug in, 17–19
half-life in estimating, 43, 45
infusion modeling of, 63–67
initial volume of distribution in, 25–27
key parameter revision in evaluating, 75–60
maximum, 51–52
minimum, 53–54
non-steady-state, *70*, 86–92
phenytoin, 401, 405, 411t, 412, 437
plasma protein binding in estimating, 12–21
and plasma protein concentration, 14–15
sampling time in estimating, 75–76, 77, *77*
sensitivity analysis in evaluating, 80–83
sirolimus, 345
steady state, 28–31, 43, 63, 83–86

timing of sampling in estimating, 75–76, 77, *77*
tissue volume distribution in, 25–27
unbound, 17–19
volume distribution in estimating, 25–27, 76–78
Plasma lithium
concentration, 366
levels, 367
Plasma protein binding, 12–21, 141t, 468
of acidic drugs, 15
of basic drugs, 15
and clearance calculations, 33–36, 123
clinical significance of, 17–19
decreased, and plasma drug concentrations, 14–15, 24
degree of, and effect on plasma drug concentrations, 17–20
drugs and fu values for, 16t
equations, 504
factors altering, clinical significance of, 17–19
free (effective) drug and, 17–19
fu values of, for selected drugs, 16t
normal, 14–15
and plasma drug concentration, relationship between, *13–14*, 14
significant, and plasma drug concentration, 12–14, *14*, 15–17
and volume of distribution, 21
Plasma volume, of average adult, 21
Pleural effusions, 264
Poor metabolizers (PMs), 156
Population pharmacokinetic model, 145
Posaconazole
adverse effects, 233
bioavailability of, 231–232
clearance, 232–233
dosing, 233
formulation of, 232
key parameters, 232
loading dose, 235–236
oral suspension formulation of, 234–235
pharmacokinetic drug interactions, 233
serum concentrations of, 231, 233
therapeutic range of, 231
time to sample, 233
volume of distribution, 232
Postconceptional ages (PCAs), 131
Potassium, loading dose of, 25–26
Premature neonates, 133
Primordial drug metabolic enzymes, 134
Propafenone, interaction with digoxin, 306
Propranolol
and first pass effect, 10
fu value of, 16t
Protein binding, valproic acid (VPA), 448–449

Pseudoallergic reaction, 468
Pseudometabolites, 471

Q

Quinidine
fu value of, 16t
increased plasma concentration, after surgery or trauma, 15
interaction with digoxin, 288, 305

R

Red man syndrome, 468, 489
Reduced exocrine function, 131
Renal clearance, 36–37, 138
Renal drug excretion, 141t
Renal elimination, 137
of drugs, 138
Renal function, 100. *See also* Dialysis therapy
changes in, 263
Cl_{Cr}, 106
dosing based on, 258
glomerular filtration rate in, 112–116
MDRD equation, 112–116
Rescue therapy, methotrexate, 269–271
Residual amniotic fluid, 131

S

Salicylic acid, fu value of, 16t
Saliva lithium concentrations, 368
Salt factor, 8–10
Sampling time, and plasma drug concentration, 75–76
effect of delayed absorption, 75, *75*
observed *vs.* average steady-state concentration, 78
Second compartment, 25
Sensitivity analysis in interpreting plasma drug concentration, 80–83
Sepsis, 218–220
Serum protein binding, 133
Short infusion modeling, 63–67, *65*
Significant two-compartmental drugs, 27
Single dose equations, 499–500
Single nucleotide polymorphisms, 155
Single-point determination, of clearance, 90–92, *90*
Sirolimus, 342–347
administration of, 342, 364–365
adverse effects, 343
bioavailability of, 344
blood concentrations of
elevated, in thrombocytopenia and leukopenia, 346
therapeutics of, 343
time to sample, 344–345
toxic, 343, 346

Sirolimus (*continued*)
   clearance of, 344
   half-life of, 344
   initial dose of, typical, 342, 344
   key parameters of, 343t, 344–345
   maintenance dose of, typical, 342, 344
   pharmacodynamics of, 343
   pharmacogenomic applications, 353–354
   sampling time for, 344–345
   therapeutics of, 343
   toxicity, 343, 346
   volume of distribution of, 344
Skin, 140t
   penetration, 132
Solubility of drug, and volume of distribution, 22
Spatial compartments, 140t
Special populations
   children, 362
   pregnancy, 363
   seniors/older adults, 362–363
Steady-state plasma concentrations, 28–31,
      63, 69
   administration rate and, 28–29
   average, 28–29
   in dosing interval calculation, 49–52
   drug clearance change and effect on, 37
   effect of changes in maintenance dose on, *41*
   given dosage regimen, 49–50
   half-life and time to reach, 44–45, *45*
   plasma level–time curve for intermittent
      dosing, *50*
Stevens-Johnson syndrome (SJS), 243
St. John's wort, 282, 306
Sulfation, 136
Sulfobutylether-cyclodextrin (SBECD) vehicle,
   226

T
Tacrolimus, 334–342
   administration of, 334–335
   adverse effects, 335
   bioavailability of, 336
   blood concentrations of
      elevated, dosing adjustments in, 338–339
      half-life of, 337
      therapeutics of, 335, 335t
      time to sample, 337
      toxic, 335
   key parameters of, 335t, 336
   pharmacogenomic applications, 353–354
   sampling time for, 337
   therapeutics of, 335, 335t
   toxicity of, 335
      patient specific, 338–339
   volume of distribution of, 336

Theophylline, 135t
   administration of, 11
   bioavailability of, 8
   concentration calculation following
      discontinuation of an infusion, 48
   loading dose of, 25
   maintenance dose of, 30
   maximum plasma concentration of, 52
   sensitivity analysis, 80–83
Therapeutic drug monitoring (TDM), 215, 259
   posaconazole, 233
   valproic acid, 452–454
   voriconazole, 225
Therapeutic orphans, 130
Third compartment pharmacokinetics, 168,
      188–190
Thyroid function, digoxin and, 301
Ticarcillin, and aminoglycoside interaction,
      170–171
Time to sample
   busulfan, 272
   fluconazole, 218
   isavuconazole, 238
   itraconazole, 224
   lithium, 362
   posaconazole, 233
   vancomycin, 472–473
   voriconazole, 228
Tissue binding, 134
   decreased, loading dose and volume of
      distribution, 24
   in loading dose calculation, 27
   in plasma drug concentration, 25–27
   slowed, and plasma drug concentration, 27
Tissue (second) compartment, 25
Tissue penetration, 362
Tissue proteins, 24
T-lymphocyte, 321
Tobramycin
   key parameters, 165t
   plasma concentrations for
      peak, 164–167
      therapeutic, 165t
   usual dose for, 164
Total body weight, 104–105
Toxic epidermal necrolysis (TEN), 243
Triazole, 213–214, 214t
   drug interactions, 214–215
   pharmacology, 214
   therapeutic drug monitoring (TDM), 215
Trileptal, 249
Two-compartment computer models, 27
Two-compartment modeling
   loading dose and plasma drug concentration
      in, 25–27

and offset of drug effect evaluation, 27
significant and non significant, 27–28
volume of distribution, 168, 284, 326

U

Units
 busulfan, 271
 methotrexate, 260
Uremic patients
 clearance in, 33
 decreased tissue binding of drugs in, 24
 free drug plasma concentration in, 17
 phenytoin pharmacokinetics in, 17–18, 24
Uridine diphosphate (UDP) glucuronidation, 233

V

Valganciclovir, 352
Valproic acid (VPA)
 administration, 447
 CYP4503A4 metabolism of, 461
 depression, 458–460
 dose-dependent changes in, 461–462
 dosing, 455–457
  forms and absorption, 447–448
  strategies, 447
  and therapeutic drug monitoring, 452–454
 Escherichia coli, 457–458
 focal epilepsy disorders, 447
 fu value of, 16t
 interactions, *253*, 451–452
  drug, 447
 key parameters, 453
 loading dose, 454
 maintenance dose, 455–456
 mechanism of action, 447
 metabolism, 457–458
  and clearance, 449–451
 phenytoin dose, 460–461
 postinfusion serum level, 454
 protein binding, 448–449
  concentration-dependent, 459
 serum level, 456–457
 steady-state concentration, 456–457, 461–462
 steady-state serum level, 461–462
 tonic–clonic seizures, 454–455
 unusual nature of, 447
 volume of distribution, 449
Vancomycin, 133, 138, 467–468
 bioavailability of, 470
 clearance, 471
 continuous renal replacement therapy, 487–488
 dosage
  adjustment, 468
  maintenance, 488–490
  regimen of, 490–493

drug monitoring, 468
 elimination rate constant, 492
 fu value of, 16t
 half-life of, 472
 hemodialysis, 486–487
 key parameters, 469
 nomograms for, 472
 prevalence of, 467
 ratio of concentrations, 493–494
 renal disease, 484–486
 serum creatinine concentration, 473–480
 steady-state peak and trough concentrations,
  492–493
 therapeutic and toxic plasma concentrations,
  480–484
  efficacy, 468
  safety, 469–470
 therapeutic drug monitoring, 468
 time to sample, 472–473
 volume of distribution of, 470, 490–491
Veno-occlusive disease (VOD), 271–272
Verapamil, interaction with digoxin, 306
Volume of distribution, 14, 20–28, *21*
 administration of drug, *21*
 amikacin, 186
 of aminoglycosides antibiotics, 166–168
  drug accumulation and patient specific,
   191–192
  expected, 183–184
  in obese patients, 166
  third compartment pharmacokinetics in,
   188–190
 apparent, 22
 busulfan, 275
 for carbamazepine, 244–245
 of creatinine, 107–109
 cyclosporine, 326
 definition, 21
 for digoxin, 283–285, 295–296
  calculating, 295
  common factors affecting, 284t
  in congestive heart failure, 288–289
  in decreased renal function, 291–293
  in thyroid disease, 283–284, 301–302
  two-compartment model for, 284, *286*
 in drug dialysis considerations, 119–121
 in estimating plasma drug concentration,
  76–78, 80–83
 factors altering and loading dose, 24
 fluconazole, 215–216
 gentamicin, 168, 176
 initial (plasma), 22, 25
 isavuconazole, 237
 itraconazole, 222
 lithium, 360

Volume of distribution (*continued*)
   and loading dose, 22–27
   methotrexate, 262
   mycophenolate, 349
   phenobarbital, 390
   phenytoin, 24, 431–432
     factors altering, 24
   posaconazole, 232
   significant and non significant, 27–28
   sirolimus, 344
   solubility of drug and, 22
   tacrolimus, 336, 344
   tobramycin, 183–184, 191–192
   two-compartment modeling of, 25–28, *26*
   valproic acid, 449
   of vancomycin, 470, 490–491
   voriconazole, 226

Voriconazole, *230*, 340
   adverse effects, 228
   bioavailability of, 225–226
   clearance, 226–227
   dosing, 229–231
   key parameters, 227
   metabolism, 228
   pharmacokinetics, 228–229
     drug interactions, 227
   serum levels, 225–226
   therapeutic range of, 225
   time to sample, 228
   volume of distribution, 226
VPA. *See* Valproic acid

W

Warfarin, fu value of, 16t

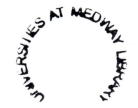